Lower Genital Tract Precancer

TO OUR WIVES AND DAUGHTERS
who have supported us unreservedly
throughout this endeavour.
They are our past, present and future.

Lower Genital Tract Precancer
COLPOSCOPY, PATHOLOGY AND TREATMENT

ALBERT SINGER PhD (Sydney), DPhil (Oxon), FRCOG
Professor of Gynaecological Research, University of London
Consultant Gynaecologist, Whittington Hospital, London

JOHN M. MONAGHAN FRCS (Ed), FRCOG
Director of Gynaecological Oncology Services, Queen Elizabeth Hospital, Gateshead
Senior Lecturer in Gynaecological Oncology, University of Newcastle upon Tyne

ASSISTANT AUTHOR
SWEE CHONG QUEK MRCOG
Research Fellow, Department of Women's Health,
Whittington Hospital, London

CONTRIBUTING AUTHOR
ALASTAIR R.S. DEERY MB, BS, FRCPath
Consultant Cytopathologist,
Royal Free Hospital, London

SECOND EDITION

b
Blackwell
Science

© 1994, 2000 by
Blackwell Science Ltd
Editorial Offices:
Osney Mead, Oxford OX2 0EL
25 John Street, London WC1N 2BL
23 Ainslie Place, Edinburgh EH3 6AJ
350 Main Street, Malden
    MA 02148-5018, USA
54 University Street, Carlton
    Victoria 3053, Australia
10, rue Casimir Delavigne
    75006 Paris, France

Other Editorial Offices:
Blackwell Wissenschafts-Verlag GmbH
Kurfürstendamm 57
10707 Berlin, Germany

Blackwell Science KK
MG Kodenmacho Building
7–10 Kodenmacho Nihombashi
Chuo-ku, Tokyo 104, Japan

First published 1994
Second edition 2000

Set by Excel Typesetters Co., Hong Kong

Printed and bound in Italy
by G. Canale & C. SpA, Turin

The right of the Authors to be
identified as the Authors of this Work
has been asserted in accordance
with the Copyright, Designs and
Patents Act 1988.

A catalogue record for this title
is available from the British Library

ISBN 0-632-04769-0

Library of Congress
Cataloging-in-publication Data

Singer, Albert.
    Lower genital tract precancer :
colposcopy, pathology, and treatment /
Albert Singer, John M. Monaghan: assistant
author, Swee Chong. —2nd ed.
        p.   cm.
    Includes bibliographical references and
index.
    ISBN 0-632-04769-0
    1. Generative organs,
Female—Precancerous conditions.
I. Monaghan, John M.   II. Chong, Swee,
III. Title.
    [DNLM: 1. Genital Neoplasms,
Female—prevention & control.
    2. Precancerous Condition—diagnosis.
    3. Colposcopy—methods.
    4. Precancerous Conditions—therapy.
WP 145 S617L 2000]
RC280.G5S56   2000
616.99′466—dc21
DNLM/DLC
for Library of Congress   99-16649
                                        CIP

DISTRIBUTORS

Marston Book Services Ltd
PO Box 269
Abingdon, Oxon OX14 4YN
(*Orders*: Tel: 01235 465500
            Fax: 01235 465555)

USA
Blackwell Science, Inc.
Commerce Place
350 Main Street
Malden, MA 02148-5018
(*Orders*: Tel: 800 759 6102
                    781 388 8250
            Fax: 781 388 8255)

Canada
Login Brothers Book Company
324 Saulteaux Crescent
Winnipeg, Manitoba R3J 3T2
(*Orders*: Tel: 204 837 2987)

Australia
Blackwell Science Pty Ltd
54 University Street
Carlton, Victoria 3053
(*Orders*: Tel: 3 9347 0300
            Fax: 3 9347 5001)

For further information on
Blackwell Science, visit our website:
www.blackwell-science.com

Contents

Preface to the Second Edition

The decision to update the first edition was taken after considering the enormous advances in aetiology, pathology, and management of diseases of the female lower genital tract. The authors approached a number of colleagues who are experts in these respective fields and who generously offered to assist in the production of this second edition. Alastair Deery enlarged the pathology and cytological aspects of the second edition and Kari Syrjänen contributed his expertise in respect of the human papillomavirus. They and other contributors helped to make the second edition more "balanced" in that it now includes extensive material on the above topics as well as a section on cytological screening that were missing from the first edition. It is imperative for the practising clinician to be aware of many of these new developments so as to help in the overall care of the patient. Knowledge of the causation of a disease will go some way towards alleviating the enormous anxiety that is generated in women who are diagnosed as having lower genital tract precancer. The brief of this text does not allow any extensive coverage of the psychological prob-lems referred to, but it is the responsibility of the clinician to be aware of these problems.

Modern technology, especially digital imaging and data management, made it imperative a colleague be found to help the senior authors incorporate these new developments into the second edition. Dr Swee Chong Quek has ably assisted us in this task and a number of these images are included in the text. He contributed the section on cytological screening and was also invaluable in the overall production.

Since the first edition, the new developments referred to above have greatly increased the profile of this subject. Clinicians are now called upon by their patients to be "expert" in all aspects of lower genital tract precancer, and it is the hope of the authors that they have succeeded in presenting a second edition that will allow them this knowledge.

Albert Singer
John Monaghan
August 1999

Preface to the First Edition

The term "precancer" has been used throughout this book. That word was chosen intentionally as it has a broad, generic connotation that changes are present in the tissue which indicate that a lesion, if not removed, will, with a high degree of likelihood, progress to invasive carcinoma. There is little doubt that the intraepithelial neoplasms of the male and female lower anogenital tract should, when they are high grade, be considered to be precancerous. The prospective follow-up studies of such lesions have established without a doubt that this categorization is appropriate. The use of the term "precancer" for the low-grade lesions is problematic, however, because it is now apparent—particularly for the uterine cervix—that some of the epithelial changes which include the morphological features of neoplasia may, in fact, be acute human papilloma virus (HPV) infections of the epithelium and that the majority of such lesions will not progress to high-grade intraepithelial neoplasia nor to invasive cancer. It is clear that lesions which are infected by the HPV types with no malignant potential will never progress to a true neoplasm and that even low-grade lesions which are caused by intermediate- or high-oncogenic risk HPV types may regress spontaneously or persist for long periods of time without progressing to a true neoplasm. In the low-grade lesions it is difficult, without HPV testing and typing, to predict the biological behaviour of the epithelial change, but the term "precancer" has still to be used because of the potential for such lesions to progress to high-grade intraepithelial disease and, subsequently, to invasive cancer.

The close relationship between precancerous lesions of the cervix, vagina, vulva and anus has long been recognized. Although the common embryonic origins of the epithelium of the vulva, lower vagina, and anus contrast with the origins of the cervix and upper vagina, these differences are all the more remarkable when the clinician studies the fascinating similarities among precancerous conditions of the entire lower genital tract. The authors have clearly illustrated the importance of a knowledge of the development of the epithelium of the lower genital tract with chapters on the development of the transformation zone with its process of metaplasia and examples of the consequences of interruption to this natural process such as when the female fetus is exposed to the effects of diethylstilboestrol (DES).

For the clinician skilled in the assessment of the cervix following the identification of an abnormal smear, this text will be invaluable in perfecting that technique. For the clinician seeking wider horizons, this text is not simply a colposcopic atlas, it is a comprehensive statement of the wide range of skills needed to diagnose and manage any or all of the precancerous conditions of the lower genital tract.

This is a text book for the modern clinician who no longer wishes to be solely a colposcopist with a limited view confined to the cervix. This text emphasizes the closely integrated relationship between molecular biology, virology, cytology, histology, and colposcopic techniques required for the development of logical and safe management methods. Our clearer understanding of the natural history of conditions covered by the term lower genital tract precancer, including a better knowledge of the capacity for spontaneous resolution exhibited by low-grade lesions, has resulted in the introduction of a wide range of conservative therapies. This logical and generally more conservative approach has removed, to a large degree, the severe overtreatment which was a characteristic of management methods of yesteryear. We have no doubt, however, that this text will not be the final word. This subject has undergone radical rethinking during the last two decades. We anticipate many more changes to come.

This illustrated textbook is a comprehensive guide to our current understanding of the diagnosis, assessment and management of all genital tract precancers and conditions which may mimic them. We commend it to the modern clinician, not only for those in training but also to those in established practice where regular updating is essential.

Albert Singer
John Monaghan
November 1993

Acknowledgements

The authors would not have been able to have completed the extensive revisions in this second edition without the generous contribution by many colleagues of photographs, diagrams and advice, not to mention encouragement.

Dr Alastair Deery, Consultant Cytopathologist, Royal Free Hospital, London, undertook the revision of Chapter 1 and contributed extensively to the pathology and cytology material, especially in Chapters 5 and 7.

Professor Kari Syrjänen, of the Department of Pathology and Forensic Medicine, University of Kuopio, Finland, contributed Chapter 2 and gave advice to the authors in respect of Chapter 1. This contribution is sincerely appreciated.

Professor Ralph M. Richart, Professor of Pathology of Columbia University, New York, assisted by Dr Thomas C. Wright Jr., assisted in the production of the first edition, some parts of which have been retained. They donated some of the histological photographs that appear throughout the first and now second edition, and on many occasions aided the authors with advice and constructive critical comments. Their contribution is acknowledged and appreciated.

Professor Ray Kaufman, of the Baylor College of Medicine, Houston, Texas, contributed material as listed below, but also gave advice and comment on various aspects of the text.

Dr Rene Cartier, of Paris, generously allowed the reproduction of many photographs and clinical details that have appeared in his classic and excellent text *Practical Colposcopy* (3rd edn), Laboratoire Cartier, Paris.

Mr Joseph Jordan with his sugical colleagues Mr Mahmood Shafi and Professor David Luesley of the Birmingham Maternity and City Hospital, Birmingham, UK, allowed the authors to use photographs of their surgical procedures as featured in Chapters 9 and 10.

Dr V. Cecil Wright of the Division of Obstetrics and Gynaecology, the University of Western Ontario, Canada, donated Figs 6.121(e–i) (from Wright, V.C., Lickrish, G.M. & Shier, R.M. *Basic and Advanced Colposcopy—a Practical Handbook for Diagnosis* (2nd edn), Biomedical Communications, Houston, 1995) and Figs 12.1–12.14.

Professor Dr Thomas Iftner of The Universitätsklinikum Tübingen (Abt. für Medizinische Virologie); Dr Linda Ho and Dr George Terry of the Department of Molecular Pathology, University College London Medical School, who provided assistance to the authors in the compilation of Chapter 2.

Listed below are the names of colleagues who have loaned the following photographic material to the authors. Their material is reproduced with sincere acknowledgement and grateful thanks.

Dr Malcolm Anderson, Department of Histopathology, Queens Medical Centre, Nottingham, UK: Figs 1.5, 1.6, 1.20, 1.30, 4.9(b–f), 4.17(b), 4.19(b,c), 4.53(b,c), 4.58, 6.23, 6.66, 6.72–6.75, 7.1(b).

Dr Simon Barton, Department of Genito–Urinary Medicine, Chelsea and Westminster Hospitals, London: Figs 9.49, 9.50, 12.3, 12.6(b), 12.8, 12.9(b), 12.11.

Dr Blanche Butler, Early Diagnostic Unit, Elizabeth Garrett Anderson Hospital, London: Figs 6.125 and 6.126 reproduced with permission from Husain, O. & Butler, B. (1988) *A Colour Atlas of Gynaecological Cytology.* Wolfe Medical Publications, London.

Dr Rene Cartier, Laboratoire Cartier, rue de Cordelières, Paris, Fance: Figs 6.7(c), 6.20, 6.43, 6.44, 6.111(c), 6.118, 6.131, 6.132, 6.134–6.146, 7.62, 12.20, 12.21.

Professor Malcolm Coppleson, King George V Memorial Hospital, Sydney, Australia: Fig. 6.127(a–d).

Mr Ian Duncan, Ninewells Hospital, Dundee, UK: Figs 7.9–7.11, 7.91, 7.92.

Professor Alex Ferenczy, The Sir Mortimer B. Davies–Jewish General Hospital Montreal, Canada: Figs 9.5(a,b), 9.22(b), 9.25, 9.29, 9.37.

Dr Ron Jones, National Women's Hospital, Auckland, New Zealand: Figs 9.3(a–d), 9.41(a).

Mr Joseph Jordan, Birmingham Maternity and City Hospitals, Birmingham, UK: Figs 9.62(a,b), 9.63(a–d). Figs 10.25, 10.26, 10.27.

Professor Jacques Hamou, Pierre and Marie Curie University of Paris, Paris: Figs 6.46–6.50, Fig. 7.50.

Professor Raymond Kaufman, Baylor College of Medicine, Houston, Texas, USA: Figs 9.5(c,d), 9.24(b,d), 9.26(a,b), 9.27(a,b), 9.39(a–c), 9.44–9.47, Figs 12.9 & 12.10.

The late Professor Per Kolstad, Norwegian Radium Hospital, Oslo, Norway: Figs 3.8, 3.9, 4.8, 6.8–6.14(c).

Professor Bert Krumholtz, Long Island Jewish Hospital, New York: Fig. 11.6.

Professor Allan Maclean, Royal Free Hospital, London: Fig. 3.7(c,d).

Dr Elizabeth Mansell, Whittington Hospital, London: Fig. 9.54(b–d).

Mrs Ann Morse, Department of Cytology, St. Mary's Hospital, London: Fig. 6.91.

Dr John Northover, Colorectal Cancer Unit, St. Mark's Hospital, London: Figs 10.15, 10.17.

Dr Ed Sawada, Towson, Maryland, USA: Fig. 12.16.

Professor Duane Townsend, Salt Lake City, Utah, USA: Figs 4.3, 4.10(b), 6.111(b), 8.5–8.7, 8.24, 8.28, 9.6–9.8, 9.48(b).

Professor Minoru Ueki, Osaka Medical College, Osaka, Japan: Figs 6.15, 6.35(b–d), 6.51(a[i] & [ii]), 6.121–6.124, 6.126, 6.128–6.130, 6.133, 6.147–6.150.

The line drawing from the first edition were all the work of Mr Patrick Elliott, Department of Medical Photography, The Royal Hallamshire Hospital, Sheffield, UK. His expert knowledge of anatomy and physiology can be seen in his excellent illustrations. A number of these illustrations are based on diagrams that appeared elsewhere and have been modified with the kind permission of the authors. Figs 7.2(b), 7.20, 7.26 and 7.64 are based on diagrams originally published by Professor V.C. Wright of the University of Western Ontario, London, Ontario, Canada; Fig. 4.2(a,b) is a modification of some diagrams originally produced by the late Dr Ellis Pixley of Perth, Western Australia; Figs 6.1e, 6.2(a,b) and 7.1(a) are modifications of ones that appeared in Cartier, R. (1993) *Practical Colposcopy*, Laboratoire Cartier, Paris; Figs 4.8 and 6.6 are modifications of ones originally published in Kolstad, P. & Stalf, A. (eds) (1982) *Atlas of Colposcopy* (3rd edn), Cambridge University Press, Cambridge, UK; Figs 6.82 and 6.83 are from the articles by Jarmulowicz *et al.* (1989) *Brit J Obstet Gynaecol* **96**,1061; while Tables 6.3 and 6.4 are from Tidbury *et al.* (1992) *Brit J Obstet Gynaecol* **99**,583; Fig. 7.67(b) is a line drawing from Baggish *et al.* (1989) *Obstet Gynecol* **74**;169; while Table 9.7 is from Ferenczy, A. (1992) In: Coppleson, M. (ed.) *Gynaecologic Oncology* Vol. I, p. 450, Churchill Livingstone, London; Tables 5.2–5.5 are modified from Morrow, C.P., Curtin, J. & Townsend, D. (eds) (1993) *Synopsis of Gynaecology* (4th edn), Churchill Livingstone, London; Figs 2.20–2.23 are from Pirog, E. & Richart, R.M. (July 1968) The Cell Cycle *Contemporary Ob Gyn*, **117**,126; while Fig. 7.104(a) is from Shepherd *et al.* (1998), *Brit J Obstet Gynaecol* **105**,912; Table 7.3(b,c) are from Fruchter *et al.* (1996), *Obstet Gynecol*. Dr Mitchell Morris, MD, Anderson Hospital, Houston, Texas, USA, allowed the publication of some data in Table 7.3. All are reproduced by kind permission of the respective authors, journals and publishers.

The final acknowledgement must be given to Mrs Madeline Cohen and her husband, Joost, of Textpertise, London, who undertook the enormous task of the typing and preliminary editing of the additional text for this second edition. Without their perseverance, patience and encouragement, the task would have been much more difficult. Our thanks also to Alice Nelson and Dr Stuart Taylor from Blackwell Science who both eventually survived the long gestation and delivery of this project with much forbearance. The authors acknowledge their assistance and encouragement.

Chapter 1
The Histopathology of Lower Genital Tract Neoplasia

1.1 Introduction

Cervical cancer has remained close to the forefront of oncologic studies for the best part of the 20th century. Among developed nations the mortality from the disease has fallen from first place among female cancers in the 1920s to eighth or ninth place in the 1990s (Miller *et al.*, 1991). Despite this, the incidence has changed little, except in those countries with effective screening programs (Hakama *et al.*, 1991). The discovery of a cytologically detectable and anatomically confirmed premalignant phase has successfully shifted the presentation of cervical squamous tumors from the clinical to the preclinical stage (IARC, 1986).

1.2 Terminology

It is critical that the terminologies used for cytologic and histologic diagnoses be similar so that they can be correlated with the colposcopic findings. It is also critical that cytologic and histologic nomenclature is based on sufficient scientific and clinical data so that the clinician can infer clinical behavior and the preferred treatment. Over the last 50 years our understanding of the etiology and pathogenesis of lower genital tract squamous neoplasia has increased enormously and, particularly in the last 15 years, progress in our understanding of the molecular events associated with lower anogenital tract neoplasia has developed rapidly. In response to this knowledge the terminology has changed, with each new classification system providing a higher degree of sophistication and reflecting the scientific thought of its day. Gradually the terminology has become more uniform and histologists' implications and clinicians' inferences have become more reliable. One of the principal trends occurring through all these changes is a gradual reduction in the number of terms used to describe the precursor lesions, with increasing emphasis upon the clinical relevance of the diagnostic terminology.

The concept of cervical cancer precursors

The concept of cervical cancer precursors dates back to 1886 when Williams (1888) noticed, next to invasive cancers, areas of epithelium that he recognized as noninvasive. It was not until Cullen (1900) better defined these noninvasive lesions, and noted that they resembled invasive cancers, that the concept of a cancer precursor became more accepted. The term "carcinoma-in-situ" (CIS) was introduced by Broders (1932) and this term has been utilized from its introduction to the present day. Smith and Pemberton (1934) reported a relationship between CIS and invasive cancer when they found that the changes described as CIS by Broders were present in a retrospective review of biopsies from patients who subsequently developed invasive cancer. This combination of histologic observations and retrospective clinical analysis led to the concept that invasive squamous cell carcinoma develops from precursor lesions that can be identified by the pathologist. This hypothesis was subsequently confirmed by a number of clinical studies in which patients with CIS were followed prospectively (Kottmeier, 1961; Koss *et al.*, 1963; McIndoe *et al.*, 1984). Once these studies had been undertaken and results published, it was generally agreed that precursor lesions had a high likelihood of developing into invasive cancer if not treated, and if the patient lived long enough.

Carcinoma-in-situ

The term "carcinoma-in-situ" was used restrictively by pathologists when it was first introduced; its use was confined to those lesions in which the full thickness of the epithelium was replaced by undifferentiated neoplastic cells. Not until exfoliative cytology began to be used was it recognized that there are a variety of atypical epithelia found in the cervix and that many of these cervical abnormalities did not have the full-thickness, highly atypical changes described for CIS. The lesions, which were less severe than CIS but still contained many of the cytologic and histologic features of that entity, were recognized to form a broad histologic spectrum, ranging from minimal deviation changes, which closely resembled the normal epithelium, through epithelia with increasingly severe atypia and disorganization, to the classical CIS. Reagan and coworkers recognized the potential importance of this "other" group of lesions and, in 1956, introduced the term "dysplasia" to designate those abnormalities with histologic and cytologic features that were intermediate between normal epithelium and CIS (Reagan & Harmonic, 1956). Walters and Regan (1956) subclassified the dysplasias into three groups—mild, moderate, and severe—depending upon the degree to which the full thickness of the epithelium was replaced by undifferentiated neoplastic cells. It was generally inferred that the higher the histologic grade, the more likely the lesion was to progress to invasive cancer and the higher the risk of developing cancer.

Precise definitions of the terms "dysplasia" and "carcinoma-in-situ" were not agreed upon until 1961 when, at the First International Congress on exfoliative cytology, the Committee on Histology Terminology for Lesions of the Uterine Cervix defined CIS as: ". . . only those cases should be classified as carcinoma-in-situ which, in the absence of invasion, show a surface lining epithelium in which throughout its whole thickness no differentiation takes place. The process may involve the lining of the cervical glands (Weid, 1961)." The Committee recognized that some of the surface cells may be flattened and that there were rare cases in which a lesion, which was otherwise characteristic of CIS, may have a greater degree of differentiation. This was noted as an exception for which no classification was made. Dysplasia, on the other hand, was defined as: "All other (than CIS) disturbances of differentiation of the squamous epithelial lining, surface and glands." It was soon realized that the definition of dysplasia was frustratingly imprecise and depended upon the degree to which the full thickness of the epithelium was replaced by poorly differentiated cells. Other terms, such as basal cell activity, basal cell hyperplasia, atypical hyperplasia, and anaplasia, were proposed but they did not enjoy much popularity, and the dysplasia/carcinoma-in-situ nomenclature became the dominant terminology. These terms were used for both cytologic and histologic diagnoses.

Terminology and management

When the terminology was originally proposed and generally accepted, the prevailing clinical management of patients with dysplasia and CIS was that patients with CIS required a hysterectomy to prevent the development of cancer, whereas patients with dysplasia, whose clinical course was not well-understood but could vary from remission to persistence and progression to CIS, were either ignored, followed, or treated by a variety of means, depending upon the clinicians' understanding and acceptance of the natural history data. However, the distinction between dysplasia and CIS was frequently based upon poorly defined and arbitrary histologic distinctions, and it gradually became clear that the enormous differences in approaches to treatment were not consistent with the unreliability of the diagnoses. In fact, a number of studies, in which pathologists interpreted a series of slides, reported that there was a high interobserver variability (Siegler, 1956; Cocker et al., 1968).

Biology and natural history

In order to better define the biology and natural history of the lesions referred to as dysplasia, a number of laboratory experiments, and a series of follow-up studies of patients with such lesions, were undertaken and the results published. It became clear that the classic two-disease configuration—dysplasia and CIS—was an artificial and arbitrary one and that there was, in fact, a continuum of change from mild dysplasia to CIS. In addition, it was found that when patients with dysplasia were followed prospectively, some cases regressed, some persisted, and some progressed to CIS. It also became clear that there was an inverse correlation of regression with histologic grade, and a direct correlation of progression with histologic grade. On the basis of these studies, a new term "cervical intraepithelial neoplasia" (CIN) was proposed (Richart, 1968). It was divided into grades 1, 2, and 3, where CIN 1 corresponded to mild dysplasia, CIN 2 to moderate dysplasia, and CIN 3 combined severe dysplasia and CIS. It was further noted that even these distinctions were arbitrary, and the concept of a continuum in the process of moving from normal epithelium through epithelial precursor lesions to invasive cancer was introduced. One of the goals of the introduction of the CIN terminology was to emphasize the concept of a single disease entity and to encourage clinicians not to treat patients based on histologic diagnosis alone, provided that the lesion was in the precursor phase (Richart, 1973). There was value in reinforcing the likely biological truth of progressive step-like changes in cancerous evolution and in abolishing some of the practical difficulties in assessing the pathologic subtleties at the severe end of the dysplastic spectrum. Many hailed and adopted the new truth (Buckley et al., 1982; Christopherson et al., 1982). However, in instinctively reaching for three grades of disease, the new classification once again ignored the histopathologic limitations and subsequent studies exposed identical levels of variability and inconsistency in the application within and between experts. The amount of high-grade disease suitable for intervention had however dramatically increased several-fold. At the milder end of the spectrum (CIN 1 and possibly CIN 2) the ground was unknowingly prepared for the subsequent confusion that would be introduced by the recognition of human papillomavirus (HPV) related epithelial changes and an infective causation.

The role of human papillomavirus (HPV)

The impact of the near synchronous publications of Meisels and Fortin (1976) and Purola and Savia (1977) of distinctive morphologic lesions in the uterine cervix with characteristic cytopathic effects (CPE) of HPV similar to those seen in genital warts (condylomata accuminata) was explosive. The typical koilocytotic vacuolated change had been earlier described under that name by Koss and Durfee (1956) but drawn even earlier as "perinuclear cavitation" by Papanicolaou (1954).

These appearances were now firmly identified in flat and endophytic (inverted) epithelial lesions, frequently asscociated with the changes previously defined as CIN. This strong associative evidence was seen to imply a viral etiology of CIN. In the last 20 years this recognition has led to breakthroughs in the understanding of this complex process, (zur Hausen, 1994, 1996; Duggan, 1996; Herrington, 1996; Franco, 1997). HPV is now detectable by molecular technology in perhaps all cervical carcinomas (Herrington, 1995) and is thought to be the principle primary cause or step in precursor development (cervical,

cervical glandular, vulval, vaginal and anal intraepithelial neoplasias, more commonly known as CIN, CGIN, VIN, VAIN and AIN respectively), in the lower anogenital tracts of men and women (Herrington, 1995).

Nomenclature of HPV lesions

A plethora of terms was spawned as a result of the new observations regarding HPV recognition in cervical dysplasia, for example flat condyloma, condyloma planum, condylomatous atypia, koilocytic atypia, warty atypia and subclinical papillomavirus infection. Confusion became rife among pathologists and clinicians. Many claimed (Fox & Buckley, 1990; Syrjänen, 1992) that the new observation of the CPE of HPV need not and should not influence the microscopic grading of CIN. This on the basis that prior to the recognition of HPV, the lesion would have been graded mild dysplasia or CIN 1 accordingly. After all the lesion grade had appeared to predict the prognosis most accurately (Östör, 1993). All low and high risk HPV types are thought to be associated with identical low-grade histologies (Franquemont et al., 1989; Willet et al., 1989; Lungu et al., 1992). Others (Al-Nafussi & Conquhoun, 1990) have stressed the overdiagnoses of CIN 1 in the presence of flat HPV changes. The convention has developed to report biopsies as showing HPV atypia without changes of CIN or HPV atypia and CIN combined.

In reality there is little disagreement that most mild dysplasias, HPV and CIN 1 or HPV alone, and indeed the majority of moderate dysplasias or HPV and CIN 2, either spontaneously regress or stay the same after prolonged follow-up (Franquemont et al., 1989; Syrjänen, 1996a,b), regardless of the histopathologic segregation.

HPV-associated cervical carcinogenesis as a continuum

From all the above it now seems that HPV-related biological changes are embedded inseparably in a morphologic continuum which stretches from hyperplasia all the way through the grades of dysplasia or CIN ending with invasive cancer. It seems likely that at a histologic level there are really only two decisions being made about any section of an abnormal biopsy; the presence or absence of HPV-related changes and the presence or absence of high-grade CIN. Let us assume that high-grade changes approximate to CIN 3 and some proportion of CIN 2.

Let us further assume that low grade changes approximate to HPV infection with accompanying epithelial regeneration. The seeming evidence of a reproducible morphologic continuum (Östör, 1993) reflects the difficulty in selecting "true" neoplastic lesions from among those which are simply infection.

Biologically there is a continuum which unfortunately is probably not reflected in a series of separate recognizable morphologic steps (beyond two perhaps). This very practical recognition of the limited reproducibility of cytologic and histologic assessments has resulted in a new nomenclature: The Bethesda System (TBS) (National Cancer Institute Workshop, 1988, 1989, 1992).

Rationalization of histologic terminology

Low- and high-grade squamous intraepithelial lesions

In parallel with the development in histopathologic terminology towards two grades of disease (Richart, 1990) a new terminology initially aimed at cytology was proposed in detail (i.e. TBS). TBS combines flat condylomatous (HPV) changes and low grade CIN (CIN 1) into LSIL (low-grade squamous intraepithelial lesion). HSIL (high-grade squamous intraepithelial lesion) corresponds to CIN 2 and CIN 3. The term lesion is substituted for neoplasia since the association of any of these morphologic grades of disease does not necessarily identify a neoplastic process. Conventionally CIN 2 and 3 are grouped together as both progress in a minor but nonetheless significant percentage of cases (Holowaty et al., 1999).

Present nomenclature

It has become clear that in the USA TBS will apply for histology as well as cytology. In most other countries CIN currently remains the most common terminology for histologic reporting. The dysplasia–CIS system is uncommonly used.

1.3 Histopathological features of CIN or SIL

Low-grade disease (mild dysplasia, CIN 1, HPV-CIN 1, LSIL) (Figs 1.1–1.3)

The principal alterations that characterize CIN include changes in the organization within the epithelium and in the cytomorphology of the cells. These changes appear to be triggered by HPV infection and represent the cytopathic effects of the virus in its replicative cycle. The morphologic changes occur because of the ability of the virus to interrupt the cell cycle, to induce polyploidy and to inhibit functional cytoplasmic differentiation (producing degenerative "koilocytotic" vacuolation). Hyperdiploid cells which have increased amounts of stainable nuclear material are hyperchromatic. Polyploid cell *populations* may contain tripolar mitoses and tetraploid metaphases (Winkler et al., 1984). Cells die and increased numbers of adjacent cells are recruited into the cycle to replace them. These cells exhibit nuclear enlargement, exaggerating previously unnoticed nuclear envelope irregularities. Nucleolar increases and dispersal become prominent among proliferating cells. Some of these features have been previously described (Fu et al., 1983; Ward et al., 1990). The most important changes at the tissue level are a retardation of the progressive maturation through the vertical layers of the normal epithelium (Fig. 1.1a) and the expansion of the proliferating parabasal or suprabasal zone associated with the presence of koilocytes (the pathognomonic cytopathic change of HPV infected cells). In low-grade lesions the atypically proliferating suprabasal cells may not occupy strata above the lower third of the epithelial thickness, though the cyto-

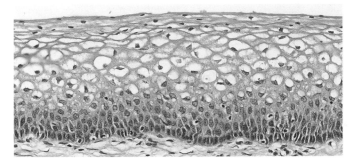

Fig. 1.1 (a) Normal cervical epithelium. The epithelium is uniform in pattern and cytology. The cells mature progressively as they move toward the surface, the nuclei become pyknotic, and glycogenation occurs.

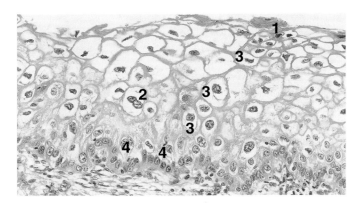

Fig. 1.1 (b) HPV infection "alone" (LSIL). There is mild, full thickness, cellular enlargement and hyperchromasia with superficial dyskeratosis accompanied by karyopyknosis (1), binucleation (2) and koilocytosis (3). In the bottom three cell layers there is variable nuclear and cell size, irregular variable condensed chromatin aggregation, degenerative nucleoplasmic clearing, nucleolar increase and some visible early koilocytes (4). These features at (4) are typical of regenerative or hyperplastic epithelial layers with some degenerative or poorly preserved features added in (e.g. nuclear clearing). They are not the features of neoplasia (see Fig. 1.6).

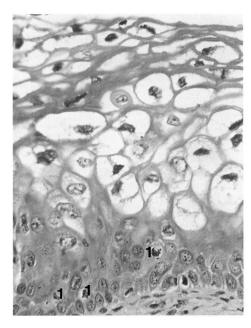

Fig. 1.2 HPV infection and CIN 1 (LSIL). The same features are present in the top three-quarters of the epithelium as in Fig. 1.1b. Now, however, the bottom four layers show more vital (better preserved) cells with the same characteristics as in Fig. 1.1b. The additional feature is visible mitoses (1). This would traditionally have been interpreted as CIN 1 (LSIL). However from a cytologic viewpoint these are no more features of neoplasia than the changes in Fig. 1.1b.

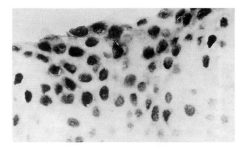

Fig. 1.3 Low-grade cervical intraepithelial neoplasia (CIN) with in-situ hybridization for human papillomavirus (HPV) DNA. Note that the nuclei are overlaid with reaction product beginning about midway in the epithelium. The nuclei that are "positive" contain a minimum of about 50 copies of HPV/cell (the minimum sensitivity level for this test).

pathic changes of HPV infection are full thickness. The presence or absence of CIN relies on the presence of morphologically recognizable neoplastic cellular features in the suprabasal population (Figs 1.1b–1.3). Polyploidy in such lesions is further evidenced by bi-, tri- or multinucleation which is another important feature of virally infected epithelium.

The observer should look for the characteristic features of HPV infection in a biopsy and then for the presence or absence of "disturbed" suprabasal layers which might allow the separation of such lesions into HPV alone or HPV and CIN 1 (Fig. 1.3). Within TBS all such lesions are ascribed to LSIL without further differentiation.

High-grade disease (moderate or severe dysplasia, CIS, CIN 2 or 3, HSIL) (Figs 1.4–1.8)

A pragmatic approach to treatment exists variably throughout the world in response to whether the precursor lesion is termed as "low-grade" or "high-grade" after biopsy. In countries where CIN terminology is operative there has

been considerable variation and difference in the placement of CIN 2 into one or other of these categories. If CIN 2 is considered high-grade, then treatment is largely obligatory. If CIN 2 is low-grade, then it may be watched or treated. Watching cytologically predicted CIN 2 (moderate dyskaryosis) results in delay in the treatment of much cytologically undetected CIN 3 (Flannelly *et al.*, 1994). In some countries (e.g. the USA) the grouping of CIN 2 lesions with CIN 3 in HSIL probably has fewer practical implications since both HPV/CIN 1 (LSIL) and CIN 2 or 3 (HSIL) are predominantly treated on consideration of the colposcopic extent or findings.

The histologic assessment of whether the suprabasal epithelial disturbance involves up to two-thirds or is practi-

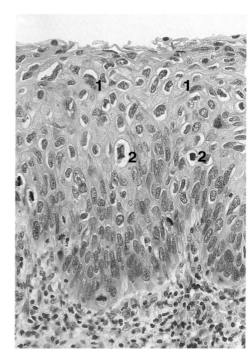

Fig. 1.4 Intermediate-grade cervical intraepithelial neoplasia (CIN 2; high-grade CIN; HSIL) and HPV infection. This is a slightly "squint" or oblique section which elongates the basal nuclei and adds to the impression of compact proliferating basal layers. The changes here are full thickness. Koilocytotic cells are confined to the upper half (1) but "truly" neoplastic cells with nuclei demonstrating rather monotypic coarse-pepper nuclear chromatin increases, without conspicuous nucleoli are present, together with mitoses, up to half way from the base (2).

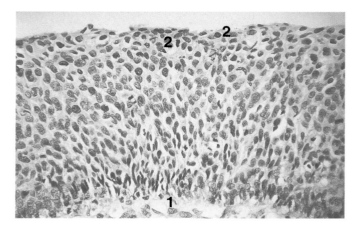

Fig. 1.6 CIN 3, (HSIL). These appearances are full thickness effacement by "small-cell," suprabasal cells exhibiting characteristic neoplastic coarse-pepper chromatin without conspicuous macronucleation. This fulfils the original criteria for carcinoma-in-situ and represents no more than 25% of today's CIN 3 (HSIL). The flat basal margin (1) may be a hint that this undoubtedly neoplastic lesion has replaced other cell populations and has restructured the epithelial-stromal interface. There is hardly detectable surface differentiation and thus no koilocytotic change. Mitoses are present close to the surface (2).

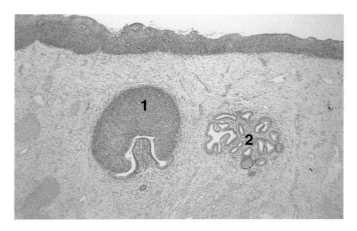

Fig. 1.7 Crypt involvement by CIN 3 (HSIL). At (2) benign uninvolved crypt profiles are seen.

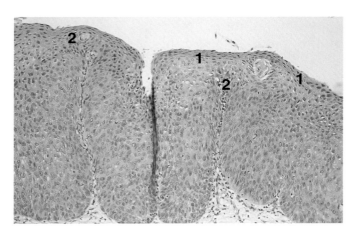

Fig. 1.5 High-grade cervical intraepithelial neoplasia (CIN 3; HSIL). Full thickness atypia, with proliferation of suprabasal cells to probably three-quarters the height within the epithelium followed by superficial maturation and flattening and minimal koilocytosis (1). There is a papillary configuration of the epithelium with high vessels (2).

cally full thickness will allow the designation of CIN 2 or 3 accordingly. The recognition of cytopathic HPV-related changes in the upper squamous layers decreases correspondingly. In Richart's original definition of high-grade CIN (Fu *et al.*, 1981) there is: (i) more hyperchromasia; (ii) mitoses occurring throughout the full epithelial thickness; (iii) the polarity of the parabasal cells is substantially altered; and (iv) a high degree of disorganized maturation and cytologic atypia is evident. These changes are thought to correspond with the occurrence of viral integration and/or amplification in cell nuclei and the development of aneuploidy, namely, abnormal chromosome numbers and DNA quantities. Along with more severe nuclear chromatin changes comes abnormal and bizarre multipolar mitoses (Fu *et al.*, 1983; Ward *et al.*, 1990). Whether these changes are clonal (i.e. arising in a single daughter cell line) or not, has not been determined. Clonality may be essential however to terming any lesion "neoplastic", since its occurrence demonstrates a survival advantage of the proliferating clone and the effacement of less genetically favored populations.

Among apparently similar histopathologic high-grade lesions only a certain, but unknown, proportion may be predominantly monoclonal or neoplastic.

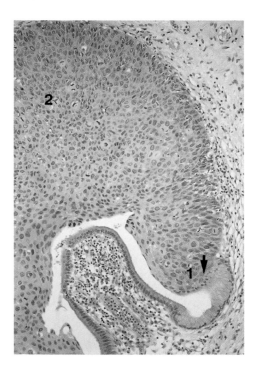

Fig. 1.8 Higher power view of involved crypt in Fig. 1.11. Note the pushing edge of the CIN 3 (HSIL) margin at (1) lifting (arrowed) the attenuated and degenerating endocervical cell layer off its basement membrane. There are numerous mitoses including tripolar metaphases (2).

1.4 Cervical glandular intraepithelial neoplasia (CGIN) and adenocarcinoma-in-situ (AIS)

Cervical glandular intraepithelial neoplasia (CGIN)

In 1953, Friedell and McKay first used the term adenocarcinoma-in-situ (AIS), to describe all precursor lesions of cervical adenocarcinoma. This term has been subsequently adopted to define all premalignant endocervical glandular lesions (Anderson, 1995; Griffin & Wells, 1995). However, consistent with the data on the pathogenesis of cervical squamous cell cancer through a series of increasingly severe dysplastic epithelial lesions; so glandular lesions with a lesser degree of dysplasia than AIS have been histologically described. To embody this concept, a variety of names have been offered for these precursors, including cervical glandular intraepithelial neoplasia (CGIN), cervical intraepithelial glandular neoplasia (CIGN) or just glandular intraepithelial neoplasia (GIN) (Brown *et al.*, 1986; Gloor & Hurliman, 1986; Cullimore *et al.*, 1992; Anderson, 1995; Wilbur, 1995). The authors prefer to adopt the term CGIN.

Histologic criteria for CGIN (Figs 1.9–1.10)

The first histologic descriptions of the lesser degrees of CGIN were provided in the late 1980s (Brown *et al.*, 1986; Gloor & Hurliman, 1986). While viewing a series of cone biopsies and hysterectomy specimens from CIN 3 and normal controls, these authors detected one case of typical

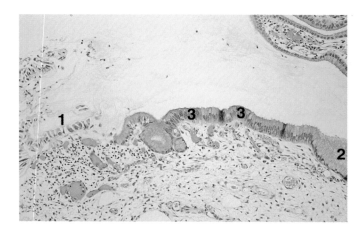

Fig. 1.9 Low-grade cervical glandular intraepithelial neoplasia (LGCGIN). On the left of this picture is "partially lifted off" ciliated columnar epithelium indicating tubal metaplasia (1). At (2) there is normal tall mucinous columnar endocervical epithelium. At (3) there is an epithelium which is very slightly irregular, where the epithelial cells appear more crowded, have retained polarity, but shift position, resulting in early pseudostratification. The nuclei are all enlarged with fine-pepper chromatin increases. The chromatin increases, the increased nuclear diameters and the nuclear (cell) crowding have resulted in a hyperchromatic appearance to this strand of epithelium.

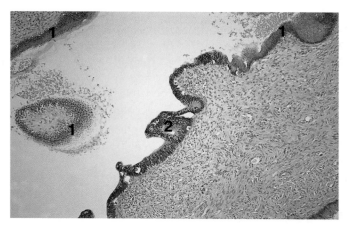

Fig. 1.10 High-grade cervical glandular intraepithelial neoplasia (HGCGIN). The epithelium on the left-hand wall of this crypt (1) is normal, and again at the upper end of the right-hand wall (1). The remainder of the right hand wall epithelium is tufted, slightly cribriform at (2), pseudostratified, hyperchromatic and contains many mitotic figures. (The differences between Fig. 1.9 and Fig. 1.10 are mainly qualitative.)

AIS and 16 additional cases, where the glandular abnormality was of lesser degree (Brown & Wells, 1986). Their observed prevalence of these minor grade lesions was 15% in the CIN 3 group and only 2% in the cervices of normal women and suggested an association with AIS, similar to that seen with CIN/CIS. The authors named these lesions as cervical glandular atypia, and subdivided them into high- and low-grades as follows: (i) low-grade lesions showing intraluminal epithelial tufting with stromal cores, abnormal glandular architecture and nuclei that are enlarged, hyperchromatic and elongated, with some limited piling up, or stratification; (ii) high-grade lesions characterized by more abnormal glandular profiles with irregular branching and budding, intraluminal papillary epithelial projections lacking stromal cores and nuclear pleomorphism, hyperchromasia, and obvious piling up or stratification (Brown & Wells, 1986) (Figs 1.9 and 1.10). In the same year, Gloor and Hurliman (1986) published their criteria for CGIN, into which they proposed to include AIS as well. Their classification is still more complex and based on both morphologic assessment and histochemical staining for mucins. It includes three grades.

In CGIN, the normal glandular epithelium is replaced by abnormal epithelium which shows loss of polarity, increased cell size, increased nuclear size, nuclear hyperchromasia, increased mitotic activity, reduction of cytoplasmic mucin expression and cellular stratification or piling (Anderson, 1995; Wilbur, 1995). A sharp demarcation from the normal glandular epithelium is usually seen in CGIN lesions. As can be anticipated from the wide intra- and interobserver variation known to bias the reporting of squamous cell cancer precursors just discussed, the reproducibility of any classification of CGIN is not high. The situation is further complicated by the lack of prospective cohort studies describing the natural history of these precancer lesions. Furthermore, there is a long list of histological mimics that should be considered in the differential diagnosis of CGIN, as has been discussed in detail elsewhere (Selvaggi & Haefner, 1997). Anderson (1995) and Griffin and Wells (1995) have suggested that CGIN be confined to two grades. High-grade CGIN would correspond to lesions previously described as AIS, and all other lesions showing lesser degrees of atypia are included in the category of low-grade CGIN. The authors fully agree with a two-tier classification of CGIN lesions. Although formal studies are still missing, we would predict that the reproducibility of this classification of CGIN into low- and high-grade categories would be considerably higher than for any attempt to use a tripartite grading.

1.5 Early invasive carcinoma (microinvasive carcinoma of the cervix)
(Figs 1.11–1.17)

The most recent staging announcement by the International Federation of Gynecology and Obstetrics (FIGO) is shown in Table 1.1a and again in Chapter 7. The previous FIGO staging is given here to allow comparison Table 1.1b.

Microinvasive carcinoma is a histological concept designating an invasive tumor with little evidenced risk of metastasis. The usefulness of the category is in affording less radical treatments for a proportion of women who nonetheless have demonstrable invasive disease. The definition needs precision. While stage I cervical carcinoma is limited to the cervix (involvement of the uterine body is excluded from consideration), Ia is restricted to include only those tumors that are diagnosed solely on microscopy and are horizontally less than 7 mm in extent and less than 5 mm in depth (see Figs 1.11 & 1.12). The 1988 staging of Ia1 (Table 1.1b) had no width restriction nor depth measurement included. Inevitably, this allowed variation in application. The correction in 1995 (Table 1.1a) has left an anomaly, however, for some lesions horizontally larger than 7 mm, but with only minimal depth of invasion

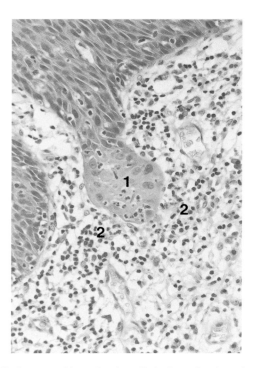

Fig. 1.11 Early stromal invasion (preclinical or microinvasion) in its earliest stage (Ia1). The sections show a differentiating tongue of malignant squamous cells (1) pushing from the epithelial margin into fibrous stroma (2) and associated with a chronic inflammatory infiltrate (3).

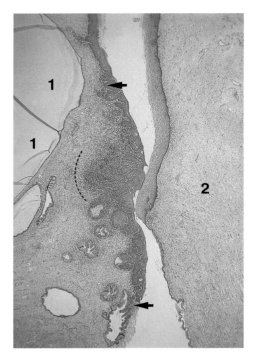

Fig. 1.12 FIGO stage Ia1 (1995), squamous carcinoma measured at 6 mm horizontally (between arrows) × 3 mm depth (dashed line) (formerly Ia2, FIGO, 1988). The intraepithelial and deeper invasive lesion is seen in association with Nabothian cyst formation (1) on the left-hand lip of the cone. The right lip is normal (2). Lesions such as this are much more frequently associated with lymphovascular space (LVS) involvement than that in Fig. 1.15 and have higher recurrence rates.

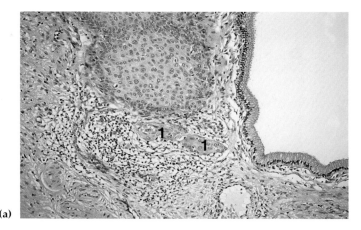

(a)

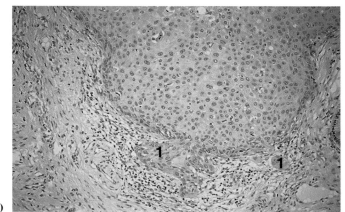

(b)

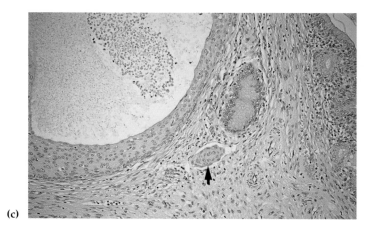

(c)

Fig. 1.13 (a) & (b) Multifocal early stromal invasion. Two foci of unmeasurable early stromal invasion (1) as seen in Fig. 1.15 but which were 9 mm apart. This is multifocal microinvasion larger than the 7 mm allowable within FIGO Ia and so is classified as Ib.

(c) Lymphovascular space (LVS) involvement is seen in less than 10% of tumors invading less than 1 mm. This is seen here (arrowed) and when present would necessitate more radical treatment. LVS involvement must be looked for in stage Ia1 and Ia2 (FIGO, 1995).

will now be classified as Ib instead of Ia1 (see Figs 1.13a & b).

The recording of lymphatic or vascular space (LVS) involvement is extended to include Ia as well as Ib. Few specialist gynecologists wish to remain conservative in treatment in the presence of Ia1 disease with LVS involvement, so this is a logical addition for audit purposes (Fig. 1.13c).

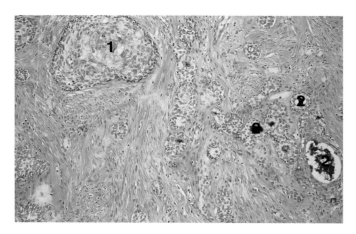

Fig. 1.14 An invasive adenosquamous carcinoma of cervix (Ib). The largest part of the tumor showed squamous differentiation as seen at (1). Basaloid small-cell areas of invasive tumor contained glandular tubule formations which stained positively for neutral mucin with AB-DPAS at (2).

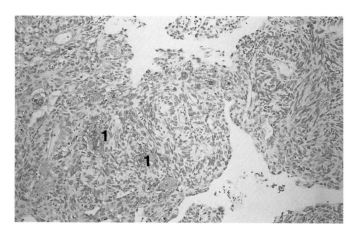

Fig. 1.15 An invasive basaloid adenosquamous carcinoma. Spindle-celled basaloid adenosquamous carcinoma of cervix (Ia2) with rosette formation morphologically, staining positively for mainly acid mucins by AB-DPAS (1).

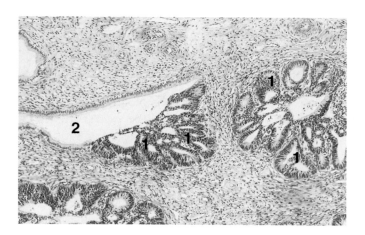

Fig. 1.16 Probable microinvasive adenocarcinoma of endocervix (Ia1). There are "budded," "back-to-back" arrangements of microtubular neoplastic glandular epithelium (1) spurring from an otherwise normal endocervical crypt (2).

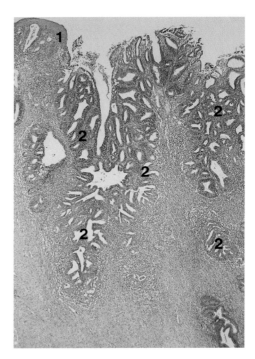

Fig. 1.17 Early invasive adenocarcinoma. Section from the transformation zone (squamocolumnar junction at (1)), revealing an occult early invasive adenocarcinoma (FIGO Ib (2)).

Table 1.1 (a) Classification and staging of cervical cancer*. FIGO (1995) staging.

Stage 0
Primary tumor cannot be assessed. No evidence of primary tumor
Carcinoma-in-situ

Stage I
Cervical carcinoma is strictly confined to the uterus (extension to corpus should be disregarded)

Stage Ia
Invasive cancer identified only microscopically. All gross lesions, even with superficial invasion, are stage IB cancers
Invasion is limited to measured stromal invasion with maximum depth of 5 mm and no wider than 7 mm†

Stage Ia1
Measured invasion of stroma no greater than 3 mm in depth and no wider than 7 mm

Stage Ia2
Measured invasion of stroma greater than 3 mm and no greater than 5 mm in depth and no wider than 7 mm

Stage Ib
Clinical lesions confined to the cervix or preclinical lesions greater than Ia

Stage Ib1
Clinical lesions no greater than 4 cm in size

Stage Ib2
Clinical lesions greater than 4 cm in size

* The classification and staging of tumors are considered not only by the Gynecology Oncology Committee of the International Federation of Gynecology and Obstetrics (FIGO), but also by the International Union Against Cancer (UICC), especially the Tumor, Nodes, Metastasis (TNM) Committee. Stages are defined by TNM or FIGO classification, with FIGO staging being conventionally used.
† The depth of invasion should not be more than 5 mm taken from the base of the epithelium, either surface or glandular, from which it originates. Vascular space involvement, either venous or lymphatic, should not alter the staging.

Table 1.1 (b) Carcinoma of the cervix: FIGO* (October 1988) staging.

Stage 0
Carcinoma-in-situ, intraepithelial carcinoma. Cases of stage 0 should not be included in any therapy statistics for invasive carcinoma

Stage I
The carcinoma is strictly confined to the cervix (extension to the corpus should be disregarded)

Stage Ia
Preclinical carcinomas of the cervix, that is those diagnosed only by microscopy

Stage Ia1
Minimal microscopically evident stromal invasion

Stage Ia2
Lesions detected microscopically that can be measured. The upper limit of the measurement should not show a depth of invasion of more than 5 mm taken from the base of the epithelium, either surface or glandular, from which it originates. A second dimension, the horizontal spread, must not exceed 7 mm. Larger lesions should be staged as Ib

Stage Ib
Lesions of greater dimensions than stage Ia2, whether seen clinically or not. Preformed space involvement should not alter the staging but should be specifically recorded to determine whether it should affect future treatment decisions

* International Federation of Gynecology and Obstetrics.
Stage 0 comprises those cases with full-thickness involvement of the epithelium with atypical cells, but with no signs of invasion into the stroma.
Stage Ia carcinoma should include minimal microscopically evident stromal invasion as well as small cancerous tumors of measurable size. It should be divided into those lesions with minute foci or invasion visible only microscopically (stage Ia1) and the macroscopically measurable microcarcinomas (stage Ia2) in order to gain further knowledge of the clinical behavior of these lesions. The term Ib occult should be omitted.
The diagnosis of both stage Ia1 and Ia2 should be based on microscopic examination of removed tissue, preferably a cone, which must include the entire lesion. As noted before, the lower limit of Stage Ia2 should be that it can be measured microscopically (even if dots need to be placed on the slide prior to measurement) and its upper limit is given by measurement of the two largest dimensions in any given section. Vascular space involvement, either venous or lymphatic, should not alter the staging, but should be specifically recorded as it may affect future treatment decisions. Lesions of greater size should be staged as Ib.

The original definition of Ia1 (with the refinement of noting the absence of LVS involvement) meant that metastatic disease was extremely rare (Burghardt *et al.*, 1991). The new stage Ia1 contains lesions that will metastasize (Copeland *et al.*, 1992). The risk is difficult to determine but may be 1–2%. Seoni *et al.* (1992) reviewed the literature which suggested a recurrence rate of 4.2% in stage Ia2. This will not change and justifies more radical treatments for this stage.

The issue of how to best make these defining measurements with any accuracy is one that is not addressed. It is unlikely that measurements on routine surgical specimens begin to approach the rigor of those within quoted studies which are used to evidence management.

The furthest depth of invasion needs to be measured to the nearest epithelial base of the surface or crypt, from which the invasion appears to arise. The width needs to be measured across all the blocks involved rather than simply the widest bit within a section of one block. This requires standardization of blocking of cone biopsies and cervices from hysterectomy specimens. Sagittal slicing to include both lips of the cervix rather than radial blocks are favored by most pathologists to maintain uniformity of thickness. If the disease is multifocal (i.e. more than a single area of invasion) then the width must include all points of invasion, even where separated by normal tissue in section (Figs 1.13a & b).

Fungating or ulcerated tumor surfaces probably preclude measurement of depth of invasion and such tumors should not be included in Ia. Their management will be individual. DPAS/Alcian Blue stains for mucin need to be performed in all cases to confirm differentiation (see Figs 1.14 & 1.15).

Whether early invasive adenocarcinoma (Figs 1.16 & 1.19) can be recognized, separated histologically from CGIN reliably and then measured remains questionable. The authors think it unlikely.

Management implications are discussed at length in Chapter 7.

1.6 Vaginal intraepithelial neoplasia (VAIN) (Figs 1.18–1.20)

Vaginal precancer can be divided into either squamous (VAIN), or glandular (VGIN) types. Both of these types may occur in association with "adenosis" (see Chapter 8). In the absence of adenosis, squamous lesions occur mainly in the upper third of the vagina most often in association with similar disease of the cervix and/or vulva.

Adenosis

The concept includes the presence of mullerian type glandular epithelium in the vagina. Sandberg (1967) discovered "occult" adenomas in 41% of postpubertal postmortem vaginas and 0% of prepubertal specimens. Similar findings were reported by Kurman (1974). Mucinous discharges are present in symptomatic cases and colposcopically the occurrence is associated with granular red spots not staining with Lugol's solution (Hart, 1976).

Clinically most occurrences have been identified in women who were exposed in-utero to diethylstilbestrol (DES) accounting for up to 90% of such exposed women in some series (Antonioli, 1975). The majority of women are affected if the exposure took place before the 8th week of pregnancy and very few if exposed after the first trimester (Sonek, 1976). More rarely, adenosis may occur sporadically without an association with DES. They all have similar histopathologic features (Robboy et al. 1986).

At biopsy endocervical glands are seen either on the surface or beneath a squamous epithelium. Tubal (ciliated) endometrial or intestinal type metaplasias occur (Hart,

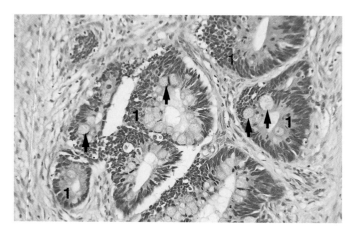

Fig. 1.18 HGCGIN/vaginal adenosis. Sporadic vaginal adenosis with extensive intestinal-type metaplasia, HGCGIN is seen here at (1) and intestinal-type or goblet-cell metaplasia is arrowed.

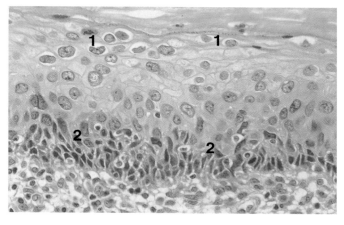

Fig. 1.19 VAIN 1 plus HPV changes. Note the koilocytes in the upper half (1). There is basal layer hyperplasia/dysplasia in the lower third of the epithelial thickness (2).

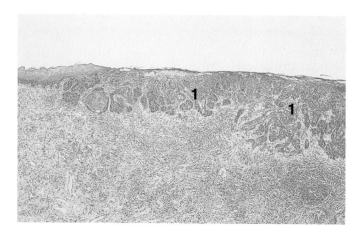

Fig. 1.20 Vaginal squamous carcinoma (1). An invasive squamous carcinoma of the vagina in a woman in her ninth decade. There was no previous history of genital tract neoplasia.

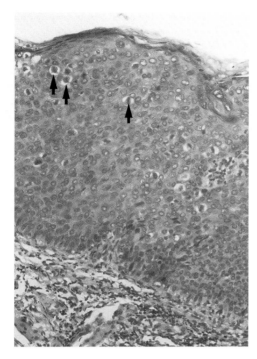

Fig. 1.21 Full thickness high-grade VIN 3 (differentiated large-cell or Bowenoid or warty-type). There is evidence of koilocytotic change in sporadic cells in the upper half of the lesion (arrowed).

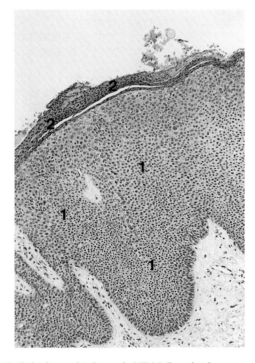

Fig. 1.22 Full thickness high-grade VIN 3 (basaloid or undifferentiated cell-type) (1). There is very superficial karyopyknosis of the atypical small basaloid squamous cells in the stratum corneum (2).

1976; Merchant, 1993). The lesions probably regress by squamous metaplasia which is very common (Robboy, 1981). VAIN 1, 2 or 3 may interrupt this process (Aho, 1991). HPV changes are usually present. Adenocarcinoma ("clear cell" adenocarcinoma) and precursor atypical lesions occur in association with tuboendometrial or intestinal metaplasias rather than with simple mucinous glands (Robboy, 1984) (Fig. 1.18).

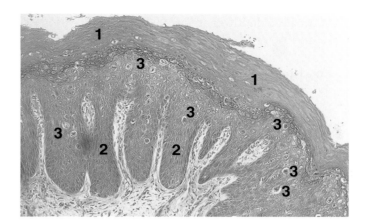

Fig. 1.23 Paget's disease. There are a sparse number of scattered macronucleolated, neoplastic, clear cells of glandular type present in a section of vulva. There is marked orthokeratosis (1), underlying vulval hyperplasia (2) with occasional included large atypical cells (3). There is no evidence of VIN.

Histopathology of vaginal intraepithelial neoplasia (VAIN)

Most cases occur in the upper third of the vagina and are usually concomitant with, or subsequent to similar lesions in the cervix (Kanbour, 1974; Aho, 1991). The same histological principles of vertical grading of severity are employed as for CIN; the mainly theoretical difference being that the target squamous epithelium is native and not metaplastic (Fig. 1.19). Treatment of high-grade lesions will usually entail local excision. Primary vaginal squamous carcinomas not associated with previous cervical neoplasia or preneoplasia do occur but are rare and usually only seen in elderly patients (Manetta, 1990) (Fig. 1.20). HPV is once again the putative causative agent.

1.7 Vulval precancer (Figs 1.21–1.22)

Vulval intraepithelial neoplasia (VIN)

Clinically seen white (leukoplakia) or red areas of thickened or excoriated vulval skin may be biopsied and variably found to include one of a range of inflammatory dermatoses, lichen sclerosis, keratosis and/or VIN. Only the latter has any significant precancerous potential.

VIN and vulval squamous cancer appear less reliably associated with HPV than CIN or VAIN. Full thickness high-grade VIN lesions may be separated into Bowenoid or differentiated types (Fig. 1.21) and suprabasal or basaloid undifferentiated types (Fig. 1.22). The latter variety shows much less association with HPV (Park *et al.* 1991).

Paget's disease

This presents as a neoplastic glandular lesion apparently arising from the intraepidermal portion of the vulval sweat glands and appearing clinically as a scaling or crusted red rash. The cells contain mucin, betraying their glandular differentiation. Invasive carcinoma is infrequently present (Curtin, 1990). Although no HPV association has been demonstrated the disease has been reported in coexistence with VIN infrequently (Hawley, 1991) (Fig. 1.23).

1.8 Related topics

The cytologic basis for the prediction of the histologic grade of squamous intraepithelial disease is discussed in Chapter 5. The epidemiology of HPV and possibilities of exploiting HPV typing in conjunction with cytology are explored further in Chapter 2. The difficulties and pitfalls of detecting glandular endocervical lesions and cytohistopathologic correlations of AIS and mimicking lesions is included in Chapter 5.

1.9 References and bibliography

Aho, M. (1991) Natural history of vaginal intraepithelial neoplasia. *Cancer* **68**,195.

Al-Nafussi, A.I. & Conquhoun, M.K. (1990) Mild cervical intraepithelial neoplasia (CIN I). A histological overdiagnosis. *Histopathology* **17**,557.

Anderson, M.C. (1995) Glandular lesions of the cervix: diagnostic and therapeutic dilemmas. *Bailliere Clin Obstet Gyn* **9**,105.

Antonioli, D.A. (1975) Vaginal adenosis. Analysis of 325 biopsy specimens from 100 patients. *Am J Clin Pathol* **64**,625.

Broders, A.C. (1932) Carcinoma in situ contrasted with benign penetrating epithelium. *J Am Med Assoc* **99**,1670.

Brown, L.J.R. & Wells, M. (1986) Cervical glandular atypia associated with squamous intraepithelial neoplasia: a premalignant lesion? *J Clin Pathol* **39**,22.

Buckley, C.H., Butter, E.B. & Fox, H. (1982) Cervical intraepithelial neoplasia. *J Clin Pathol* **35**,1.

Burghardt, E., Girardi, F., Lakonsen, M. *et al.* (1991) Microinvasive carcinoma of the uterine cervix (FIGO Stage IA). *Cancer* **67**,1037.

Christopherson, W.M. & Gray, L.A. Sr. (1982) Dysplasia and preclinical carcinoma of the uterine cervix. Diagnosis and Management. *Semin Oncol* **9**,265.

Cocker, J., Fox, H. & Langley, F.A. (1968) Consistency in the histological diagnosis of epithelial abnormalities of the cervix uteri. *J Clin Pathol* **21**,67.

Copeland, L.J., Silva, E.G., Gershenson, D.M. *et al.* (1992) Superficially invasive squamous cell carcinoma of the cervix. *Gynecol Oncol* **45**,307.

Cullen, T.S. (1900) *Cancer of the Uterus.* Appleton and Company, New York.

Cullimore, J.E., Luesley, D.M. & Rollason, T.P. (1992) A prospective study of colonization of the cervix in the management of cervical intraepithelial glandular neoplasia (CIGN) — a preliminary report. *Br J Obstet Gynaecol* **99**,314.

Curtin, J.P. (1990) Paget's disease of the vulva. *Gynecol Oncol* **39**,374.

Duggan, M.A. (1996) Human papillomaviruses in gynecological cancer. *Curr Opin Obstet Gynecol* **8**,56.

Duggan, M.A., Benoit, J.L., McGregor, S.E. *et al.* (1994) Adenocarcinoma in situ of the endocervix: human papillomavirus determination by dot blot hybridization and polymerase chain reaction amplification. *Int J Gynecol Pathol* **13**,143.

Duk, J.M., Aalders, J.G., Fleuren, G.J., Krans, M. & de Bruijn, H.W.A. (1989) Tumor markers CA 125, squamous cell carcinoma antigen, and carcinoembryonic antigen in patients with adenocarcinoma of the uterine cervix. *Obstet Gynecol* **73**,661.

Flannelly, G., Anderson, G., Kitchener, H.C. *et al.* (1994) Management of women with mild and moderate dyskaryosis. *BMJ* **308**,1399.

Fox, C.H. (1967) Biologic behaviour of dysplasia and carcinoma-in-situ. *Am J Obstet Gynecol* **99**,960.

Fox, H. & Buckley, C.H. (1990) Current problems in the pathology of intra-epithelial lesions of the uterine cervix. *Histopathology* **17**,1.

Franco, E.L. (1997) Understanding the epidemiology of genital infection with oncogenic and nononcogenic human papillomaviruses: a promising lead for primary prevention of cervical cancer. *Cancer Epidem Biomarker Prev* **6**,759.

Franquemont, D.W., Ward, B.E., Andeerson, W.A. & Crum, C.P. (1989) Prediction of "high risk" cervical papillomavirus infection by biopsy morphology. *Am J Clin Pathol* **92**,577.

Friedell, G.H. & McKay, D.G. (1953) Adenocarcinoma in situ of the endocervix. *Cancer* **6**,887.

Fu, Y.S. (1979) Nuclear DNA and histologic studies of genital lesions in diethylstilbestrol-exposed progeny. I. Intraepithelial squamous abnormalities. *Am J Clin Pathol* **72**,503.

Fu, Y.S., Braun, L., Shah, K.U., Lawrence, D.W. & Robboy, S.J. (1983) Histologic, nuclear DNA and human papillomavirus studies of cervical condyloma. *Cancer* **52**,1705.

Fu, Y.S., Reagan, J. & Richart, R.M. (1981) Definition of precursors. *Gynecol Oncol* **12**,220.

Gloor, E. & Hurliman, J. (1986) Cervical intraepithelial glandular neoplasia (adenocarcinoma in situ and glandular dysplasia). *Cancer* **58**,1272.

Govan, A.D.T., Haines, R.M., Langley, F.A., Taylor, C.W. & Woodcock, A.S. (1968) Changes in the epithelium of the cervix uteri. *J Obstet Gynaecol Br Commonw* **73**,883.

Griffin, N.R. & Wells, M. (1995) Premalignant and malignant glandular lesions of the cervix. In: Fox, H. and Wells, M. (eds) *Haines and Taylor Obstetrical and Gynaecological Pathology*, 4th edn, p. 323. Churchill Livingstone, New York.

Hakama, M., Maguus, K., Petterson, F., Storm, H. & Tulinium H. (1991) Effect of organised screening on the risk of cervix cancers in the Nordic countries. In: Miller, A.B. *et al.* (eds) *Cancer Screening*. UICC, Geneva.

Hart, W.R. (1976) Histopathologic spectrum of vaginal adenosis and related changes in stilbestrol-exposed females. *Cancer* **37**,763.

Hawley, I.C. (1991) Extramammary Paget's disease of the vulva with dermal invasion and vulva intra-epithelial neoplasia. *Histopathology* **18**,374.

Herrington, C.S. (1994) Human papillomaviruses and cervical neoplasia I: classification, virology, pathology and epidemiology. *J Clin Pathol* **47**,1066.

Herrington, C.S. (1995) Human papillomaviruses and cervical neoplasia II: interaction with other factors. *J Clin Pathol* **48**,1.

Herrington, C.S. (1996) Control of HPV replication: implications for squamous neoplasia. *J Pathol* **178**,237.

Holmquist, N.D., McMahan, C.A. & Williams, O.D. (1967) Variability in classification of carcinoma in situ of the uterine cervix. *Arch Pathol* **84**,334.

Holowaty, P., Miller, A.B., Rohan, T. & To., T. (1999) Natural history of dysplasia of the uterine cervix. *JNCI* **91**(3),252.

Hörding, U., Daugaard, S. & Visfeldt, J. (1997) Adenocarcinoma of the cervix and adenocarcinoma of the endometrium: distinction with PCR-mediated detection of HPV DNA. *APMIS* **105**,313.

IARC. (1986) Working Group on Cervical Cancer Screening. Summary Chapter 1a. In: Hakama, M., Miller, A.B. & Day, N.E. (eds) *Screening for Cancer of the Uterine Cervix*. IARC, Lyon. Scientific Publications no. **76**,133.

Ikenberg, H., Runge, M., Göppinger, A., Pfleiderer, A. (1990) Human papillomavirus DNA in invasive carcinoma of the vagina. *Obstet Gynecol* **76**,432.

Ismail, S.M., Colclough, A.B., Dinnen, J.S. *et al.* (1990) Reporting cervical intraepithelial neoplasia (CIN). Intra- and interpathologist variation and factors associated with disagreement. *Histopathology* **16**,371.

Jaworski, R.C., Pacey, N.F., Greenberg, M.L. & Osborn, R.A. (1988) The histologic diagnosis of adenocarcinoma in-situ and related lesions of the cervix uteri. *Cancer* **61**,1171.

Jones, M.H., Jenkins, D., Cuzick, J. *et al.* (1992) Mild cervical dyskaryosis: safety of cytological surveillance. *Lancet* **339**,1440.

Kanbour, A.I. (1974) Carcinoma of the vagina following cervical cancer. *Cancer* **34**,1838.

Korn, A.P., Judson, P.L. & Zaloudetz, C.J. (1998) Importance of atypical glandular cells of uncertain significance in cervical cytologic smears. *J Reprod Med* **43**,774.

Koss, L.G. & Durfee, G.R. (1956) Unusual patterns of squamous epithelium of the uterine cervix; cytologic and pathologic study of Roilocytotic atypia. *Ann NY Acad Sci* **63**,1245.

Koss, L.G., Stewart, F.W. & Foote, F.W. *et al.* (1963) Some histological aspects of behaviour of epidermoid carcinoma in situ and related lesions of the uterine cervix. *Cancer* **16**,1160.

Kottmeier, H.L. (1961) Evolution et traitement des epitheliomas. *Rev Fr Gynecol Obstet* **56**,821.

Kurman, R.J. (1974) The incidence and histogenesis of vaginal adenosis. An autopsy study. *Human Pathol* **5**,265.

Lee, K.R., Manna, E.A. & Jones, M.A. (1991) Comparative cytological features of adenocarcinoma in situ of the uterine cervix. *Acta Cytol* **35**,117.

Leminen, A., Paavonen, J., Vesterinen, E. *et al.* (1991) Human papillomavirus types 16 and 18 in adenocarcinoma of the uterine cervix. *Am J Clin Pathol* **95**,647.

Lungu, O., Sun, X.W., Felix, J. *et al.* (1992) Relationship of human papillomavirus type to grade of cervical intraepithelial neoplasia. *J Am Med Assoc* **267**,2493.

Maini, M., Lavie, O., Comeerci, G. *et al.* (1998) The management and follow-up of patients with high-grade cervical glandular intraepithelial neoplasia. *Int J Gynecol Cancer* **8**,287.

Manetta, A. (1990) Primary invasive carcinoma of the vagina. *Obstet Gynecol* **76**,639.

McIndoe, W.A., McLean, M.R., Jones, R.W. & Mullins, P.R. (1984) The invasive potential of carcinoma in situ of the cervix. *Obstet Gynecol* **64**,451.

Meisels, A. & Fortin, R. (1976) Condylomatous lesions of the cervix and vagina. I. Cytological patterns. *Acta Cytol* **20**,505.

Merchant, W.J. (1993) Intestinal metaplasia in stilboestrol-induced vaginal adenosis. *Histopathology* **23**,373.

Miller A.B., Chamberlain, J., Day, N.E., Hakama, M. & Protock, P.C. (1991) *Cancer Screening*. UICC, Geneva.

Nasiell, K., Roger, V. & Nasiell, M. (1986) Behavior of mild cervical dysplasia during the long term follow-up. *Obstet Gynecol* **67**,665.

National Cancer Institute Workshop. (1988) The 1988 Bethesda system for reporting cervical/vaginal cytologic diagnoses. *J Am Med Assoc* **262**,931.

National Cancer Institute Workshop. (1989) The 1988 Bethesda system for reporting cervical/vaginal cytologic diagnoses. *J Reprod Med* **34**,779.

National Cancer Institute Workshop. (1992) The revised Bethesda system for reporting cervical/vaginal cytologic diagnoses: Report of the 1991 Bethesda Workshop. *Anal Quant Cytol Histol* **14**,161.

Östör, A.G. (1993) Natural history of cervical intraepithelial neoplasia—a critical review. *Int J Gynecol Pathol* **12**,186.

Papanicolaou, G.N. (1954) *Atlas of Exfoliative Cytology*. The Commonwealth Fund, New York.

Park, J.S., Jones, R.W., McLean, M.R., Currie, J.L., Woodruff, J.D., Shah, K.V. *et al.* (1991) Possible etiologic heterogeneity of vulvar intraepithelial neoplasia. A correlation of pathologic characteristics with human papillomavirus detection by in situ hybridization and polymerase chain reaction. *Cancer* **67**(6),1599.

Petersen, O. (1956) Spontaneous course of cervical precancerous conditions. *Am J Obstet Gynecol* **72**,1063.

Purola, E. & Savia, E. (1977) Cytology of gynecologic condyloma acuminatum. *Acta Cytol* **21**,26.

Quinn, M.A. (1997) Adenocarcinoma of the cervix. Are there arguments for a different treatment policy? *Curr Opin Obstet Gynecol* **9**,21.

Reagan, J.W. & Harmonic, M.J. (1956) The cellular pathology in carcinoma in situ; a cytohistopathological correlation. *Cancer* **9**,385.

Reagan, J.W., Seidemann, I.L. & Saracusa, Y. (1953) Cellular morphology of carcinoma in situ and dysplasia or atypical hyperplasia of the uterine cervix. *Cancer* **6**,224.

Richart, R.M. (1968) Natural history of cervical intraepithelial neoplasia. *Clin Obstet Gynecol* **10**,748.

Richart, R.M. (1973) Cervical intraepithelial neoplasia: a review. In: Sommers, S.C. (ed.) *Pathology Annual*, p. 301. Appleton–Century–Crofts, East Norwalk, CT.

Richart, R.M. (1990) A modified terminology for cervical intraepithelial neoplasia. *Obstet Gynecol* **75**,131.

Richart, R.M. & Barron, B.A. (1969) A follow-up study of patients with cervical dysplasia. *Am J Obstet Gynecol* **105**,386.

Riotton, G., Christopherson, W.M. & Lunt, R. (eds) (1973) *International Histological Classification of Tumors, No. 8. Cytology of the Female Genital Tract*. World Health Organization, Geneva.

Robby, S.J., Szyfelbein, W.M., Goellner, J.R., Kaufman, R.H., Taft, P.D., Richard, R.M. *et al.* (1981) Dysplasia and cytologic findings in 4589 young women enrolled in diethylstilbestrol-adenosis (DESAD) project. *Am J Obstet Gynecol* **140**(5),579.

Robboy, S.J. (1984) Atypical vaginal adenosis and cervical ectopion. Association with clear cell adenocarcinoma in diethylstilbestrol-exposed offspring. *Cancer* **54**,869.

Robboy, S.J., Hill, E.C., Sandberg, E.C & Czernobilsky, D. (1986) Vaginal adenosis in women born prior to the diethylstilbestrol era. *Human Pathol* **17**,488.

Robertson, A.J., Anderson, J.M., Beck, J.S., Burnett, R.A., Howatson, S.R., Lee, F.D. *et al.* (1989) Observer variability in histopathological reporting of cervical biopsy specimens. *J Clin Pathol* **42**,231.

Sandberg, E.C. (1967) The incidence and distribution of occult vaginal adenosis. *Trans Pac Coast Obstet Gynaecol Soc* **35**,36.

Saurel, J. (1996) Adenocarcinoma in situ du col uterin. Aspects cytologiques et histologiques. *Ann Pathol* **16**,374.

Selvaggi, S.M. & Haefner, H.K. (1997) Microglandular endocervical hyperplasia and tubal metaplasia: pitfalls in the diagnosis of adenocarcinoma on cervical smears. *Diagn Cytopathol* **16**,168.

Seoni, B.U., Nadji, M., Averette, H.E. *et al.* (1992) Microinvasive carcinoma of the cervix. *Cancer* **70**,2121.

Shingleton, H.M., Gore, H., Bradley, D.H. & Soong, S.J. (1981) Adenocarcinoma of the cervix I. Clinical evaluation and pathologic features. *Am J Obstet Gynecol* **139**,799.

Shroyer, K.R. (1993) Human papillomavirus and endocervical adenocarcinoma. *Hum Pathol* **24**,119.

Siders, D.B., Parrott, M.H. & Abell, M.R. (1965) Gland cell prosoplasia (adenosis) of vagina. *Am J Obstet Gynecol* **91**,190.

Siegler, E.E. (1956) Microdiagnosis of carcinoma in situ of the uterine cervix. A comparative study of pathologists' diagnoses. *Cancer* **9**,463.

Smith, G.V. & Pemberton, F.A. (1934) The picture of very early carcinoma of the uterine cervix. *Surg Gynecol Obstet* **59**,1.

Sonek, M., Bibbo, M., Wied, G.L. (1976) Colposcopic findings in offspring of DES-treated mothers as related to onset of therapy. *J Reprod Med* **16**(2),65.

Syrjänen, K.J. (1992) Genital human papillomavirus (HPV) infections and their associations with squamous cell cancer: reappraisal of the morphologic, epidemiologic and DNA data. In: Fenoglio-Preiser, C.M., Wolff, M. & Rilke, F. (eds) *Progess in Surgical Pathology*, p. 217, Vol. XII. Field & Wood, New York.

Syrjänen, K.J. (1996a) Spontaneous evolution of intraepithelial lesions according to the grade and type of the implicated HPV. *Eur J Obstet Gynecol Reprod Biol* **65**,45.

Syrjänen, K.J. (1996b) Natural history of genital human papillomavirus infections. In: Lacey, C. (ed.) *Papillomavirus Reviews. Current Research on Papillomaviruses*. Leeds Medical Information, Leeds University Press, Leeds.

Tabbara, S., Sieh, A.D., Andersen, W. *et al.* (1992) The Bethesda classification for squamous intraepithelial lesions: histologic, cytologic and viral correlates. *Obstet Gynecol* **79**,338.

Tamimi, H.K. & Figge, D.C. (1982) Adenocarcinoma of the uterine cervix. *Gynecol Oncol* **13**,335.

Ward, B.E., Burkett, B.A., Peterson, C. *et al.* (1990) Cytological correlates of cervical papillomavirus infection. *Int J Gynecol Pathol* **9**,297.

Walters, W.D. & Reagan, J.W. (1956) Epithelial dysplasia of the uterine cervix in pregnancy. *Am J Clin Pathol* **26**,1314.

Weid, G.L. (1961) *Proceedings of the First International Congress on Exfoliative Cytology*. J.B. Lippincott, Philadelphia.

Wilbur, D.C. (1995) Endocervical glandular atypia: a "new" problem for the cytologist. *Diagn Cytopathol* **13**,463.

Willet, G.D., Kurman, R.J. & Reid, R. (1989) Correlation of the histological appearance of intraepithelial neoplasia of the cervix with human papillomavirus types. *Int J Gynecol Pathol* **8**, 18.

Williams, D.R. (1987) A retrospective review of adenocarcinoma in situ and glandular atypia of the uterine cervix. *Br J Obstet Gynaecol* **94**,699.

Williams, J. (1888) *Cancer of the Uterus: Harveian Lectures for 1886.* H.K. Lewis, London.

Winkler, B., Crum, C.P. & Fujli, T. (1984) Koilocytotic lesions of the cervix: the relationship of mitotic abnormalities to the presence of papillomavirus antigens and nuclear DNA content. *Cancer* **53**,1081.

Wolff, M. & Rilke, F. (eds) (1992) *Progress in Surgical Pathology*, p. 217. Field & Wood.

zur Hausen, H. (1991) Human papillomaviruses in the pathogenesis of anogenital cancer. *Virology* **184**,9.

zur Hausen, H. (ed.) (1994) Human pathogenic papillomaviruses. *Curr Top Microbiol Immunol* **186**,1.

zur Hausen, H. (1996) Papillomavirus infections — a major cause of human cancers. *Biochim Biophys Acta* **1288**,F55.

Chapter 2
Human Papillomaviruses in Pathogenesis of Lower Genital Tract Neoplasia

2.1 Introduction

Before the late 1970s, the meagre interest in human papillomavirus (HPV) infections was focused on external genital warts (*condylomata acuminata*), suspected to be a sexually transmitted disease (STD) since antiquity, and convincingly proved to be so in 1954. The late 1970s witnessed a major breakthrough by the light microscopic description of koilocytosis (the cytopathic effect of HPV, regularly present in exophytic condylomas) in the flat epithelial lesions as well, thus linking HPV with the precancer lesions of the uterine cervix and other genital mucosa (Meisels & Fortin, 1976; Purola & Savia, 1977). Since 1978, it has been well-recognized that HPV infections are frequently associated with genital precancer lesions; cervical intraepithelial neoplasia (CIN); vulvar intraepithelial neoplasia (VIN); vaginal intraepithelial neoplasia (VAIN); penile intraepithelial neoplasia (PIN); anal intraepithelial neoplasia (AIN) and frankly invasive squamous cell carcinomas (Syrjänen et al., 1987; zur Hausen, 1994, 1996). Together with the currently characterized and pending viral types, the number of different HPV types exceeds 100 at the time of writing, and no end to this listing is in sight. According to a recently adjourned expert panel, the evidence is sufficient to warrant the statement that distinct high-risk HPV types (16 and 18) are definitely carcinogenic agents to humans, conveying a significant risk for the development of an invasive cervical (and other genital) squamous cell cancer (IARC, 1995).

Apart from the molecular and clinical studies, significant new data to support the causal role of HPV in genital carcinogenesis have been obtained by epidemiologic means. Using different approaches, these studies have provided data on the prevalence and incidence of HPV infections, the risk factors predisposing the women to HPV infections and genital precancer lesions, as well as on the determinants of progression of these precancer lesions towards an invasive disease. Of special importance from the epidemiologic point of view is the mode of transmission of this virus by sexual contact, thus conferring a potential risk for the development of genital precancer lesions in both sexual partners. Recently, other possible modes of HPV transmission have been suggested (Cason, 1996; Puranen et al., 1996). These include a vertical transmission from an infected mother to her newborn baby. Such data have important implications in the planning of effective measures for early detection and prevention of HPV infections (Franco, 1997).

Another key issue in understanding the epidemiology of HPV infections is the assessment of their natural history by prospective follow-up without therapeutic intervention. In such cohort studies, decisive evidence on the inherent progressive potential of HPV lesions has been obtained. Equally important, however, is the documented spontaneous regression established for a substantial proportion of cervical HPV infections in such studies. Indeed, the natural history of cervical HPV infections seems to be identical with that of the precancer lesions, as established by a number of large cohort studies going back several decades (Östör, 1993; Syrjänen, 1996a,b). This provides further strong evidence implicating the role of HPV in cervical carcinogenesis.

2.2 Characteristics of human papillomaviruses

Because viruses are obligate intracellular parasites, they cannot survive extended periods outside their target cells. However, they must be sufficiently stable in the environment to keep alive until they find a susceptible host. The first step in viral pathogenesis is to enter that susceptible host by using any of the available portals of entry, including the skin, mucosa of the eyes, oral cavity, upper gastrointestinal tract, respiratory tract, urogenital mucosa or anal canal. Not unexpectedly, HPV infections can be readily demonstrated at all these sites (Syrjänen et al., 1987; zur Hausen, 1996).

HPV is a DNA virus that has a double-stranded, tightly coiled, circular genome of about 8000 Da (zur Hausen, 1994, 1996; de Villiers, 1997). When the capsid is fully assembled, it forms an icosahedral structure. A complete virion measures approximately 55 nm in diameter (Fig. 2.1). HPV has been classified into more than 100 types by DNA homology. The genetic structure of individual types is similar and the genome can be subdivided into three regions:

1 The upper regulatory region (URR), containing binding sites for factors which regulate gene expression and DNA replication.

2 The early region, coding for proteins which regulate viral transcription (E2); viral DNA replication (E1, E2); cell proliferation (E5, E6, E7); and virus release (E4).

3 The late region, which codes for the two proteins forming the viral capsid (L1 and L2) (Fig. 2.2).

It is generally assumed that the initial HPV infection in

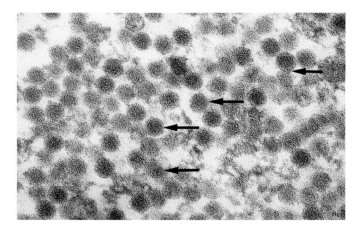

Fig. 2.1 Transmission electronmicroscopic view of papillomavirus particles (arrowed). (Original magnification × 100 000.)

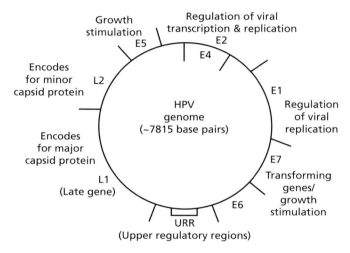

Fig. 2.2 Schematic drawing of the HPV genome organization.

the squamous epithelium requires that the virus be in the form of a complete virion, i.e. a central core of DNA surrounded by its protein coat. Once it enters the host, for example through the genital mucosa, the steps of viral pathogenesis within the individual target cells include the following: adsorption, penetration, uncoating, transcription, translation, replication, assembly, and release. Details of many of these steps are still poorly understood, and an in-depth discussion about these molecular events clearly falls outside the scope of this chapter (zur Hausen, 1996).

The replication of HPV is closely geared to the differentiation of the cervical epithelium. The initial infection occurs in the basal layer of undifferentiated stem cells. At this stage, only early HPV proteins are synthesized. These include:

1 E5, E6 and E7 proteins for the induction of a transient host DNA synthesis thereby providing the environment and macromolecules essential for viral DNA replication.

2 E1 and E2 proteins for the replication of viral DNA.

The synthesis of the early proteins is switched off as the cells are displaced upwards through the epithelium and differentiate. The viral structural proteins, L1 and L2, are synthesized in the superficial epithelium prior to exfoliation and are assembled into capsids enclosing viral DNA. The progeny virions are released from the infected cells and this is accompanied by cytoskeletal collapse induced by another viral gene product, E4.

Infected cells may not be able to differentiate fully as a result of either: (i) functional interference of cell cycle regulating proteins, caused by viral gene expression (e.g. interaction between HPV 16 E6 with cellular protein p53, interaction between HPV 16 E7 with cellular protein pRB); or (ii) overproduction of E5, E6 and E7. When this occurs the host DNA synthesis continues unchecked and leads to rapidly dividing undifferentiated cells with morphologic characteristics of CIN 3. It is thought that accumulated chromosomal breakages, rearrangements, deletions and other genomic mutations in these cells lead to cells with invasive capability and ultimately to cervical malignancy.

Papillomaviruses are strictly species-specific, and named according to their host (zur Hausen, 1994, 1996). It was agreed in 1979 that HPVs would be named by number, and in their order of discovery. The previous criteria of HPV typing by 50% homology in their hybridization pattern were revised in the early 1990s, and classification is currently based on direct sequencing of certain regions of the viral genome (zur Hausen, 1994, 1996). At present, more than 80 different HPV types have been officially identified, and together with the types pending characterization, the total number of HPV types currently exceeds 100 (de Villiers, 1997). Of these recognized HPV types, over 30 are known to infect the anogenital mucosa of both sexes (Table 2.1).

It has become clear that HPVs can be divided into three groups based on their oncogenic potential:

1 Low or no oncogenic potential. This includes HPV types 6, 11, and the 40s other than 45.

2 High oncogenic potential. This group includes types 16, 18, 45, 56, and probably some of the more recently characterized types.

3 Intermediate oncogenic potential, which includes the types 31, 33, 35, 51, and 52 (Lörincz *et al.*, 1992; de Villiers, 1997).

The typical manifestations and the oncogenic potential of the HPV types infecting the genital mucosa are described in Table 2.1.

2.3 Manifestations of genital HPV infections

Successful transmission of genital HPV infections seems to depend upon the access of the virus into epithelial cells capable of dividing. The only such cells in the squamous epithelium are those of the basal layer. Thus, HPV infection probably occurs upon exposure of the basal cells to infectious virus particles as a result of minor traumas of the epithelium, for example, due to sexual intercourse. After an established viral infection, two possible pathways may ensue:

1 the HPV genome persists in a latent form in the basal and parabasal cells without noticeable changes in the target epithelium; or

Table 2.1 Anogenital HPV types and their clinical manifestations.

HPV type	Clinical disease	Oncogenic potential
6	Condyloma accuminata, flat condylomas, CIN 1, laryngeal papillomas	Benign
11	Condylomata acuminata, flat condylomas, CIN 1, laryngeal papillomas, conjunctival papillomas, sino-nasal papillomas	Rarely malignant
16	CIN 1–2, Bowenoid papulosis, Bowen's disease, cervical, vulvar, oral, sino-nasal, ocular, laryngeal, and anal carcinomas	Malignant
18	CIN 1–3, cervical, vulvar, anal, and laryngeal cancers	Malignant
31	CIN 1–3, carcinomas	Malignant
33	CIN 1–3, carcinomas	Malignant
35	CIN 1–3, carcinomas	Malignant
39	Bowenoid papulosis, CIN, carcinomas	Malignant
41	Condylomata, CIN 1	Benign
42	Flat condylomata, Bowenoid papulosis	Benign
43	CIN 1–2	Benign?
44	Condylomata acuminata	Benign
45	Condylomata, CIN, carcinomas	Malignant
51	CIN 1–3, carcinomas	Malignant
52	Condylomata acuminata, CIN 1–3, carcinomas	Malignant
53	CIN 1–3	Rarely malignant
54	Genital condylomata	Benign
55	Bowenoid papulosis	Rarely malignant
56	CIN 1–3, carcinomas	Malignant
57	CIN, nasal papillomas, oral papillomas	Benign
58	Genital condylomata, CIN	Benign
59	VIN	Benign?
60	CIN	Benign?
61–64	VAIN	Benign?
66	Carcinomas	Malignant
67–68	VIN	Benign?
69	CIN	Benign?
70	Vulvar papilloma	Benign
71	VAIN	Benign?

Data compiled from different sources.

Table 2.2 Diagnostic criteria of the different HPV infections.

Diagnostic technique	Findings by the different diagnostic techniques in:		
	Clinical infection	Subclinical infection	Latent infection
Colposcopy	Conclusive	Inconclusive	Negative
Pap smear	Conclusive	Inconclusive	Negative
Histology	Conclusive	Inconclusive	Negative
Hybridization	Conclusive	Conclusive*	Conclusive*
PCR	Conclusive	Conclusive	Conclusive
Serology	Unclear	Unclear	Unclear

*May remain negative, depending on the sensitivity of the technique.

1 Condyloma acuminatum.
2 Giant condylomata acuminatum or Buschke–Löwenstein tumor.
3 Flat condyloma.
4 Papulosis (pigmented papulosis) lesions.
5 Bowenoid papulosis (Gross & von Krogh, 1997).

Although there is no clear-cut association between the macroscopic and microscopic appearance and the HPV type involved, practically all exophytic condylomata (and benign flat condylomata) are induced by HPV 6 and 11, whereas the high-risk HPV types 16 and 18 have been isolated from papulosis/pigmented papulosis, Bowenoid papulosis (Gross & von Krogh, 1997) and flat CIN lesions.

Clinical infections (predominately condylomata)

HPVs do not significantly deviate from most other viruses in that they are clearly capable of inducing both clinical, subclinical and latent infections (zur Hausen, 1996; Gross & van Krogh, 1997). Unfortunately, there is some confusion in the literature concerning the definitions of these three manifestations. In particular, the term subclinical HPV infection is used to mean different things by different authors (Roman & Fife, 1989; Syrjänen, 1996a,b). A proper evaluation requires the division of the different manifestations of HPV infections strictly into three categories (clinical, subclinical, latent) by taking into account the molecular biological data as well as utilizing all the diagnostic tools available to categorize these lesions, as defined in Table 2.2.

Accordingly, in a *clinical* HPV infection, the lesion should be readily apparent by all the generally used clinical diagnostic means, i.e. colposcopy, peroxidase–antiperoxidase (pap) smear test and biopsy. Much has been written with abundant illustrations of the clinical manifestations of genital HPV infections, making a detailed description of these lesions unnecessary in this context (Syrjänen *et al.*, 1987; IARC, 1995; Mindel, 1995; Gross & Barrasso, 1997; Gross & von Krogh, 1997, Burghardt *et al.*, 1998). It is generally agreed that clinically manifest genital HPV lesions include the following distinct morphologic entities: condyloma acuminatum (exophytic genital wart); giant condyloma; flat condyloma; endophytic (inverted) condyloma;

2 an active infection of the parabasal cells is established.

In the latter case, HPV stimulates the proliferation of the basal cells (and the synthesis of early HPV proteins as discussed above), leading to formation of a visible epithelial lesion, for example a genital wart. In such an active replicative infection, the number of viral particles increases substantially during the life-cycle of the epithelial cell until the cell containing large numbers of complete virions is exfoliated at the epithelial surface. As with many other viruses, this productive HPV infection is associated with viral cytopathic effects (CPE), and it is these CPEs which create the typical histologic and cytologic changes recognizable as morphologic manifestations of an HPV infection on light microscopy. In the genital tract of both sexes, five morphologically distinct clinical HPV lesions can be encountered:

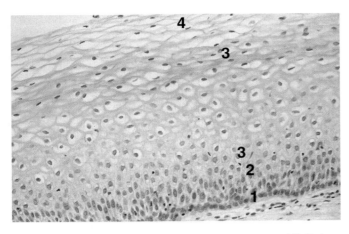

Fig. 2.3 Normal squamous epithelium of the ectocervix. All distinct cell layers (basal (1), suprabasal (2), intermediate (3) and superficial (4)) are clearly distinguished in this well-glycogenated epithelium.

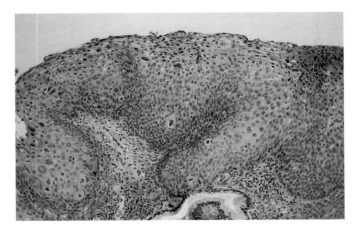

Fig. 2.5 A typical endophytic condyloma associated with CIN 2 (HPV-CIN 2). The acanthotic epithelium shows a dysplastic change extending to one-half to two-thirds of the epithelial thickness, with some highly abnormal (multipolar) mitotic figures. The uppermost one-third of the epithelium is occupied by characteristic koilocytes. This abnormal epithelium shows an endophytic growth pattern, extending down to underlying connective tissue and endocervical glands, giving the lesion an inverted appearance.

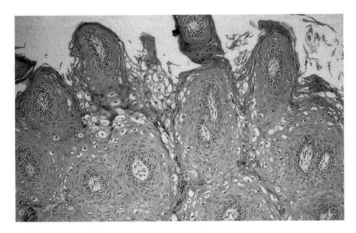

Fig. 2.4 A typical benign exophytic condyloma acuminatum. The lesion is characterized by extensive papillomatosis and koilocytosis, as well as a thin layer of dyskeratotic (parakeratotic) superficial cells. No signs of dysplasia are present.

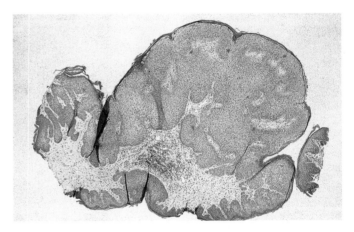

Fig. 2.6 A benign papulosis lesion of the female external genitalia. This acanthotic focus of epithelium has a rounded papular outline, clearly distinct from the classical condyloma acuminatum. The markedly acanthotic epithelium is covered by a thin layer of parakeratotic superficial cells, giving the lesion an acetowhite appearance on colposcopy. No signs of dysplasia are present, but small foci of superficial koilocytes are detectable.

Bowenoid papulosis; papulosis; and pigmented papulosis. The accurate diagnosis of these clinical HPV lesions does not usually pose any major problems, provided that proper colposcopy and cytopathology facilities are available (Figs 2.3–2.14).

Subclinical HPV infections (SPI)

As mentioned above, the term *subclinical* HPV infection is used to mean different things by different authors. According to some authors, all lesions visualized only after the application of acetic acid are called subclinical. To others, subclinical HPV infections are those lesions that are not visible on routine inspection, but become visible on colposcopy after acetic acid, and which on histology contain typical HPV-induced changes (Roman & Fife, 1989). Yet others use this term interchangeably with a flat condyloma (Schneider, 1990). Syrjänen (1996a,b) believes that the term subclinical HPV infection should be reserved for lesions which become visible only on colposcopy after acetic acid, and which on light microscopy, show minor epithelial

changes not consistent with typical flat condylomata (Table 2.2). Representative examples are seen in Figs 2.15–2.16.

It is clear that subclinical HPV infections may significantly contribute to the clinical disease. If correctly categorized, all subclinical HPV infections should contain HPV DNA when subjected to hybridization or polymerase chain reaction (PCR) (Table 2.2). In some patients, subclinical infection may be the only feature of HPV, but it may also be associated with condylomata acuminata or other common lesions at various genital sites. Its appearance at a site where previous condylomata have been treated and healed is suggestive of a persistent HPV infection (Gomez-Rueda *et al.*, 1994). The mechanisms by which such persis-

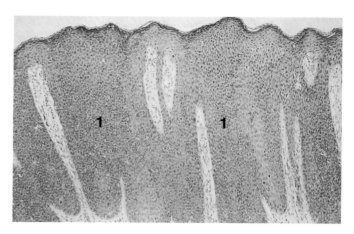

Fig. 2.7 A classical Bowenoid papulosis lesion of the vulva. This acanthotic focus of epithelium is flat, giving the gross appearance of a macule. The full thickness of the epithelium is composed of highly abnormal cells of the basaloid type (1), and extensive mitotic activity is present. No cytopathic effects (CPEs) of HPV are detectable, but using *in situ* hybridization, this lesion contained HPV 16 DNA, localized in scattered cells of the most superficial layers. (Toluidine blue.)

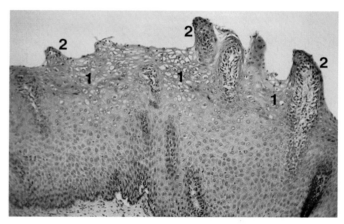

Fig. 2.8 A flat HPV lesion with completely even surface contour. Notice the extensive koilocytotic change in the intermediate layers of the epithelium (1). It is important to recognize that there are no signs of CIN in this lesion, as evidenced by the regular layer of the basal cells (2).

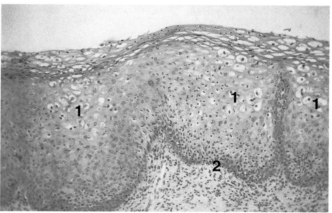

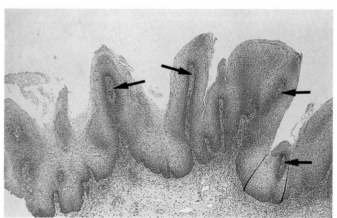

Fig. 2.9 Another flat HPV lesion with extensive small spikes (or asperities) on its surface. Koilocytotic change (1) is clearly discernible, and no signs of CIN are present. Notice the small blood (2) vessels extending close to the surface within the connective tissue core of each individual spikes, giving this lesion a punctate appearance on colposcopy.

Fig. 2.10 Yet another distinct morphologic manifestation of HPV infection, known as spiked condyloma, in the vagina. This lesion extending laterally on the vaginal wall has a spiked appearance on colposcopy (see Chapter 12, p. 311), due to the numerous papillary structures covered by koilocytotic squamous epithelium and supported by a connective tissue core with abundant blood vessels (arrowed). Notice a completely different growth pattern to that of the lesion depicted in Fig. 2.7.

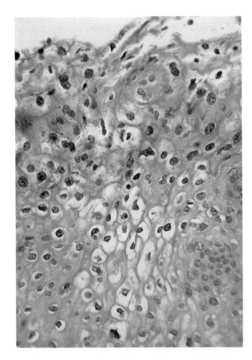

Fig. 2.11 A medium-power detail from the superficial layers of a highly proliferative flat condyloma to illustrate the typical appearance of the koilocytotic cells. Marked nuclear changes are obvious, characterized by increased size, variable shape, hyperchromasia, binucleation, and karyopyknosis (in most superficial cells). These abnormal nuclei are surrounded by extensive cytoplasmic clearing (koilocytosis), giving the typical light microscopic morphology.

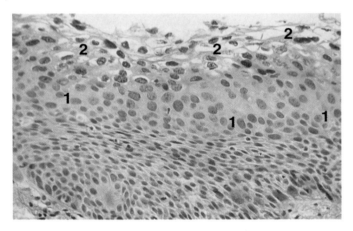

Fig. 2.12 Another flat HPV lesion associated with CIN 2 (HPV-CIN 2). One-half to two-thirds of the epithelial thickness are occupied by basaloid type of transformed cells (1), with few mitotic figures. There is a sharp border between this dysplastic layer and the uppermost one-third of the epithelium, which is composed of extensive koilocytosis (2). This is a frequent finding in these flat HPV-CIN lesions.

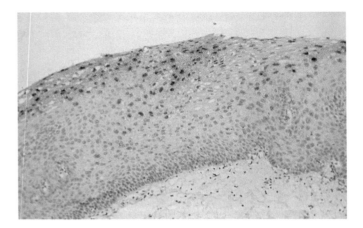

Fig. 2.13 A flat HPV lesion subjected to *in situ* hybridization (ISH) with 35S-labeled HPV-DNA probes. Intense positive signals (black spots) signifying a high copy-number infection of HPV 11 are superimposed on the intermediate and superficial layer cells with typical koilocytotic morphology. Low-risk HPV types are regularly found in these benign flat HPV lesions by using ISH or other hybridization techniques. (ISH, hematoxylin counterstaining.)

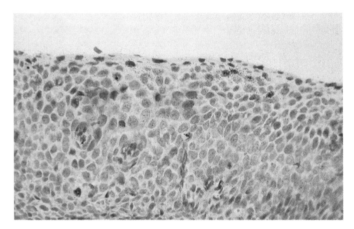

Fig. 2.14 A high-grade CIN 3 lesion examined for the presence of HPV-DNA by using ISH with 35S-labeled HPV-DNA probes. No morphologic evidence (CPE) of HPV exists in this lesion, the full thickness being composed of anaplastic basaloid-type of cells. However, weak positive signals (black spots) signifying a low copy-number infection of HPV 16 are found, superimposed on a few scattered cells close to the lesion surface. In lesions like this, ISH or other HPV tests are the only reliable means to document the HPV involvement, as demonstrated in this case. (ISH, hematoxylin counterstaining.)

tent HPV infections develop into clinical disease are not fully understood, but they are probably associated with an altered host immune response.

Latent HPV infections

By virological definition, latent viral infections represent cases where viral genome (DNA or RNA) is present in an otherwise normal target tissue. Accordingly, the term *latent*

HPV infections should be reserved for the cases where HPV-DNA is found in biopsies which by all histologic criteria are classifiable as normal epithelium (Syrjänen, 1992). The assessment of whether epithelium is normal or not should always be based on careful histopathologic examination. This is often of a directed punch biopsy and it is important to realize that there is an associated inherent false negative rate. There is little doubt that HPV genomes may persist in epithelial cells without inducing any cytopathic changes. HPV-DNA has been identified in cervical smears from colposcopically and cytologically healthy women. Latent infections which are presumed to be non-infectious probably represent the largest reservoir for genitoanal HPV infections (Gross & von Krogh, 1997). It is speculated that periodic activation and phenotypic expres-

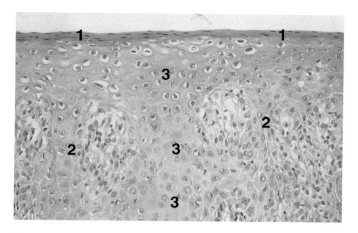

Fig. 2.15 This and the next photomicrograph (Fig. 2.16) demonstrate examples of a subclinical HPV infection. In this biopsy from an acetowhite lesion on the introitus, a thin layer of superficial (1) parakeratotic cells is seen, responsible for the acetowhite reaction. The epithelium is acanthotic, extending as narrow streaks (2) downwards. The intermediate layer is composed of squamous cells (3) with varying degrees of cytoplasmic vacuolization. In contrast to true koilocytes, however, these vacuolized cells lack the nuclear abnormalities shown in Fig. 2.11. The nuclear size is not altered compared with that of the non-vacuolized counterparts, and the nuclei have retained their normal staining properties (i.e. they are not hyperchromatic). This lesion was negative with ISH, but contained HPV 11 DNA on PCR amplification.

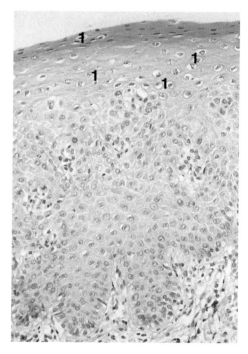

Fig. 2.16 Another biopsy from the vagina, showing subtle epithelial (1) changes consistent with a subclinical HPV infection. Observable changes are very much like those in Fig. 2.15. Again, cells with vacuolized cytoplasm are seen, but they lack the nuclear abnormalities of true koilocytes. This lesion was positive with ISH, containing HPV 42 DNA in some of the vacuolized cells close to the lesion surface.

sion of small infectious foci within the field of latent infection could represent a source of HPV for most of the sexually transmitted HPV-associated diseases. So far it is not clear, whether these latent infections may also be residuals of the lesions having regressed spontaneously.

2.4 Prevalence of genital HPV infections

The revived interest in HPV as a potential etiologic agent for cervical neoplasia arose from the morphologic examination of both pap smears and cervical biopsies, in which the CPEs of HPV were identified with or without concomitant dysplastic changes (Meisels & Fortin, 1976; Purola & Savia, 1977). These morphologic reports were the first to provide evidence for the presence of HPV in a substantial proportion of cervical cancer precursors. It took considerably longer, however, before data on the prevalence of genital HPV infections in women with no cervical lesions started to emerge.

It is well-established that genital HPV infections peak in the 20–29 years age group (Syrjänen *et al.* 1990a). This group is not generally covered by the national screening program in Finland (Fig. 2.17). To assess the prevalence figures among these young women, a special mass-screening was undertaken in 1985–86 which was focused on an unselected cohort of 22-year-old women in Kuopio province, i.e. a birth cohort of 1963 (*n* = 2.013 women) (Syrjänen *et al.*, 1990b). In two successive years, the same cohort of women was screened using routine pap smears. The prevalence of HPV infection among these women was 3% in the first year and 7% in the subsequent year. These data could be then used to calculate the annual incidence, as discussed below.

The prevalence data obtained in our mass-screening as discussed above could be directly used to calculate the annual incidence of cervical HPV infections in this population of sexually active young women. The crude annual incidence was 7.0%. The prevalence figures for those attending both rounds of screening and for those attending only once indicated that the non-attenders had some 25% higher risk of HPV infection than the attenders. Adjusting for this source of bias increased the annual incidence to 8% in this age group (Syrjänen *et al.*, 1990b). Noteworthy is the fact that these figures only apply to clinical HPV infections detectable by conventional pap smears. Undoubtedly, the application of PCR would certainly result in significantly higher incidence rates, while revealing the subclinical and latent HPV infections as well.

Incidence rates of HPV infections

The incidence data on cervical HPV infections from the studies utilizing PCR technology are emerging only recently (van Doornum *et al.*, 1992). These authors assessed the prevalence, incidence and risk factors of HPV infections in a prospective cohort of 162 women and 85 men attending an STD clinic in Amsterdam. The incidence of HPV infection proved to be as high as 47.1 and 50.5 per 100 person-years in women and men, respectively. It is noteworthy, however, that this cohort represents a selected group of high-risk STD patients with multiple sexual partners, and

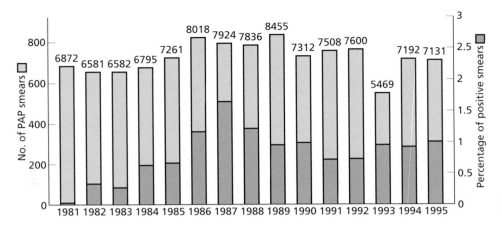

Fig. 2.17 Prevalence of HPV infection in Kuopio mass-screening 1981–95.

as such does not reflect the true incidence among the general population. In a Brazilian cohort study, the incidence of new cervical HPV infections seemed to be dependent on HPV type (Franco & Monsonego, 1997). Accordingly, the incidence of infections by the low-oncogenic HPV types was 7.9/1000 women per month, compared with 9.2 for the high-risk types. Taken together for the low- and high-risk types, these data implicate an incidence of 1.71% per month of new infections in women who were HPV-negative at enrollment. The majority of these infections proved to be transient, however (Franco & Monsonego 1997). Further studies on the true incidence of genital HPV infections in the general population are clearly needed.

2.5 Transmission of genital HPV infections

Sexual transmission

Following the demonstration that external genital warts are a sexually transmitted disease by Barrett & Silbar (1954), this mode of transmission has been regarded as the most important in sexually active adults (Oriel, 1981). The data confirming this concept are derived from different epidemiologic approaches. Reference has already been made to the studies which show that HPV is virtually absent in women with no previous sexual experience, i.e. in virgins and nuns (Rylander *et al.*, 1994; Critchlow & Koutsky, 1995). With increasing sexual experience, the risk of contracting HPV infections seems to increase (Syrjänen *et al.*, 1984). Indeed, recent data suggest that this risk increases in parallel with the number of sexual partners, for example from 17% in women with one partner up to 83% in women with five partners, respectively (Critchlow & Koutsky, 1995). Similar observations have been reported by other authors (Kataja *et al.*, 1992, 1993; Moscicki, 1996). At present, the evidence implicating the number of sexual partners as one of the most significant risk factors for genital HPV infections is compelling (IARC, 1995).

To interfere with the sexual transmission of HPV, it is of prime importance to assess the reservoirs of this virus in both sexes. Recent data suggest that the epithelium of the male genital tract (i.e. penis, urethra and prostate) might act

as such a reservoir (Hillman *et al.*, 1993; Rotola *et al.*, 1994; Baken *et al.*, 1995). In recent years, studies have been completed, searching for HPV reservoirs in asymptomatic males by Southern blot or PCR. These have been summarized (Mindel, 1995; Gross & von Krogh, 1997) and it seems to be established beyond doubt that HPV-DNA exists in these apparently normal mucosal sites of the penis, urethra and prostate. The existence of such a reservoir, in turn, is the prerequisite for sexual transmission of HPV, and for the subsequent detection of HPV-associated precancer lesions and identical HPV types in both sexual partners (Mindel, 1995). The latter issue is controversial, however, because HPV type-concordance figures between sexual couples have been reported as both low and high (Monsonego *et al.*, 1993; Hippeläinen *et al.*, 1994).

Vertical transmission

Of the non-sexual routes of HPV transmission, the perinatal (or antenatal) vertical transmission from an infected mother to her newborn baby is of particular clinical relevance. Mounting evidence from different types of approaches (including the detection of HPV in the oral mucosa and larynx, serum antibodies to genital HPV in children as well as HPV-DNA in amniotic fluid) is now suggesting that this kind of vertical transmission of HPV might be an important route of spreading the virus (Pakarian *et al.*, 1994; Cason, 1996; Puranen *et al.*, 1996). This mode of transmission would also feasibly explain how this virus gets access into the oral mucosa as well as that of the upper aerodigestive tract (nasal cavity, paranasal sinuses, larynx, trachea, bronchus, and esophagus), where HPV-DNA has been well-documented in both benign and malignant tumors (Syrjänen *et al.*, 1987). Firm evidence for this kind of maternal-to-baby transmission was recently provided by the sequence data confirming the identity of the viruses found in both baby and mother (Cason, 1996; Puranen *et al.*, 1996).

2.6 Risk factors for genital HPV infections

Elucidation of the risk factors for the etiologic agent (HPV) is mandatory to identify the populations at risk for cancer precursors, to be able to target the efforts of primary prevention appropriately (Franco, 1997). For such an assessment, different epidemiologic approaches are available.

The major risk factor for genital HPV infections is sexual behavior, particularly having multiple sexual partners. On the other hand, the role of other factors (e.g. cigarette smoking, oral contraceptives and pregnancy) is less clear even after the vast amount of effort put into these analyses (Xi & Koutsky, 1997). Almost irrespective of the target population, the risk factors predisposing women to this infection remain the same, with some minor modifications.

These risk factors were classified into five distinct categories:

1 Sexual behavior.
2 Smoking habit.
3 Reproductive history.
4 Nutritional factors.
5 Immunosuppression.

All the above cited studies analysed the risk factors which were classifiable into one or more of these categories. The studies differed in three aspects: (i) the target population analyzed; (ii) the in-depth penetration of the interviewing; and (iii) the test used to detect HPV (IARC, 1995; Franco, 1997; Xi & Koutsky, 1997). In the more recent studies, PCR was used for HPV-DNA detection, thus reducing the variability in the detection techniques, which was considered to be a problem in the earlier studies. Standardized statistical techniques used to evaluate the results using the OR (odds ratios) with 95% CI (confidence interval) approach, allow a comparison between studies. Taken together, all these data unequivocally support the notion that sexual intercourse is the main mode of transmission of genital HPV infections among adults, and sexual promiscuity (expressed by different characteristics) seems to be the most significant risk factor for genital HPV infections (Xi & Koutsky, 1997). Not unexpectedly, these same risk factors have been shown to predispose the women to cervical cancer and its precursors.

2.7 HPV and cancer precursors

A number of different epidemiologic approaches are available to search for the evidence of HPV as a risk factor for cervical cancer and its precursors. Such approaches include: (i) descriptive epidemiologic studies; (ii) case reports and case series; (iii) cohort studies; and (iv) case-control studies. The merits and limitations of these different types of studies have been discussed (IARC, 1995; Schiffman, 1995; Holly, 1996; Franco, 1997).

The number of case-control studies using PCR amplification is continuously increasing, with new studies being reported almost monthly. This makes any attempted complete listing of these works inevitably obsolete (IARC, 1995; Mindel, 1995; Gross & von Krogh, 1997). Using a similar type of meta-analysis as for the non-PCR studies, the IARC monograph lists these PCR-based case-control studies published up to 1995 (IARC, 1995). After that, a continuous flow of studies with similar case-control design and PCR testing for HPV have been reported (Olsen et al., 1995; Cuzick et al., 1996; de Sanjose et al., 1996; Kjaer et al.,

1996; Wang & Lin, 1996). Due to the technical differences, the comparison of these PCR-based case-control studies is problematic, as evidenced by the wide range of variability in the odds ratios (IARC, 1995). It should be also remembered that these PCR studies are by no means free from the sources of bias due to misclassification in the CIN grading, as discussed above for the other categories of case-control studies. In summary, however, these PCR-based case-control studies provide, notwithstanding, evidence implicating that infections by the oncogenic HPV types are a significant risk factor for all grades of CIN, in particular high-grade CIN 3 (IARC, 1995; Franco & Monsonego, 1997).

2.8 HPV infections and the risk for cervical cancer

Cervical cancer remains the second most common female malignancy worldwide, second only to breast cancer; and the most frequent malignancy in the developing countries (Parkin et al., 1993). Thus, it represents a major public health problem with almost 500 000 new cases and some 200 000 deaths attributed to this malignancy every year worldwide. The epidemiology of cervical cancer is an extensive and complex topic which is impossible to account in full detail here. Because of the fact that an invasive cervical cancer only develops through the well-defined precursor lesions, the epidemiologic approaches used to analyze the risk factors for cervical cancer are identical to those described above for CIN. Thus, data can be obtained from: (i) descriptive studies; (ii) case reports and case series; (iii) cohort studies; and (iv) case-control studies (IARC, 1995; Franco, 1997; Franco & Monsonego, 1997).

Case reports and case series

A large number of studies on extensive series of cervical carcinomas almost unanimously confirm the detection of the oncogenic types of HPV-DNA in the vast majority of these lesions. Indeed, some of the largest studies using state-of-art PCR technology detected HPV-DNA in over 95% of cervical carcinomas (Bosch et al., 1995), raising the question of whether HPV-DNA-negative cervical carcinomas do exist (Bosch et al., 1997). This remains to be determined by additional studies using high sensitivity level PCR tests applied to optimally collected and preserved cancer samples.

Cohort studies

A large number of prospective cohort studies have been conducted for cervical precancer lesions in the last few decades. Undoubtedly, these studies have significantly contributed to our current understanding of the biology of this disease, and taught us to recognize dysplasia and CIS as potential cancer precursors (Koss et al., 1963; Richart, 1973; Spriggs, 1981; Nasiell et al., 1986). Good as many of these classical studies are, there are several methodologic and conceptual problems encountered in many of them, as recently discussed in detail (Östör et al., 1993; Duffy et al., 1994).

Table 2.3 Comparison of the natural history of CIN and genital HPV lesions.

Lesion	Regression (%)	Persistence (%)	Progression to CIS (%)	Progression to invasive cancer (%)
CIN 1	57.0	32.0	11.0	1.0
CIN 2	43.0	35.0	22.0	5.0
CIN 3	32.0	<56.0	–	>12.0
HPV-NCIN	79.9	14.6	5.2	0.0
HPV-CIN 1	65.1	20.8	14.2	0.0
HPV-CIN 2	58.6	18.6	21.4	0.0
HPV-CIN 3	11.6	9.3	79.1*	0.5†

Table compiled from the data reviewed by Östör (1993), and from the figures of Kuopio Prospective Follow-up Study (1981–98) (Syrjänen *et al.*, 1996a,b).
* Progression based on colposcopy (lesion severity and extent) and histology (progress from severe dysplasia to CIS in two subsequent biopsies). HPV-NCIN: HPV lesion without CIN.
† One lesion progressed to invasion in less than 3 years.

2.9 Natural history

The prospective cohort studies reported over the past 40 years were subjected to an extensive critical review by Östör (1993) (Table 2.3). This impressive paper is an excellent source of information, subsequently complemented by a number of more recent reviews (Syrjänen, 1996a,b).

Natural history of cervical HPV infections

By the end of 1970s, the number of case reports and case series of CIN lesions had provided emerging evidence implicating HPV involvement in the development of these lesions, when analyzed using morphology and immunohistochemistry. Prompted by these data, a prospective cohort study was started in Finland in October 1981, and is ongoing at the time of publication. During the 18 years of its existence, the results of this extensive cohort study have been reported in a series of original publications and reviews (Kataja *et al*, 1992, 1993; Syrjänen *et al.*, 1985, 1992; Syrjänen, 1996a,b). It soon became apparent that cervical HPV lesions in individual women could undergo any of four possible options:

1 Regression.
2 Persistence.
3 Progression.
4 Recurrence.

These are summarized in Fig. 2.18.

The proportion of women classifiable into these four categories is the indicator of the natural history of the disease at any one time, as shown in Fig. 2.18. In this respect, the extent of the follow-up time is a crucial discriminator of the lesions into regression, persistence and progression categories.

From these data, two important patterns emerge in the disease course, when individual women are followed-up for prolonged periods: (i) regression trends; and (ii) progression trends (Fig. 2.19). Importantly, the effect of the follow-up time on these two outcomes is entirely different. The rate of spontaneous regression increases in parallel with the extent of the follow-up time, from 24.8% at 25 months of mean follow-up; to 39.7% at 45 months; further to 54% at 57 months; and up to 63.8% after 83 months. Thereafter, the increase in the proportion of lesions undergoing spontaneous regression increases very slowly, to 66.4% at 96 months, and reaching 68.9% after 110 months of the mean observation period. This should have important implications in interpreting the follow-up data of different cohort studies, the majority of which only run for a relatively short time (Östör, 1993).

From the clinical viewpoint, even more important than spontaneous regression is the progression of HPV lesions to CIN 3/CIS. In contrast to the increasing regression rates with time, no such increase is observed in the progression rates. In fact, the progression rate remains unchanged (around 14%) after 25 months of the mean follow-up time until the currently reached 110 months. In practical terms, this means that the lesions destined to clinical progression do so quite rapidly, almost invariably during the first 2 years from the start of the follow-up.

CIN and HPV have an identical natural history

Based on the figures derived from the review of over 100 follow-up studies conducted for cervical precancer lesions (Östör, 1993), and by compiling the latest (110-month) data from the Finnish prospective cohort study for genital HPV infections (Kataja *et al.*, 1992, 1993; Syrjänen, 1996a,b), the estimates for regression, persistence and progression can be made for these lesions, as depicted in Table 2.3. The figures for CIN and HPV lesions are in many respects almost identical. This applies particularly to the figures for the lower grade lesions CIN 1 and 2, which are practically identical for both regression and progression. These data also clearly show that lesions without evidence of CIN (Syrjänen, 1992), run an even more benign clinical course than CIN 1, progression to CIN 3 being a rare event (5.2%). This may warrant a distinction of these HPV lesions from CIN 1 (Syrjänen, 1992; 1996a,b). The progression rates of CIN 2 and HPV-CIN 2 show high concordance (22% and 21.4%, respectively). Clearly, CIN 2 seems to be an intermediate category with the progression rate approximately twice that of CIN 1, and regression clearly less than CIN 1. In our cohort, HPV-CIN 2 lesions behave much more like HPV-CIN 1 in their progression rate, and particularly their regression rate (58.6% and 65.1%, respectively). This speaks in favor of the predominantly low-grade nature of HPV-CIN 2 lesions, rather than advocating their categorization into high-grade squamous intraepithelial lesions (HSIL), as is the case in The Bethesda System (Kurman *et al.*, 1991). Grouping CIN 2 with CIN 3 into the HSIL leads to a group of lesions, 40% of which will spontaneously regress (Syrjänen *et al.*, 1992).

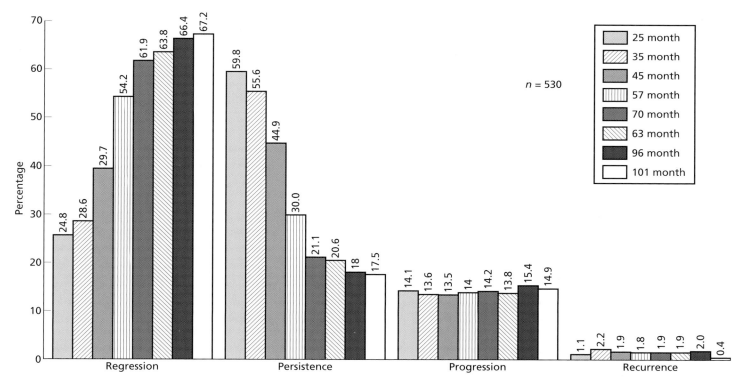

Fig. 2.18 Summary of the natural history of cervical HPV lesions (Kuopio Prospective Follow-up Study 1981–98).

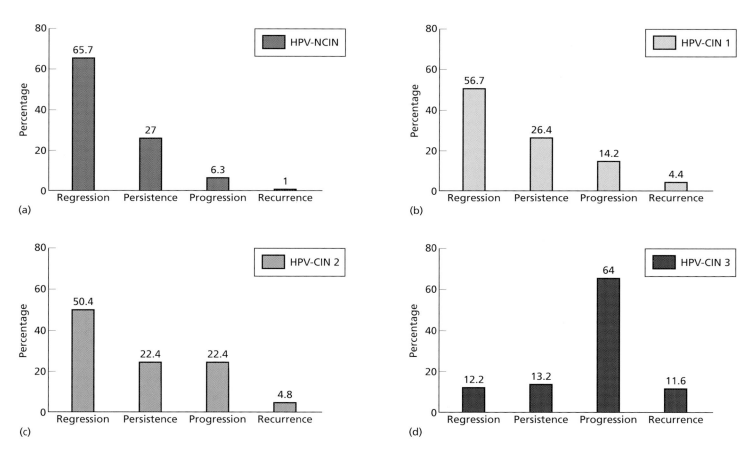

Fig. 2.19 Natural history of cervical HPV lesions prospectively followed up since 1981.

2.10 Molecular pathways of HPV oncogenesis

The normal cell cycle

Cellular division requires all cell components, including genetic information to be duplicated before being partitioned between the two progenitor cells. These events referred to as the "cell cycle" are composed of four stages:

1 *Stage 1*: The replication of chromosomal DNA during the S phase (DNA synthesis).
2 *Stage 2*: The segregation of this replicated chromosomal DNA during mitosis M phase.
3 *Stage 3*: Gap phase G1.
4 *Stage 4*: Gap phase G2.

Both the M and the S phase are separated by G1 and G2.

During the G1 phase an opportunity exists for the exit from the cell cycle of non-dividing cells which reside in the G0 or quiescent state. These stages are seen in Fig. 2.20.

Tissue growth and cellular proliferation are coordinated and regulated by an array of cell specific-growth factors. These growth factors and nutrients act during the initial stages of G1, at which stage the cell is extremely sensitive.

The coordination of all the processes involved with the progression of the cell cycle is controlled by a group of regulatory proteins called cyclin-dependent kinases (CDKs). These are enzymes that phosphorylate a wide range of proteins via inhibition or activation. These CDKs are active throughout the cell cycle, but their activity varies in specific phases, and depends very much on a non-covalent association with activating proteins called cyclins. These are labile proteins that appear for a brief period during certain phases of the cycle. A specific cyclin (which is lettered A through to E in Fig. 2.21) is produced and associated with a CDK during specific phases of the cycle, and it is found that cyclins not only activate CDKs but also affect their localization at a subcellular level within the cell, aiding such movements of these forms from cytoplasm to nucleus. The individual cyclins can be rapidly degraded after completion of the cycle step. These processes can be seen in Fig. 2.21.

Growth factors are concerned with the synthesis of D-type cyclins of which there are three, namely D1, D2 and D3, with D-cyclins binding CDK4 and CDK6 and involved in the initiation of progression of the G1 cycle (Fig. 2.21). One of the cyclins (cyclin D-CDK4) and CDK6 target a retinoblastoma tumor suppression protein (pRB). Normally this protein is present in complexes with the transcription factors referred to as E2Fs shown in Fig. 2.22; these transcription factors are proteins that regulate gene transcription necessary for entry into the S phase of a cycle. In this form, the E2Fs in combination with pRB are inactive, but phosphorylation of pRB by cyclin D-CDKs results in the release of E2F and allows the mitotic cycle to progress. The cyclin E-CDK complex further pushes the cell into the S phase by phosphorylation of the proteins involved in the DNA synthesis initiation.

Once the cell has entered the S phase, this latter cyclin is rapidly degraded to be replaced by the accumulation of cyclin A, whose role is the regulation of DNA replication and the progression of the cell cycle through the G2 to the M phase. Cyclin B levels rise during this phase (Fig. 2.21) and peak during the mitosis phase. A cyclin B-CDK complex also plays a major role in most parts of mitosis, including chromosome condensation, nuclear membrane breakdown and cytokinesis.

There must be an internal regulation so that the progression of the cell cycle is equally balanced between the positive forward action of the CDKs and the negative suppressing action of the cyclin-dependent kinase inhibitors (CKIs). The most well-known of these CKIs are best seen in Fig. 2.23 and are p16, p27, and p21 ("p" representing "protein" and molecular weights represented by a number). p16 binds specifically CDK4 or CDK6 and by this action prevents the progression of the G1 phase. p27 production is dependent on the activity of transforming growth factor B (TGF-B) or cell–cell contact. By this action contact inhibition, or the cessation of the proliferation of

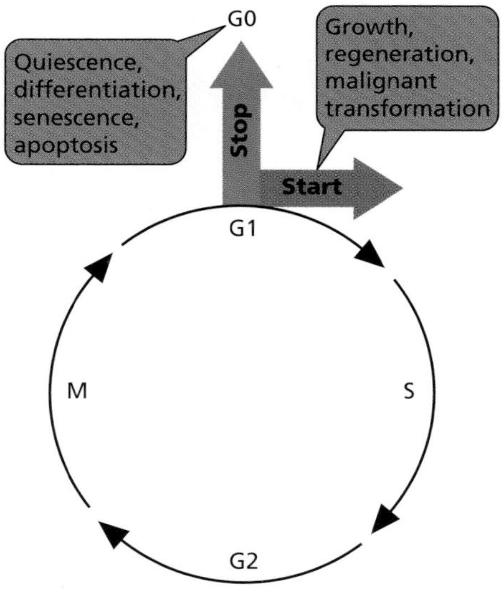

Fig. 2.20 The cell cycle.

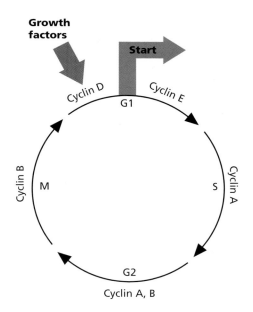

Fig. 2.21 Cyclins of the cell cycle.

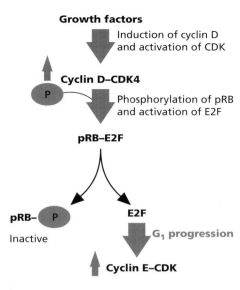

Fig. 2.22 Retinoblastoma protein (pRB) and the cell cycle.

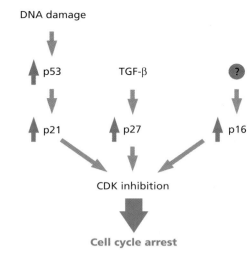

Fig. 2.23 CDK inhibitors: p21, p27, p16.

cells after contact occurs. It further inhibits multiple cyclin-CDK complexes, and its expression is induced by the p53 tumor suppressing protein which is developed in response to DNA damage (Fig. 2.23). There are high levels of p21 in senescent cells (G0) stage. p53 holds a pivotal role in protecting the genetic information of the cell from damaging outside influences. As a result of DNA damage there is an accumulation of p53, which causes a transient arrest of the cell cycle, thereby permitting the cell to repair its DNA. This in turn increases the expression of p21, which as explained above inhibits a wide range of CDKs and therefore may halt the cell cycle at any stage. If it is found that the DNA is damaged irreparably, then p53 induces the expression of other proteins (Bax) that drive the cell towards apoptosis (Fig. 2.20). Any alterations of p53 will lead to inappropriate replication of damaged DNA or abnormal chromosomal segregation during mitosis, which eventually can lead to malignant transformation due to the effects of accumulation and propagation of DNA coding errors (Pirog & Richart, 1998).

The effect of HPV/host cell interaction —a prerequisite for neoplasia

Malignant changes in the cell usually take several separate mutations in cell cycle controlling genes at various levels of control within the cell cycle. Such mutations in regulatory genomes fall into two categories: first, mainly alterations in positive mechanisms of proliferation; or second, the inactivating mutation of the genes controlling the negative or cessation signals involved in the cell cycle. The genes involved in the positive progressive movement of the cycle are called proto-oncogenes, and once mutated their expression is enhanced or activated during an inappropriate phase of the cycle. They are then called oncogenes, and becomes the uncontrollable driving force for cellular proliferation. The most common activating mutation involves proto-oncogenes is amplification. An example can be seen when there is an over-expression of the cyclin D1 protein which instead of being broken down during the

G1 phase remains and continues to produce activation in this phase, therefore destabilizing the normal cell cycle (Fig. 2.20).

The second form of regulatory genomic control involves the inactivating mutation of tumor suppressor genes which produce a "negative" effect on the cell cycle. Any disruption of their function may lead to the uncontrolled proliferation of the cell, and this is best seen when mutations occur in the p53 gene.

With this background, it can be easily seen how HPV can affect a cell to produce neoplasia by the inactivation of p53 protein. This, and consequent cellular events induced by HPV are seen in Fig. 2.24. The HPV, to achieve its aim, must replicate within the host cell and in some way disrupt the DNA synthesis mechanism thereby further removing cell cycle control. The p53 "damage" is induced by an E6 oncoprotein of the HPV 16, which increases the p53 level by reducing its destruction. This carcinogenic-type E6 protein, by its binding and inactivation of host tumor supressor protein p53, will prevent the normal host pathway of genetic damage repair and programmed cell death (apoptosis) from proceeding. Furthermore, the E7 HPV 16 oncoprotein binds and inactivates tumor suppressor protein pRB and its related members, thereby liberating the E2S transcription factors which play a key role in promoting host cell (and thereby also viral) DNA synthesis. E7 also binds and activates cyclin complexes such as p33cdk2 that control progression through the cell cycle. Thus, E7 pushes normally quiescent cells through the cell cycle while E6 removes the cell's failsafe mechanism of apoptosis which normally activates in cases where there is massive DNA damage or unscheduled cell cycle progression. The combined effect is a mutator phenotype where the cell constantly cycles and incorporates any spontaneous mutation that may occur. This explains the long but variable development time of cervical carcinoma, as it depends on the chance occurrence of additional mutations that permit premalignant cells to destroy the basement membrane, and migrate through the body to form extensive localized disease and metastasis.

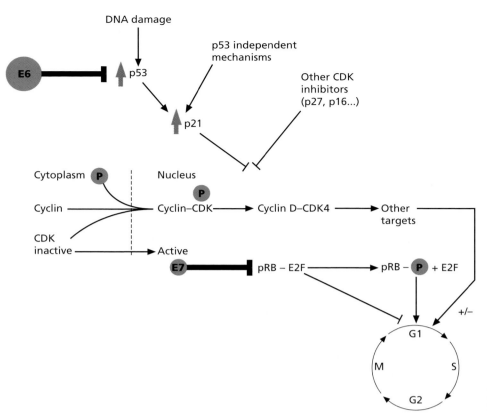

Fig. 2.24 E6 and E7 involvement in cell cycle regulation. P, phosphorylation.

It has recently been reported that an increased susceptibility of p53 protein to degradation by the E6 protein derived from oncogenic HPV results from polymorphism at codon 72 of the p53 gene which leads to the substitution of arginine for proline in the gene product (Storey *et al.*, 1998). If this were so it would suggest that there were two p53 isoforms that were functionally different and therefore could provide a marker to detect women at increased risk of developing cervical cancer. Storey and his group found that the frequency of the arginine encoding allele was significantly higher in normal tissue from 30 women with cervical cancer than in 41 healthy controls, with 76% of cancer cases being homozygous for the arginine polymorphism compared with 37% of controls. Zehbe *et al.* (1999) in studying 142 Italian and Swedish women have found similar results. However, three other studies have failed to find any such association. Rosenthal *et al.* (1998) studied 50 women with cervical cancer and 150 controls, and found that individuals homozygous for the arginine variant of codon 72 of the p53 gene were not at increased risk of cervical cancer, while Lanham *et al.* (1998) found no difference in the frequency of the homozygous arginine genotype in 38 women with cervical cancer and 265 women with CIN when compared with 250 controls. They also found no difference in the allele distribution when stratified according to CIN. When exclusion of the CIN cases without HPV 16 or 18 was performed, it did not affect the alternate allele distribution. Strickler *et al.* (1998) examining Jamaican women of African descent failed to find any strong relationship of cervical cancer with p53 arginine homozygocity.

In summary, it is the E6 and E7 of the carcinogenic HPV types (HPV 16, 18, 31 etc) that are the motors of malignant progression. Infection by these HPVs in contrast to infection by the other HPV types can lead to immortalization of cells at a high rate. *In vitro* culture of these immortalized cells can grow artificial tissue fragments that resemble CIN 3 and HPV-DNA frequently integrates into the host genome's cancers in such a way that the E2 repressor protein is deleted. In cases where HPV integration is not detected, mutations can be shown in the E2 protein, or in repressive factors that allow the continuous overproduction of the E6 and E7 oncoproteins. These events involving E6 and E7 in disruption of the cell are seen in Fig. 2.24 and it is obvious that the development of any future therapeutic agents must depend on interference with the continued production of E6 or E7 within the cell, or the possible restoring of pRB or p53 activity.

2.11 The role of oncogenic HPV detection in the prevention of lower genital tract precancer

The detection of oncogenic HPV plays an increasingly important part in cytology and colposcopy services. It can be used as an adjunct to both cytology and colposcopy, in a primary screening role, or in managing women presenting with minor cytologic abnormalities and although discussed briefly below, they are considered in Chapters 5 & 7.

As an adjunct to cytology in primary screening

The detection of oncogenic HPV DNA in primary screening has been evaluated in several large-scale studies (Koutsky *et al.*, 1992; Meijer *et al.*, 1992; Cuzick *et al.* 1995). In relation to cytologic screening, the detection of HPV16, 18, 31 and 33 DNA by type-specific PCR increases the sensitivity and provides additional specificity for prediction of high-grade lesions. Persistent oncogenic HPV-DNA in a normal population has also been found to be a good indicator of the presence of cervical pathology (Meijer *et al.*, 1992; Nobbenhuis *et al.*, 1999). At present hybrid capture techniques are more commonly used as objective standardized kits are available.

For the purpose of primary screening the detection of oncogenic HPV-DNA may be useful in:

1 Identification of high-grade lesions in women presenting with mildly abnormal or normal cytology.

2 Identification of women with normal cytology who are at increased risk of developing high-grade lesions which are associated with oncogenic HPV-DNA (Koutsky *et al.*, 1992).

Melkert *et al.* (1993) showed that in women with normal smears the prevalence of all HPV types is age-related, decreasing from 20% in women aged between 20 and 25 years to 4.5% in women aged over 30 years. High-risk HPV types decrease from 7% in women aged between 20 and 25 years, to less than 2% in women aged over 30 years. Similar age-dependent prevalence rates have been found by others: Bauer *et al.* (1991) and Evander *et al.* (1995). These observations suggest that HPV infections are very common among young women and that these infections very frequently clear spontaneously. In the women aged over 30 years with normal cytology, the HPV clearance and acquisition rates have been estimated at between 30% and 40%; and 0.5% per year respectively (Rozendaal *et al.*, 1996; J.M.M. Walboomers, personal communication).

Walboomers and his group (1999 and personal communication) have recently shown that among a cohort group of 1622 women with normal cytology but who had a positive HPV test at baseline, the risk of developing CIN 3 after a follow-up period of 4–6 years was 116 times more than those women who had a negative high-risk HPV test. Their data show that for women with normal cytology and an HPV high-risk negative test, the risk of developing a severe lesion is very low. The sensitivity of the high-risk HPV positive test was 90% for the detection of CIN 3 in the future, while the specificity was 95%. This means that HPV and cytology testing together can much better identify the high-risk population than cytology alone.

As an adjunct to colposcopy in the management of women presenting with mild or borderline dyskaryosis (ASCUS/AGUS)

Currently the major component of hospital colposcopy referrals comprises women with two abnormal smears, graded up to mild dyskaryosis—low-grade squamous intraepithelial lesions (LSIL) only approximately 20–35% of whom will have CIN 3 (Cox *et al.*, 1995; Hatch *et al.*, 1995; Wright *et al.*, 1995; Cobalin *et al.*, 1998). However, a recent study in North California (Kinney *et al.*, 1998) has shown that atypical squamous cells of undetermined significance (ASCUS) was the most common abnormal Papanicolaou diagnosis representing 3.6% of the total number of 46000 women. Of the total number of cases of histologically confirmed high-grade cervical intraepithelial neoplasia

present in the population, the largest proportion (38.8%) was in women showing these ASCUS smears. This combined with atypical glandular cells of undetermined significance and LGSIL accounted for 68.6% of cases of histologic high-grade lesions diagnosed in this routine screening population. This ASCUS group subsequently had HPV DNA testing (hybrid capture, HCII, Digene Corporation, MD), repeat pap smears and colposcopy with histologic evaluation. Manos *et al.* (1999) found that of 973 women, 65 (6.7%) had high-grade SIL or cancer. Of this group, 89.2% were tested positive for high-risk oncogenic HPV and the specificity of the test was 64.1%. The corresponding repeat pap test result was abnormal in 76.2% of cases. Hence the sensitivity of HPV-DNA testing was found to be as good, if not better than repeat pap tests. They calculated that the use of an HPV-based algorithm in which HPV-positive women would have immediate colposcopy, and repeat pap tests performed on all the others, would result in an overall sensitivity of 96.9% for the detection of high-grade SIL.

In this group of women presenting with these minor smears, overtreatment inevitably occurs, primarily because the outcome of a persistent minor cytologic abnormality in association with a large colposcopic lesion cannot be reliably predicted. Furthermore, repeat colposcopy visits are required for those women who are judged not to require treatment but whose cytology still remains mildly abnormal.

A comparison of the sensitivity and specificity of detection of high grade lesions by abnormal cytology and/or HPV-DNA positivity has been reported in a number of studies (Mansell *et al.*, 1994; Cox *et al.*, 1995; Hatch *et al.*, 1995; Ferris *et al.*, 1998). Relative to cytology, the detection of oncogenic HPV-DNA in this group of women improves both sensitivity and specificity in identification of these high-grade lesions, many of which are of small volume. In general, oncogenic HPV 16, 18, 31 and 33 positivity as detected by type-specific PCR provides additional specificity and presence of multiple oncogenic HPV types as detected by hybrid capture (Digene Corporation, MD) or consensus PCR/SHARP provides additional sensitivity over cytology alone.

HPV-DNA testing is of value in targeting clinical resources to those who are at risk of high-grade lesions because:

1 Oncogenic HPV-DNA positivity helps to identify the at least one third of high grade lesions which are missed in this group by colposcopy and punch biopsy when they are initially referred. Negative colposcopy in women with repeated low-grade cervical cytologic abnormalities can present a problem. A recent study by Fait *et al.* (1998) clearly showed the ability of HPV-DNA testing to identify CIN lesions in women with negative colposcopic findings. They used a hybrid capture technique (HCII, Digene Corporation, MD) together with electrodiathermy removal of the transformation zone (LEEP) in 166 women with repeated low-grade cytology and who were referred for colposcopy. A highly significant correlation between a positive result for high-risk oncogenic HPV-DNA and the subsequent identification of high-grade CIN (CIN 2/3) was

found. They therefore suggest that HPV-DNA testing may be used to triage these women in respect of colposcopic tissue sampling.

2 Persistent oncogenic HPV-DNA positivity occurs in 20% of women who require no treatment on colposcopy. However, persistent infection is predominantly associated with HPV 16–18 and a consequent high risk (30%) of developing high-grade lesions within 2 years (Londesborough et al., 1996). Recently Harmsel et al. (1999) have shown that persistent infection over an 18-month period with HPV 16 is associated with a higher risk of developing CIN and when found is usually of a high-grade nature. In their study they showed that even a single positive HPV test (using PCR) predisposed women to considerable risk of developing CIN, but that the CIN that develops in persistent HPV 16 infection is of a more severe nature than in women infected for a short period only.

2.12 HPV type and type variant as determinants of the natural history

Recently, it has become obvious that a wide variety of sequence variants of common oncogenic prototype HPVs (e.g. HPV 16 and HPV 18) exist in distinct populations and ethnic groups (Ho et al., 1993). Using a catalog of HPV 16 E6 and L1 nucleotides, PCR-based oligonucleotide probe systems were recently developed, capable of distinguishing these HPV 16 class and subclass variants (Wheeler et al., 1997; Yamada et al., 1997). The major HPV 16 variants detected so far include European prototype (E-P), Asian (As), Asian-American (AA), and African (Af1 and Af2) lineages (Ho et al., 1993). In addition, E-G131, an E-class variant, and AA-G183, an AA-class variant, were also identified (Wheeler et al., 1997). Emphasis has been repeatedly made to utilize these techniques in large-scale epidemiologic studies on HPV 16 prevalence, transmission and natural history, with special emphasis on the associations between these HPV 16 variants, host-immune responses, and cervical neoplasia (Hildesheim, 1997; Terry et al., 1997; Yamada et al., 1997). It might well be that the outcome of HPV infections depends not only on the virus type itself or its receptor, but on specific HPV class and subclass variants and their presentation to T-cells by different HLA class I and II allele variants. Thus, a feasible approach to solve this issue would be to pool the data on both HLA typing and HPV type variant analyses in CIN (and cancer) patients (Hildesheim, 1997). Taken together, the current data are convincing to substantiate the concept that the high-risk HPV 16 infection is a distinct risk factor predisposing the cervical precancer lesions to clinical progression significantly more often than infections by other HPV types. Viral load seems to increase this probability of progression (Villa, 1997). The data on the other high-risk types of the 40s, 50s and 60s series are still too scanty to permit definite conclusions. Whether HPV type and type variants have any prognostic significance in invasive cervical cancer is a more controversial issue (Yamada et al., 1997), with highly contradictory reports being reported (Ji et al., 1991; Burger et al., 1996b; Viladiu et al., 1997).

A number of studies have shown that a specific HPV E6 variant, L83, was associated with persistence and progression of cervical neoplasia (Londesborough et al., 1996; Zehbe et al., 1998a). Recently a most intriguing study was presented by Zehbe et al. (1998b) who showed that the oncogenicity of this L83V polymorphism varied in different populations. His group compared E16 variants in preinvasive and invasive cervical lesions in Italian and Swedish women and found that the distribution in cervical lesions of all three E6 polymorphisms examined (L83V, multivariant, and prototype) showed striking differences between the two populations examined. They found that the HPV 16 E6 prototype had low oncogenicity in the Swedish population, decreasing from 50% in CIN to 6% in invasive cervical cancer. In contrast, the Italian cases showed that the E6 prototype was equally distributed between CIN and invasive cancer, indicating that the oncogenicity of specific E6 variants is related to the population examined.

These findings could be interpreted as showing that the genetic differences between the two populations are involved in determining the potential risk of E6 polymorphism. Another explanation is that this phenomenon could be associated with a cellular immune response. Different haplotypes of the major histocompatibility complex, which in themselves are population related, may recognize the E6 variant with different frequencies and could result in either persistence or regression of the viral infection. Alternatively, as Zehbe et al. (1998b) have suggested, polymorphism of E6-binding cellular targets may influence the neutralization by the E6 oncoprotein.

It would seem that in future, more epidemiologic studies will be forthcoming that will identify additional risk factors which may contribute to the development of cervical cancer such as HPV 16 E6 polymorphism.

2.13 References and bibliography

Baken, L.A., Koutsky, L.A., Kuypers, J. et al. (1995) Genital human papillomavirus infection among male and female sex partners: prevalence and type-specific concordance. J Infect Dis **171**,429.

Barrett, T.J. & Silbar, J.D. (1954) Genital warts—a venereal disease. J Am Med Assoc **154**,333.

Bauer, H.M., Ting, Y., Green, C.E. et al. (1991) Genital human papillomavirus infection in female university students as determined by a PCR based method. JAMA **265**,472.

Becker, T.M., Stone, K.M. & Alexander, E.R. (1987) Genital human papillomavirus infection. A growing concern. Obstet Gynecol Clin North Am **14**,389.

Becker, T.M., Wheeler, C.M., McGough, N.S. et al. (1994) Sexually transmitted diseases and other risk factors for cervical dysplasia among southwestern Hispanic and non-Hispanic white women. JAMA **271**,1181.

Bosch, F.X., Manos, M.M., Munoz, N. et al. (1995) Prevalence of human papillomavirus in cervical cancer: a worldwide perspective. International Biological Study on Cervical Cancer (IBSCC) Study Group. J Natl Cancer Inst **87**,796.

Bosch, F.X., Munoz, N. & de Sanjose, S. (1997) Human papillomavirus and other risk factors for cervical cancer. Biomed Pharmacother **51**,268.

Burger, M.P., Hollema, H., Pieters, W.J., Schroder, F.P. & Quint, W.G. (1996a) Epidemiological evidence of cervical intraepithelial neoplasia without the presence of human papillomavirus. Br J Cancer **73**,831.

Burger, R.A., Monk, B.J., Kurosaki, T. et al. (1996b) Human

papillomavirus type 18: association with poor prognosis in early stage cervical cancer. *J Natl Cancer Inst* **88**,1361.

Burghardt, E., Pickel, H. & Girardi, F. (eds) (1998) *Colposcopy Cervical Pathology*, 3rd edn, p. 24. 1998. Thieme, Stuttgart.

Campion, M.J., McCance, D.J., Cuzick, J. & Singer, A. (1986) Progressive potential of mild cervical atypia: prospective cytological, colposcopic, and virological study. *Lancet* **2**,237.

Cason, J. (1996) Perinatal acquisition of cervical cancer-associated papillomaviruses. *Br J Obstet Gynaecol* **103**,853.

Chuang, T.-Y., Perry, H.O., Kurland, L.T. & Ilstrup, D.M. (1984) Condyloma acuminatum in Rochester, Minn. 1950–1978.1. Epidemiology and clinical features. *Arch Dermatol* **120**,469.

Cobalin, M.H., Cobalin, C.G., Burke, L. *et al.* (1998) Incidents and predictors of cervical dysplasia in patients with minimally abnormal Papanicolaou smears. *Obs Gynaecol* **92**(3),356.

Cooper K. (1996) Nonisotopic in situ hybridization in the detection of integrated HPV 16/18 in cervical cancers. *Hum Pathol* **27**,745.

Cox, J.T., Lorincz, A.T., Schiffman, M.H. *et al.* (1995). Human papillomavirus testing by hybridcapture appears to be useful in triaging women with a cytological diagnosis of atypical squamous cells of undetermined significance. *Am J Obstet Gynecol* **172**,946.

Critchlow, C.W. & Koutsky, L.A. (1995) Epidemiology of human papillomavirus infection. In: Mindel A. (ed.) *Genital Warts. Human Papillomavirus Infection*, p. 53. Edward Arnold, Kent.

Cuzick, J., Sasieni, P. & Singer, A. (1996) Rick factors for invasive cervix cancer in young women. *Eur J Cancer* **32A**,836.

Cuzick, J., Terry, G. Ho, L., Hollingworth, T. & Anderson, M. (1994) Type-specific human papillomavirus DNA in abnormal smears as a predictor of high-grade cervical intraepithelial neoplasia. *Br J Cancer* **69**,167.

Cuzick, J., Szarewski, A., Terry, G., Ho, L., Hanby, A., Maddox, P. *et al.* (1995) Human papillomavirus testing in primary cervical screening. *Lancet* **345**,1533.

de Brux, J., Cochard, I.B. & Kaeding, M.H. (1981) Epidemiologie morphologie evolution des condylomes cervicaux. *Gynecology* **32**,314.

de Brux, J., Orth, G., Croissant, O., Cochard, B. & Ionesco, M. (1983) Lesions condylomateuses du col uterin evolution chez 2466 patientes. *Bull Cancer* **70**,410.

de Sanjose, S., Bosch, F.X., Munoz, N. *et al.* (1996) Socioeconomic differences in cervical cancer: two case-control studies in Colombia and Spain. *Am J Public Health* **86**,1532.

de Villiers, E.M. (1997) Papillomavirus and HPV typing. *Clin Dermatol* **15**,199.

Duffy, S.W., Rohan, T.E. & McLaughlin, J.R. (1994) Design and analysis considerations in a cohort study involving repeated measurement of both exposure and outcome: the association between genital papillomavirus infection and risk of cervical intraepithelial neoplasia. *Stat Med* **13**,379.

Evander, M., Edlund, K., Gustafsson, A. *et al.* (1995) Human papillomavirus infection is transient in young women: a population based cohort study. *J Inf Dis* **171**,1026.

Fait, G., Daniel, Y., Kupferminc, M.J., Lessing, J.B., Niv, J., Baram, A. (1998) Does typing of human papillomavirus assist in the triage of women with repeated low-grade, cervical cytologic abnormalities? *Gynecol Oncol* **70**,319.

Ferris, D.G., Wright, T.C., Litaker, M.C. *et al.* (1998) Triage of women with ASCUS and LSIL on pap smear reports; management by repeat pap smear, HPV DNA testing, or colposcopy. *J Fam Prac* **46**(2),125.

Franco, E.L. & Monsonego, J. (eds) (1997) *New Developments in Cervical Cancer Screening and Prevention*. Blackwell Science, Oxford.

Franco, E.L. (1997) Understanding the epidemiology of genital infection with oncogenic and nononcogenic human papillomaviruses: a promising lead for primary prevention of cervical cancer. *Cancer Epidem Biomarker Prev* **6**,759.

Gomez-Rueda, N., Garcia, A., Vighi, S. *et al.* (1994) Epithelial alterations adjacent to invasive squamous carcinoma of the vulva. *J Reprod Med* **39**,526.

Gross, G. & Barrasso, R. (eds) (1997) *Human Papilloma Virus Infection. A Clinical Atlas.* Ullstein–Mosby, Berlin, Wiesbaden.

Gross, G. & von Krogh, G. (eds) (1997) *Human Papillomavirus Infections in Dermatovenereology.* CRC Press, Boca Raton, CA.

Hakama, M. (1997) Screening for cervical cancer: experience from the Nordic Countries. In: Franco, E. & Monsonego, J. (eds) *New Developments in Cervical Cancer Screening and Prevention*, p. 190. Blackwell Science, Oxford.

Harmsel, B.T., Smedts, F., Kuijpers, J. *et al.* (1999) Relationship between human papillomavirus type 16 in the cervix and intraepithelial neoplasia. *Obstet Gynecol* **93**(1),46.

Hatch, K.D., Schneider, A. & Abdel-Nour, M.W. (1995) An evaluation of human papillomavirus testing for intermediate- and high-risk types as triage before colposcopy. *Am J Obstet Gynaecol* **172**,1150.

Hildesheim, A. (1997) Human papillomavirus variants: implications for natural history studies and vaccine development efforts. *J Natl Cancer Inst* **89**,752.

Hillman, R.J., Ryait, B.K., Botcherby, M. & Taylor-Robinson, D. (1993) Changes in HPV infection in patients with anogenital warts and their partners. *Genitourin Med* **69**,450.

Hippeläinen, M., Yliskoski, M., Syrjänen, S. *et al.* (1994) Low concordance of genital human papillomavirus (HPV) lesions and viral types in HPV-infected women and their male sexual partner. *Sex Transm Dis* **21**,76.

Ho, L., Chan, S.-Y., Burk, R.D. *et al.* (1993) The genetic drift of human papillomavirus type 16 is a means reconstructing prehistoric viral spread and the movement of ancient human populations. *J Virol* **67**,6413.

Holly, E.A. (1996) Cervical intraepithelial neoplasia, cervical cancer and HPV. *Annu Rev Public Health* **17**,69.

IARC (1995) *Monographs on the Evaluation of Carcinogenic Risks to Humans. Papillomaviruses*, p. 1, Volume 64. IARC, Lyon.

Ji, H.X., Syrjänen, S., Klemi, P. *et al.* (1991) Prognostic significance of nuclear DNA content and human papillomavirus (HPV) type in invasive cervical cancer. Polymerase chain reaction (PCR) and flow cytometric analysis. *Int J Gynecol Cancer* **1**,59.

Kataja, V., Syrjänen, S., Mantyjarvi, R., Yliskoski, M., Saarikoski, S., Syrjänen, K. (1992) Prognostic factors in cervical human papillomavirus (HPV) infections. *Sex Transm Dis* **19**,154.

Kataja, V., Syrjänen, S., Yliskoski, M. *et al.* (1993) Risk factors associated with cervical human papillomavirus (HPV) infections: a case-control study. *Am J Epidemiol* **138**,735.

Kinney, W.K., Manos, M. Hurley, L. & Ransley, J. (1988) Where's the high grade cervical neoplasia? The importance of minimally abnormal Papanicolaou diagnoses. *Obstet Gynaecol* **91**(6),973.

Kjaer, S.K., de Villiers, E.M., Caglayan, H. *et al.* (1993) Human papillomavirus, herpes simplex virus and other potential risk factors for cervical cancer in a high-risk area (Greenland) and a low-risk area (Denmark)—a second look. *Br J Cancer* **67**,830.

Kjaer, S.K., Engholm, G., Dahl, C. & Bock, J.E. (1996) Case-control study of risk factors for cervical squamous cell neoplasia in Denmark. IV: role of smoking habits. *Eur J Cancer Prev* **5**,359.

Koss, L.G., Stewart, F.W., Foote, F.W. *et al.* (1963) Some histological aspects of behavior of epidermoid carcinoma in situ and related lesions of the uterine cervix. *Cancer* **16**,1160.

Koutsky, L.A., Galloway, D.A. & Holmes, K.K. (1988) Epidemiology of genital human papillomavirus infection. *Epidemiol Rev* **10**,122.

Koutsky, L.A., Holmes, K.K., Critchlow, C.W. *et al.* (1992) A cohort study of the risk of cervical intraepithelial neoplasia grade 2 or 3 in relation to papillomavirus infection. *N Engl J Med* **327**,1272.

Kurman, R.J., Malkasian, G.D., Sedlis, A. & Solomon, D. (1991) From Papanicolaou to Bethesda: the rationale for a new clinical cytologic classification. *Obstet Gynecol* **77**,779.

Kurman, R.J., Schiffman, M.H., Lancaster W.D. *et al.* (1988) Analysis of individual human papillomavirus types in cervical neoplasia: a possible role for type 18 in rapid progression. *Am J Obstet Gynecol* **159**,293.

Lanham, S., Campbell, I., Watt, P. & Gornall, R. (1998) p53 polymorphism and risk of cervical cancer. *Lancet* **352**,1631.

Londesborough, P., Ho, L., Terry, G., Cuzick, J., Wheeler, C., Singer, A.

(1996) Human papillomavirus (HPV) genotype as a predictor of persistence and development of high grade lesions in women with minor cervical abnormalities. *Int J Cancer* **69**,364.

Lörincz, A.T., Reid, R., Jenson, A.B. *et al.* (1992) Human papillomavirus infection of the cervix: relative risk associations of 15 common anogenital types. *Obstet Gynecol* **79**,328.

Manos, M.N., Kinney, W.K., Hurley, L.B. *et al.* (1999) Identifying women with cervical neoplasia—using human papillomavirus DNA testing for equivocal Papanicolaou results. *JAMA* **281**(17),1605.

Mansell, M.E., Ho, L., Terry, G., Singer, A. & Cuzick, J. (1994). Semi-quantitative human papillomavirus DNA detection in the management of women with minor cytological abnormality. *Br J Obs Gynaecol* **101**,807.

Meijer, C.J., van den Brule, Snijders, P.J. *et al.* (1992) Detection of human papillomavirus in cervical scrapes by the polymerase chain reaction in relation to cytology: possible implications for cervical cancer screening. In: Munoz, N., Bosch, F.X., Shah, K.V. (eds) The epidemiology of human papillomavirus and cervical cancer. *IARC Sci Publ* **119**,271.

Meisels, A. & Fortin, R. (1976) Condylomatous lesions of the cervix and vagina. I. Cytologic patterns. *Acta Cytol* **20**,505.

Melkert, P.J.W., Hopman, E., Brule, A.J.C. *et al.* (1993) Prevalence of HPV in cytomorphologically normal cervical smears as determined by the polymerase chain reaction is age-dependent. *Int J Cancer* **53**,919.

Mindel, A. (ed.) (1995) *Genital Warts. Human Papillomavirus Infection.* Edward Arnold, Kent.

Mitchell, H., Drake, M. & Medley, G. (1986) Prospective evaluation of risk of cervical cancer after cytological evidence of human papilloma virus infection. *Lancet* **i**,573.

Mitchell, M.F., Hittelman, W.N., Hong, W.K., Lotan, R. & Schottenfeld, D. (1994) The natural history of cervical intraepithelial neoplasia: an argument for intermediate endpoint biomarkers. *Cancer Epidemiol Biomarkers Prev* **3**,619.

Monsonego, J., Zerat, L., Catalan, F. & Coscas, Y. (1993) Genital human papillomavirus infections—correlation of cytological, colposcopic and histological features with viral types in women and their male partners. *Int J STD AIDS* **4**,13.

Moscicki, A.B. (1996) Genital HPV infections in children and adolescents. *Obstet Gynecol Clin North Am* **23**,675.

Nasiell, K., Roger, V. & Nasiell, M. (1986) Behavior of mild cervical dysplasia during long term follow-up. *Obstet Gynecol* **67**,665.

Nobbenhuis, M.A., Walboomers, J.M.M., Helmerhorst, T.J., Rozendaal, L., Remmink, A.J., Risse, E.K. *et al.* (1999) Relation of human papillomavirus status to cervical lesions and consequences for cervical-cancer screening: a prospective study. *Lancet* **354**,20.

Olsen, A.O., Gjoen, K. Sauer, T. *et al.* (1995) Human papillomavirus and cervical intraepithelial neoplasia grade II–III: a population-based case-control study. *Int J Cancer* **61**,312.

Oriel, J.D. (1981) Genital warts. *Sex Transm Dis* **8**,326.

Östör, A.G. (1993) Natural history of cervical intraepithelial neoplasia—a critical review. *Int J Gynecol Pathol* **12**,186.

Pakarian, F., Kaye, J. & Cason, J. (1994) Cancer associated human papillomaviruses: perinatal transmission and persistence. *Br J Obstet Gynaecol* **101**,514.

Palefsky, J.M. & Holly, E.A. (1995) Molecular virology and epidemiology of Human papillomavirus and cervical cancer. *Cancer Epidem Biomark Prev* **4**,415.

Parkin, D.M., Pisani, P. & Ferlay, J. (1993) Estimates of the worldwide incidence of 18 major cancers in 1985. *Int J Cancer* **54**,594.

Pirog, E.C. & Richart, M. (1998) The cell cycle. *Contemporary OB/GYN* **43**(7),117.

Poka, R. & Czegledy, J. (1997) HPV- and node status in cervical cancer: long-term results. *Eur J Obstet Gyn Reprod Biol* **71**,169.

Puranen, M. Yliskoski, M., Saarikoski, S., Syrjänen, K. & Syrjänen, S. (1996) Vertical transmission of human papillomavirus (HPV) from infected mothers to their newborn babies and persistence of the virus in childhood. *Am J Obstet Gynecol* **174**,694.

Purola, E. & Savia, E. (1977) Cytology of gynecologic condyloma acuminatum. *Acta Cytol* **21**,26.

Reid, R., Greenberg, M.D., Lorincz, A., Jenson, A.B., Laverty, C.R., Husain, M. *et al.* (1981) Should cervical cytologic testing be augmented by cervicography or human papillomavirus deoxyribonucleic acid detection? *Am J Obstet Gynecol* **164**,1461.

Richart, R.M. (1973) Cervical intraepithelial neoplasia. *Pathol Annu* **8**,301.

Roman, A. & Fife, K.H. (1989) Human papillomaviruses: are we ready to type. *Clin Microbiol Rev* **2**,166.

Rosenthal, A.N., Ryan, A., Al-Jehani, R.M. *et al.* (1998) p53 codon 72 polymorphism and risk of cervical cancer in UK. *Lancet* **352**,871.

Rotola, A., Costa, S., Monini, P. *et al.* (1994) Impact of sexual habits on the clinical evaluation of male HPV infection. *Eur J Epidemiol* **10**,373.

Rozendaal, L., Walboomers, J.M.M., Van der Linden, J.C. *et al.* (1996) PCR based high risk HPV test in cervical cancer screening gives objective risk assessment of women with cytomorphologically normal cervical smears. *Int J Cancer* **68**,766.

Rylander, E., Ruusuvaara, L., Almströmer, M.W., Evander, M. & Wadell, G. (1994) The absence of vaginal human papillomavirus 16 DNA in women who have not experienced sexual intercourse. *Obstet Gynecol* **83**,735.

Schiffman, M.H. (1995) The epidemiology of cervical carcinogenesis. *Cancer* **76**,1888.

Schneider, A. (1990) Latent and subclinical genital HPV infections. *Papillomavirus Rep* **1**,2.

Sebbelov, A.M., Svendsen, C., Jensen, H., Kjaer, S.K. & Norrild, B. (1994) Prevalence of HPV in premalignant and malignant cervical lesions in Greenland and Denmark: PCR and in situ hybridization analysis on archival material. *Res Virol* **145**,83.

Spriggs, A.I. (1981) Natural history of cervical dysplasia. *Clin Obstet Gynaecol* **8**,65.

Storey, A., Thomas, M., Kalita, A. *et al.* (1998) Role of a p53 polymorphism in the development of human papillomavirus-associated cancer. *Nature* **393**,229.

Strickler, H., Manns, A., Rattray, C., Brown, C. & Reiss, M. (1998) p52 polymorphisms at position 72 and development of cervical cancer. *Int J Gynecol Cancer* **8**,439.

Syrjänen, K., Gissmann, L. & Koss, L.G. (eds) (1987) *Papillomaviruses and Human Disease.* Springer-Verlag, Heidelberg.

Syrjänen, K., Hakama, M. Saarikoski, S. *et al.* (1990b) Prevalence, incidence and estimated life-time risk of cervical human papillomavirus (HPV) infections in nonselected Finnish female population. *Sex Transm Dis* **7**,15.

Syrjänen, K., Kataja, V., Yliskoski, M. *et al.* (1992) Natural history of cervical HPV lesions does not substantiate the biologic relevance of the Bethesda system. *Obstet Gynecol* **79**,675.

Syrjänen, K., Väyrynen, M., Castren, O. *et al.* (1984) Sexual behaviour of women with human papillomavirus (HPV) lesions of the uterine cervix. *Br J Vener Dis* **60**,243.

Syrjänen, K., Väyrynen, M., Saarikoski, S. *et al.* (1985) Natural history of cervical human papillomavirus (HPV) infections based on prospective follow-up. *Brit J Obstet Gynaecol* **92**,1086.

Syrjänen, K., Yliskoski, M. Kataja, V. *et al.* (1990a) Prevalence of genital human papillomavirus (HPV) infections in a mass-screened Finnish female population aged 20–65 years. *Int J STD & AIDS* **1**,410.

Syrjänen, K.J. (1979) Histological and cytological evidence of a condylomatous lesion in association with an invasive carcinoma of uterine cervix. *Arch Geschwulstforsch* **49**,436.

Syrjänen, K.J. (1992) Genital human papillomavirus (HPV) infections and their associations with squamous cell cancer: Reappraisal of the morphologic, epidemiologic and DNA data. In: Fenoglio-Preiser, C.M., Wolff, M. & Rilke, F. (eds) *Progress in Surgical Pathology*, p. 217. Field & Wood, New York.

Syrjänen, K.J. (1996a) Spontaneous evolution of intraepithelial lesions according to the grade and type of the implicated HPV. *Eur J Obstet Gynecol Reprod Biol* **65**,45.

Syrjänen, K.J. (1996b) Natural history of genital human papillomavirus infections. In: Lacey, C. (ed.) *Papillomavirus Reviews.*

Current Research on Papillomaviruses, p. 189. Leeds Medical Information, Leeds University Press, Leeds.

Terry, G., Ho, L. & Cuzick, J. (1997) Analysis of E2 amino acid variants of human papillomavirus types 16 and 18 and their associations with lesion grade and HLA DR/DQ type. *Int J Cancer* **73**,651.

van Doornum, G.J., Hooykaas, C., Juffermans, L.H. *et al.* (1992) Prevalence of human papillomavirus infections among heterosexual men and women with multiple sexual partners. *J Med Virol* **37**,13.

Viladiu, P., Bosch, F.X., Castellsague, X. *et al.* (1997) Human papillomavirus DNA and antibodies to human papillomaviruses 16 E2, L2, and E7 peptides as predictors of survival in patients with squamous cell cervical cancer. *J Clin Oncol* **15**,610.

Villa, L.L. (1997) Human papillomaviruses and cervical cancer. *Adv Cancer Res* **71**,321.

Walboomers, J.M., Jacobs, M.V., Manos, M.M., Bosch, F.X., Kummer, J.A., Shah, K.V. *et al.* (1999) Human papillomavirus is a necessary cause of invasive cervical cancer worldwide. *J Pathol* **189**,12.

Wang, P.D. & Lin, R.S. (1996) Risk factors for cervical intraepithelial neoplasia in Taiwan. *Gynecol Oncol* **62**,10.

Wheeler, C.M., Parmenter, C.A., Hunt, W.C. *et al.* (1993) Determinants of genital human papillomavirus infection among cytologically normal women attending the University of New Mexico student health center. *Sex Transm Dis* **20**,286.

Wheeler, C.M., Yamada, T., Hildesheim, A. & Jenison, S.A. (1997) Human papillomavirus type 16 sequence variants: identification by E6 and L1 lineage-specific hybridization. *J Clin Microbiol* **35**,11.

Wright, T.C., Sun, X.W. & Koulos, J. (1995) Comparison of management algorithms for the evaluation of women with low-grade cytological abnormalities. *Obs Gynaecol* **85**,202.

Xi, L.F. & Koutsky, L.A. (1997) Epidemiology of genital human papillomavirus infections. *Bull Inst Pasteur* **95**,161.

Yamada, T., Manos, M.M., Peto, J. *et al.* (1997) Human papillomavirus type 16 sequence variation in cervical cancers: a worldwide perspective. *J Virol* **71**,2463.

Zehbe, I., Voglino, G., Delius, H., Wilahderr, E. & Tomasino, M. (1998b) Risk of cervical cancer and geographic variations of human papillomavirus 16 E6 polymorphism. *Lancet* **352**, 1441.

Zehbe, I., Wilander, E., Delius, H. & Tomasino, M. (1998a) Human papillomavirus 16 E6 variants are more prevalent in invasive cervical carcinoma than the prototype. *Cancer Res* **58**,829.

Zehbe, I., Voglino, G., Wilander, E., Genta, F., Tomasino, M. (1999) Codon 72 polymorphism and its association with cervical cancer. *Lancet* **354**,218.

zur Hausen, H. (ed.) (1994) Human pathogenic papillomaviruses. *Curr Top Microbiol Immunol* **186**,1.

zur Hausen, H. (1996) Papillomavirus infections — a major cause of human cancers. *Biochim Biophys Acta* **1288**,F55.

Chapter 3
Examination for Cervical Precancer
Use of colposcopy

3.1 Introduction

In the detection of cervical intraepithelial neoplasia (CIN), both exfoliative cytology and colposcopy are essential diagnostic aids. Alterations from the normal pattern, revealed during exfoliative cytology, will have alerted the clinician to the possibility of an abnormality existing on the cervix. Use of the colposcopy, providing magnified and illuminated vision, enables the examiner to locate any precancerous epithelium on the cervix.

In this chapter the tissue basis for colposcopy, and the colposcopic examination will be discussed.

3.2 Tissue basis for colposcopy

To interpret correctly the colposcopic appearance of normal and precancerous tissue a knowledge of the histopathologic changes that occur within the cervical epithelium and its stroma is required. It is essential that examiners are able to visualize what they have seen of the living tissues and to extrapolate that image to what is present in the fixed or stained tissue specimen under the microscope.

The colposcopic appearances are a summation of various factors. These include the following.
1 The architecture of the *epithelium* and possible variations in its thickness and formation.
2 The composition of the underlying *stroma*.
3 The *surface configuration* of the tissue.

The image seen through the colposcope is therefore based on the reciprocal relationship between these three morphologic characteristics. The epithelium acts as a filter through which both the reflected and the incident light must pass to produce the final colposcopic picture. The epithelium is colorless, whereas the stroma is colored by the blood vessels it contains. The redness of the stroma is transmitted back to the observer, with modifications depending on the characteristics of the epithelium through which the light must pass.

As seen in Fig. 3.1, as the light passes through the *normal epithelium* it will be altered, depending upon a number of characteristics of the epithelium. The thickness, architecture and resultant density of the epithelium will all produce alterations. The reflected light from the underlying stroma will impart a pink appearance to the normal epithelium. In Fig. 3.2, the epithelium is *abnormal (atypical)* (1) and has an increased thickness and altered architecture, with the result that the reflected light imparts

on opaque appearance especially after the application of acetic acid.

The role of the epithelium

Various epithelial types modify the general features of the

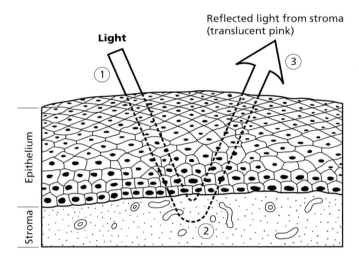

Fig. 3.1 Normal epithelium.

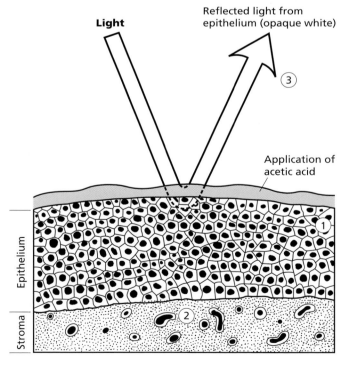

Fig. 3.2 Abnormal (atypical) epithelium (CIN).

colposcopic appearance described above. In the normal cervix, glycogen-containing squamous epithelium, which is present during reproductive life, is thick and multilayered and acts as an effective filter, imparting a pink to reddish appearance when viewed colposcopically. The columnar epithelium is thin, contains mucus, and is highly translucent, resulting in a dense red colposcopic appearance. Within the bounds of the transformation zone, defined as the area in the columnar epithelium where a new squamous (metaplastic) epithelium forms, will be found metaplastic epithelium at various stages of development. It may be thinner than the normal squamous epithelium, devoid of glycogen, and appear reddish. Very rapidly regenerating epithelium, as seen in immature squamous metaplastic tissue, may adopt an opaque appearance. Abnormal epithelium contains the CIN stages, some of which will be precancerous. It differs from normal epithelium in that it is more cellular, with a higher nuclear content. The result is an opaque appearance, which has sometimes been described as deep red mixed with a dirty gray of whitish discoloration.

The atrophic or postmenopausal, or indeed the prepubertal, squamous epithelium is thinner than normal squamous epithelium and devoid of glycogen. The stromal blood supply is reduced and, as seen later (Chapter 4), is characterized by a pale red colposcopic appearance.

The role of the stroma

When inflammatory infiltration occurs within the stroma, the resultant colposcopic appearance of the epithelium may be altered. The result may be a grayish white or yellowish appearance, dependent purely upon the degree of stromal inflammatory infiltration.

The role of the surface configuration

This is determined by the surface shape and by the variations in thickness of the epithelium. The surface shape can be either smooth or papillary. Columnar epithelium, for example, is represented colposcopically as grapelike villi that, when pronounced, become conglomerated into the so-called columnar ectopy.

Vascular patterns also become evident through the surface, as will be discussed later (Chapter 5). The capillaries may shine through the epithelium, either appearing as red dots on a white or opaque background, giving rise to so-called punctation, or arborizing within the stromal papillary ridges that subdivide the surface epithelium and thereby forming discrete fields, the so-called mosaic epithelium.

An addition to the colposcopic image may occur when white patches, which can be seen by the unaided eye, appear on the surface epithelium. This so-called leukoplakia is due to a thick keratin covering that may overlie both histologic normal and abnormal epithelium. When production of the latter is sufficiently exuberant, the surface may adopt an even more irregular appearance with resultant obvious ridging and folding, and the develop-

ment of the so-called microexophytia or mountain-range appearance of invasive cancer.

The combination of variable degrees of epithelial maturity, alterations in surface contour, and in blood-vessel patterns, as described above, results in variation in the appearance of both normal and abnormal epithelia. There is no single appearance which can be called pathognomic, especially for the abnormal epithelium; these changes therefore allow grading systems to be adopted (see Chapter 6). Coppleson *et al.* (1986) described three grades of the abnormal (atypical) epithelium that they believed both to be diagnostic and to carry "prognostic correlations of practical significance." This helps in the identification of lesions that are insignificant or significant in respect of management; the former with minimal neoplastic potential, where invasion is years away (if it ever occurs), and the latter with a neoplastic potential with a high malignant potential. This grading system will be described later, together with the Reid Colposcopic Index.

3.3 The colposcopic examination

The colposcope

The colposcope is a microscope providing illuminated magnification which allows the cervix to be viewed at between six- and 40-fold magnification. Originally developed by Hinselmann in the 1920s, it has gained popularity only in the last two decades in Western Europe and North and South America. It is either mounted on a free, movable stand, as shown in Fig. 3.3, or can be attached to a wall, ceiling, or the actual colposcope couch.

The colposcope lens has a focal length ranging between 200 and 300 mm; this establishes a comfortable working distance for the observer. Occasionally, the objective can be less, i.e. 125 mm; this is used predominantly when the saline method of colposcopy, a technique to demonstrate the vascular patterns within the surface epithelium (see Chapter 6), is employed.

The colposcope is binocular and has eye-piece lenses (3 in Fig. 3.3a) that have a magnification range from six- to 12-fold. As seen in Fig. 3.3 there are accessories to the colposcope itself. On most machines there is a tilting mechanism, a fine focus, binocular eyepieces, and a side arm that allows either a still or video camera to be attached.

Another attachment sometimes used is a green filter; this may be inserted between the light source and the objective lens of the colposcope. It will absorb red light so that blood vessels become much darker and appear black and is used in particular when the saline technique is employed.

The examination

Colposcopic examination is usually conducted with the patient placed in a modified lithotomy position on a suitable couch. The couch shown in Fig. 3.3a makes use of a heel rest rather than the knee crutches that are sometimes employed. An instrument tray is placed beside the couch and on this tray are instruments that are essential

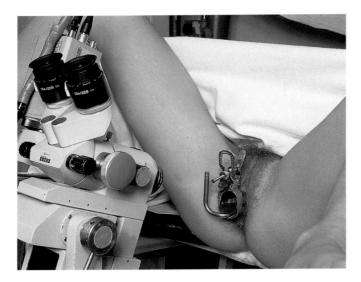

Fig. 3.3(a)

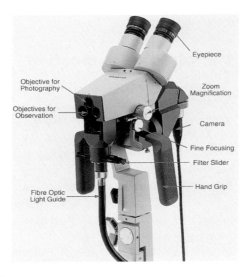

Eyepiece

Objective for
Photography

Zoom
Magnification

Objectives for
Observation

Camera

Fine Focusing

Filter Slider

Fibre Optic
Light Guide

Hand Grip

Fig. 3.3(b)

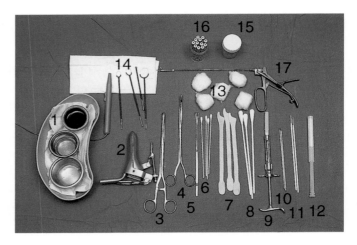

Fig. 3.4 A typical tray used in colposcopy: 1, pots with solution (acetic acid, saline, and Lugol's iodine); 2, vaginal speculum; 3, sponge-holding forceps; 4, Desjardin's endocervical forceps; 5, three-pronged probe for retraction; 6, cotton-tipped fine swab sticks; 7, Aylesbury cytology spatula; 8, larger cotton-tipped swab sticks; 9, local anesthetic syringe; 10, silver nitrate sticks for hemostasis; 11, endocervical brushes; 12, antibiotic cream; 13, cotton swabs; 14, diathermy electrodes for diagnosis or treatment; 15, Monsell's solution (ferric subsulfate); 16, local anesthetic ampules; 17, Eppendorfer cervical biopsy forceps.

for colposcopy. The legend to Fig. 3.4 lists instruments that are used in the examination. Most important is the bivalve speculum, which may vary in width and length to allow the easy placement of the cervix between the blades. Occasionally the patulous walls of the vagina may fall in and obscure the view; in this situation a rubber condom, or the finger of a glove with the end cut off, can be placed around the blade, thereby keeping the vaginal walls away from the central viewing area. Lateral wall retraction, provided by attachments to the speculum or held by an attendant, can also be used to hold back patulous vaginal walls.

Before examining the cervix, the vulva and vagina are inspected. This is important as there is a small, but increased risk of vulvar and vaginal neoplasia in women with cervical disease. The vulva can be examined with the naked eye, but the vagina should be viewed through the sixfold magnification of the colposcope. It is not usually necessary to take a cervical smear before examination, but if it is necessary then it must be remembered that this could interfere with the surface epithelium. Abrasions and bleeding could be caused.

When the speculum has been inserted and the cervix

manipulated between the ends of the blades, the epithelia that are visualized are predominantly those on the ectocervix. Once the blades of the speculum have been opened, not only the ectocervix but also part of the endocervix becomes visible. This is shown in Fig. 3.5a and b. In Fig. 3.5a the speculum is fully opened and the cervix is in what is referred to as the "apparent view." The endocervix with its columnar epithelium comes fully into view. The metaplastic squamous epithelium on the ectocervix, existing between points 1 and 4, is clearly seen. When the speculum is removed into the lower vagina, imitating the normal *in vivo* situation, the so-called "real view" becomes obvious. This view (Fig. 3.5b) shows how the endocervical tissues have retracted and all that is "outside" on the ectocervix is the metaplastic squamous epithelium (between points 1–4). As will be discussed later, this epithelium has indeed developed as a result of the exposure of columnar epithelium to the effect of the vaginal environment (i.e. pH) during certain periods, such as pregnancy.

It is usual to find a small amount of vaginal discharge, mixed with cervical mucus, covering and obscuring the area to be examined. A dry swab is normally used to remove the secretions. In Figs 3.6 and 3.7a, this procedure has taken place: the vaginal and cervical secretions (Fig. 3.6) have been removed, allowing the cervix to be more easily visualized (Fig. 3.7a).

Visualization of the endocervix can be optimized if the examination is conducted at the mid-cycle. The profuse outflowing of clear cervical mucus allows an uninterrupted view of the endocervical tissues, as can be seen in Fig. 3.7b. The endocervix is marked at (1) and an area of atypical (abnormal) epithelium seen at (2) and (3).

After the patient has been placed in the modified lithotomy position, the cervix is exposed, as shown in

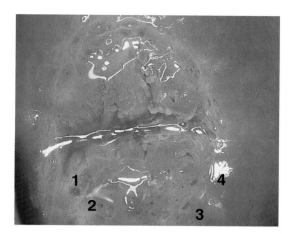

Fig. 3.5(a)

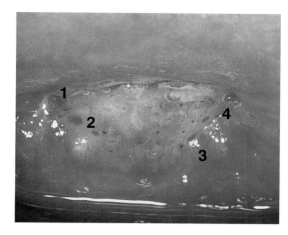

Fig. 3.5(b)

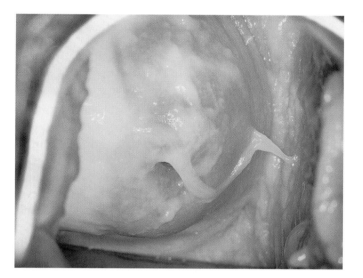

Fig. 3.6

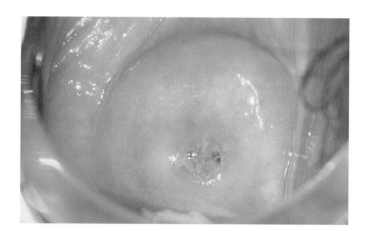

Fig. 3.7(a)

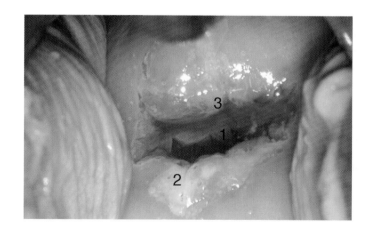

Fig. 3.7(b)

Fig. 3.3, using a bivalve speculum. Solutions of acetic acid (3 or 5%) or normal saline are then applied to the cervix. Other solutions, such as Lugol's iodine (1%), can also be applied.

Acetic acid technique

In the acetic acid technique, strengths of between 3 and 5% acetic acid are used; the solution is applied with either a cotton ball or spray. The acetic acid causes the tissues, especially the columnar and abnormal epithelia, to become edematous. Abnormal (atypical) epithelium adopts a white or opaque appearance, as described previously, which is then quite easy to distinguish from the normal epithelium, which appears pink. The acetic acid seems to act by causing the coagulation of epithelial and stromal cytokeratins in a reversible event.

There also seems to be swelling of the tissues and recently Maddox et al. (1994) have shown an increase in the keratin filament proteins in epithelium which stains white with acetic acid. These keratin filament proteins, called cytokeratin, seem to be increased in association with cellular swelling caused by acetic acid in this type of epithelium. There are 20 different cytokeratin polypeptides (Smedts et al., 1993) and Maddox and his group have shown that there is a significant increase in cytokeratin 10; they believe that it is an essential requirement for the formation of the so-called acetowhite epithelial change.

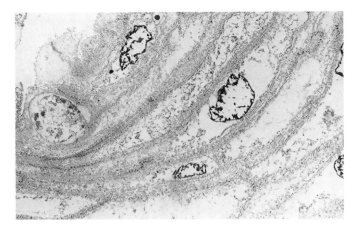

Fig. 3.7 (c) Transmission electron micrograph (EM) of superficial nucleated epithelial cells (cervical intraepithelial neoplasia) with precipitated nucleoprotein and cytoplasmic vacuolation.

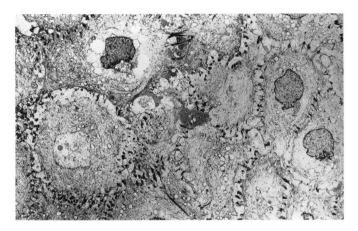

Fig. 3.7 (d) Transmission showing swelling of the cells and separation of desmosomes.

The appearance of white areas within the atypical transformation zone following the application of 3 or 5% aqueous acetic acid solution is one of the basics of colposcopy. An explanation for this phenomenon recognizes that acetic acid is a frequent component of tissue fixatives, and will rapidly penetrate through tissue. Its effect within the nucleus of cells is to precipitate nucleoprotein (Fig. 3.7c). The cytoplasm undergoes vacuolation, the cell becomes

swollen and desmosomes are separated (Fig. 3.7d). When acetic acid is applied to normal squamous epithelium, the penetration through the sparsely nucleated surface, and intermediate layers produces little precipitation. The parabasal and basal cells of the epithelium contain more nucleoprotein, but this is not sufficient to obscure the color of the underlying cervical stroma with its rich network of subepithelial vessels, and the epithelium looks pink. When acetic acid is applied to areas of CIN, the precipitated nucleoprotein within the neoplastic cells obscures the underlying vessels, the light is reflected and the epithelium appears white—acetowhite epithelium. With low-grade CIN the acid must penetrate into the lower half of the epithelium and the onset of "white" is delayed. High-grade or full-thickness CIN will give an almost instant response and will appear markedly "white". The effect is slowly reversed because the acid is buffered and nucleoprotein no longer precipitated. The appearances are not unique for neoplasia, and will be seen on other occasions when there is increased nucleoprotein present, for example during metaplasia, healing, and with the presence of virus or viral products.

It is usual to allow some time for the various changes within the epithelium to appear (Figs 3.8 & 3.9). The cervix painted with a 5% solution will obviously respond quicker than one painted with a 3% solution. The effects will wear off in about 50–60 seconds. It is usual for a small amount of acetic acid to be left in the posterior fornix and by using small swab sticks it is possible to wash the cervical epithelium continuously, thereby maintaining the characteristics produced by the acetic acid. This is readily seen in Figs 3.10 and 3.11. In Fig. 3.10 the cervix has had no acetic acid applied to it, whereas in Fig. 3.11, 40 seconds after acetic acid application a whitish appearance has been produced.

Saline technique

The saline technique, expounded by the late Professor Kolstad of Oslo, Norway, involves the application of a cotton-wool swab, soaked in physiologic saline, to the cervix (Kolstad & Stafl, 1982). This allows the subepithelial

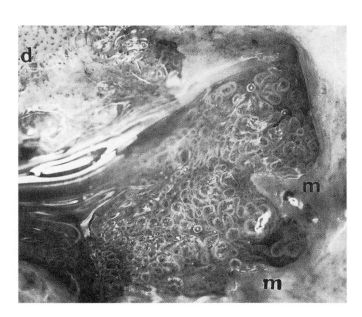

Fig. 3.8 The transformation zone before the application of acetic acid: d, dysplasia; m, metaplasia.

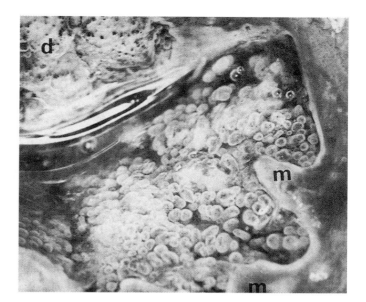

Fig. 3.9 After the application of 3% acetic acid, the edematous columnar villi are seen in the central part of the picture; the metaplastic tissue (m) appears opaque and the dysplastic (d) area has a pronounced whiteness with small vessel punctation.

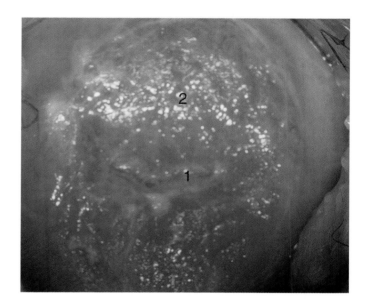

Fig. 3.10 In this figure a large ectropion (normal transformation zone) exists, with the endocervix at (1) and the ectocervix at (2).

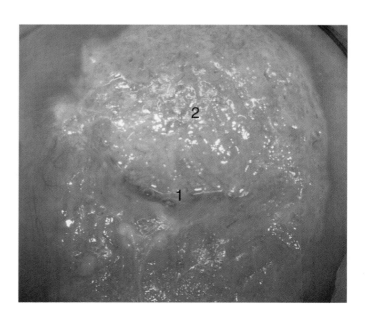

Fig. 3.11 In this figure, after the application of 5% acetic acid, the squamous (metaplastic) epithelium that covers the ectocervix at (2) appears opaque and the area is clearly distinct from the surrounding pink squamous epithelium.

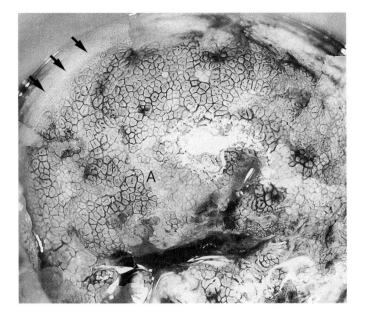

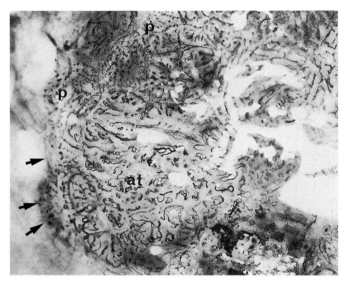

Fig. 3.12 An atypical transformation zone showing a large area of mosaic epithelium characterized by large intercapillary distances. This is clearly seen at (A) and the original squamocolumnar junction is arrowed.

Fig. 3.13 Atypical vessels (at) are clearly seen within the transformation zone with two areas of punctation (p). The sharp edge of the transformation zone is arrowed.

angioarchitecture to become obvious. A green filter must be used to identify the red vessels that appear dark and stand out most clearly. This allows the various vascular features of the atypical (abnormal) epithelium to be clearly visualized (Figs 3.12 & 3.13). The subject is discussed in Chapter 6.

Decontamination of colposcopy clinic equipment

Human papillomavirus (HPV) and human immunodeficiency virus (HIV) are associated with serious genital tract pathology. This has made it imperative that the decontamination of any equipment used in the colposcopy clinic, is 100% reliable. Before the choice of instruments is made, one of the parameters which must be assessed is the ease with which decontamination may be accomplished. The hazard to the patient arises from the flora of the vagina and contamination with blood or serum. Whilst bacteria are easily dealt with largely by cleaning, the hazard posed by the blood-born viruses (hepatitis A and C, and HIV), and the local viral pathogens (HPV and HSV) are perhaps more emotive.

The rules that should be followed are simple:

1 All equipment in contact with the patient must be cleanable, usually with hot water and detergent, to remove visible soil.

2 Once cleaned, it must be capable of undergoing a disinfecting process.

(a) This is preferably a moist heat process such as autoclaving.

(b) A second line approach is the use of a disinfectant with proven bacterial and virucidal properties, such as gluteraldehyde.

The local disinfection policies should be observed and local expert guidance sought.

There is also value in using disposable instruments, especially vaginal speculi. However, this is an expensive exercise and there is no reason why, if the above decontamination procedures and principles are followed, concern should arise either in the patient or in the colposcopist.

3.4 New developments in colposcopy

Video colposcopy, image management and electronic databases

Video colposcopy is a new method for the examination of the lower genital tract. It utilizes a video colposcope which comprises a video camera and colposcope with an electronic green filter, motorized zoom magnification and fine focus controls, combined in one unit (Fig. 3.14). Because of the omission of eyepieces, the observer examines the cervix on a high resolution video monitor. A modified colposcopy technique is utilized to assist depth perception as the system does not allow for the traditional stereoscopic view. The potential advantages of such a system include enhanced teaching for trainees and improved patient education (as is the case with traditional colposcopes attached to video systems). In addition the system may appeal to clinicians who are uncomfortable with the use of a binocular colposcope (Ferris, 1997). Such a system has been used in the assessment of a technique termed "video colpography" for secondary screening (Etheridge, 1997). The principle is essentially the same as cervicography except that instead of using a still photograph, a moving image is examined. A video recording using a camera equipped with a macro lens and autofocus is made of the cervix and vaginal fornices after the application of 5% acetic acid. The recording can then be assessed by a colposcopist and an impression formed.

A number of image management systems are now available which are able to set up a database so that images can be captured and stored digitally for documentation or teaching purposes. Many of them allow annotations directly onto the image (e.g. biopsy sites) (see Fig. 3.15) and will also make area measurements where necessary. In addition, electronic filters can be utilized to highlight particular areas and de-emphasize others if needed. These images can be accessed for comparison to follow the progression or regression of lesions over time, and a printout obtained if required.

Many of the image management systems are also combined with a colposcopy database so that patient information and clinical data can be entered to facilitate patient management and clinic administration. Reports can be generated automatically, greatly assisting in the collection of data for audit or training purposes.

3.5 References and bibliography

Coppleson, M., Pixley, E. & Reid, B. (eds) (1986) Colposcopic appearances of the atypical transformation zone. In: *Colposcopy*, 3rd edn, p. 254. Charles C. Thomas, Springfield.

Etheridge, I.J., Dunn J., Shafi, M.I. *et al.* (1997) Video colpography: a technique for secondary cervical screening. *Br Obstet Gynaecol* **104**,150.

Fait, G., Daniel, Y., Kupfermine, M.J. *et al.* (1998) Does typing of human papillomavirus assist in the triage of women with repeated low grade cytologic abnormalities? *Gynecol Oncol* **70**,319.

Ferris, D.G. (1997) Video colposcopy. *J Lower Genit Tract Dis* **1**,15.

Kolstad, P. & Stafl, A. (eds) (1982) Methods of colposcopic examination. In: *Atlas of Colposcopy*, 3rd edn, p. 34. Churchill Livingstone, Edinburgh.

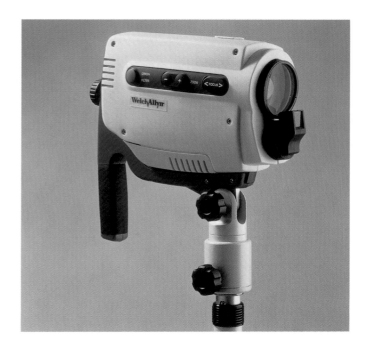

Fig. 3.14 A Welch Allyn video-colposcope.

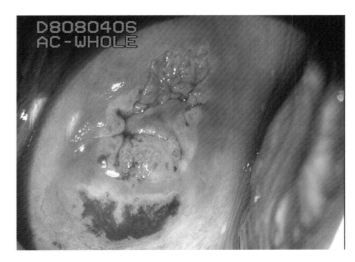

Fig. 3.15(a)

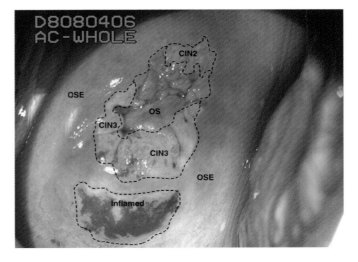

Fig. 3.15(b)

Maddox, P., Szarewski, A., Dyson J. & Cuzick, J. (1994) Cytokeratin expression and acetowhite change in cervical epithelium. *J Clin Pathol* **47**(1),15.

Manos, M.N., Kinney, W.K., Hurley, L.B. *et al.* (1999) Identifying women with cervical neoplasia—using human papillomavirus DNA testing for equivocal Papanicolaou results. *JAMA* **281**(17),1605.

Smedts, F., Ramaekers, F.C.S. & Vooijs, P. (1993) The dynamics of keratin expression in malignant transformation of cervical epithelium; a review. *Obstets Gynecol* **82**(3),465.

Chapter 4
Colposcopy of the Normal Cervix
A prerequisite to establish the diagnosis of cervical precancer

4.1 Introduction

Together with cytology, colposcopy is an important pre-requisite for the diagnosis of cervical precancer. The gynecologist, alerted by abnormal cytology or by a suspicious appearance to the cervix in the presence of negative cytology, is directed toward colposcopy, which facilitates an assessment of the distribution of precancerous epithelium within the cervix. As will be shown later, not only will the colposcope allow localization of the lesion but it will also aid in the selection of a biopsy site. It helps the clinician to select the treatment for cervical intraepithelial neoplasia (CIN), evaluate the very common subclinical papilloma-virus infections (SPI), manage effectively the abnormal smear in pregnancy, and evaluate any extension of the pre-cancerous lesion into the vagina. It does, however, require that the gynecologist has an understanding of the funda-mental and varied physiologic processes that occur within the cervix at different times in a woman's life. Thus, this chapter will not only detail the developmental anatomy and natural history of the different epithelial types but also examine them at times such as during adolescence, preg-nancy, and the menopause. This allows a better under-standing for the later study of the neoplastic changes that develop within the physiologic epithelium.

4.2 Cervical epithelium: natural history

The cervical epithelium is derived in fetal life from the Mul-lerian epithelium and the vaginal plate. The latter structure is attached to the urogenital sinus, which is believed to rep-resent a modified Wolffian duct epithelium. There are two types of epithelium that exist in the fetal cervix: the colum-nar epithelium, derived from the Mullerian epithelium, and squamous epithelium, originating from the vaginal plate epithelium. These join at a fixed point at or just inside the cervical orifice (Forsberg, 1976); this point of union is called the *original squamocolumnar junction*. Present during fetal life, and thus deserving the term "original", these two types of epithelium are referred to as the *original columnar* and *original squamous*. The columnar epithelium continues cephalad to the endometrium and extends caudally for a variable distance to border with the original squamous epithelium. The squamous epithelium is highly differenti-ated, stratified, and in turn extends upward from the junc-tion with the vulvar epithelium cephalad to its contact with the columnar epithelium. In some fetuses, the area between the original columnar and squamous epithelia is taken up by a third type of epithelium called the *original metaplastic epithelium*. This metaplastic epithelium seems to be of the same type and configuration to that found at other periods in the female's life, such as during adolescence and preg-nancy, times when the cervix is subjected to hormonal changes that induce epithelial modifications.

It seems as though the hormonal changes present at such times result in columnar epithelium becoming exposed on the vaginal surface to an acidic environment; this event ap-pears to be the stimulus for metaplastic transformation. The increase in estrogen secretion in late pregnancy, which also influences the cervix at puberty, seems to produce expan-sion of the cervical body. An eversion process takes place in which the columnar epithelium of the endocervix is expo-sed to the ectocervical acidic milieu (Singer, 1976a). Ex-amination using a vaginal speculum reveals a red area surrounding the external cervical os in later life; this corre-sponds to the area of everted endocervical tissue. Various terms have been used to describe this everted area: most commonly erosion, but alternate terms, such as erythrop-lakia, ectopy, and transformation zone, have also been used.

The term *transformation zone*, that area enclosed by the original squamocolumnar junction, amply describes this region in which transformation between columnar and squamous epithelium occurs. The epithelium induced by the transforming process of metaplasia is called the meta-plastic epithelium. It appears, as described above, in late fetal life, during adolescence, and in pregnancy. It is some-times referred to as the typical, physiologic, or normal transformation zone. Within the transformation zone, a third type of epithelium, namely *abnormal* or *atypical epithe-lium*, develops; this is easily recognized colposcopically, and is related to the neoplastic process. It has distinctive colposcopic features, and within its tissues can be found not only physiologic epithelium but also the precursors and cursors of invasive squamous carcinoma of the cervix. The transformation zone containing this abnormal or atypical epithelium is called the *atypical transformation zone*. These epithelia are depicted in Fig. 4.1.

The changes of transformation alter the appearance of the cervix at various stages in the female's life. In the prepubertal cervix there is minimal eversion compared with that occurring after puberty. In pregnancy, eversion with transformation dramatically alters the morphology of the different epithelial types. In contrast, during the menopausal era, there is inward retraction of the epithelium. All these periods will be discussed in more detail later.

4.3 Cervical epithelium: topography

The original squamocolumnar junction, the permanent point of meeting between original squamous and columnar epithelia, outlines the lateral border of the transformation zone. It is fixed, but moves in relation to the whole cervix when eversion of the endocervical columnar epithelium occurs, as happens during adolescence and pregnancy. Figure 4.2a shows the likely positions of this junction; (1) corresponds to the view of the cervix as seen colposcopically in Fig. 4.3. In this position the squamocolumnar

junction is situated within the endocervix and the whole of the ectocervix is covered with original squamous epithelium. Position (2) in Fig. 4.2a corresponds to the general view in Fig. 4.4; the transformation zone is now obvious. The junction seems to exist halfway between the endocervical limit and the vaginal fornix. This appearance is also typical of the so-called ectropion or ectopy. The

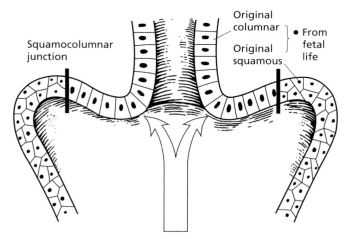

1 **Original epithelia**

Squamocolumnar junction

Original columnar
Original squamous

• From fetal life

2 **Metaplastic squamous epithelium**
Typical transformation zone

• Late fetal life
• Adolescence
• Pregnancy

3 **Abnormal (atypical) epithelium**
Atypical transformation zone

• Adolescence
• Pregnancy
• ? Other times

Includes (immature metaplastic squamous epithelium)
Cervical intraepithelial neoplasia 1–3, early invasion

Fig. 4.1

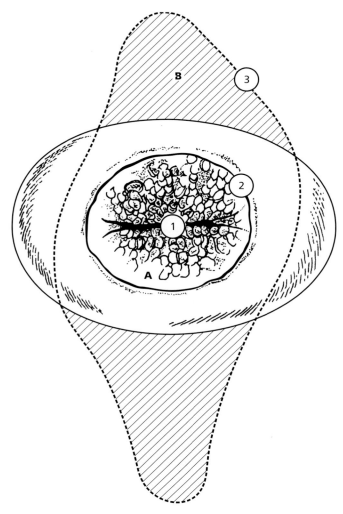

Fig. 4.2(b)

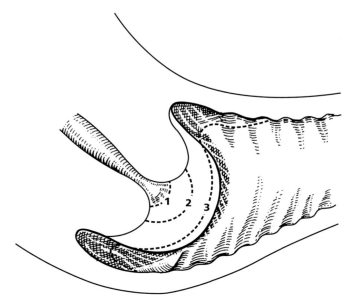

Fig. 4.2(a)

Fig. 4.3 (*Above opposite*) The cervix showing the squamocolumnar junction (1) in the endocervix, with original squamous epithelium (2) covering the ectocervix.

Fig. 4.4 (*Centre opposite*) The squamocolumnar junction (3) is at the mid-distance point between the endocervix and vaginal fornix. The original columnar epithelium is at (1), with a small island of metaplastic squamous epithelium at (2). Original squamous epithelium is at (4).

Fig. 4.5 (*Below opposite*) Colpophotograph showing an extensive transformation zone. The endocervical canal is at (1) with islands of metaplastic epithelium at (2) within areas of original columnar epithelium. The squamocolumnar junction is at (3) with a small longitudinal strip of immature squamous metaplastic epithelium (stippled) medial to this line, and extends posteriorly in the 6-o'clock position into the posterior vaginal fornix (toward 4). The original squamous epithelium is at (5). This condition is also called an ectropion or ectopy.

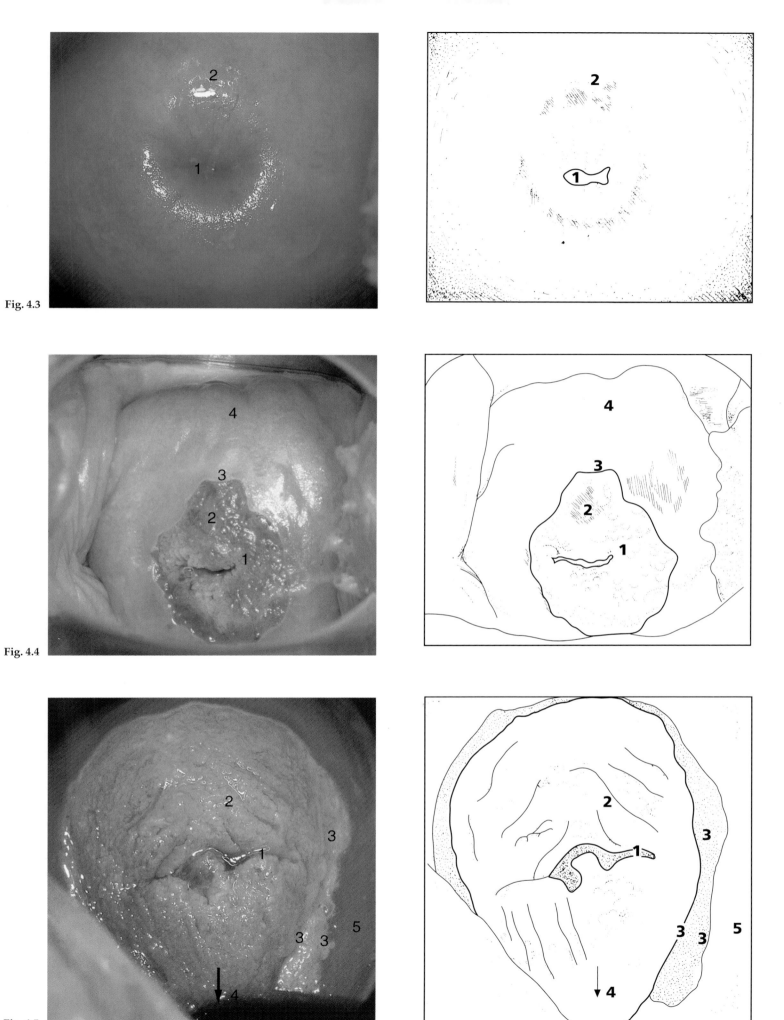

Fig. 4.3

Fig. 4.4

Fig. 4.5

transformation zone in this situation is composed mainly of original columnar epithelium, although some small areas of metaplastic squamous epithelium have already developed.

Position (3) in Fig. 4.2a corresponds to the general colposcopic view in Fig. 4.5. In this situation, most of the ectocervix is covered by columnar epithelium and, as shown, may extend onto the vaginal fornix. The large transformation zone, with its basically columnar epithelium (Fig. 4.5), will very quickly develop metaplastic epithelium, owing to its exposure to the vaginal acidic secretions that bathe the ectocervix (Coppleson & Reid, 1966). Figure 4.2b shows this situation; a physiologic transformation zone exists on the ectocervix and this is marked (A), the endocervix is at (1), and the original squamocolumnar junction is at (2). At (3) is the line of the squamocolumnar junction in a situation where columnar epithelium has extended onto the vaginal vault. This Mullerian duct epithelium extends into this situation in about 4% of normal females and is also found in those who have been exposed, during intrauterine existence, to nonsteroidal estrogens (see Chapter 11). Such changes are also seen in cases of gynatresia.

4.4 Cervical epithelium: colposcopic appearances

The cervical epithelia have distinctive colposcopic appearances and each will be described separately.

Original columnar epithelium

Colposcopically the original columnar epithelium exists in two general forms of arrangement. In the first relatively coarse subdivision it appears as two or three mounds or cushions which are called *rugae* on either lip of the cervix (around 2 in Fig. 4.6a). Within the endocervix this arrangement is present in the form of longitudinal folds [(1) in Fig. 4.6b] from which emanate smaller folds directed obliquely towards the internal os. Because of their general pattern, said to resemble the trunk and branches of a tree, they have been called *arbor vitae*. They have also been referred to as palmate folds or *plicae palmatae*. The regular arrangement of these folds can be seen clearly on a cross-section of the endocervix.

In the second, much finer, grouping the folds are present as small pendulous areas resembling bunches of grapes [2 in Figs 4.6 and 4.9]. The basic subunit of the epithelium is the villus. This is usually ovoid, about $0.15 \times 1.5\,mm$ in diameter, or sometimes appearing as a flattened mound or circumvallate type of up to $2\,mm$ in diameter. Each villus is separated from the next by an intervillus crypt (Fig. 4.6b). The terminal capillary loop in each villus is seen colposcopically and a detailed description of the angiographic as well as the ultrastructural appearance is found in Section 4.5. The tissue is present either by itself or, more commonly, in combination with metaplastic squamous epithelium. Figure 4.6a shows the small individual grape-like villi present in the endocervical canal as well as on the ectocervix [in positions (1) and (2)]. The squamocolumnar junction is at (3) and the original squamous epithelium is at (4).

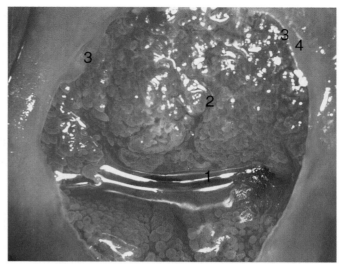

Fig. 4.6(a)

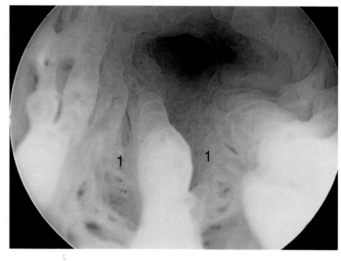

Fig. 4.6(b)

Fig. 4.6 (a) The "apparent" view of the transformation zone. (b) View of the endocervix. The light foreground is reflection artefact.

Original squamous epithelium

The original squamous epithelium [(4) in Fig. 4.6a] is clearly identified as a smooth, usually featureless covering of the cervix; its uniform pink color contrasts with the redness of the original columnar epithelium. It joins the latter at the original squamocolumnar junction, shown at (3).

Transformation zone

The zone in which transformation will occur during fetal life, adolescence, and pregnancy is termed the typical or normal transformation zone. It is characterized by the presence of metaplastic epithelium, which may extend not only across the ectocervix but to within the endocervical canal.

Transformation is more prominent at the squamocolumnar junction in an area where columnar epithelium is everted and exposed to the vaginal environment as seen in Figs 4.6a and 4.7. In Fig. 4.6a the endocervical canal has been everted to show the transformation zone on the ectocervix. However, this is an artificial view, which has been called the "apparent view", because as the speculum is removed into the lower vagina, so the columnar epithelium of the transformation zone recedes into the endocervical canal [positions (1) and (2) in Fig. 4.7]. In the *in vivo* situation (Fig. 4.7), no exposure to the vaginal environment has occurred and therefore no transformed epithelium (i.e. metaplastic epithelium) has developed. This is called the "real view". The squamocolumnar junction is at (3) with the original squamous epithelium at (4). The columnar epithelium, being highly specialized and sophisticated, is preserved within the endocervical canal, away from the degrading influence of the vaginal environment ((1) and (2) in Fig. 4.7).

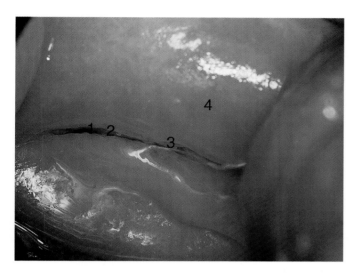

Fig. 4.7 The "real" view of the transformation zone.

Mechanisms involved in squamous metaplastic transformation

Various theories exist as to how the squamous epithelium develops from the columnar epithelium. At the turn of the century, Myer's theory of healing of "the erosion" was preeminent. It suggested that there were wedge-shaped offshoots from the surrounding original squamous epithelium, and that these undermined and then detached the columnar epithelium, uprooting it from its base (Myer, 1910). It seems difficult to understand how this theory was accepted, and it has been replaced in modern times by the concept that metaplasia arises from cellular elements either within the columnar region or from the stroma.

Squamous metaplasia is preceded by the appearance of new cell types underneath the columnar epithelium, the so-called subcolumnar cells. These cells multiply and form a layer that eventually produces a normally differentiating squamous epithelium. The columnar epithelium sometimes remains atop these new squamous elements. They are eventually shed. These cells are believed to be pluripotent and are sometimes referred to as reserve cells (Fluhmann, 1961). They are believed to replace continually the endocervical columnar epithelium that is lost in day-to-day wear.

It has also been suggested that these cells may originate from the stroma. These would appear to be blood-borne monocytic-type cells that appear within the subcolumnar

area and eventually develop in a similar manner to that described above for reserve cells (Song, 1964).

Morphologically, reserve cells have a somewhat similar appearance to the basal cells of the original squamous epithelium, in that they have round nuclei and little cytoplasm. During metaplastic development, the reserve cells multiply and form a layer that may be several cells thick; this gives rise to a distinct morphologic entity of reserve cell hyperplasia (Burghardt, 1991).

Recent information concerning the role of reserve cells in the formation of metaplastic epithelia is forthcoming from a study by Smedts *et al.* (1993) of the cytokeratins of eukaryotic cells. The intermediate filament proteins, which are the important constituents of cytokeratin, are involved in providing internal stability within the cell as well as involvement in transport functions and gene regulation of the structure. It seems from the study, that reserve cells, by virtue of their specific keratin characteristics, would seem to be the progenitor cell of both immature squamous metaplasia and endocervical columnar cells. These reserve cells, according to the observations of Smedts and co-workers, tend to display a bidirectional keratin pattern comprising keratins typical of both squamous and simple types of differentiation, reflecting the bipotential nature of the cells. Likewise, in their studies of mature squamous metaplastic epithelium, they found that the keratin expression was identical to that found in ectocervical epithelium, with the exception of one cytokeratin (17), which is sporadically expressed in the basal layers of the ectocervical epithelium. Furthermore, they found the keratin expression is not compartmentalized as strictly as in the ectocervical noncornifying epithelium. This probably means that the mature squamous metaplastic epithelium, even though it seems mature, based on morphologic criteria, is not yet fully matured based on its keratin phenotype.

Associated with this stage is the thickening and fusing of the endocervical villi, a development that can be seen both histologically and colposcopically (Fig. 4.8a–e).

4.5 Squamous metaplastic epithelium

It has been suggested by many investigators that the behavior of squamous metaplasia "holds the key to the understanding of cervical oncogenesis" (Coppleson & Reid, 1967). This dynamic process can be followed sequentially by colposcopic observation and would seem to involve three distinct phases.

Colposcopic stages of development

In stage 1, there is a loss of translucency of the top of the villus, and the vascular structures within the villus become indistinct. This is shown in Fig. 4.8a and corresponds to tissue seen at position (2) in Fig. 4.9a. A histologic examination of the area will demonstrate a reduction in mucus content of the epithelial cells, which become flattened and cuboidal. This stage is followed by the appearance of multilayered undifferentiated epithelium, caused by the rapid division of the reserve cells. These eventually cap the villus and extend into the clefts between two adjacent villi, as

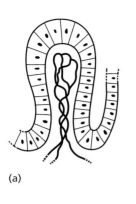
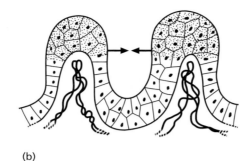
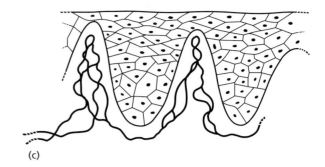

(a)   (b)   (c)

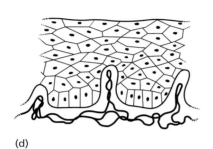
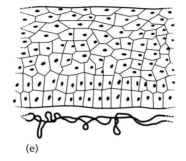

(d)   (e)

Fig. 4.8 (a)–(e) The normal process of squamous metaplasia. The villi of columnar epithelium are replaced by metaplastic epithelium. The capillary structures of the stroma in the villi are compressed and reduced in height, ultimately forming a network under the epithelium; this is indistinguishable from the capillary network of normal squamous epithelium (modified from Kolstad & Stafl, 1982).

shown in Fig. 4.8b; colposcopically, this is represented by the tissue in position (3) in Fig. 4.9a.

Stage 2 is an extension of stage 1. More mature areas of squamous epithelium appear, in which individual opaque villi appear to be fused; the origin of the new surface is still apparent in this tissue [Fig. 4.8c and the area between positions (3) and (4) in Fig. 4.9a]. Minute humps are also present and these represent the tips of the old villi.

In stage 3, there is near obliteration of the original structure. This produces a smooth surface with multilayered and undifferentiated epithelium, into which has been incorporated the original vascular structures that existed in relation to the stromal core of the now fused villi. This is represented in Fig. 4.8d and e, and in area (4) of Fig. 4.9a.

In this colpophotograph (Fig. 4.9a), the original squamous (1) and columnar (2) epithelium with the original squamo-columnar junction (6) are seen. There are also many gland openings arrowed in the area of (5) and are associated with the intermediate forms of the process.

Colposcopically, features of this process can be easily seen. Firstly, the process starts at the tips of the villi, suggesting that the stimulus to this change is found in the external environment provided by the vagina. This influence seems to be the acidic pH of the vagina (Coppleson & Reid, 1986a). Secondly, the essential process is an in-situ transformation, so that the new epithelium emerges from beneath, and not by an ingrowth from, the original squamous epithelium (Burghardt, 1991). Thirdly, the process proceeds from patches of already fused villi that are present within the unchanged columnar epithelium. The end result is a combination of epithelial patches, and this produces a superficial homogeneity, providing the covering to the transformation zone.

Histologic features of development

As squamous metaplasia progresses, reserve cells undergo maturation giving rise to recognizable immature squamous

metaplasia (Fig. 4.9b). While columnar cells remain on the surface of the newly developing squamous epithelium the metaplasia is said to be "incomplete". This is seen in Fig. 4.9c where there are residual glands and mucin containing columnar cells (1) on the surface of the developing squamous epithelium (2). At this stage stratification is not apparent or may be just visible. This is shown in Fig. 4.9d and e (high power) where the OSE is to the left again, incomplete squamous metaplasia at (1) and stroma at (2). The squamocolumnar junction is marked by a solid arrow. As the process continues further the epithelium loses its columnar surface and the mature squamous epithelium appears. This is shown in Fig. 4.9f. The solid arrow separates the OSE (1) with its usual pale glycogenated squamous layers from the metaplastic epithelium (2). There is striking epithelial scalloping or irregularity of the lower half of the epithelium (3) as a result of the intercalated

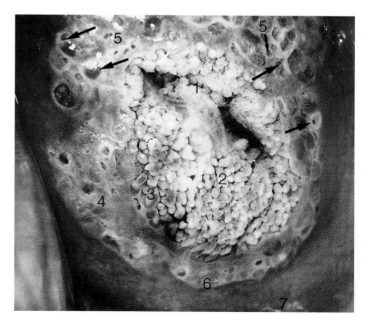

Fig. 4.9(a)

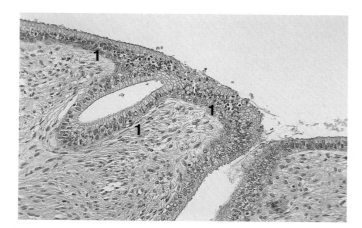

Fig. 4.9 (b) A single layer of "reserve cells" appearing conspicuously beneath the columnar mucinous endocervical cells (1). The origin of these cells is uncertain, but at this stage their detailed keratin signature already identifies them as parabasal or suprabasal squamous cells. They are present over the papillary surface and within the endocervical crypts or troughs. Their monotypic single layer occurrence at one moment suggests a threshold crossed or a switch tripped over.

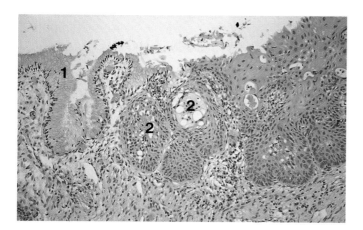

Fig. 4.9 (c) A later stage of still incomplete squamous metaplasia with normal endocervical epithelium on the left at (1). Within the developing squamous epithelium there are residual columnar-lined surfaces (2) with endocervical cells.

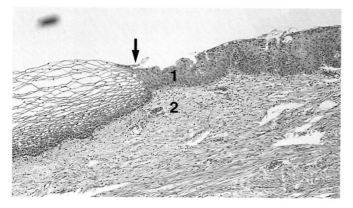

Fig. 4.9(d)

stromal papillae which were originally sited between the endocervical crypts and still contain capillary vascular channels. The new epithelium is very often darker with reduced glycogen levels and may remain so.

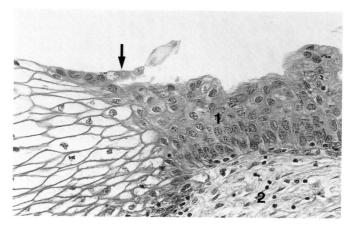

Fig. 4.9(e)

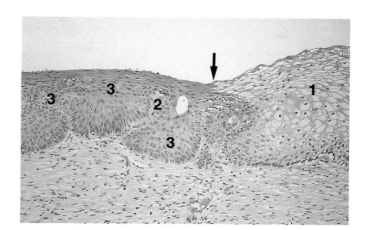

Fig. 4.9(f)

Stimulus to development

The metaplastic process is stimulated by changes in the vaginal pH. It seems as though, especially in pregnancy, the vaginal pH causes destruction of the overlying columnar epithelium and generation of the reserve or subcolumnar cells (Coppleson & Reid, 1966). This can be seen in Fig. 4.10a and b. In both these cervixes, the metaplastic process is more intense the more peripheral the tissue is within the transformation zone. In Fig. 4.10a, the original columnar epithelium at (1) contrasts with the immature squamous epithelium formed at (3). In Fig. 4.10b, the intensity of the metaplastic process is apparent at the top of the villous process (3), again representing the portion of tissue most exposed to the vaginal pH. In Fig. 4.10c the metaplastic process extends to the region of the internal os (1). Its upper extent is arrowed with the columnar epithelium appearing above this point and in the intervening so-called crypt spaces (2). This eversion process occurs predominantly in adolescence and during pregnancy, and shows the proclivity of the resultant exposed columnar area to undergo metaplasia.

The process of eversion with squamous metaplasia formation can easily be seen by close observation of the transformation zone in apparent and real views; these views imitate the normal eversion process. These processes are clearly displayed in Figs 4.11–4.13.

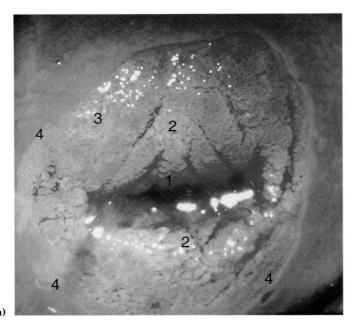

Fig. 4.10(a)

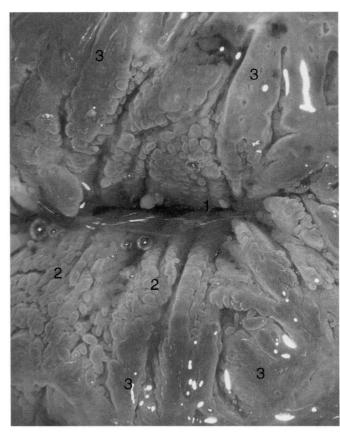

Fig. 4.10(b)

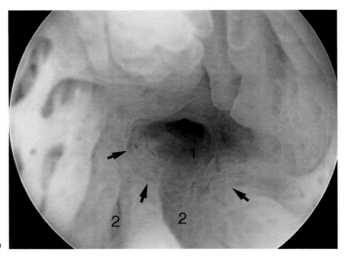

Fig. 4.10(c)

Fig. 4.10 (a) The cervix of an adolescent (16 years) showing all the stages of squamous metaplasia. The endocervix with its original columnar epithelium is at (1). At position (2) is seen stage 2 of squamous metaplasia development with fusion of the villi, and at (3) this has extended to fusion of all the villi. Immature squamous epithelium is present, adjacent and medial to the squamocolumnar junction at (4). Between (2) and (3) it can be seen that the villous structure of the original columnar epithelium has been gradually lost until the surface has become flat with the development of more peripheral immature epithelium. This has developed in an area that is more exposed to the effect of the vaginal pH. The pallor of this immature epithelium (3) contrasts with the redness of the previous columnar epithelium (1). With further maturity, this pallor will be lost as the epithelium becomes thicker. (b) An area of the ectocervix showing the tendency for the metaplastic process to develop in areas exposed to the vaginal pH. Original columnar epithelium is seen at (2), emanating from the endocervix at (1) with early squamous metaplasia developing at (3) in the exposed areas atop the villous processes.

In Fig. 4.11, the cervix is seen in the apparent view, with the original columnar epithelium at (1), the original squamocolumnar junction marked with a dashed line, and the upper limit of the metaplastic process, the so-called *new squamocolumnar junction*, at (2). The original squamocolumnar junction is at (3), with original squamous epithelium at (4). Between positions (2) and (3), the squamous epithelium is pale and immature. As the speculum

is withdrawn into the lower vagina (Figs 4.12 & 4.13), imitating the *in vivo* position (real view) of the epithelial types, it can be seen that the original columnar epithelium recedes into the canal and all that is exposed on the ectocervix is immature squamous metaplastic epithelium (positions 2–3).

In Fig. 4.12, there is still some original columnar epithelium (1) exposed and the new squamocolumnar junction (2) remains obvious. However, upon full retraction (Fig. 4.13) this junction is within the endocervix, leaving the newly developed immature squamous epithelium present on the ectocervix (between positions 2–3); this represents the area most in contact with the vaginal pH.

Colposcopic representations of squamous metaplastic epithelium

The squamous metaplastic epithelium is present in most cervixes between late fetal life and the menopause, with periods of development primarily related to late fetal life, menarche, and the first pregnancy (Singer, 1975). In all these eras, exposure of the original columnar epithelium to the vaginal acidity is preceded by the eversion process induced by estrogen stimulation.

The process develops at variable speed within these three periods and may be associated with rapid growth. One may see development from an immature epithelium containing between eight and 10 cells to a mature epithelium that is some three to five times thicker. This process can be halted at any stage between the immature and the mature, and so in any given cervix there may be a combination of these varying degrees of maturity. There seem to be three distinct colposcopic representations to the metaplastic process within the transformation zone, and these corre-

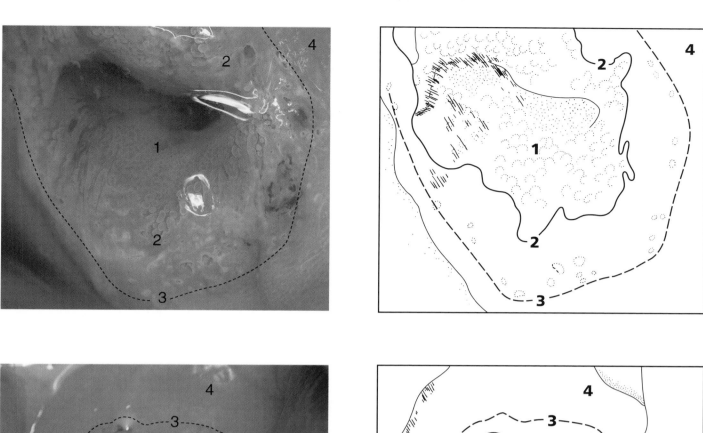

Fig. 4.11

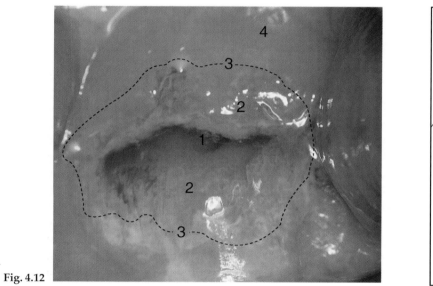

Fig. 4.12

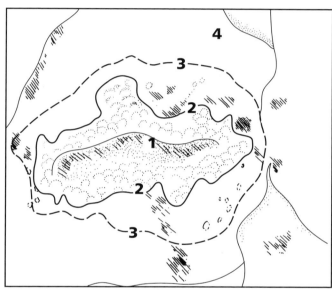

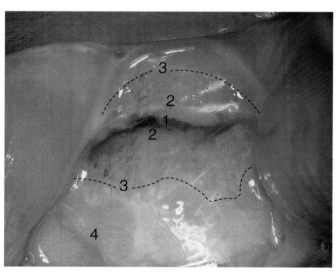

Fig. 4.13

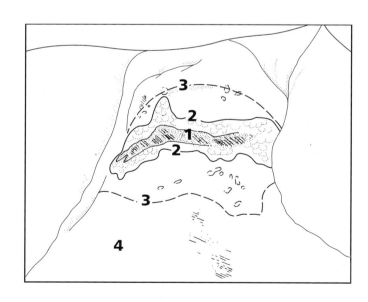

spond to the stages of development described on p. 48. They are as follows.

1 An early or immature stage found commonly in adolescents; the villi become opaque at their tips and successively fuse to produce patches of fingerlike processes that, in turn, fuse as the process spreads (Fig. 4.10a). The pallor of this immature epithelium contrasts with the redness of the previous columnar epithelium. Representations of this early stage can be seen in Figs 4.14 and 4.15a.

2 An intermediate or well-developed stage in which the epithelium is thicker and has lost its pallor with maturity. The more mature areas of metaplastic epithelium can be found more caudally in relation to the original squamocolumnar junction, where the vaginal acidity is more intense (Figs 4.10a & 4.15–4.17).

3 The mature or fully developed metaplastic epithelium, whose maturity sometimes makes it difficult to distinguish between the metaplastic and original squamous epithelia. Associated with this mature stage are gland openings or Nabothian follicles. These two features arise from alterations to the preexisting clefts of the cervix; the former are associated with patency and the latter with occlusion of the clefts (Figs 4.18–4.20).

The overall appearance of the transformation zone is a mixture of all these metaplastic types. Recognition of them is important as some of their changes may well be difficult to differentiate from the atypical or abnormal epithelium associated with cervical precancer.

As a female ages, the transformation zone, which has undergone change during adolescence and pregnancy, adopts a more mature appearance in that the line of separation of the metaplastic epithelium from the original squamous epithelium is hard to see because both tissues develop a similar color pattern. The only way to differentiate between mature metaplastic epithelium and original squamous epithelium is in the situation of the gland openings. During the replacement of the columnar epithelium

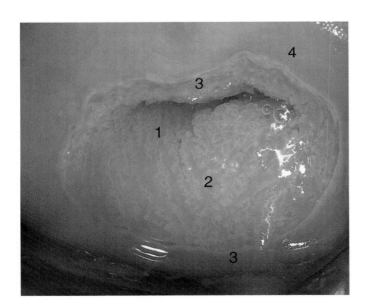

Fig. 4.14 An early stage in the transformation process is seen in this cervix of an adolescent (16 years). The characteristic villous pattern of the original columnar epithelium (1) has been replaced by several smooth areas of immature metaplastic squamous epithelium at (2). The original squamocolumnar epithelium is at (3) and the original squamous epithelium is at (4).

by squamous epithelium, mostly on the exposed ectocervical surface, the recesses of the glands or crypts remain intact with their mouths open. Usually the metaplastic squamous epithelium extends to the edges of these crypts or gland openings (Fig. 4.10b). Very occasionally, it penetrates into the gland openings, which are usually circular. These gland openings therefore signify the lateral margins of the transformation zone (Burghardt, 1991).

Figures 4.18, 4.19a, and 4.20 clearly show the similarity in pink tone between the mature metaplastic and the original columnar epithelia in three females in the fourth decade of life. The gland openings can clearly be seen.

Histologically, it may be extremely difficult to tell where the division exists between the mature metaplastic epithelium and the original columnar epithelium. Sometimes there is an obvious histologic division between the two, as seen in Fig. 4.19b and c. Occasionally in mature metaplastic epithelium overlays a nabothian cyst, within the transformation zone and close to this junction (see Fig. 4.19d and position (5) in Fig. 4.15d). Occasionally, acanthotic epithelium is seen medial to this junction.

4.6 Colposcopy of the adolescent cervix

Adolescence, the period of life extending from puberty to full physical maturation, has an important effect on the cervical epithelium. During that time, regular menstruation, coitus, and pregnancy may occur and with the latter two come the first opportunities for environmental factors to influence the morphology and possibly induce neoplastic change. Indeed, the age at first intercourse and the number of sexual partners are independent risk factors for cervical neoplasia.

Epidemiologic evidence (Brinton *et al.*, 1987; Reeves *et al.*, 1989) suggests that the risk of neoplasia is related to the age at first intercourse and multiple sexual partners indicating that intercourse at an early age may increase sensitivity to the effects of a sexually transmitted agent, most likely human papilloma virus (HPV). This contention is supported by other evidence (Peters *et al.*, 1986) that the interval between the menarche and first intercourse appears to be more important than the age at first intercourse or the age at first regular intercourse, thus linking the risk of neoplasia to "sexual" age rather than chronologic age. The profound effect of HPV, a virus which is the major etiologic agents in cervical neoplasia, has been discussed in Chapter 2 and its effect on the cervical epithelium will be demonstrated.

During the 2 to 3 years preceding puberty there is an alteration in the ratio of the dimensions of the body and cervix of the uterus. Prior to this period, the cervix constitutes the bulk of the organ, but by puberty the body increases to such a size that both parts are of equal size. It is probable that the original cervical epithelia undergo simultaneous changes during this increasingly active peripubertal period, but the exact nature of these morphologic alterations is controversial (Singer, 1976a).

The adolescent cervix is easily accessible to colposcopic monitoring, and therefore the epithelial alterations induced by the physical factors of puberty and pregnancy and by behavioral events (i.e. coitus) can be studied. Examination

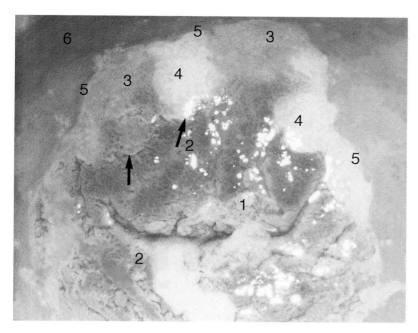

Fig. 4.15(a)

Fig. 4.15 (a) In this transformation zone of the early metaplastic process in the cervix of a 16-year-old female, various stages of development can be seen. The original columnar epithelium is at (2) with some opaqueness already developing in the columnar villi at (1). However, at (3) immature metaplastic epithelium has already developed with a typical pallor. It can be easily differentiated from the redness of the original columnar epithelium (2). A line (arrowed) has developed between the metaplastic process and the columnar epithelium and this represents the new squamocolumnar junction. This signifies the upper extent of the metaplastic process. At (4), there exists a faint micropapillary surface contour that is indicative of the effect of human papillomavirus (HPV). This transformation zone with its abnormal (atypical) epithelium [at (4)] would be labeled an atypical transformation zone. The original squamocolumnar junction can be clearly seen at (5).

(b) Shows the early stages of the metaplastic process. Original columnar epithelium has been replaced on the anterior lip by an increasing opaqueness at the tips and successive fusion of the original columnar epithelium. These features are at (1) and (2) respectively. At (3), a finger-like projection in relation to the original squamo-columnar junction indicates the presence of an intermediate or well-developed stage of the metaplastic process with the epithelium being thicker and having lost its pallor with maturity. The original squamo-columnar junction is dotted.

The evolution of the metaplastic process is clearly seen in (c) with the columnar epithelium in several areas being modified. Villi are becoming opaque, confluent and undergoing fusion indicating the latter phases of metaplasia. Mature metaplastic epithelium seem to form a finger-like process at (2) and a border between it and the recently fused immature metaplastic squamous epithelium is arrowed. This more mature epithelium is thicker and has lost its pallor.

In (d), which is of the posterior lip, similar features to the anterior lip can be seen but a rim of true metaplastic epithelium is present at (4) with the original squamo-columnar junction peripheral and marked by a dotted line. Regular shaped vessels are present at (5) in relation to a small retention cyst (Nabothian follicle).

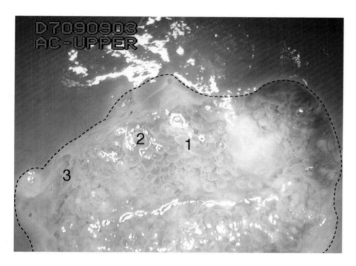

Fig. 4.15(b)

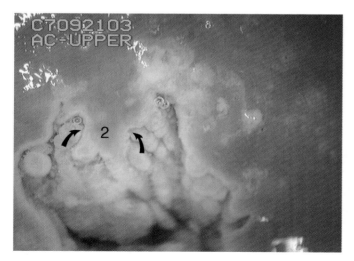

Fig. 4.15(c)

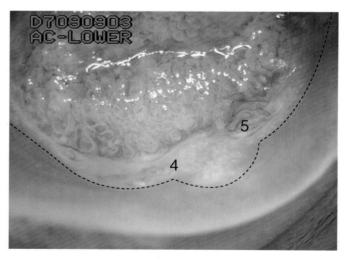

Fig. 4.15(d)

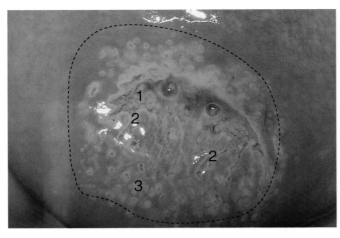

Fig. 4.16 This cervix of a 16-year-old adolescent shows how quickly the conversion from immature to mature squamous epithelium can occur. There are a few villous structures representing the original columnar epithelium at (1); the new squamocolumnar junction, representing the cephalic limit of the metaplastic process, is present at (2); and in the area associated with (3) there is already the smooth surface of a mature metaplastic epithelium that is interrupted here and there by glandular structures. This picture represents progression to an intermediate stage, or possibly even a mature end-stage, of the process. The original squamocolumnar junction is represented by the broken line.

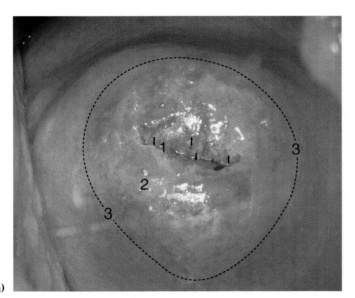

Fig. 4.17(a)

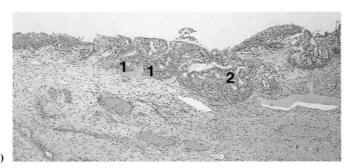

Fig. 4.17(b)

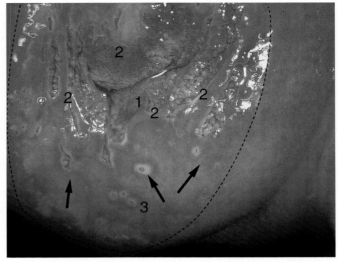

Fig. 4.18(a)

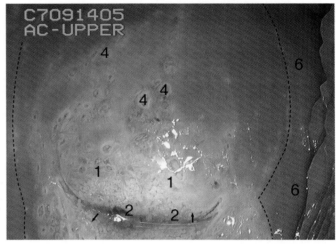

Fig. 4.18(b)

Fig. 4.18 (a) Colpophotograph of a mature transformation zone in a 38-year-old female. The native columnar epithelium is at (1) within the endocervix and the new squamocolumnar junction can easily be seen at (2). Mature metaplastic squamous epithelium is present at (3). Within this area are small gland openings (arrowed). The dotted line marks the original squamocolumnar junction, and the native squamous epithelium is lateral to this line.

(b) A photograph of immature transformation zone showing the characteristic pallor of the immature epithelium that contrasts with the redness of a previous columnar epithelium. This epithelium is seen at (1). Areas of columnar epithelium in the early stages of metaplasia are seen within the endocervical canal at (2) abutting the new squamo-columnar junction arrowed. Numerous gland openings are seen at (4) and the original squamo-columnar junction with the presence of the 'last gland' seen as a dotted line. The original squamous epithelium is at (6).

Fig. 4.17 (*Left*) (a) This cervix of a 23-year-old female shows intermediate and mature stages of the metaplastic process with remnants of the original columnar epithelium present at (1). The new squamocolumnar junction is just visible within the endocervical canal (and arrowed), but the vast majority of the transformation zone is taken up by a smooth metaplastic squamous epithelium (2), which, in parts, is indistinguishable from the original squamous epithelium. The original squamocolumnar junction is at (3) (dashed line).

This photomicrograph (b) corresponds to biopsies taken from the area between positions (1) and (2) in (a). The metaplastic epithelium is incomplete (1) and is seen underlying degenerate columnar endocervical cells. The glandular architecture is still clearly visible (2).

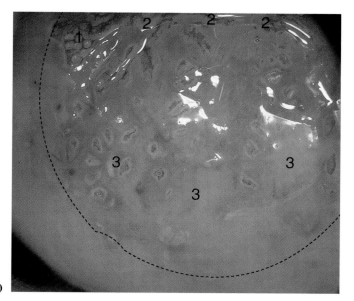

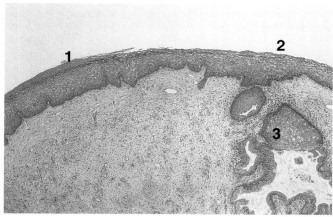

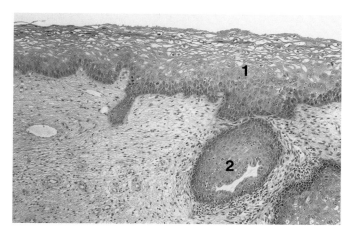

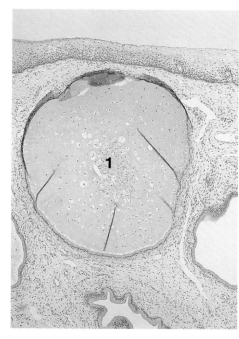

Fig. 4.19 (a) Colpophotograph of the mature transformation zone in a 39-year-old female. There is some original columnar epithelium at (1) within the endocervix, but the new squamocolumnar junction is seen at (2) extending toward the endocervix. At (3) there is mature metaplastic squamous epithelium with numerous gland openings. Close inspection will reveal the presence of columnar epithelium, surrounded by metaplastic squamous epithelium. The dotted line signifies the original squamocolumnar junction. It is difficult to distinguish between the original squamous epithelium, which is lateral and outside this line, and the metaplastic epithelium, within the line. Maturation has occurred with aging and differentiation between the two is difficult; only the presence of gland openings indicates where the squamous metaplastic process has taken place. (b) Histologic section showing the border between original squamous epithelium (1) and squamous metaplasia (on the right) at (2). The metaplastic epithelium is of a mature type and involves superficial gland crypts with metaplasia (3) occurring within them. (c) A high-power view of the mature metaplastic epithelium (1), showing crypt involvement (2). (d) Histologic section revealing occasional crypt occlusion by immature metaplastic squamous epithelium and formation of Nabothian cyst (1). The cyst contents are the product of continued mucous cell secretions.

of virginal and sexually active adolescents allows the role played by coitus to be appreciated.

The frequency of epithelial type

The menarche and the onset of sexual behavior influence the type of epithelium found within the adolescent cervix. These two events seem to promote the formation of metaplastic squamous epithelium. A number of studies have monitored this development and one such study is presented here (Singer, 1975). The cervixes of sexually active adolescents were compared with those of virgins (Table 4.1). The presence of early (immature) squamous metaplasia was found to account for just over half of the epithelial composition of the adolescent transformation zone. Within the virginal cervix metaplasia was present, indicating that coitus was not the only stimulus to metaplasia. The presence of abnormal (atypical) epithelium was assessed colposcopically.

There are four distinct patterns of epithelial distribution within the adolescent cervix. In the first, the ectocervix medial to the squamocolumnar junction is completely covered by original columnar epithelium, but completely retracts into the endocervix when a speculum, used to view the cervix, is removed. This is a very uncommon finding.

The second pattern, also very uncommon, involves the ectocervix being totally, or nearly totally, covered by

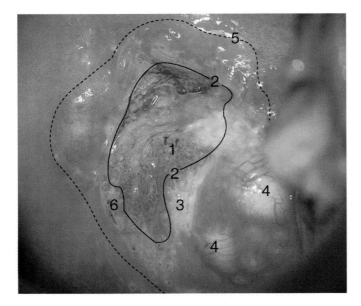 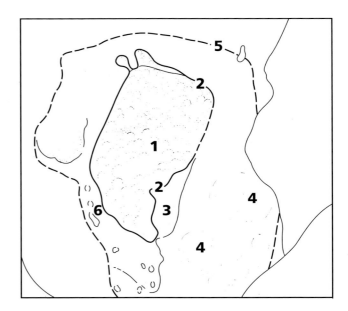

Fig. 4.20 Colpophotograph showing a mature transformation zone with many epithelial types. The original squamocolumnar junction is marked by the dotted line and (5). The original columnar epithelium at (1) extends within the endocervix, and some metaplastic squamous epithelium appears as a small gray patch at (3). The new squamocolumnar junction is present as a firm line at position (2). The area between (2) and (5) represents the transformation zone. Various changes during adolescence and pregnancy have shaped the ultimate composition of this zone to give this appearance in midadult life. There are two other noteworthy structures within the transformation zone. First, the Nabothian follicles at (4) have developed as a result of obstruction to the glandular clefts or crypt openings (see Figs 4.18 & 4.19a). They have developed into retention cysts. Two large cysts can be seen at positions (4), but smaller ones also appear lateral to these. Second, gland openings are present in position (6). These are minor compared with those shown in Figs 4.18 and 4.19a, but they signify the lateral margins of the transformation zone. In this figure they abut the edge of the original squamocolumnar junction (dotted line).

Table 4.1 Epithelial composition of the adolescent transformation zone as assessed by colposcopy.

		Total area (mm²)	Native columnar	Early squamous metaplasia*	Mature squamous metaplasia†	Atypical epithelium
Virgins (n = 40)	Mean	170	90	51	27	2
	Range	(112–240)	(45–137)	(32–73)	(10–52)	(0–3)
	Per cent	–	53	30	16	1
Sexually promiscuous adolescents (n = 170)	Mean	117	14	65	25	13
	Range	(72–132)	(8–26)	(33–84)	(12–32)	(9–27)
	Per cent	–	12	56	21	11

Differences in the amounts of native columnar epithelium and of early metaplastic epithelium between the two groups was significant ($P < 0.01$). From Singer (1975) with kind permission of the editor of *Br J Obstet Gynaecol*.
* Early squamous metaplasia was diagnosed colposcopically when there was an increase in pallor, fusion of the native columnar villi, and smooth opaque surfaces were seen either as tongues or islands of tissue.
† Mature metaplasia was diagnosed colposcopically when there was epithelium with a characteristic reddish hue, associated gland openings, and cytic inclusions (Nabothian follicles).

original squamous epithelium; the squamocolumnar junction is wholly, or nearly completely, situated within the endocervix. The third and very common pattern is that of a typical or normal transformation zone in which an area comprising both original columnar epithelium and metaplastic squamous epithelium exists (Figs 4.21–4.23). In the fourth and final pattern, the two epithelial types are associated with colposcopically atypical epithelium within what is defined as an atypical transformation zone.

4.7 Cervical epithelium during pregnancy and puerperium

Pregnancy and delivery have a profound effect on the cervical epithelium and the subepithelial tissues. Changes that occur in pregnancy prepare the cervix for the enormous physiologic task that it must perform during labor, when its diameter alone increases 10-fold. There are few organs in the body that exhibit the ability to undergo such dramatic

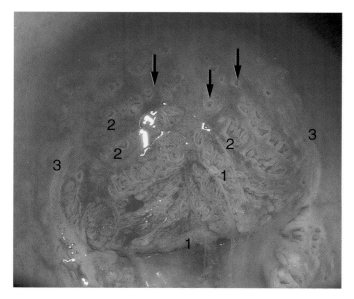

Fig. 4.21 Cervix of a 14-year-old adolescent showing the presence of a normal (typical) transformation zone with areas of original columnar epithelium and patches of newly developed immature metaplastic squamous epithelium. The original columnar epithelium is at (1) within the endocervix, and areas of recently formed metaplastic epithelium are at (2) within the transformation zone. The original squamocolumnar junction is within the area of position (3). Numerous gland openings can be seen in the outer half of the transformation zone (arrowed).

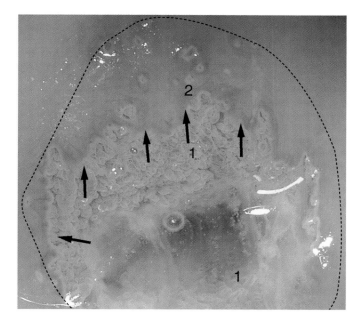

Fig. 4.23 The cervix of a 16-year-old adolescent. Original columnar epithelium is at (1) within the endocervix and the new squamocolumnar junction is arrowed. Metaplastic squamous epithelium has developed within the original columnar epithelium and this can be seen at (2). Some gland openings can also be seen within this tissue. The original squamocolumnar junction is indicated by a dotted line.

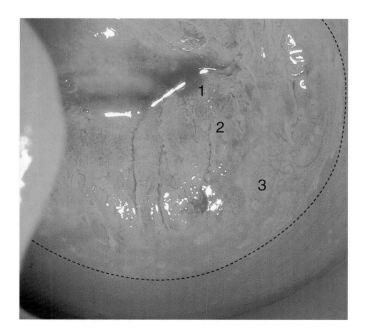

Fig. 4.22 The cervix of a sexually active 15-year-old adolescent. The original columnar epithelium is at (1). Early squamous (immature) metaplasia is seen developing at (2), with fusion of some of the columnar villi. Their original form can still be made out underneath the new metaplastic squamous epithelium. A more advanced stage of squamous metaplasia is seen at (3); again, the form of the original columnar epithelium is just visible as a type of mosaic structure at point (3). The original squamocolumnar junction is marked by a dotted line and there is a sharp differentiation between the two forms of metaplasia, i.e. metaplastic squamous epithelium and original squamous epithelium (outside the original squamocolumnar junction).

changes in so short a time. Furthermore, the relative infrequency of long-term damage emphasizes the physiologic resilience of this organ.

The epithelium bears the brunt of the increasing hormonal and metabolic changes that occur in the cervicovaginal region as pregnancy progresses. It is therefore not surprising that dynamic alterations occur in its structure, and these alterations can be easily monitored by use of the colposcope. Subepithelial tissues, comprising smooth muscle, fibrillar and cellular components, ground substance and collagen fibers in a gelatinous matrix, also undergo intense change. These changes are no less dramatic than those occurring in the epithelium, but cannot be so efficiently monitored.

Ultrastructure and biomechanic properties of subepithelial tissues

The subepithelial tissues, composed predominantly of elastic tissue with a small amount of smooth muscle, have recently undergone intense study (Leppert & Yu, 1991). When studied under scanning electron microscopy (SEM), the elastic tissue, composed of collagen and elastin, has been shown to be composed of two distinct structures: fibrils and thin sheets of elastic membranes. The fibrils are arranged into fishnet-like structures, while within the thin elastic membranes there are fenestrations and pits with diameters of some 3–5 μm. In the Leppert & Yu (1991) study, the concentration of the insoluble elastin was found to be approximately 1.4% of the dry, defatted tissues of the cervix, while the total collagen was estimated to be between 64 and 72%. The orientation of the elastic tissues within the cervix has been described in detail by Leppert et al. (1986), who have shown that they are orientated from the external os to the periphery and from there in a band upwards towards the internal os, where they become sparse in that area of the cervix which contains the greatest amount of smooth muscle, just below the internal os.

The tensile strength and firmness of the cervix is derived from the collagen which is the predominant protein of the extracellular matrix. Minamoto et al. (1987) have described four types of collagen within the dense fibrous tissue of the cervix which, at term, is broken down by the enzyme collagenase. It would seem that the cells involved in this degeneration during the process of dilatation are not resident fibroblasts, as previously had been assumed, but rather polymorphonuclear leukocytes that migrate from blood vessels within the cervix (Osmers et al., 1992). Not surprisingly, there is an elevation in serum collagenase levels during the ripening process at term, and in active labour it increases further.

Assessment of the biochemical and muscular contractile ability of the cervix has shown no significant difference in these physical properties (Petersen et al., 1991) between tissues taken from the distal and proximal parts of the cervix or between circular and longitudinally arranged elastic tissues. Petersen et al. (1991) concluded that the passive biomechanical strength of the cervix markedly exceeds the active muscular contractile ability and this is explained by a high collagen concentration and a low content of smooth muscle within the cervical tissues.

Physiologic mechanisms operating in the cervix during pregnancy

Two physiologic mechanisms operate in the cervix and its epithelium during pregnancy. These are:
1 The endocervical epithelium is subjected to two types of process that draw it into closer contact with, and thereby expose it to, the vaginal environment. These involve either an eversion of the endocervical canal epithelium, or a gaping of the external cervical os. In both instances the vaginal environment, or more precisely the pH of the vaginal secretions, gains access to this previously protected epithelium (Figs 4.24–4.30).
2 As a result of these two processes, a stimulus induces within the now exposed epithelium, which is usually the original columnar epithelium, the development of squamous epithelium by metaplastic formation. These stages are illustrated in Fig. 4.30.

The frequency and extent of these changes depend primarily upon parity (Coppleson & Reid, 1966; Singer, 1975). For example, eversion is more common in the primiparous, while gaping predominates in the multiparous cervix. The formation of metaplastic squamous epithelium is more likely to occur during the first pregnancy than during subsequent gestations. The method of delivery also influences these changes. Although in epidemiologic studies the age at first pregnancy has been suggested as a risk factor in the etiology of cervical neoplasia, it would seem that this event is related to the age at first sexual intercourse and the

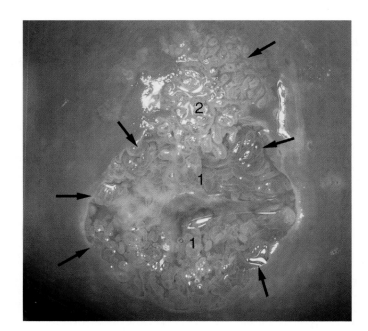

Fig. 4.24

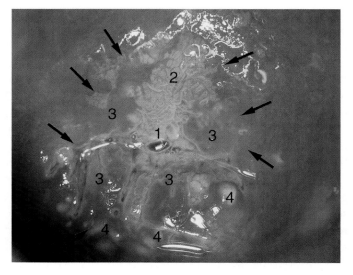

Fig. 4.25

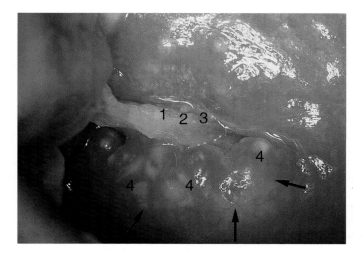

Fig. 4.26

number of sexual partners (Armstrong *et al.*, 1992). However, the profound physiologic events, especially the formation of squamous metaplasia, may influence the development of neoplasia. Indeed, Reid (1992) has shown that there is a phagocytic effect of the subepithelial stromal cell on exogenous DNA (e.g. male gamete, viral DNA) during formation of squamous metaplasia. In the following section, it will be shown that the effects of vaginal delivery also significantly affect the morphology and, in turn, the natural history of the cervical epithelium, especially if this has been affected by a neoplastic process.

4.8 The effect of vaginal delivery on the cervical epithelium

Types of epithelial injury caused by delivery

The passage of the fetus through the dilated cervix produces gross, easily recognizable injury to the epithelial and subepithelial areas (Wilbanks & Richart, 1967). Sequential observations have shown the presence of four specific types of lesion that occur immediately postpartum (Singer, 1975) (Figs 4.31–4.33). They include: (i) ulceration—an area recognized colposcopically and histologically by the absence of the original overlying cervical epithelium (Fig. 4.31); (ii) laceration—an area defined by a linear separation or tear within the epithelium and which extends into the stroma (Fig. 4.32); and (iii) bruising—an area of subepithelial hemorrhage discoloration, which ranges from small petechial hemorrhages to an area of gross contusion (Fig. 4.33). In this condition it is possible to envisage the alteration of the natural history of any neoplastic epithelium affected by these changes. In this example, an area of abnormal (atypical) epithelium [(2) in Fig. 4.33], corresponding to a major-grade neoplastic lesion, was involved by a hematoma; sequential observation 6 months later showed complete removal of most of this lesion. It has recently been shown in a study of smears in the postpartum period (Adhoot, 1998) that high-grade squamous intraepithelial cells had an increased frequency of spontaneous regression women delivered vaginally compared with those delivered by caesarean section (48% regression in 59 women delivered vaginally vs. 0% regression in 12 delivered abdominally). The fourth change is the formation of yellow areas—dis-

tinctly colored tissue regions that are usually associated with the edges of a deep laceration composed histologically of structureless necrotic tissue with an inflammatory cell infiltrate.

Healing of these lesions is very rapid with a covering of immature squamous metaplastic epithelium appearing within 5–7 days. Singer (1975) suggested that the subepithelial stromal cells, migrating into the traumatized areas of the cervix within 72 hours of delivery, were the progenitor cells of the new epithelium. However, recent evidence (Smedts *et al.*, 1993) favors a role for reserve cells as the progenitor cell for the immature metaplastic tissue in the non-pregnant situation; their role in the healing of puerperal cervical injuries has yet to be defined.

4.9 The cervical epithelium during the menopause

Changes in the appearance of the cervix after the menopause follow a less regular pattern than that seen in earlier life. They tend to result from the female's hormonal status. When estrogen levels fall, atrophy will result. This simple picture is complicated because the eventual appearance of the postmenopausal cervix depends upon the results of numerous changes, such as pregnancy and infections, that have been sustained by the cervix.

The transformation zone tends to retract within the endocervix in up to 40% of women over the age of 50. There is considerable variation in the degree to which this inversion occurs (Crompton, 1976). As seen in Fig. 4.34, the transformation zone, marked as the area between point (A) and the squamocolumnar junction (SCJ), retracts into the canal after the menopause.

The squamous epithelium, be it original or metaplastic, becomes atrophic after the menopause; it becomes thinner, and stratification, which is a feature in younger women, disappears (Figs 4.35–4.36). The degree of atrophy at this time varies. Some females show very little tendency for atrophic change, or indeed for retraction.

The degree of glycogenation may be demonstrated by applying Schiller's iodine solution. Prior to the menopause, the normal mature squamous epithelium is well glycogenized and stains mahogany brown. When atrophy occurs, glycogenation is lost and the epithelium stains light yellow. This loss of glycogenation is not uniform, and it is estimated that in approximately 20% of females the squamous epithelium remains well glycogenated for several years after the menopause.

When the vascular epithelium becomes atrophic, the underlying capillary network becomes more easily visible colposcopically (Fig. 4.37). The thinness of the epithelium means that the delicate subepithelial capillaries are much more readily traumatized; petechial hemorrhages are often seen, particularly after a smear has been taken. The arterioles in the cervical connective tissue of the postmenopausal cervix extend toward the surface epithelium after dividing into many large capillaries, giving a candelabra effect. These vessels still maintain a normal branching system, and are distinct from the atypical vessels within cervical

Figs 4.24–4.26 (*Opposite*) Colpophotographs of a primigravid cervix at (Fig. 4.24) 12 and (Figs 4.25 & 4.26) 36 weeks of gestation, taken as (Figs 4.24 and 4.25) "apparent" and (Fig. 4.26) "real" views. The latter imitates the *in vivo* position of the cervical epithelium and from this the extent of the eversion process can be gauged. In the real views the original squamocolumnar junction (arrowed in Fig. 4.26) has extended outward into an ectocervical position as pregnancy progresses; this has resulted in the metaplastic squamous transformation (2) and (3) of the exposed columnar epithelium (1), which in the nonpregnant state resides within the endocervix (1). Nabothian follicles (4) have developed within the area occupied by the new metaplastic squamous epithelium.

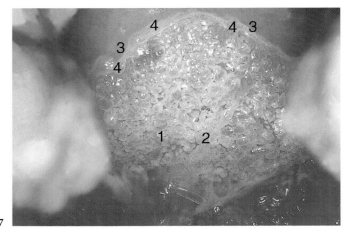

Fig. 4.27

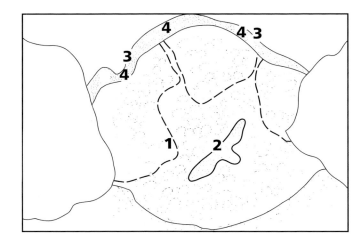

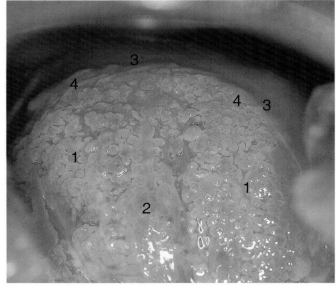

Fig. 4.28

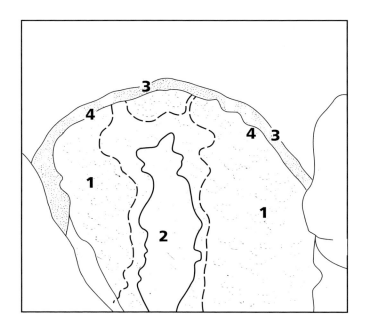

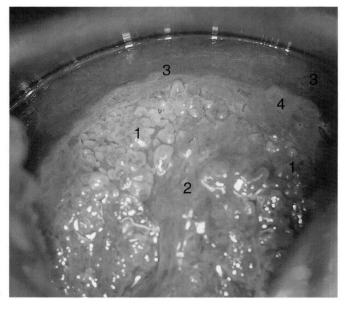

Fig. 4.29

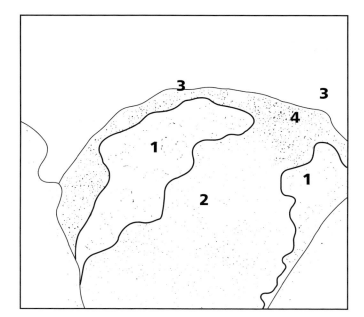

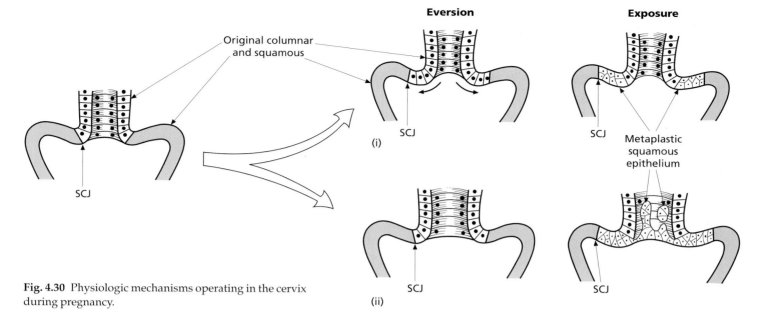

Fig. 4.30 Physiologic mechanisms operating in the cervix during pregnancy.

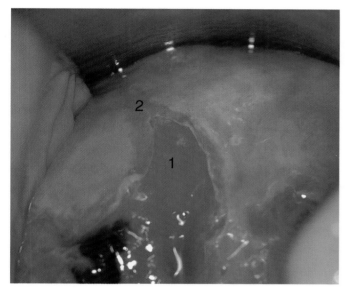

Fig. 4.31 Anterior cervical lip in a primigravida 36 hours after a normal delivery. The epithelium is missing over a large area (1), and healing by metaplastic squamous epithelium, confirmed on biopsy, has already occurred over the upper part of the lesion (2). This lesion is classed as an ulceration.

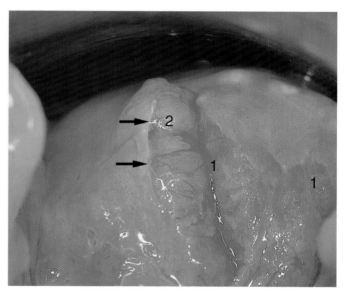

Fig. 4.32 Anterior lip of the cervix in a primigravida 24 hours after a normal delivery. Large lacerations (1), extending into the cervical stroma, radiate from the cervical canal. In one of the lacerations, a small Nabothian follicle (2) is visible. Epithelium that has been abraded from the covering of these Nabothian follicles is arrowed.

Figs 4.27–4.29 (*Opposite*) Colpophotographs of a primigravid cervix at (Fig. 4.27) 12, (Fig. 4.28) 26, and (Fig. 4.29) 36 weeks of pregnancy. At *12 weeks*, the cervix is mainly composed of original columnar epithelium (1), with a small island of metaplastic squamous epithelium (2). By *26 weeks*, this island (2) has enlarged principally by fusion of the adjacent columnar villi. Metaplasia is still developing within the original columnar epithelium at (1), and is in the second stage of the metaplastic process where there is already fusion between the columnar villi. At *36 weeks*, the new metaplastic epithelium (2) has extended to the squamocolumnar junction (3). Some columnar villi have not undergone complete metaplastic transformation and are seen in an arrested stage at (1). An area of metaplastic squamous epithelium has developed adjacent to the squamocolumnar junction, giving rise to the theory that this epithelium grows inward and covers the original columnar epithelium. This rim of tissue (4) is already visible by 12 and 26 weeks. The sequence shown here clearly demonstrates the island formation of the new metaplastic epithelium that extends outward toward the original squamocolumnar junction. The tissue types have the same labels in all three photographs.

neoplasia (Figs 4.37a & b). The problems associated with cytologic screening in the postmenopausal era will be discussed in Chapter 5.

4.10 The oral contraceptives and their effect on the cervix

The oral contraceptives have an effect on the cervix and usually cause the formation of columnar epithelium on the ectocervix. This condition has been called ectopy or ectropion (Figs 4.38–4.41). The squamocolumnar junction is situated outside the external os on the ectocervix (Jordan & Singer, 1976; Baader, 1981; Burghardt, 1991). Occasionally, the columnar epithelium extends to the vaginal fornix. This has to be differentiated from the condition of vaginal adenosis, in which columnar epithelium appears isolated

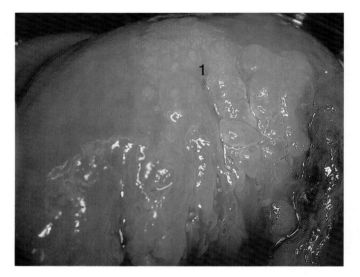

Fig. 4.33 Colpophotograph of an atypical transformation zone (2), 48 hours after delivery. A hematoma occupies this lateral area. Biopsy of the atypical epithelium (1) prior to pregnancy revealed histologic evidence of a cervical intraepithelial neoplasia (CIN) 3.

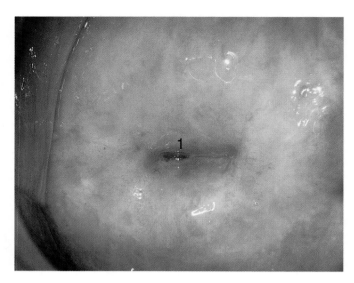

Fig. 4.35 The cervix of a 58-year-old woman, 10 years postmenopausal. The transformation zone has completely retracted within the endocervical canal (1). The ectocervix is covered with atrophic epithelium.

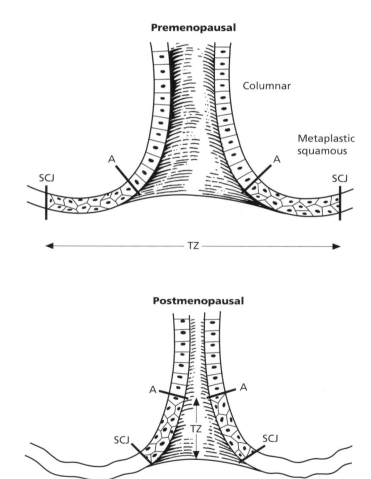

Premenopausal

Columnar

Metaplastic squamous

A   A

SCJ   SCJ

TZ

Postmenopausal

A   A

TZ

SCJ   SCJ

Fig. 4.34

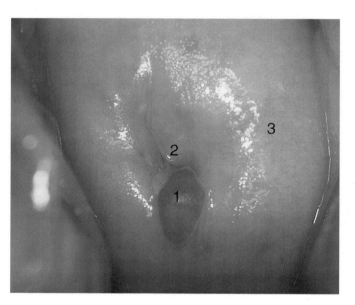

Fig. 4.36 This colpophotograph of the transformation zone 8 years after the menopause shows the transformation zone to have completely retracted within the endocerical canal (2). A small benign polyp has appeared at (1). A very fine capillary pattern is present at (3) on the ectocervix. This is not an unusual finding in the postmenopausal cervix, where distinctly separated, fine caliber, capillary loops radiate toward the external os. Most of these loops appear to be inclined obliquely toward the surface.

in the fornices as well as in the midst of the vaginal epithelium. In ectopy, the surface columnar epithelium and the whole mucosa, including glands and supporting stroma, is displaced outward, as occurs in pregnancy and menarche. It is not always possible to see the original squamocolum-nar junction on the surface. However, its true position is permanently marked by the position of the last gland, which can be diagnosed on a histologic section. It is obvious that these changes, which impart an exophytic appearance to the cervix, can be confused with the early changes of clinical carcinoma of the cervix. It is only by the use of colposcopy that differentiation can be made between a perfectly benign effect, resulting from the oral contraceptive steroids, and malignant changes. Histologically, the

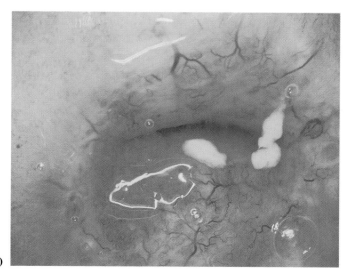

Fig. 4.37(a)

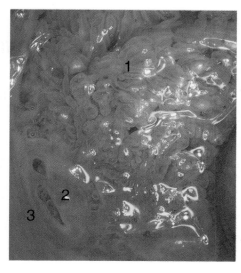

Fig. 4.38 Typical colposcopic findings of oral contraceptive usage; the columnar villi are enlarged and have adopted a small capillary loop pattern at (1). Squamous metaplastic epithelium appears at (2) and the squamocolumnar junction is at (3). Biopsy of the area around (1) showed the pattern characteristic of microglandular hyperplasia.

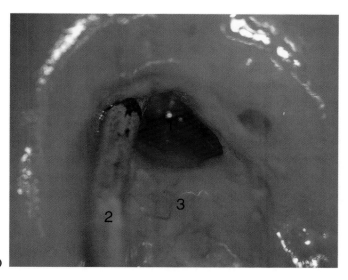

Fig. 4.37(b)

Fig. 4.37 (a) A postmenopausal cervix with normal branching capillaries. The candelabra appearance of these capillaries results from the atrophic nature of the epithelium; it shows a larger terminal vessel with irregular branching patterns. The branches decrease in diameter to terminate in a fine meshlike capillary network. There is no suggestion of any abnormal vascularity.

(b) In this colpophotograph, the transfromation zone extends into the endocervical canal (1). A probe is shown opening up the canal (2), and the mature squamous metaplastic epithelium with normal branching vessels is seen at (3). The new squamocolumnar junction, indicating the upper extent of the transformation zone, is high in the cervical canal and cannot be seen.

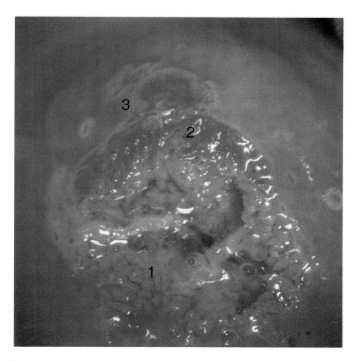

Fig. 4.39 Colpophotograph of the cervix of a young woman who is taking oral contraceptive steroids. There is some swelling of the columnar villi at (1) within the endocervix, and further clumping at (2). Small, irregular polypoid structures are present. Some immature metaplastic epithelium is already developing at (3), and there is a gland opening in that area. This pattern of the columnar epithelium may also be called an ectopy or ectropion.

condition of microglandular endocervical hyperplasia (MEH) is a classic accompaniment to this condition (Figs 4.42 & 4.43). It is a combination of cellular changes within the endocervix and results from progestogenic influences on the epithelium (Taylor *et al.*, 1967; Govan *et al.*, 1969; Wilkinson & Dufour, 1976). The condition can also be seen in women who are pregnant, or who have cervical polyps (Lowe & Slavin, 1987).

Cervical smears taken from women on the pill also vary considerably; they range from smears that have an almost atrophic pattern, with predominantly parabasal cells, to those where there is a well-estrogenized pattern, with predominantly superficial squamous cells (Anderson *et al.*, 1992b). Females on high-dose progestogen pills have a very thickened cervical mucus, and usually present with unsatisfactory smears, owing to an excessive degree of clumping and folding of the cells and the presence of large numbers

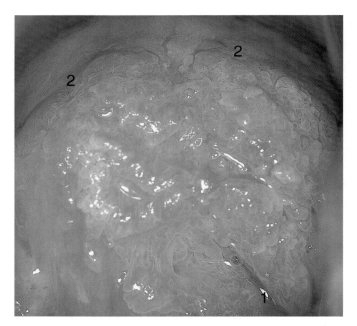

Fig. 4.40 The development of ectopy or ectropion, with the columnar epithelium situated on the ectocervix in young women taking oral contraceptive steroids. The endocervical canal is at (1) and the original squamocolumnar junction at (2). In between, there are columnar villi that are clumped and present as irregular but small polypoid structures. These look quite abnormal to the naked eye and imitate the appearance of malignancy. Colposcopy allows the benign nature of this lesion to be confirmed.

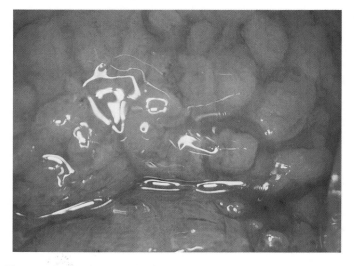

Fig. 4.41 Colpophotograph of the cervix of a female who has been taking an oral contraceptive for 15 years. The individual columnar villi are grossly enlarged and fused, giving a polypoid appearance. There is an apparent eversion of these columnar villi, which protrude from the endocervical canal; this results in an ectropion or ectopy.

of Doderlein bacilli. In such cases the use of colposcopy becomes important.

4.11 The congenital transformation zone

In many young women there exist areas of epithelium that are usually situated on the caudal side of a more recently formed transformation zone that stain intensely white with acetic acid, and have a fine, regular mosaic or punctated

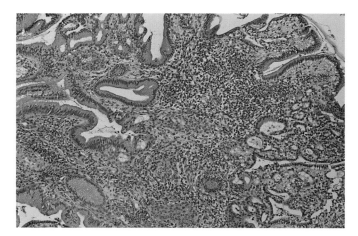

Fig. 4.42

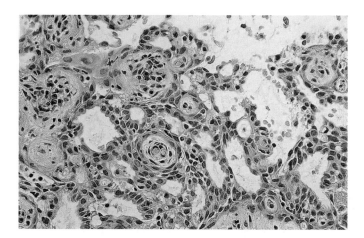

Fig. 4.43

Figs 4.42 and 4.43 The histology of a biopsy taken from the cervix of a woman with a history of long-term oral contraceptive usage; microglandular endocervical hyperplasia (MEH) is evident. Figure 4.42 shows a low-power view and Fig. 4.43 a part of this view at higher magnification. Multiple, and apparently complex, superficial cervical crypts are present, and numerous small glandular spaces are lined by regular cuboidal cells. The nuclei are uniform and vesicular, with occasional nucleoli. Mitotic figures are not present here, but can sometimes be found. Vacuoles also appear in an extracellular position. The stromal cells are present between the glandular elements and these have the appearance of reserve cells. Two important features of MEH are the presence of irregular nuclei and the virtual absence of mitotic figures. These should be kept in mind when this condition is to be differentiated from invasive carcinoma.

appearance. The epithelium is nonglycogenated and it seems as though this epithelium represents a form of immature squamous metaplasia. Some authors believe that it represents squamous metaplasia occurring in late fetal life (Linhartova, 1970; Pixley, 1976; Coppleson & Reid, 1986b; Borgno et al., 1988) and have therefore called the area within which this epithelium is found, the congenital transformation zone (Anderson, 1991; Anderson et al., 1992a). It has many similarities with the squamous metaplasia found later in life; maturation of the squamous epithelium is incomplete and there may be disorders of maturation that can be in the form of either excessive surface maturation with accompanying keratinization or delayed and incomplete maturation of the deeper layers.

There is also a characteristic histologic pattern (see Fig. 4.48b and c, on p. 67, in which there is thickening of the stromal papillae, with an arborizing network of stromal ridges subdividing the surface epithelium into discrete fields; this produces a type of mosaic or crazy-paving appearance (Burghardt, 1991; Anderson *et al.*, 1992b). Hyperkeratosis and parakeratosis (layers of keratinized cells that retain their nuclei although these become pyknotic) are very often present on the epithelial surface, and the characteristic leukoplakia, which is a colposcopic feature of the zones, occurs as a result of the thickness of these layers (Anderson *et al.*, 1992b).

The areas containing these changes have been found in the virginal cervix and also in some fetal cervixes. They show a number of patterns, which are as follows.

1 A triangular shape that extends onto the anterior and posterior lips of the cervix and vagina, and is caudal to a more recently formed transformation zone (Figs 4.44a & b).

2 Isolated areas in the anterior or posterior vaginal vaults, with a tenuous connection to the squamocolumnar junction. Such areas may show evidence of patchy keratosis (Figs 4.45–4.47).

3 An irregular area that projects transversely from the cervix, extends into the lateral vaginal fornix, and is still contained within the limits of the transformation zone (Fig. 4.48a).

These conditions are benign, but their very bizarre nature can be disconcerting to the inexperienced colposcopist who may interpret them as indicative of cervical precancer. Because they may also contain colposcopic features of abnormal (atypical) epithelium (i.e. acetowhiteness, punctation and mosaic vascular changes), the transformation zone is designated atypical (see Chapter 6). Some examples of the various patterns are displayed in Figs 4.44–4.48a in which a combination of abnormal (atypical) epithelia, indicative of not only the congenital transformation zone but also instances of subclinical papillomavirus infection (SPI) (Figs 4.49–4.53) are seen. It is not uncommon to find the two types of epithelium coexisting in young women (Coppleson & Pixley, 1992). Difficulty can be encountered when abnormal cervical cytology is found in such a situation especially if the grade of abnormality is of a low-grade nature. The epithelial changes, i.e. abnormal (atypical) and SPI, are striking and the inexperienced colposcopist is

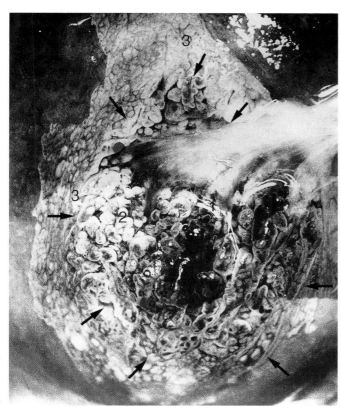

Fig. 4.44(a)

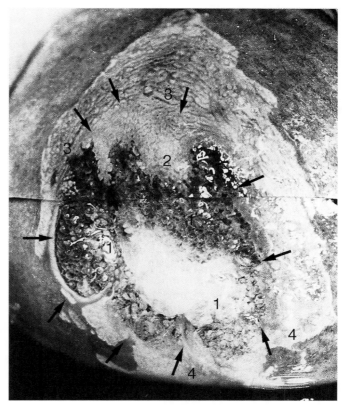

Fig. 4.44(b)

Fig. 4.44 The first pattern of the congenital transformation zone shows regular fine mosaic epithelium that extends anteriorly and posteriorly onto the vaginal fornices. In (a) the endocervical canal is at (1), and early metaplastic epithelium is developing within the original columnar epithelium at (2). The original transformation zone with its concentric boundary, identified as the original squamocolumnar junction, is arrowed. The fine and regular mosaic epithelium of the congenital transformation zone (3) is caudal to this line and extends anteriorly, laterally, and posteriorly onto the vaginal fornices. In (b) original columnar epithelium exists at (1) and the original squamocolumnar junction, marking the lateral boundaries of

the transformation zone, is arrowed. At (2), there is an area of acetowhite smooth epithelium, indicative of immature metaplasia. Caudal to the original squamocolumnar junction are elements of the congenital transformation zone. On the anterior lip at (3) there exists a fine, regular mosaic and punctated area that extends laterally and posteriorly in the form of patchy keratotic tissue. Biopsies from these tissues in areas (3) and (4) show a very acanthotic type of epithelium. This is characterized by markedly elongated stromal papillae with the clasic stromal ridges subdividing the surface epithelium into discrete fields, resulting in the mosaic appearance. Keratinization is seen on the surface, particularly in area (4).

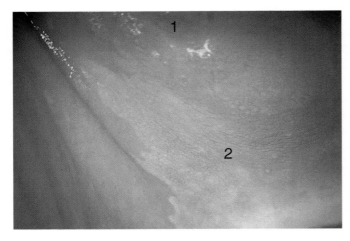

Fig. 4.45 The congenital transformation zone extending into the posterior fornix at (2). The cervical transformation zone, just below the endocervix, is seen at (1).

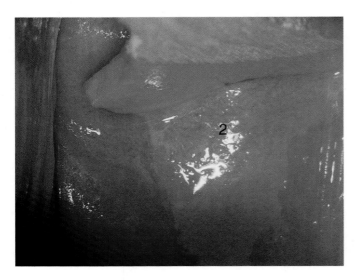

Fig. 4.46 An example of the congenital transformation zone with the triangular area of very fine and regular mosaic epithelium staining white with the application of acetic acid (2); the transformation zone extends into the posterior fornix. The lack of glycogenation will result in this epithelium appearing sharp white with the application of Schiller's iodine solution.

likely to mistake these changes for high-grade disease. In such circumstances, multiple punch biopsies are recommended with due care being taken in the histologic analysis of the tissues.

4.12 Summary: the normal (typical) transformation zone

Before moving on to consider in the next chapter abnormal (atypical) colposcopic changes within the transformation zone, it is worthwhile summarizing the recognizable characteristics of the typical (normal) transformation zone. There are three types of epithelium that are easily recognizable and have characteristic histologic and morphologic appearances. These are:
1 The original squamous and columnar epithelia.
2 The metaplastic squamous epithelium.

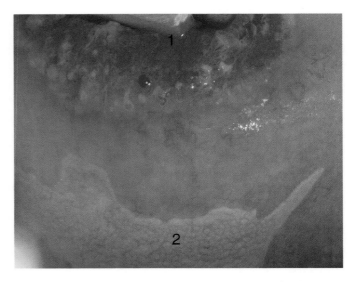

Fig. 4.47 An area of very fine and irregular epithelium (2) that is most likely related to the transformation zone seen at (1). However, the epithelium at (2) is in an area of original squamous epithelium and it may be that this is another form of the congenital transformation zone. It would need to be differentiated from vaginal intraepithelial neoplasia (VAIN) and the only method of diagnosis is by punch biopsy and the resultant pathology.

3 The abnormal (atypical) epithelium or, under the new international classification, abnormal colposcopic findings.

Figure 4.54 shows the topographic pattern of the typical or normal transformation zone. The squamocolumnar junction, which has a fixed position on the cervix, may be placed at any point across the ectocervix or endocervix, and in 4% of cases occurs in the vaginal fornix. The metaplastic squamous epithelium is seen within this squamocolumnar junction line and develops during certain periods of life (such as late fetal life, menarche, and pregnancy) by an alteration within the original columnar epithelium. This results in the formation, by the process of metaplasia, of the second type of epithelium, the so-called metaplastic squamous. The process is a physiologic one that occupies a short period of days or weeks. Metaplasia may occur rapidly or be arrested in one of its various developmental stages, thereby leading to a variable colposcopic appearance.

Within the area of the squamocolumnar junction occur all the dynamic physiologic and pathologic processes that are found in the human cervix. There is also evidence that during the early stages of metaplasia, the epithelium may be vulnerable to a genetic change that results in a cell population that somehow acquires a neoplastic potential. It is also now accepted that HPV produces some minor abnormal changes outside the transformation zone. However, the major part of the neoplastic potential results in the third type of epithelium, which has distinctive morphologic characteristics and is found within the transformation zone with essentially the same topographic distribution as that of the original and metaplastic epithelium. In this state the transformation zone is called the atypical transformation zone. Some other classifications use the terms doubtful or suspicious zone to describe such changes. Figure 4.54 shows the topographic relationship of both the normal and abnormal (atypical) epithelia within their respective zones;

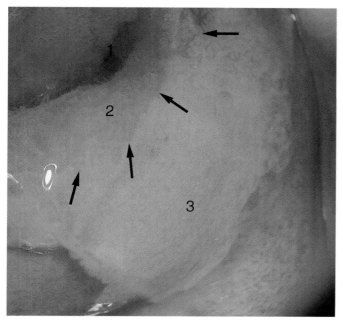

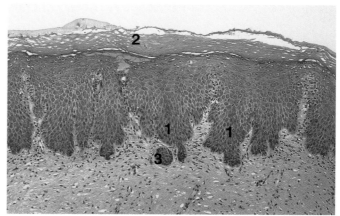

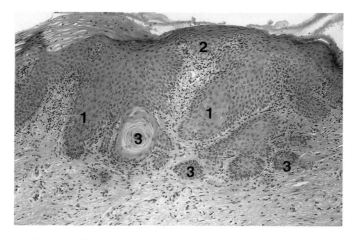

Fig. 4.48(b)

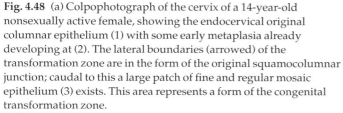

Fig. 4.48(a)

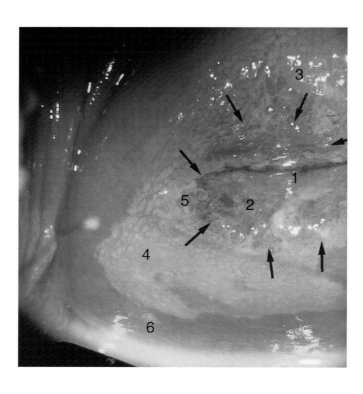

Fig. 4.48(c)

Fig. 4.48 (a) Colpophotograph of the cervix of a 14-year-old nonsexually active female, showing the endocervical original columnar epithelium (1) with some early metaplasia already developing at (2). The lateral boundaries (arrowed) of the transformation zone are in the form of the original squamocolumnar junction; caudal to this a large patch of fine and regular mosaic epithelium (3) exists. This area represents a form of the congenital transformation zone.

(b) A punch biopsy from an area of mosaic epithelium similar to that seen in Fig. 4.45. It shows the typical acanthotic appearance (1) of the congenital transformation zone. The epithelium also shows some mild parakeratosis (2). The stromal papillae are elongated, and

vessels extend between them and toward the surface, giving rise to the fine mosaic pattern seen colposcopically. Buds of squamous epithelium are visible at (3).

(c) This biopsy taken from an area designated a congenital transformation zone shows acanthotic rete pegs (1) with parakeratosis at (2). The epithelium is completely benign. Epithelial buds with pearl formation are present at (3).

Fig. 4.49 Colpophotograph of the cervix of a 14-year-old nonsexually active female, showing original columnar epithelium within the endocervix at (1) and early immature metaplasia developing at (2). The outline of the transformation zone is arrowed at the original squamocolumnar junction. Caudal to this junction—on the anterior lip at (3)—there is a triangular area of very fine mosaic epithelium that is indicative of the congenital transformation zone. Another such area exists on the posterior cervical lip where it extends onto the vaginal fornix in area (4). However, the presence of a small condyloma at (5) and a "satellite" lesion at (6) suggests subclinical papillomavirus infection (SPI). In this cervix there is a mixture of features of both the congenital transformation zone and SPI. Biopsy of the area at (4), shown in Fig. 4.50, reveals the presence not only of acanthotic rete pegs but also the histologic features similar to human papillomavirus infection.

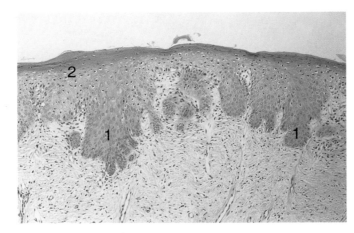

Fig. 4.50 Photomicrograph showing acanthotic rete pegs (1) that are indicative of the congenital transformation zone and associated with extremely thickened epithelium with vacuolated cells that appear like koilocytes (2). These appearances mimic HPV infection closely. This type of morphology appears in a biopsy taken from area (4) in Fig. 4.49.

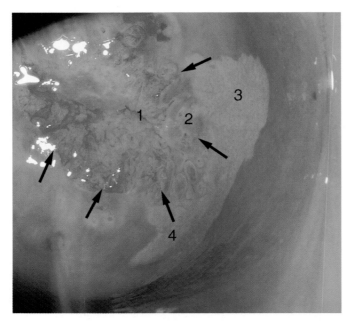

Fig. 4.51 The cervix of a 14-year-old sexually active female. The endocervical columnar epithelium at (1) abuts an area of early immature metaplasia at (2). The outline of the original squamocolumnar junction is arrowed. Caudal to this area is a localized patch of fine regular mosaic epithelium that is indicative of the congenital transformation zone (3). However, its upper border is irregular, and with an associated satellite lesion visible at (4) is highly suggestive of subclinical papillomavirus infection (SPI). Biopsy of this area shows the presence of acanthosis with thickened rete pegs, but there is also evidence of SPI.

Fig. 4.53 (*above right*) Colpophotograph of a sexually active 17-year-old female; original columnar epithelium is present within the endocervix at (1) and there is very active immature squamous epithelium at various sites within the transformation zone (2). At (3), there is an area of very fine and regular mosaic epithelium that represents the congenital transformation zone; this is separated from the physiologic transformation zone by the dashed line. However, on

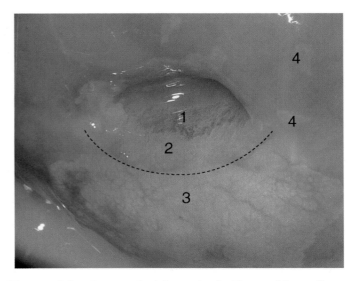

Fig. 4.52 Colpophotograph of the cervix of a 15-year-old sexually active female; this shows another example of the occurrence of both a congenital transformation zone and subclinical papillomavirus infection (SPI). The endocervical original epithelium is at (1), and an area of active immature squamous metaplasia is present at (2). The probable original squamocolumnar junction is indicated by the dotted line. Caudal to this line, and extending into the posterior vaginal fornix, is an area of fine mosaic epithelium (3). Although indicative of the congenital transformation zone, its irregular outline and the presence of some larger areas of mosaic epithelium and of some satellite lesions (4) suggest the presence of an associated area of SPI. Punch biopsies confirm the colposcopic impression.

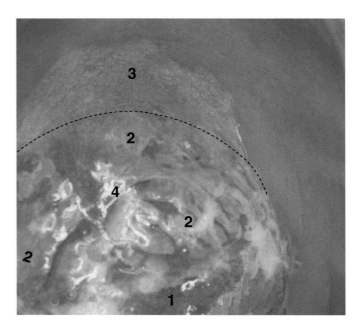

close examination, within the transformation zone there are certain areas visible that appear to possess shiny white epithelium (4), which, although accentuated by the flash reflections, suggest human papillomavirus (HPV) infection. Biopsy of the area at (4) reveals the presence of acanthotic rete pegs with associated thickened epithelium, koilocytosis, and other characteristics of subclinical papillomavirus infection (SPI). This case again demonstrates the difficulty of differentiating between epithelium that is colposcopically suggestive of the congenital transformation zone and epithelium that is infected by HPV. Although these changes represent abnormal (atypical) epithelium, they are of a very minor nature, and final diagnosis can only be determined from biopsy and the resultant pathology.

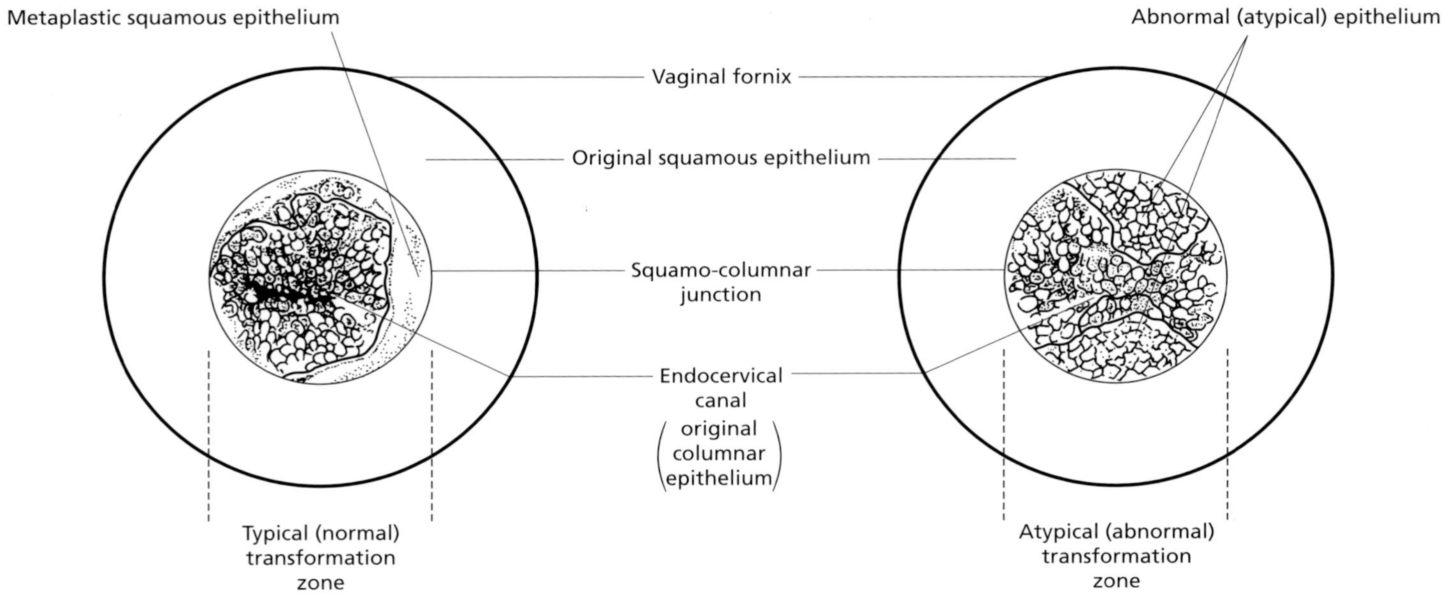

Fig. 4.54

the only difference between the two is that there is a distinctive morphologic pattern to the abnormal (atypical) epithelium compared with that found in the presence of metaplastic squamous epithelium. With this relationship explained, a description of the precancerous lesions of the cervix will become easier to understand.

4.13 References

Adhoot, D., Van Nostrand, K.M., Nguyen, N.J. *et al.* (1998) The effect of delivery on regression of abnormal cervical cytologic findings in the postpartum period. *Am J Obstet Gynecol* **178**(6),1116.

Anderson, M.C. (1991) The cervix, excluding cancer. In: Anderson, M.C. (ed.) *Female Reproductive System*. This is Vol. 6, 3rd edn, in the series *Systemic Pathology*, edited by Symmers, W. St C. Churchill Livingstone, Edinburgh.

Anderson, M.C., Jordan, J., Morse, A. & Sharp, F. (1992a) Congenital transformation zone. In: Anderson, M.C. *et al.* (eds) *Text and Atlas of Integrated Colposcopy*, p. 78. Chapman and Hall Medical, London.

Anderson, M.C., Jordan, J., Morse, A. & Sharp, F. (1992b) Oral contraceptive changes. In: Anderson, M.C. *et al.* (eds) *Text and Atlas of Integrated Colposcopy*, p. 99. Chapman and Hall Medical, London.

Armstrong, B.K., Muñoz, N. & Bosch, F.X. (1992) Epidemiology of cancer of the cervix. In: Coppleson, M. (ed.) *Gynaecological Oncology*, 2nd edn, p. 11. Churchill Livingstone, Edinburgh.

Baader, O. (1981) Hormonell bedingte kolposkopische befund. *Arch Gynäkol* **232**,17.

Borgno, G., Bersani, R., Micheletti, L. & Barbero, M. (1988) Colposcopic findings before sexual activity. *Cervix Lower, Female Gen Tract* **6**,69.

Brinton, L.A., Hamman, R.F., Huggins, G.R. *et al.* (1987) The sexual and reproductive risk factors for invasive squamous cell cervical cancer. *J Natl Cancer Inst* **79**,23.

Burghardt, E. (1991) *Colpscopy, Cervical Pathology, Textbook and Atlas*, 2nd edn. Georg Thieme Verlag, Stuttgart.

Coppleson, M. & Pixley, E.C. (1992) Colposcopy of the cervix. In: Coppleson, M. (ed.) *Gynaecological Oncology* 2nd edn, p. 314. Churchill Livingstone, Edinburgh.

Coppleson, M. & Reid, B. (1966) The colposcopic study of the cervix during pregnancy and the puerperium. *J Obstet Gynaecol Br Commonw* **73**,375.

Coppleson, M. & Reid, B. (1967) *Pre-Clinical Carcinoma of the Cervix Uteri; Its Origin, Nature and Management*. Pergamon, Oxford.

Coppleson, M., & Reid, B. & Pixley, E. (eds) (1986a) Natural history of squamous metaplasia. In: *Colposcopy*, 3rd edn, p. 82. Charles C. Thomas, Springfield.

Coppleson, M., & Reid, B. & Pixley, E. (eds) (1986b) The vaginal transformation zone. In: *Colposcopy*, 3rd edn, p. 408. Charles C. Thomas, Springfield.

Crompton, A.C. (1976) The cervical epithelium during the menopause. In: Jordan, J. & Singer, A. (eds) *The Cervix*, p. 128. W.B. Saunders, Philadelphia.

Fluhmann, C.F. (1961) *The Cervix Uteri and Its Diseases*, p. 30. W.B. Saunders, Philadelphia.

Forsberg, J.G. (1976) Morphogenesis and differentiation of the cervico-vaginal epithelium. In: Jordan, J. & Singer, A. (eds) *The Cervix*, p. 3. W.B. Saunders, Philadelphia.

Govan, A.D., Black, W.P. & Sharp, J.L. (1969) Aberrant glandular polypi of the uterine cervix associated with contraceptive pills, pathology and pathogenesis. *J Clin Pathol* **22**,84.

Jordan, J. & Singer, A. (1976) The effect of oral contraceptive steroids upon epithelium and mucus. In: Jordan, J. & Singer, A. (eds) *The Cervix*, p. 192. W.B. Saunders, Philadelphia.

Kolstad, P. & Stafl, A. (1982) *Atlas of Colposcopy*, 3rd edn, p. 58. Churchill Livingstone, Edinburgh.

Leppert, P.C., Cerreta, J.M. & Mandl, I. (1986) Orientation of elastic fibers in the human cervix. *Am J Obstet Gynecol* **155**(1),219.

Leppert, P.C. & Yu, S.Y. (1991) Three-dimensional structures of uterine elastic fibers; scanning electron microscopic studies. *Connect Tis Res* **27**(1),15.

Linhartova, A. (1970) Congenital ectopy of the uterine cervix. *Int J Obstet Gynaecol* **8**,653.

Lowe, D. & Slavin, G. (1987) Non-neoplastic conditions of the cervix. In: Fox, H. (ed.) *Obstetrical and Gynaecological Pathology*, Vol. 1, 3rd edn, p. 237. Churchill Livingstone, Edinburgh.

Minamoto, T., Arai, K., Hirakawa, S. & Nagai, Y. (1987) Immunohistochemical studies on collagen types in the uterine cervix in pregnant and non-pregnant states. *Am J Obstet Gynecol* **156**(1),138.

Myer, R. (1910) Die Epithelentwicklung der Cervix und Portio Vaginalis Uteri und die Pseudoerosio Congenita. *Arch Gynäkol* **91**,579.

Osmers, W.D., Raff, M.W. & Alderman-Grill, B.C. (1992) Origin of cervical collagenase during parturition. *Am J Obstet Gynecol* **166**(5),1455.

Peters, P.K., Thomas, D., Hagan, D., Mack, T. & Henderson, B. (1986) Risk factors for invasive cervical cancer among Latinas and non-Latinas in Los Angeles county. *J Natl Cancer Inst* **77**,1036.

Petersen, L.K., Oxlund, H., Uldbjerg, N. & Forman, A. (1991) *In vitro* analysis of muscular contractile ability and passive biomechanical properties of uterine cervical samples from non-pregnant women. *Obstet Gynecol* **77**(5),772.

Pixley, E.C. (1976) Basic morphology of the pre-pubertal and youthful cervix, topographic and histologic features. *J Reprod Med* **16**,221.

Reeves, W.C., Brinton, L.A., Garcia, M. *et al.* (1989) Human papillomavirus infection and cervical cancer in Latin America. *N Engl J Med* **320**,1437.

Reid, B. (1992) Carcinogenesis. In: Coppleson, M. (ed.) *Gynaecological Oncology*, 2nd edn, p. 95. Churchill Livingstone, Edinburgh.

Singer, A. (1975) The uterine cervix from adolescence to the menopause. *Br J Obstet Gynaecol* **82**,81.

Singer, A. (1976a) The cervical epithelium during puberty and adolescence. In: Jordan, J. & Singer, A. (eds) *The Cervix*, p. 87. W.B. Saunders, Philadelphia.

Singer, A. (1976b) The cervical epithelium during pregnancy and the puerperium. In: Jordan, J. & Singer, A. (eds) *The Cervix*, p. 105. W.B. Saunders, Philadelphia.

Smedts, F., Ramaekers, F.C.S. & Vooijs, P. (1993) The dynamics of keratin expression in malignant transformation of cervical epithelium; a review. *Obstets Gynecol* **82**(3),465.

Song, A. (1964) *The Human Uterus: Morphogenesis and Embryological Basis for Cancer.* Charles C. Thomas, Springfield.

Taylor, H.B., Irey, N.S. & Norris, H.J. (1967) Atypical endocervical hyperplasia in women taking oral contraceptives. *J Am Med Assoc* **202**,637.

Wilbanks, G.D. & Richart, R.N. (1967) The puerperal cervix, injuries and healing, a colposcopic study. *Am J Obstet Gynecol* **97**,1105.

Wilkinson, E. & Dufour, D.R. (1976) Pathogenesis of microglandular hyperplasia of the cervix uteri. *Obstet Gynecol* **47**,189.

Chapter 5
Cytology and Screening for Cervical Precancer

5.1 Introduction

The history of histopathologic classifications of cervical precursor lesions and similar lesions elsewhere in the genital tract has been described in Chapter 1. High-grade cervical intraepithelial neoplasia (CIN) is considered by pathologists to include probable neoplastic lesions that have a high likelihood of being true precursors of invasive disease. Likewise, colposcopists may be able to separate lesions with certain appearances into those that are at high risk or low risk of progression to malignancy. Cytologists must use the cellular patterns within smears to predict low- or high-grade lesions in a complementary fashion.

The clinician colposcopist ultimately evaluates the data from the interlinked techniques and decides the management.

5.2 Cytological classifications

Papanicolaou

At first glance, the nomenclature for cervical squamous cytology seems to have barely changed since 1943 (Papanicolaou, 1954). "Dyskaryotic" squamous cells (with abnormal nuclear appearances) when present in cervical and/or vaginal vault smears and displaying different degrees of cytoplasmic maturation were proved to predict histologic dysplastic lesions. "Perinuclear cavitation" was described and linked with superficial and intermediate squamous cell dyskaryosis and seen to commonly regress spontaneously (Papanicolaou, 1954). This "cavitation" was later referred to as koilocytosis by Koss *et al.* (1956). These changes were then identified as human papillomavirus (HPV)-associated cytopathic effects (CPEs) by Meisels and Fortin (1976); Purola and Savia (1977).

Superficial and intermediate cell dyskaryosis generally predicted mild or moderate dysplasias or low-grade abnormalities as these were then thought. Without specifically describing the representative nuclear abnormalities, the drawings of Hashime Muruyama and a few scattered descriptive phrases can be brought together to reflect Papanicolaou's early view: that dyskaryosis chiefly affected the nucleus and consisted of nuclear enlargement, irregularity of shape, hyperchromasia and multinucleation (Papanicolaou, 1954). Parabasal dyskaryosis was an indication of carcinoma-in-situ and pleomorphic or bizarre whole cellular forms, e.g. "snake cell" or "tadpole cell" types were typical indicators of malignancy.

For general cytology, Papanicolaou had developed a five-grade system of classifying cells, using Roman numerals I–V, ranging from:

I   Negative.
II   Atypical but not neoplastic cells.
III Suspicious of neoplastic cells.
IV   Strongly suggestive of neoplastic cells.
V   Malignant cells.

This system became widely used in many areas of cytologic detection of tumors. The same system was applied for cervical cytology but was differentially modified by different users in different countries (Koss, 1992).

The recognition of HPV CPEs in 1976 brought on confusion in the histopathologic assessment of lower grades of dysplasia or CIN and should probably have been more smoothly incorporated into the cytologic spectrum of cellular changes.

Such was the histopathologic enthusiasm, however, for the new CIN orthodoxy (Richart, 1968) that many refused to accommodate HPV-associated atypia within the "neoplastic" changes so recently described. This practice engendered the belief, still rife today, that there is an early stage of koilocytotic nuclear atypia that is separable and distinguishable from dyskaryosis, though this was never discernible by Papanicolaou who invented the term.

Koilocytes with, of course, variably abnormal nuclei from mild to severe hyperchromasia, limited or striking nuclear irregularity, multinucleation and almost any degree of maturity from superficial to deep intermediate, can be demonstrated in nearly all CIN lesions with which they are inextricably and causally linked.

Most countries operating a version of the five-grade Papanicolaou system would advocate referral of the patient at grade 3 (mild dyskaryosis). Koilocytotic cells "without dyskaryosis" are variably included in grades 2 or 3 in different countries.

British Society for Clinical Cytology (BSCC) classification

Various attempts have been made to bend the cytologic appearances to a direct correlation with the CIN system. Possibly the most successful terminology is that introduced by a BSCC working party in 1986 (Evans *et al.*, 1986).

Dyskaryotic nuclei without regard for other cellular

features are considered to be separable into mild, moderate and severe categories which then predict CIN 1, 2, or 3. A borderline grade was introduced which was similar to pap grade II and which received "clarification" by a working party of the national health service (NHS) Screening Programme in 1994 (BSCC, 1994). This category largely consists of HPV infection "without dyskaryosis." This fateful decision has ensured that a very considerable portion of high-grade CIN receives long periods of surveillance or is lost to follow-up while masquerading in smears as HPV changes, prior to referral. Waltzer *et al.* (1986) found 29.9% of 41 patients with borderline nuclear changes (BNC) had CIN at punch biopsy. Soutter (1986) found 37% had disease. Stewart (1993) found CIN in 31%. Usnam (1998) found CIN in 34% and 84.6% of this CIN was high grade (CIN 2 and CIN 3). This effect of delaying treatment for high-grade lesions is heightened since it is program policy within the NHS to refer only after a second mildly dyskaryotic smear predicting CIN 1. Giles (1989) studied a group of 200 women with predominantly a single mildly dyskaryotic smear nearly 10 years ago. The author was the cytologist in that study and all HPV changes were considered to be inseparable from mild dyskaryosis predicting CIN 1 in that study. Up to a third of these patients had high grade disease (CIN 2 or 3) on biopsy close to the time of initial cytology.

The BSCC classification is an unevidenced refinement of Papanicolaou's work but it disregards the essential assessment of the maturity of the exfoliated cell. If the gradation of nuclear dyskaryosis was proportional, then it might be thought that successful automated scanning by nuclear densitometry would have quickly followed, but unfortunately this is not so.

The Bethesda System (TBS) (see Table 5.1)

In 1988, the National Cancer Institute (NCI) in the USA convened a group of pathologists to develop a standardized system of nomenclature (National Cancer Workshop, 1988). The result of these deliberations are known as "The Bethesda System" (TBS) for reporting cervical/vaginal cytologic diagnoses (National Cancer Workshop, 1992a,b).

This system has essentially three categories of findings:
1 Normal cytology.
2 Atypical squamous cells of uncertain significance (ASCUS).
3 Cellular changes suggesting:
(i) a low-grade squamous intraepithelial lesion (LSIL);
(ii) a high-grade squamous intraepithelial lesion (HSIL).
The fundamental differences from many pap system usages and the BSCC classification are:
1 At the low-grade end of the spectrum in TBS, koilocytotic atypia is seen as indistinguishable from mild dyskaryosis and incorporated seamlessly in LSIL.
2 The high-grade end incorporates predictions for CIN 2 and CIN 3.
3 A new borderline area is created that does not include HPV changes and is therefore quite different in content from both "borderline nuclear changes" (BSCC) and pap grade II (where HPV may be incorporated).

The terminology recognizes the frequency of regression

Table 5.1 Systems for the classification of cytology.

Historical (pap) grade	BSCC	Bethesda	
0	Unsatisfactory	Inadequate	
I	Negative	Within normal limits	
II (+HPV)	Borderline (+HPV)	ASCUS AGCUS }	(–HPV)
		LSIL	(+HPV)
III (+HPV)	Mild dyskaryosis	LSIL	
	Moderate	HSIL	
IV	Severe dyskaryosis	HSIL	
V	Severe dyskaryosis? Invasion	HSIL	

and refers to predicted "lesions"; not neoplasia. In use, the new system appears to have seen a major expansion of the inconclusive smear result, namely atypical squamous cells of uncertain significance (ASCUS) or atypical glandular cells of uncertain significance (also known as AGCUS) (see later). However, this is probably more a consequence of the recent frequency of litigation for false-negative assessment in the USA, rather than any criticism of the classification. A summary of both classifications is given in Table 5.1.

5.3 Cytological reporting

Normal cytology

Normal cytology varies according to the functional status of the cervix, that is, premenopausal, postmenopausal or postpartum; proliferative, secretory or menstrual phase; oral contraceptive pill use; IUCD use; and the presence or absence of viral, bacterial, fungal or parasitic infections. Whether the pattern of cells is predominantly exfoliative or due to direct scrape or brush recovery is indeterminable. A "normal" smear might usually contain mature orangeophilic squamous cells with a low nuclear : cytoplasmic ratio and a nucleus less than 6 μm diameter; intermediate or navicular glycogenated cells; parabasal squamous cells with high nuclear : cytoplasmic ratios; columnar mucinous endocervical cells; mucus trails; neutrophils; perhaps macrophages; perhaps endometrial cells; recognizable metaplastic squamous cells and lactobacilli. This list is routine but not exhaustive. If no dyskaryosis is present the smear report is normal or negative (Fig. 5.1).

A variety of regenerative and degenerative nuclear and cytoplasmic changes may be seen in normal smears accompanied even by occasional mitoses and sometimes dramatic nuclear and cellular enlargements; multinucleation; irregular coarse hyperchromasia; margination or "beading" of the nuclear envelope by chromatin aggregation; nucleolation and irregular nucleolar dispersal. All such changes need to be assessed and filtered out as due to reactive physiological changes separate from dyskaryosis, predicting dysplasia or CIN or SIL (Fig. 5.2). Poor cytologic assessments in those with little aptitude and/or experience will inflate the various borderline categories and reduce cytological specificity.

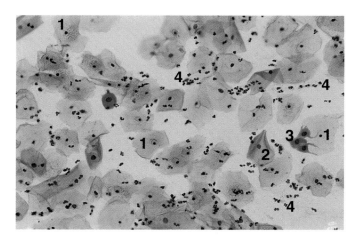

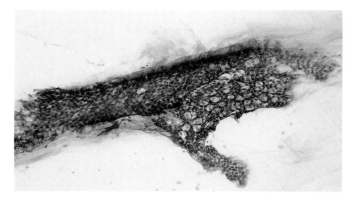

Fig. 5.2(a)

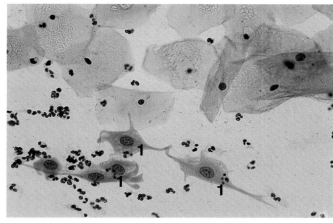

Fig. 5.2(b)

Fig. 5.1 Normal smear stained with Papanicolaou stain. The principal cell type is an eosinophilic/orangeophilic mature cell with a less than 6 µm diameter nucleus (1). An occasional intermediate layer (middle layers) squamous cell is present (2). Metaplastic cells are present with cytopoietic processes that suggest migration (3). There are neutrophils in the background (4).

Fig. 5.2 (a) A sheet of endocervical cells. Endocervical cells have been thought by many to be a necessary component of a "satisfactory" smear. This patient however had vaginal adenosis (sporadic, non-DES associated) and the "portholes" seen in the epithelial honeycomb are goblet cells indicating benign intestinal type metaplasia.
(b) High-power view of metaplastic squamous cells with processes.

Smear adequacy

Adequacy is not defined by the variety of cell types that are present. The total squamous cellularity is extremely variable. Endocervical and metaplastic squamous cells were seen in the majority of Papanicolaou's vaginal swabs or aspirates and so do not reliably indicate direct endocervical canal sampling (Figs 5.2a, b). Nonetheless their presence or absence in smears seems to have been the subject of much historical cytologic debate concerning adequacy. Provided that the smear taker is confident that he/she has visualized the cervix and placed the sampler correctly and that:
1 The smear is not obscured by blood or overlying neutrophilic exudate or artefact (Fig. 5.3);
2 The smear is not purely composed of endocervical cells;
3 The smear is properly fixed in alcohol without air drying;
4 The smear is not overly thick due to poor spreading technique (Fig. 5.4);
then the smear is likely to be adequate. Different sampling devices may provide marginally different yields under otherwise good conditions for the procurement of abnormal cells (Fig. 5.5).

Atrophic smears

Atrophic smears may present particular difficulties for cytologic assessment, whether postmenopausal or postnatal. Infection and therefore inflammatory changes may alter the cellular morphologies resulting in increased numbers of small orangeophilic or cyanophilic or amphophilic cells with pyknotic nuclei, that imitate some patterns of maturing dyskaryosis (Fig. 5.6). The estrogen lack produces thin epithelia which yield rafts of cohesive parabasal cells (Fig. 5.7a) or trails of "stripped" parabasal nuclei (Fig. 5.7b) mimicking dyskaryosis.

The cellularity of the smear is often low and the retracted transformation zone may be poorly or not represented. This is the basis for treating such patients briefly

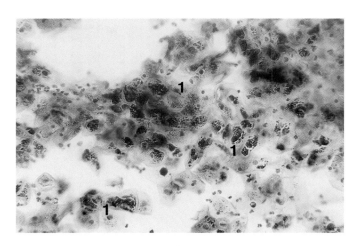

Fig. 5.3 A smear where the bulk of the squamous cell nuclei are obscured by "cornflake" artefact (1). This appearance has been said to be due to the incomplete removal of the polyethylene glycol component of some smear fixatives during processing. A more likely explanation is of air entrapment following the premature evaporation of the clearing agent immediately prior to mounting.

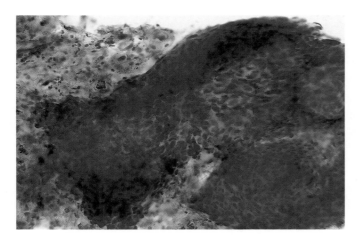

Fig. 5.4 A thick obscured smear.

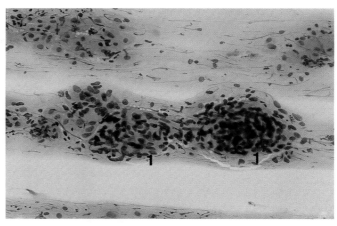

Fig. 5.7(a)

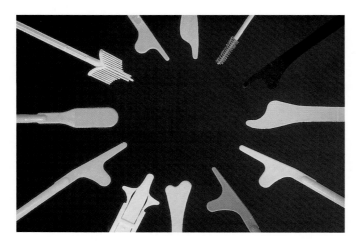

Fig. 5.5 A variety of wooden and plastic spatulas. All of these devices may be used to take smear samples. A critical component is the sampling technique used which requires correctly passing a speculum and visualizing the cervix.

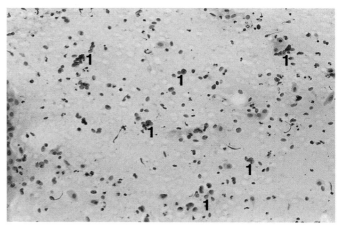

Fig. 5.7(b)

Fig. 5.7 (a) An atrophic postmenopausal smear with clumps of suprabasal squamous cells in trails (1). Normal maturation is absent and such cells can mimic dyskaryotic suprabasal cells predicting severe disease. (b) An atrophic postmenopausal smear with numerous stripped or isolated parabasal nuclei (1). These appearances are so "expected" that sometimes stripped small-cell squamous dyskaryosis or even stripped isolated atypical glandular epithelial cells can be overlooked.

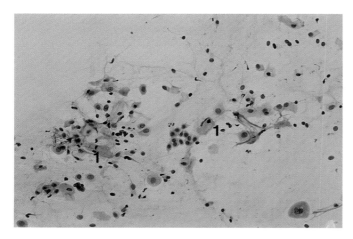

Fig. 5.6 An atrophic smear with included karyopyknotic orangeophilic cells (1) whose nuclear: cytoplasmic ratio must be very carefully assessed to avoid missing sometimes high-grade abnormalities. These are normal.

Borderline abnormalities

In the BSCC nomenclature, the category of "borderline nuclear changes" (BNC) appears largely to refer to "HPV-associated nuclear atypia". This is also true of the way in which some countries use the pap grade II category. In the report (BSCC, 1994), prepared for the NHS Cervical Screening Programme in Britain, there are example slide fields given. Compare Figs 5.8 and 5.9 from that report, said to predict CIN 1 and HPV, with Figs 5.10 and 5.11, thought to show examples of HPV associated BNC. In the author's view, these are merely quantitative sample differences and in the context of a partial sample (as in the cervical smear) have no biological or pathologic validity as separate qualitative appearances.

In that same document (BSCC, 1994), mild dyskaryosis is defined as permitting a nuclear:cytoplasmic area ratio of up to 50%. However, a quick calculation of the diameter ratio reveals that this could be as much as 75% in such a

with estrogens and retaking a smear to ensure adequacy by increasing the smear yield and decreasing the cytologic difficulties introduced by immature and inflamed cell populations.

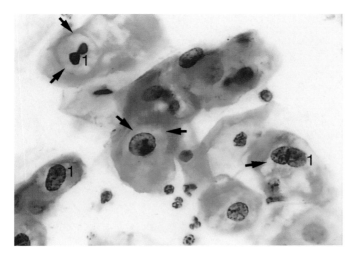

Fig. 5.8 Mild dyskaryosis with koilocytosis. Many of the cells show perinuclear clearing of the cytoplasm with a hard margin to the vacuole (arrowed). These are typical koilocytes. Several of the cells also have features of mild dyskaryosis (1).

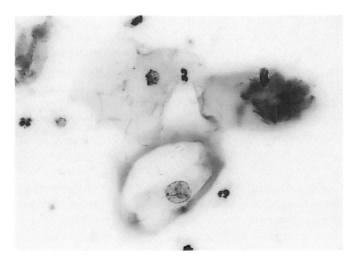

Fig. 5.11 Borderline nuclear changes with koilocytosis. Contrast the cell below centre of field, in which there is an increased nuclear: cytoplasmic ratio, smooth nuclear outline, and fine, evenly dispersed chromatin with that in Fig. 5.9 in which there is mild dyskaryosis. (*Author's view*: actually a dyskaryotic enlarged nucleus with chromatin clearing and incomplete nuclear envelope as a result of degenerative superimposed changes.)

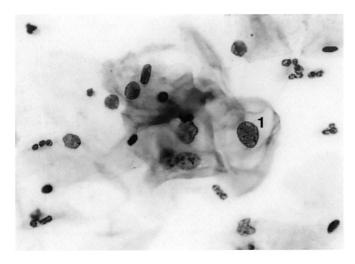

Fig. 5.9 Mild dyskaryosis with koilocytosis. The cell to the right of centre is another example of a cell with mild dyskaryosis and koilocytosis (1).

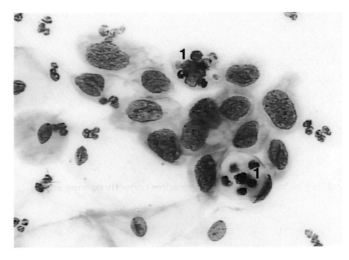

Fig. 5.12 Dyskaryosis in metaplastic squames. Mild and moderate dyskaryosis is present. Note that two of the cells contain ingested polymorphs (1). (*Author's view*: severe parabasal dyskaryosis predicting CIN 3 (HSIL). Compare with Fig. 5.13.)

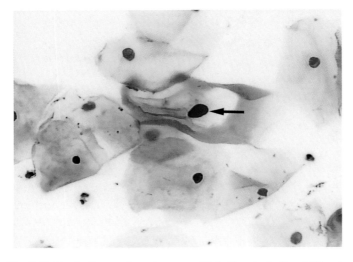

Fig. 5.10 Borderline nuclear changes with koilocytosis. In addition to the perinuclear halo with condensed cytoplasmic rim, typical of a koilocyte, in the cell indicated by the arrow there is nuclear enlargement, slight nuclear irregularity, and pyknosis. (*Author's view*: actually nuclear enlargement, hyperchromasia and irregularity equates to dyskaryosis.)

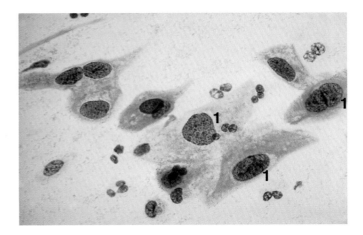

Fig. 5.13 Intermediate and parabasal squamous dyskaryosis. These show coarse-pepper chromatin patterns predicting CIN 3 (HSIL) (1). The histology of this case revealed a large volume CIN 3 (HSIL) lesion with some slight surface differentiation. Compare this figure with Fig. 5.12.

definition, which would indicate parabasal dyskaryosis predicting CIN 3. In that report, Fig. 5.12 is said to be "mild to moderate" dyskaryosis, presumably utilizing the above area definition. However, these cells fulfil the author's criteria for predicting CIN 3 (see Fig. 5.13).

The intent of the category appears to be as a holding category for inconclusive appearances, yet up to two-thirds of women with such HPV smears will prove to have CIN lesions at biopsy around the time of these smears. Other markers for significant cervical disease are oddly excluded or included in this borderline category without evidence or discussion (parakeratotic appearances and tuboendometrioid metaplasias respectively) (see Figs 5.14–5.21). The problems introduced by misplacing certain specific glandular atypias in this category will be discussed later under AGCUS. These abnormalities cannot be evidenced except by cone biopsy and are completely inappropriate for a "holding category."

In summary, the impact of the guidelines in that report (BSCC, 1994) are to promote disease surveillance and delay referral.

ASCUS seems tame by comparison and mainly incorporates reactive or regenerative and degenerative cellular combinations. Accordingly, inexperienced cytologists will defensively abuse the category and confine all their indecision into this basket. About 20 to 25% of laboratory reports in the USA may be in this category. The size of the category, however, is not so dissimilar to the numbers of "inflammatory smears" (without recognized specific infections) that

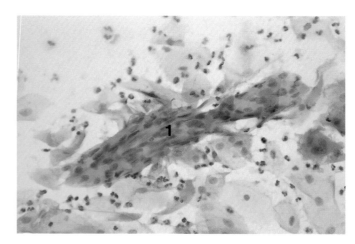

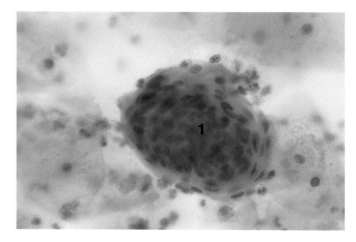

Fig. 5.15 A "raft" of parakeratotic squames (1). This feature of underlying parakeratosis in the absence of dyskaryosis has the same implications as the "whorl" in Fig. 5.14. (Permission from: The benign squamous pearl—Papanicolaou revisited. From Deery, A.R.S. (1989) *J Path* **157**,176A.)

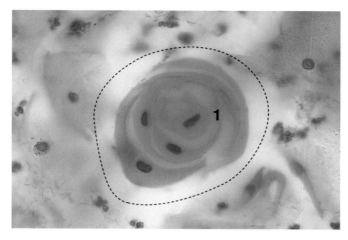

Fig. 5.16 A squamous "core" with centrifugal differentiation or flattening (1). (Permission from: The benign squamous pearl—Papanicolaou revisited. From Deery, A.R.S. (1989) *J Path* **157**,176A.)

Fig. 5.14 A squamous "whorl" with centripetal differentiation (1). This is a feature of parakeratosis. In the age group 25–45 where the cervix has not been biopsied or treated, the commonest cause is HPV infection, together with any associated degree of CIN or even invasive keratotic carcinoma. (Permission from: The benign squamous pearl—Papanicolaou revisited. From Deery, A.R.S. (1989) *J Path* **157**,176A.)

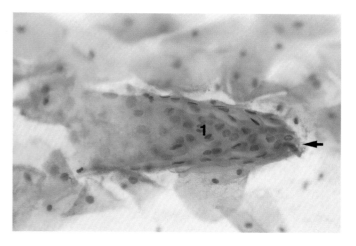

Fig. 5.17 A squamous "spike" (1) with a pointed end (arrowed) and bi-directional flattening. (Permission from: The benign squamous pearl—Papanicolaou revisited. From Deery, A.R.S. (1989) *J Path* **157**,176A.)

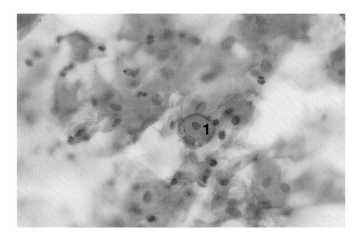

Fig. 5.18 A squamous "button" (1). This consists of a dyskeratotic squamous cell with either a ghost or preserved nucleus, encircled or entrapped by a second squamous cell with a crescentic nucleus and encircling cytoplasmic arms. The central cell is still within the extracellular space. All of these appearances Figs 5.14–5.18 may appear in the same smear in combination and in the absence of dyskaryosis. Nonetheless they reveal a parakeratotic CIN/HPV lesion of whatever grade in the majority of cases. TBS and BSCC (BNC) ignore these appearances in smears. (Permission from: The benign squamous pearl—Papanicolaou revisited. From Deery, A.R.S. (1989) *J Path* **157**,176A.)

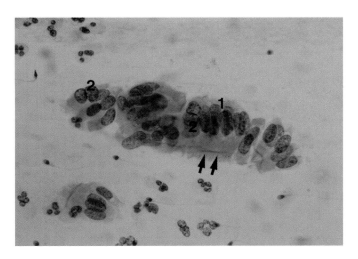

Fig. 5.19 Ciliated or tubal metaplasia (1) with fused terminal bars and ciliated tufts (arrowed). There is some multinucleation and minimal atypia (nuclear hyperchromasia and enlargement).

were being reported in some British laboratories in the mid-1980s prior to the introduction of the BSCC's "borderline nuclear changes." Indeed, one or two laboratories almost immediately achieved this level of "borderline smears" upon adoption of the new terminology.

Dyskaryotic cellular changes

The common feature of a dyskaryotic cell nucleus is an increase in nuclear size, perhaps between 1¼ to 1½ times normal, squamous nuclear diameters of equivalent maturity squamous cells. The nuclei are usually hyperchromatic (Fig. 5.22), but because this is exfoliative cytology and therefore entails devitalization and loss of nuclear stain

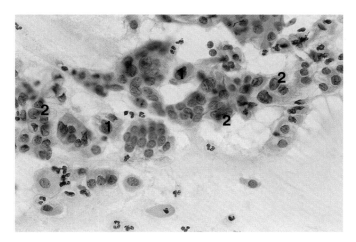

Fig. 5.20 Tubal metaplasia with cellular multinucleation, nuclear overlays (1), hydropic nuclear changes (2) and some nuclear envelope irregularities. These appearances are a common occurrence and a potent source of false-positive squamous dyskaryosis, CGIN, AGCUS or BNC reports.

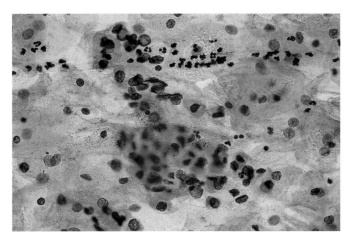

Fig. 5.21 Tubal metaplasia with more obscured features making misinterpretation more likely. Several examples of such metaplasia have been mistakenly described as borderline nuclear changes.

stoichometry, the nuclei may be euchromatic or even hypochromatic, so-called "pale cell dyskaryosis" (Fig. 5.23) (Smith & Turnbull, 1987). It is the increased nuclear size that screeners scanning cells with a × 10 objective, usually detect first. The next most important criterion is probably the amount of cytoplasm or overall cell size and thirdly the degree of orangeophilia or cyanophilia. These allow assessment of cell maturity and in an exfoliative cell pattern predict the maturation achieved by cells from the epithelial surface.

The presence of dyskaryotic orangeophilic mature cells with an appropriate low nuclear:cytoplasmic ratio (Fig. 5.24) will generally predict CIN 1. The occurrence of mainly immature cyanophilic parabasal cells with a high nuclear:cytoplasmic ratio will predict CIN 3 (Fig. 5.25). In between patterns find their way into estimated CIN 2 (Fig. 5.26). The nuclei are not usually more irregular or folded or more nucleolated than normal squamous cells. They may well exhibit mitoses or apoptosis. Higher grade nuclei may often appear more fragile and may "strip" from their

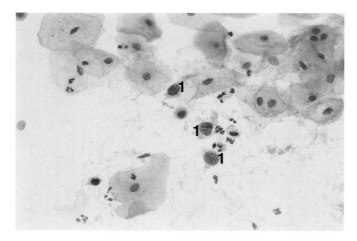

Fig. 5.22 "Typical" severe dyskaryosis. A few hyperchromatic dyskaryotic, suprabasal squamous cells predicting CIN 3 (1) (HSIL) (see Fig. 5.23).

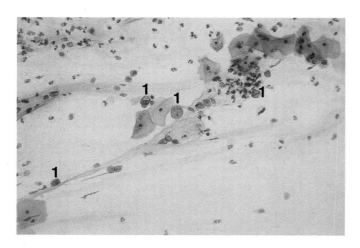

Fig. 5.23 "Pale-cell dyskaryosis". A few degenerate, hypochromatic dyskaryotic, stripped suprabasal squamous cells predicting CIN 3 (HSIL) ("pale cell dyskaryosis") (1) (c.f. Fig. 5.22).

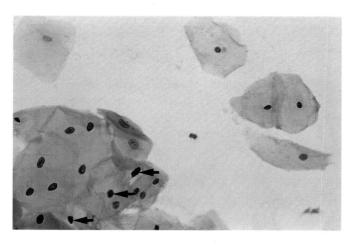

Fig. 5.24 "Typical" mild dyskaryosis. A few mildly dyskaryotic mature squamous cells are present in the lower left hand quadrant predicting the presence of CIN 1 (LSIL) (arrowed).

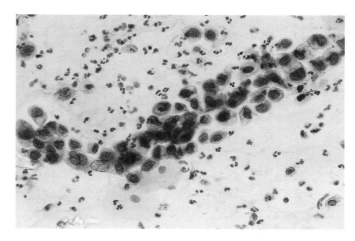

Fig. 5.25 Severe dyskaryosis. A loose slightly dyshesive trail of parabasal dyskaryotic cells predicting CIN 3 (HSIL).

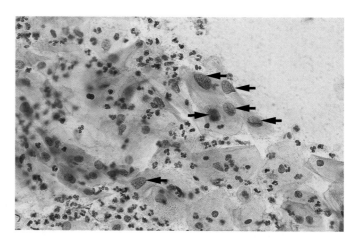

Fig. 5.26 Moderate dyskaryosis. Dyskaryotic intermediate squamous cells are present with atypical enlarged nuclei predicting CIN 2 (HSIL) (arrowed).

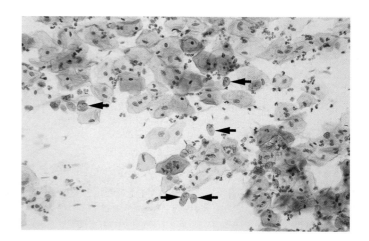

Fig. 5.27 "Stripped" severe dyskaryosis. Several scattered dyskaryotic cells are present including stripped nuclei predicting CIN 3 (HSIL) (arrowed).

cytoplasm more frequently (Fig. 5.27). Macronucleolation may be seen in the most anaplastic, high-grade intraepithelial lesions (Fig. 5.28).

Koilocytotic changes commonly accompany such dyskaryosis, along with individual cell keratinisation (dyskeratosis), and multinucleation. In high-grade lesions,

such accompanying changes usually are restricted to intermediate and superficial cells with parabasal cells left largely unaffected (Fig. 5.29).

Patterns of dyskaryosis that may be most typical include:
1 Dispersed scanty attached superficial, koilocytotic, dyskaryotic cells, in CIN 1/HPV (Fig. 5.30).
2 Trails of monomorphic dyskaryotic intermediate cells

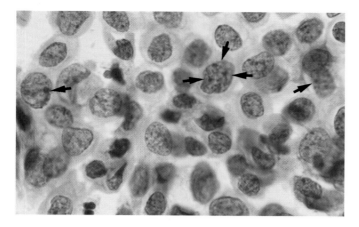

Fig. 5.28 "Nucleolated" severe dyskaryosis. Severely dyskaryotic parabasal cells with coarse-pepper chromatin, increased nuclear envelope folding or irregularity and early macronucleolation with anisonucleolinosis (arrowed).

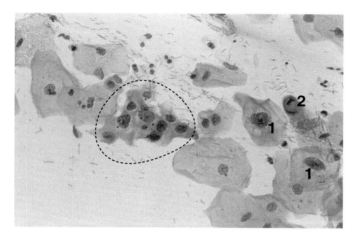

Fig. 5.29 Combined moderate dyskaryosis/HPV (LSIL and HSIL). On the right are two superficial intermediate squamous cells with koilocytotic changes and dyskaryotic nuclei (1) and a dyskeratotic cell "button" (2). These cells suggest CIN 1 and HPV infection (LSIL). However, in the center, left field are dyskaryotic, overlapped and even stripped deep intermediate nuclei (circled) indicating at least CIN 2 (HSIL). This is the worst area and generates the report of HSIL with HPV changes. (Histologically there were areas of CIN 1, 2 and 3.)

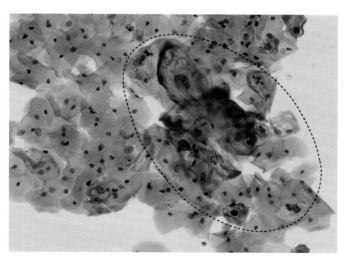

Fig. 5.30 Typical mature mild dyskaryosis. Overlapped superficial intermediate squamous cells exhibiting koilocytotic changes, multi or binucleation and dyskaryosis indicating CIN 1 and HPV infection (LSIL) are enclosed in a circled area.

without further differentiation characteristic of CIN 2 (Fig. 5.31).

5 Clumped cohesive groups of dyskaryotic parabasal cells with trails of similar cells in typical CIN 3 (Fig. 5.32).

6 "Sprinkle pattern" scantly cellular parabasal dyskaryosis in another smear version of CIN 3 (Fig. 5.33).

7 Karyopyknotic but high nuclear:cytoplasmic ratio, orangeophilic, keratinized cells in loose rafts from maturing CIN 3 (Fig. 5.34).

Some other patterns and features occur, but less commonly.

Cytologic indications of invasion

The principal and most reliable pattern of possible invasion in a cervical smear is the presence of an ulcerative "diathesis." This is the presence of pleomorphic, keratinized and parabasal squamous cells with often pale, degenerate nuclei, together with inflammatory cell exudate, necrotic (ghost) tumor cells and fresh blood (Fig. 5.35). Lesser comedo-like crypt CIN 3 lesions can mimic these appearances in smears, however (Fig. 5.36). "Fiber cells" (Fig. 5.37) may hint of early invasion and reflect either surface flattening in large cell, keratinizing CIN 3 (Fig. 5.38) or marginal focal differentiation accompanying microinvasion in HSIL (Fig. 5.39).

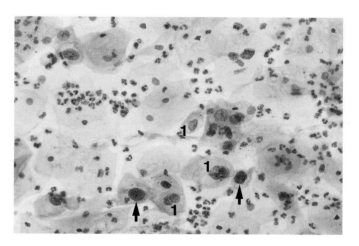

Fig. 5.31 Typical moderate dyskaryosis. Dyskaryotic intermediate squamous cells (arrowed) with some hints of HPV changes (1) predicting at least CIN 2 (HSIL).

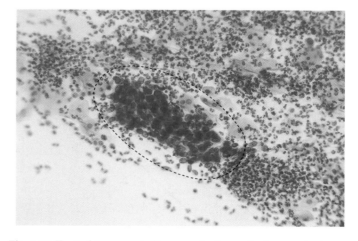

Fig. 5.32 Typical "aggregated" severe dyskaryosis. An aggregate (scrape microbiopsy) of dyskaryotic parabasal cells sitting in a trail of neutrophilic exudate and predicting CIN 3 (HSIL) (circled).

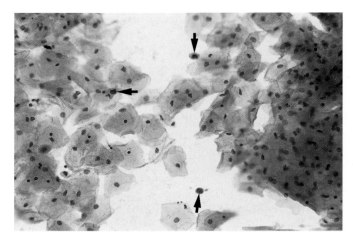

Fig. 5.33 "Sprinkle-pattern" severe dyskaryosis (author's term). "Sprinkle pattern" parabasal dyskaryosis indicating CIN 3 (HSIL) (arrowed). This pattern has been identified as a common source of screener error.

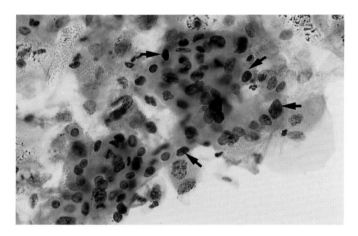

Fig. 5.34 "Maturing" severe dyskaryosis. Severely dyskaryotic dense karyopyknotic, orangeophilic cells, predicting maturing or large cell CIN 3 (HSIL) (arrowed).

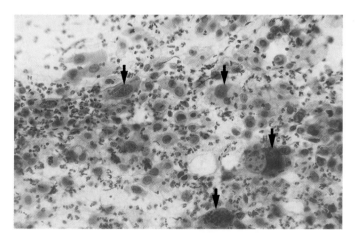

Fig. 5.35 The presence of diathesis (arrowed) is strongly suggestive of an underlying invasive squamous carcinoma (arrowed). But see Fig. 5.36 (the histology from this case).

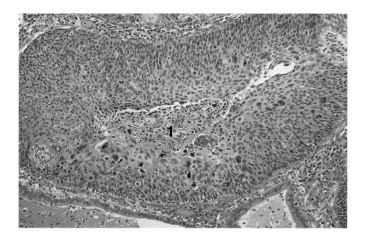

Fig. 5.36 Central crypt necrosis in CIN 3 (HSIL). In screened populations where numbers of invasive cancers are few, central comedo-necrosis in crypts (1) filled with differentiating large cell CIN 3 (HSIL) can produce an exfoliative "diathesis" in the corresponding smear (Fig. 5.35).

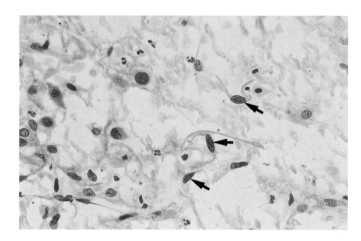

Fig. 5.37 Fiber-cells. Dyskaryotic parabasal cells indicating CIN 3 (HSIL) and dyskaryotic plump spindle cells **whose nuclei override the cytoplasmic margins in the short cellular axis** (arrowed). The occurrence of these cells are predictive of early invasion in the majority of cases (see Figs 5.38 & 5.39).

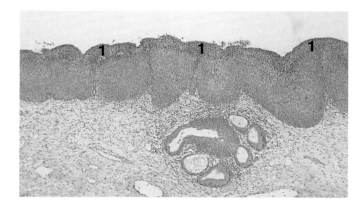

Fig. 5.38 CIN 3 (HSIL) with superficial differentiation (1) and "fiber-cell" formation in the corresponding smear. There was no apparent microinvasion (see Fig. 5.37).

5.4 Clinical referral

In certain countries cytologic report includes guidelines for referral to colposcopy or other gynecologic services. Different guidelines apply according to levels of patient anxiety, expectations of intervention, available colposcopic resources and clinical and social perceptions of disease significance.

In general, smears predicting CIN 2 or worse will be accompanied by advice for referral to colposcopy. Across Europe, referral will occur after one or sometimes two mildly dyskaryotic, pap class III or LSIL smears. Persistent

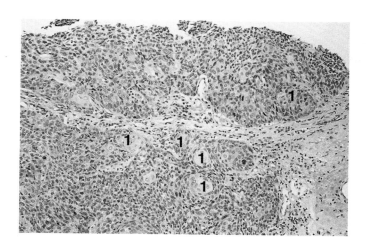

Fig. 5.39 Section of an early invasive (Ia1) squamous carcinoma with focal "pearls" of squamous differentiation at whose eddying margins "fiber-cells" are seen (1). If these exfoliate from the surface they are potent indicators of underlying differentiation in otherwise high-grade lesions. Focal differentiation is an association of microinvasion. (see Fig. 5.37.)

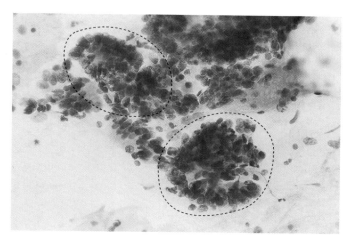

Fig. 5.40 Cervical glandular intraepithelial neoplasia (CGIN). Rafts and linked rosettes of hyperchromatic, crowded, columnar cells with retained polarity or orientation, fine-pepper chromatin increase, but little pleomorphism or nucleolation (circled). These features indicate CGIN. Same case as Figs 5.41 and 5.42. The histology can be seen in Figs 5.43 and 5.44.

borderline, ASCUS or pap class II smears (either two or three) will usually also earn referral.

Adjunctive analysis of high-risk HPV status, some argue, might assist the segregation of patients with low-grade smear abnormalities (Cuzick *et al.*, 1992; Londsborough *et al.*, 1996) (see Chapter 2). Others have found no advantage of such testing over repeat cytology, however (Bavin *et al.*, 1993). Recently Nobbenhuis *et al.* (1999) showed that persistent high risk HPV infection is necessary for development and maintenance of CIN 3. A 6-year study of 18–55 year old screened women indicated that mild–moderate dyskaryosis in smears should be referred only after a second HPV (high risk) positive test; severe dyskaryosis indicating immediate referral.

5.5 Cytodiagnosis of cervical glandular intraepithelial neoplasia (CGIN)/ adenocarcinoma-in-situ (AIS)

An outline of the histology of these precursor glandular lesions has been given in Chapter 1. The author believes a two-grade segregation of these lesions is supportable on morphologic grounds.

Cytologic criteria for CGIN have been espoused by Bousefield *et al.* in 1980 and then Anderson (1992); Wilbur (1995); Saurel (1996): Lee (1997); Siziopikou (1997). It is probably not possible to separate the cytologic appearances into two grades of disease. Only one grade CGIN/AIS is detectable cytologically. The distinction between AIS and invasive carcinoma is usually achievable, however, despite contrary views (Anderson, 1995). The introduction of BSCC "borderline nuclear changes in glandular cells" and AGCUS in the USA provides, for many, a convenient, if ultimately unhelpful, dumping ground when trying to sort these appearances.

High-grade CIN/AIS

Within smears, typical changes of AIS are recognized

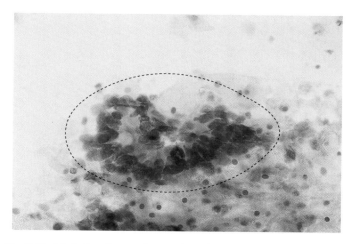

Fig. 5.41 A tubule of hyperchromatic endocervical cells with altered, crowded microarchitecture (circled). These nuclei have increased nuclear diameters relative to normal endocervical nuclei (approx. $1^1/_2 \times$) in the same preparations. CGIN is predicted reliably. There are no features to suggest invasion.

within rafts, rosettes, or papilliform and cribriform arrangements of tall, hyperchromatic columnar, glandular epithelial cells with retained peripheral orientation and cellular trailing or "feathering" (Figs 5.40–5.42). Crowding of cells with nuclear overlap is evident and the increase in nuclear size by comparison with those of normal endocervical glandular cells is in the range ×1½ to ×2. Nucleolation is not a feature. Mitoses are frequent (Figs 5.43 & 5.44).

Despite these fairly characteristic appearances, cytologic screening misses the vast majority of such cases. For although the relative prevalence of adeno Ca/squamous Ca of cervix is perhaps 1:5, the AIS/CIN 3 ratio varies between 1:26 (Boon *et al.*, 1981) and 1:239 (Christophereson, 1979). Most AIS is encountered incidentally after smear referral with squamous dyskaryosis (Maini *et al.*, 1998). Hence, many such cone biopsies reveal combined disease (Figs 5.45–5.47). This is probably illusory and explained as a consequence of the lesion's incidental finding in a group being mostly correctly referred for CIN.

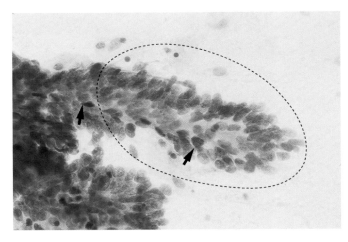

Fig. 5.42 Papilliform fronds with so-called "feathering" (circled) or trailing of fragile, altered, hyperchromatic, neoplastic nuclei so commonly associated with columnar cell dysplasia in early neoplasia. (These same features are seen in adenomatous dysplasia (neoplasia) in Barrett's oesophagus and in colonic adenomas and in ampullary lesions in the duodenum.) Mitoses are present (arrowed). Endocervical cells with mitoses should always be referred and *not* allocated to a "borderline" category.

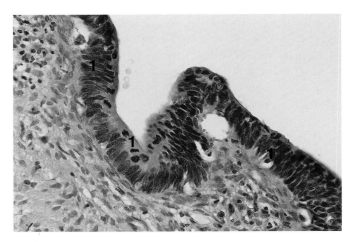

Fig. 5.43 High-grade CGIN (1). This section is from the cone biopsy of the case shown in Figs 5.40–5.42. There were no features at colposcopy to suggest disease.

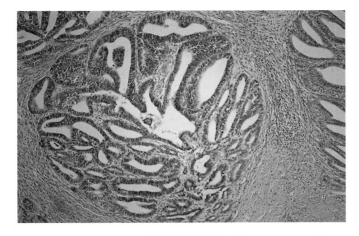

Fig. 5.44 A further section of HGCGIN. This shows more complex, crowded glands lined by neoplastic epithelium. There was no invasion. No CIN was present.

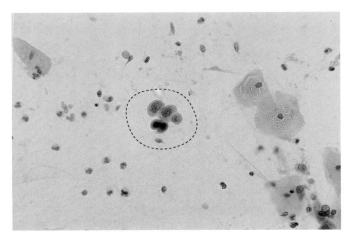

Fig. 5.45 Severely dyskaryotic parabasal cells suggesting CIN 3 (HSIL) (circled). (See also Figs 5.46 and 5.47. from the same patient.)

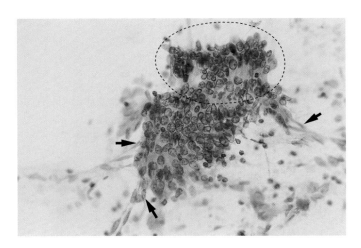

Fig. 5.46 Atypical, crowded, hyperchromatic enlarged columnar mucinous epithelial cells with a cribriform area of small linked tubular rosettes at the north-west pole (circled). There is "feathering" or trailing of abnormal nuclei at the edges of the sheet (arrowed). This is CGIN. (See also Figs 5.45 and 5.47.)

AGCUS/borderline glandular cells

Korn *et al.* (1998) described the prevalence of both adenocarcinoma/AIS and SIL in a population of women referred with AGCUS. They compared this with similar studies performed and showed that between 0% and 28% of women in the various reviewed studies had adenocarcinomas or AIS. Between 10% and 81% of patients had SILs only or in addition. This paper supports an aggressive biopsy based approach for the assessment of patients with AGCUS. The same approach should be advised for "borderline nuclear changes in glandular cells".

Atypical metaplasia

Tubal or tuboendometroid metaplasia (Selvaggi, 1997) and perhaps cervical endometriosis are potent mimics of CGIN and will be the cause of some false-positive cytologic assessments (Figs 5.19–5.21 & Fig. 5.48). Ciliated cells were thought a normal component of endocervix by Papanicolaou and Traut (1954) and Koss (1992). They are in fact a feature of tubal metaplasia and the finding of such metaplasia in cervical smears is common in the absence of previous

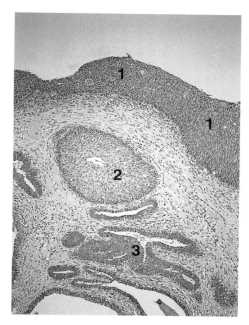

Fig. 5.47 Combined CIN 3 (HSIL) (1) with extension into crypts (2) and (HG) CGIN at (3). This case was correctly predicted cytologically. Such combined lesions are said to be present in approximately 50% of cases of CGIN/AIS. This seems to be a consequence of incidental but low levels of histologic recognition of CGIN in patients, correctly referred with predicted CIN. In the author's laboratory most CGIN is pure, with only 10% having CIN as well (almost the same incidence as the normal population in the same age cohorts).

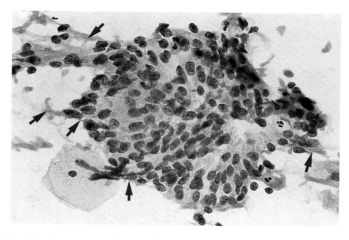

Fig. 5.48 Endometrioid metaplasia. A crowded sheet of slightly overlapped cuboidal/columnar glandular cells with "crumbly" chromatin and a hint of "feathered" edges (arrowed). These smear appearances were associated with endometrioid metaplasia in the subsequent LLETZ cone biopsy. (False-positive cytology.)

conization. The presence of, and correct recognition of, benign atypia in association with tubal metaplasia in cervical smears does not exclude the possible associated presence of CGIN for which it may be a marker (Figs 5.49–5.51) (author's observations). Colposcopic evaluation of any or all of these glandular appearances is unhelpful (Maini *et al.* 1998) and excisional biopsy must be considered.

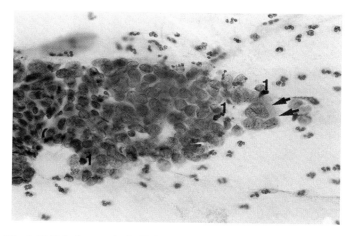

Fig. 5.49 Tubal metaplasia/CGIN. A sheet of glandular epithelial cells is present. At the right-hand tip of the sheet a small syncytial group of ciliated, hydropic, tubal epithelial cells is visible indicating tubal metaplasia (arrowed). The remainder of the cells within this microbiopsy indicate CGIN. There are mitoses (1), occasional rosettes and crowded, overlapped, enlarged hyperchromatic nuclei throughout. Because of devitalization of the cells most of the nuclear chromatin is "pale." The appearances predict combined CGIN and tubal metaplasia.

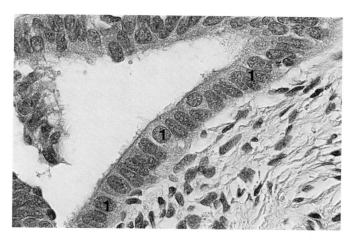

Fig. 5.50 Tubal metaplasia. Block B, step 1 from LLETZ cone biopsy showing part of a crypt containing tubal-type epithelial lining (1).

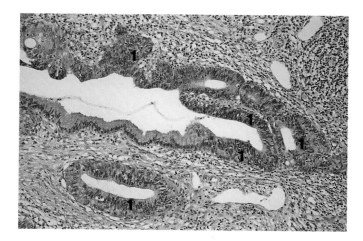

Fig. 5.51 HGCGIN. Block D, step 2 and an irregular crypt-like space is seen with crowding, pseudostratification or piling up of the hyperchromatic cells with papillary tufts and mitoses indicating (HG) CGIN (1). This lesion disappeared at step 4 and was not present in any other of five blocks. CGIN is frequently small making it difficult for the pathologist to locate. Both smears and cones in these cases should be reserved for "specialist pathologist" opinions.

5.6 Cytologic features of adenocarcinoma

The features of adenocarcinoma are usually more severe than for CGIN with loss of polarity within cellular clusters, more masked cellular and nuclear enlargement, nucleolation and individual cell necrosis (Figs 5.52 & 5.53). These features coupled with an awareness of the patient's age should assist at least the suggestion in smears.

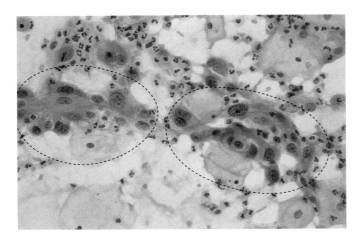

Fig. 5.52 Malignant, macronucleolated, loose clustering of adenocarcinoma cells (circled) in a smear. The critical challenge for the cytologist is to decide between "reactive" (?Borderline ?AGCUS ?ASCUS) or "malignant" changes. Further identification of glandular or squamous differentiation is largely academic.

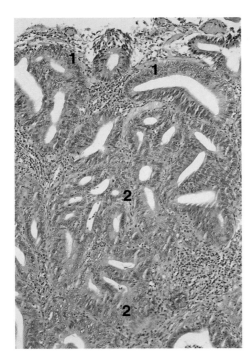

Fig. 5.53 Histology from the case shown in Fig. 5.52. This shows invasive adenocarcinoma with in-situ (1) and invasive appearances (2). The area at (2) is populated by macronucleolated vesicular large glandular epithelial cells quite different from the typical hyperchromatic, elongated nuclei, seen lining the glandular profiles at (1).

5.7 Screening for cervical cancer

Introduction

Cervical cancer is the second leading cause of death for women world-wide, and the leading cause of death from cancer among women in developing nations.

Each year there are approximately 437 000 new cases of invasive cancer diagnosed (representing 12% of new cases of cancer in women) and in excess of 200 000 deaths from the disease (Pisani *et al.*, 1993). Three-quarters of cases are in the developing world where there is no established screening program. Until such time that primary prevention is feasible, perhaps by means of a vaccine against human papillomavirus (HPV), screening remains the only practical way of reducing the mortality from cervical cancer.

Screening can detect the well-recognized premalignant stages of cervical cancer and appropriate treatment of them will prevent progression to invasive disease. Cervical cancer is therefore largely but not entirely preventable with effective screening and appropriate treatment and should therefore be afforded high priority in national cancer control programs.

Cytologic screening

The concept of using exfoliative cytology for the detection of cancer was first described by Papanicolaou in 1928. The present technique of sampling the cervix using a spatula or brush has been modified from the method first described by Ayre in 1948. Widespread introduction of Papanicolaou smear screening began in the USA in the 1950s and was introduced in the UK in 1964 on an opportunistic basis. The screening programs in place in many countries involve obtaining a cervical smear from women at intervals ranging between 1 and 5 years; with referral of women with smear abnormalities for colposcopy and subsequent treatment if necessary.

Effectiveness

There has never been a prospective controlled trial to determine the effectiveness of cytologic screening. However its effectiveness has been evaluated on the basis of several non-experimental case control and cohort studies. In British Columbia, high levels of screening resulted in the reduction of both incidence of; and mortality from squamous carcinoma of the cervix (Boyes, 1981). In the Nordic countries, an 80% reduction in cervical cancer deaths has been seen in the age groups exposed to intensive screening (Singer, 1995) and a strong correlation exists between the intensity of the screening program and the reduction in risk of cervical cancer (Laara *et al.*, 1987). A large study coordinated by the International Agency for Research on Cancer (IARC Working Group, 1986) showed that total eradication of cervical cancer was an unrealistic goal, and that the maximum protection afforded after a negative smear is about 90%; this remaining high for several years afterwards. In the UK, where the population coverage now exceeds 80% following the introduction of a computerized call and recall system in 1988, there has been more than a 20% reduction in incidence since 1986 with mortality rates falling by 7% a year (Sasieni *et al.*, 1995; Office for National Statistics, 1996).

Countries with well-established screening programs have generally been able to demonstrate a reduction in mortality from squamous cervical cancer but not so for adenocarcinoma, which now constitutes a much larger proportion of cervical cancer, particularly in younger women. The propensity for frankly malignant change in adenocarcinoma-in-situ is unknown, but it is thought to progress through a shorter latent phase and the resulting malignancy more prone to rapid spread. Population studies have found no effects of cervical cancer screening on either the incidence or mortality from adenocarcinoma of the cervix (Sigurdsson, 1995; Van Wijngaarden *et al.*, 1995).

Accuracy

Despite the cervical smear being responsible for the 60–70% reduction in mortality from cervical cancer in well-screened areas, the test itself and indeed the cytologists who interpret the test have come under intense scrutiny and criticism. Most of this is directed at the false-negative smear. This false-negative rate for a single smear examination has been variously reported to range from 10% to 50% (Ferenczy *et al.*, 1996) and reflects the sensitivity of the test. The majority of this error rate is due to poor sampling of the cervix due to inadequate technique or equipment, failure to transfer abnormal cells to the glass slide (preparation error) or because the lesion was not exfoliating cells—the so called "sampling false-negative". The remainder of the error is probably due to inaccuracies in laboratory reporting where abnormal cells are present on the glass slide but are either not detected or incorrectly classified—the so called "screening false-negative". It is important to realize that however good a screening test may be, it can never be 100% sensitive and so will miss a proportion of cases.

The specificity of the cervical smear depends on the cytology classification system used and the threshold for referral to colposcopy. In the USA, the specificity has effectively decreased since the introduction of The Bethesda System, which introduced a new category of ASCUS (atypical squamous cells of undetermined significance) (National Cancer Institute Workshop, 1992). Broadly equivalent cytologic categories include morphologic changes bordering on mild dyskaryosis, atypical cells, minor atypia and minimal atypia. If a particular screening program requires the referral of this category to colposcopy, the overall increase in sensitivity will be mitigated by a higher false-positive rate and a lower effective specificity (Quek *et al.*, 1998). This is a major problem in developed countries where large numbers of women, most of whom are not at risk of cervical cancer, are unnecessarily investigated. This represents a waste of valuable resources and will almost certainly require additional tests other than cytology to distinguish those women who are truly at risk (Duncan, 1997).

5.8 Improvements to cervical screening

Improvements to cervical screening may broadly be achieved in two ways:
1 Improving cytologic screening.
2 The use of additional tests (adjunctive tests).

Improving cytological screening

The accuracy of cytologic screening is dependent on:
1 Sampling techniques.
2 Slide preparation.
3 Cytologic interpretation.

5.9 Sampling techniques

Sampling techniques are a significant source of smear error (Morell *et al.*, 1982; Mitchell *et al.*, 1990). An important area that is often overlooked is ensuring the competence of the smear taker. They need to have the right skills both to improve the experience for the woman and to ensure that the smears meet the technical criteria for examination. To this end, regular training/retraining of smear takers and audit of the extent of inadequate smears has been recommended (The performance of the NHS cervical screening program in England; National Audit Office, 1998).

A variety of sampling devices is available (see Fig. 5.5) but surprisingly little work has been done to evaluate how different devices contribute to the sampling error (Beeby *et al.*, 1993; Metcalf *et al.*, 1994). Hutchinson *et al.* (1994) found that a significant proportion of the cells collected is never transferred to the slide but is discarded with the device. Using a variety of devices, they found that the available epithelial cells transferred to the slides ranged from a mere 6.5% using a cotton swab/spatula, 8.4% with a Cervex brush, 18.1% with a Cytobrush®/spatula, to 62.5% using a plastic spatula alone. More recently, Sasieni (1996) showed in a meta-analysis that more abnormalities were detected using an extended tip spatula such as the Aylesbury, and various combinations of devices such as the Aylesbury and Cytobrush.

Slide preparation—thin layer technology

Another problem is the fact that the conventional smears are usually of variable thickness and may be obscured by mucus, blood and other debris. This results in cell and nuclear overlap, causing problems with detection and interpretation. Several techniques have been described using thin-layer techniques (Figs 5.54–5.56). Another development utilizes a fluid-based medium for the preparation of cytology slides. These systems should reduce the number of inadequate smears, allow more efficient screening either by conventional or automated screening systems (see later), and have the added advantage that the residual cell suspension can be used for other adjunctive tests (e.g. HPV typing and testing) (McGoogan & Reith, 1996). The ThinPrep® pap test (Cytyc Corporation, Boxboro, MA) is a system that produces a thin, even layer of cervical cells. A plastic sampling device is used to collect the cells in the

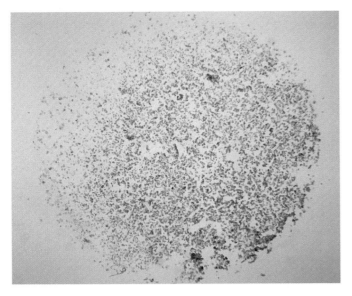

Fig. 5.54 Thin-layer cytology. A low power of a cytocentrifuge (low acceleration centrifuge thin layer) of a randomized cervical spatula smear taken into RPMI 1640. Approximately 1000 cells are present (six fields under ×10 objective covers the area).

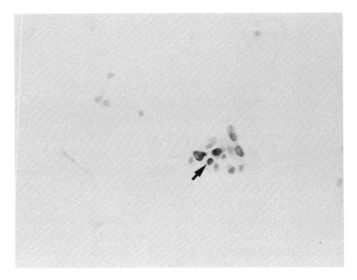

Fig. 5.56 Thin-layer immunocytochemistry. Higher power of parallel cytocentrifuge from the same case revealing MIB1 (cell cycle associated marker marking cells in G_1, G_2 and S phases) immunocytochemical nuclear staining of some of a group of parabasal dyskaryotic cells (arrowed). MIB1 detects approximately 60–70% of CIN 3 (HSIL) lesions morphologically predictable from Papanicolaou-stained parallel preparations and is not a substitute for careful observation. (Unpublished observations by author [A.D.].)

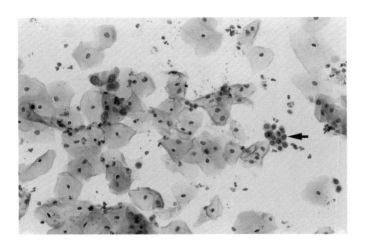

Fig. 5.55 Thin-layer cytology. Higher power of the cytocentrifuge preparation showing aggregates of parabasal dyskaryotic cells suggesting CIN 3 (HSIL) (arrowed).

5.10 Cytologic interpretation

The failure to detect, or the misinterpretation of abnormal cells present on a smear is another source of error. This may be due to a number of reasons including poor training, poor quality control and cytotechnician exhaustion. Manual screening of cervical smears is a time consuming and fatiguing task which is subject to psychologic habituation as more than 90% of the slides examined will be normal. Moreover the test is entirely dependent on human judgement. Internal and external quality control of cytology laboratories should therefore be an important part of the screening program (Koss, 1989). In the UK, guidelines and expected standards relating to cytology have been published by the National Health Service Cervical Screening Programme (Herber, 1995; Pritchard, 1996). The US Congress enacted the Clinical Laboratory Improvements Amendments in 1988 which legislated proficiency testing for cytotechnicians as well as limiting their caseload.

Automation in screening

Automated systems for cervical screening can potentially eliminate much of the tedium and habituation associated with manual screening. These systems have been in development for several decades but earlier attempts were hampered by the fact that they could not reliably process conventionally prepared smears because of the variable thickness of the smears and the cell and nuclear overlap. In addition, the early computer classification schemes which made use of algorithmic "rules" were unable to deal with the many degrees of abnormalities which represent a diverse set of morphologies (Mango, 1994). Recent advances in this field have resulted in more sophisticated

usual manner but instead of smearing it on a glass slide, this is immersed and rinsed in a vial of buffered preservative solution which is subsequently filtered to separate mucus and debris. The prepared cells are then collected on the filter membrane by means of a gentle vacuum and transferred to a glass slide for cytologic interpretation (Fig. 5.57). This technique has been shown to increase the detection of squamous intraepithelial lesions (CIN) (Corkhill et al., 1997) as well as significantly improving the quality of the smear, thus reducing the sampling false-negative rate (Lee, 1997). Other systems that utilize thin-layer technology include CytoRich (Roche Image Analysis Systems) and Megafunnel (Shandon).

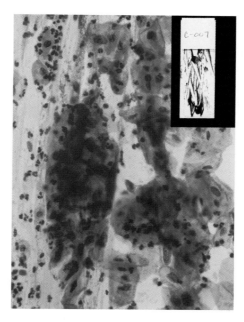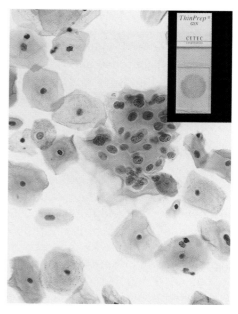

Fig. 5.57 (a & b) Pictured here is a photo comparison of slides from the ThinPrep® pap test (b) vs. a conventional pap smear (a). Both slides were prepared from one patient sample and are shown at the same magnification. The ThinPrep® pap test relies on fluid-based technology and the cell sample is dispersed and filtered to reduce mucus, blood and inflammation, resulting in a thin, even layer of the cervical cells. With a conventional pap smear, cervical cells are "smeared" directly onto a slide.

Fig. 5.57(a)

Fig. 5.57(b)

algorithms which have made automated screening of conventionally prepared smears a reality. At present the objectives of these systems are to automate the search for abnormality rather than to perform a diagnosis. However, it seems likely that as these systems continue to become more sophisticated and image processors become more precise, they will eventually be able to screen as well, if not better than a trained cytotechnician, and handle a much larger workload.

Neural networks have provided significant advantages over standard algorithmic computer classification methods. They are ideal for highly variable pattern recognition as they do not rely on rules but rather mimic the human brain's ability to "learn" (Mango, 1994). This technology is incorporated into the Papnet® Cytological Screening System* (Neuromedical Systems, Inc., Suffern, New York, USA). Rather than attempting automated diagnosis of cell abnormalities, this process presents fields of view containing abnormal cells or cell clusters to trained human observers on a high resolution monitor (Fig. 5.58a & b) (Koss *et al.*, 1994). Papnet has been proposed as a supplementary test to improve cervical smear screening accuracy, particularly to reduce the false-negative rate. In a trial involving the analysis of 9666 smears reported as negative by manual screening, Papnet rescreening identified 464 (4.8%) abnormal smears (Ferenczy *et al.*, 1996). This represents a 30% increase over average historical detection of 12.7% (Hutchinson *et al.*, 1994). In a large multicenter study involving more than 20 000 smears, Papnet assisted screening was compared with conventional manual screening. It was found that Papnet assisted screening was at least as reliable as the manual method in identifying abnormal smears but was able to perform the task in one-third of the time (approximately 3 vs. 10 minutes).

The AutoPap System (Neopath Inc., Redmond, WA, USA) uses an image processor which systematically scans the slide and runs the resultant images through a series of interpretation algorithms to determine the final results. The device designates a score for each slide based on the

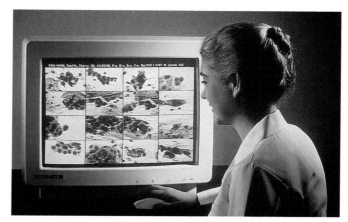

Fig. 5.58(a)

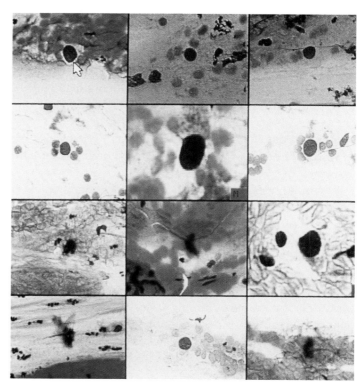

Fig. 5.58(b)

likelihood that an abnormality exists. Clinical trials using this system as a rescreening device shows a five-fold improvement over manual methods in detecting previously missed abnormal cells (Wilbur *et al.*, 1998).

It is likely that these systems which are able to process conventionally prepared smears will perform even better with thin-layer preparations.

5.11 Adjunctive tests

Despite all the techniques described above to improve cytologic screening, there remains an "irreducible" false-negative rate inherent to the smear test (Kreiger & Bibbo, 1997). In addition there is the problem of the increasing numbers of women with minor cytologic abnormalities, a significant proportion of whom will have CIN requiring treatment. A number of studies have reported that of women with ASCUS smears, between 6% and 7% will harbor histologically high-grade CIN (HSIL or CIN 2/3) (Cox *et al.*, 1995; Wright *et al.*, 1995; Kinney *et al.*, 1998). In women with mild dysplasia or LSIL, between 17% and 26% have high-grade CIN (HSIL or CIN 2/3) (Campion *et al.*, 1986; Lonky *et al.*, 1995; Wright *et al.*, 1995). The referral of all these women to colposcopy would put an enormous burden on existing services and result in unnecessary colposcopy visits. It has been suggested that the maximum benefits of cytology have already been achieved in well-screened populations, and new or additional methods are needed to make further significant improvements (Van Wijngaarden *et al.*, 1995; Reid *et al.*, 1991). A number of adjunctive tests to cytology have been used in an attempt to further improve primary screening or to act as a triage for women with minor smear abnormalities to either colposcopy or continued cytologic surveillance. Among the adjunctive tests used are:

1 HPV-DNA testing.
2 Cervicography.
3 TruScan* (formerly The PolarProbe).
4 Visual inspection based techniques.

HPV-DNA testing

It is now established through many epidemiologic and in vitro studies that HPV plays a major role in cervical carcinogenesis (see Chapter 2). More than 100 genotypes exist of which about 20 infect the cervix. Types 16, 18, 31, 33, 35, 39, 45, 51, 52, 56, 58, 59 and 68 are termed high risk and are associated with cervical cancer.

Two main tests are available: polymerase chain reaction (PCR) and hybrid capture (HC) Although there are other methods of HPV-DNA detection, these two have been shown to be most useful for routine clinical utility. At the time of writing PCR is only available as a laboratory protocol and requires a high degree of technical expertise and stringent controls to prevent contamination. Hybrid capture is the more commonly used of the two and is an objective quantitative test available as a standardized kit (Hybrid Capture II Assay, Digene Corp.). It employs RNA probes complementary to the 13 high-risk HPV types as

well as five low-risk types. HPV-DNA present in a sample is denatured and hybridized to the RNA probes. These RNA-DNA hybrids are then captured on to microtiter plates with monoclonal antibodies. A second monoclonal antibody conjugated to alkaline phosphatase is then reacted with the captured hybrids followed by the addition of a chemoluminescent substrate. As the alkaline phosphatase conjugate cleaves the chemoluminescent substrate, light is emitted which can be detected with a luminometer and the amount of light is proportional to the amount of HPV-DNA in the original sample (Fig. 5.59).

The test can detect the presence of HPV-DNA in concentrations as low as 0.2 pg/mL. However, to optimize sensitivity and specificity for management, particularly in the triaging of women with minor smear abnormalities, it is usually set to give a positive result with concentrations of 1.0 pg/mL (corresponding to 5000 copies of the HPV genome) and above.

The use of HPV-DNA testing for primary screening has been assessed in a number of trials, some of them still ongoing at the time of publication (Table 5.2). The cumulative results from these trials (using Hybrid Capture, HCII, Digene Corp.) involving over 23 000 women showed that HPV testing had a sensitivity of 90% for high-grade CIN compared with 67% for the pap smear (Lorincz, 1999).

HPV-DNA testing as triage

One suggested scheme for triage would be to subject women with minor cytologic abnormalities to HPV-DNA testing within 3–6 months of the initial smear. If thin-layer slides had been used, HPV-DNA testing could be performed on the residual cell suspension thus saving the woman a return visit. A positive result for high-risk HPV types would warrant referral to colposcopy, whilst a negative result could be followed-up cytologically.

A number of clinical trials involving women with ASCUS or LSIL smears using hybrid capture assay for HPV-DNA (using first generation HCI assay, Digene Corp.) show that the sensitivity of the test for detecting CIN 2 or more was

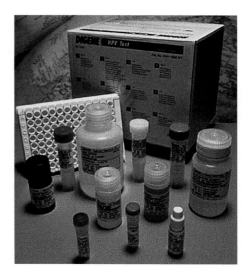

Fig. 5.59(a)

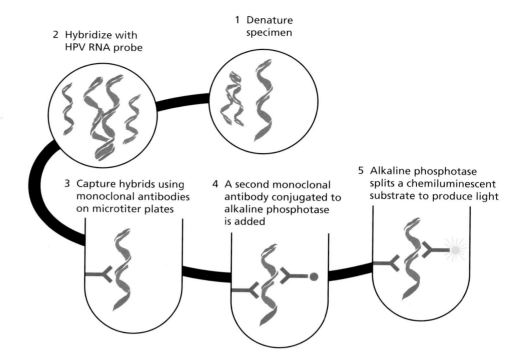

Fig. 5.59 (b) Hybrid capture for HPV DNA detection.

1 Denature specimen

2 Hybridize with HPV RNA probe

3 Capture hybrids using monoclonal antibodies on microtiter plates

4 A second monoclonal antibody conjugated to alkaline phosphotase is added

5 Alkaline phosphotase splits a chemiluminescent substrate to produce light

Table 5.2 Comparison of the sensitivity of HPV-DNA detection and conventional pap smear for cervical cancer screening. Presented at the 17th International Papillomavirus Conference, Charleston, January 1999 (Lorincz, 1999).

Principal investigator	Country	Total women screened	Sensitivity for disease (CIN 2/3)	
			HPV (%)	Pap smear (%)
Birembaut	France	1 200	97	75
Cuzick	UK	2 988	95	75
Ratnam	Canada	2 098	86	37
Schiffman/NCL	Costa Rica	10 049	89	77
Shah	Zimbabwe	2 206	81	44
Walboomers/Meijer	The Netherlands	2 070	95	84
Wright	South Africa	2 719	86	78
Cumulative results		23 330	90	67

equivalent to that of repeat cytology. However the combination of hybrid capture and repeat cytology was better than either test alone, achieving a sensitivity of over 95% for clinically important cervical disease (Cox et al., 1995; Hatch et al., 1995; Wright et al., 1995; Ferenczy et al., 1996; Hall et al., 1996; Lorincz et al., 1996). The second generation HCII assay has been shown to be capable of achieving an even better sensitivity (Ferris, 1998; Manos et al., 1999).

In the USA, a large nationwide study was launched in 1997, known as the ASCUS/LSIL Triage Study (ALTS), to investigate the optimum management of women with ASCUS and LSIL smears. The two principal aims of the study are: (i) to determine if "watchful waiting" which involves repeating smears every 6 months is a reasonable alternative to immediate colposcopy; and (ii) to determine if HPV-DNA testing can reliably predict which types of cells will revert to normal and which will progress to high-grade disease. In addition the women will also be interviewed to seek their views on which approach they find most acceptable. The results of this study are awaited with great interest.

HPV-DNA testing as an adjunctive test to cytology

Several large clinical trials to assess the utility of HPV-DNA testing as an adjunctive test to cytology for primary screening are underway. The ideal adjunctive test would improve detection rates for high-grade CIN and reduce the referral rate to colposcopy by allowing HPV-DNA negative women with minor cytologic abnormalities to be followed by cytologic surveillance.

A preliminary study by Cuzick et al. (1995) compared PCR (for HPV types 16, 18, 31 and 33) with cytology on 2009 women attending for routine screening. In this study HPV-DNA testing was shown to be more sensitive than cytology (75% vs. 33%) for high-grade disease (CIN 2/3) and had a similar positive predictive value for CIN 2/3 as moderate dyskaryosis.

Cervicography

Cervicography is the process of obtaining a high resolution

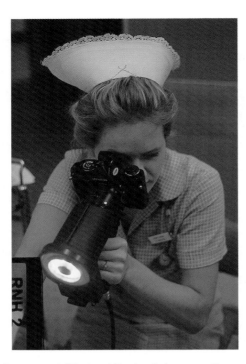

Fig. 5.60 Cerviscope® (National Testing Laboratory, Fenton, MO, USA).

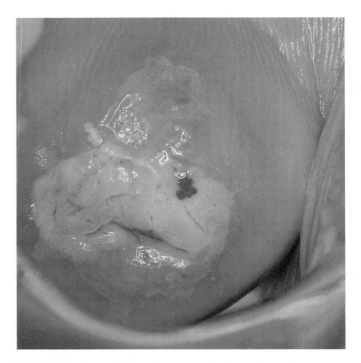

Fig. 5.61 Cervicograph showing an atypical transformation zone (using a cerviscope as pictured in Fig. 5.60).

photograph, using a cerviscope (Fig. 5.60), of the cervix under magnification after the application of 3–5% acetic acid. The photograph is viewed on a screen by a trained assessor who then examines it for any abnormalities (Fig. 5.61). The technique was developed in 1981 (Stafl, 1985) and was proposed as a new or adjunctive method for cervical cancer screening.

As a screening tool, cervicography has been shown to have a better sensitivity than cytology in the detection of CIN (Ferris *et al.*, 1993; Kesic *et al.*, 1993) but suffers from poor specificity. The test has not been widely used mainly because of its high false-positive rate ranging from 8.2% to 61.0% (median 42.1%) (Nuovo *et al.*, 1997). In a system where any abnormality detected by cervicography would result in referral to colposcopy, this poor specificity would lead to costly and unnecessary referrals. Other problems include the expense associated with cerviscopes, the need for adequate analysis facilities and the subjectivity of the test. There is significant interobserver variability, making the performance of the test highly dependent on the assessor's experience (de Sutter *et al.*, 1998).

Cervicography may have a role in triaging women with minor cytologic abnormalities. A study examining the use of cervicography combined with repeat cytology in women with minor cytologic abnormalities showed that the combination had a sensitivity of 97% for the detection of high-grade CIN (CIN 2/3) in women with an initial smear showing LSIL (CIN 1). This was higher than the sensitivity of either of the two tests alone (cytology 78%, cervicography 89%). The corresponding sensitivity for an initial ASCUS smear was 91% (Eskridge *et al.*, 1998).

At the Whittington Hospital, London, cervicography was used to triage women with minor smear abnormalities

for a period from 1988. A retrospective review of the 1436 women with minor smear abnormalities showed that cervicography had a sensitivity of 91% for the detection of high-grade CIN (CIN 2 or above). All the cases missed by cervicography were of small volume disease. The specificity however was only 51% but this was offset by the fact that this was a very high-risk population with 21% of the women having CIN 2 or more.

A recent randomized study by Autier *et al.* (1999) comparing the ability of combined cytology and cervicography with cytology alone found that the addition of cervicography did not significantly reduce the number of precancer lesions when examined a year later.

The usefulness of cervicography is dependent on the local referral practice for abnormal smear results. Where all women with low-grade smears are referred for colposcopy, the use of cervicography as an adjunct should reduce the number of colposcopies performed and allow for the detection of high-grade abnormalities missed by the smear. However if low-grade smears are followed up by watchful waiting with repeat cytology, cervicography, with its high false-positive rate will substantially increase the use of colposcopy.

TruScan* (formerly called The PolarProbe)

TruScan* is a portable optoelectronic system which has been designed for the detection of cervical cancer and precancer. It provides an instantaneous and objective assessment of the cervix without requiring tissue for histologic or cytologic analysis. It makes use of the principle that cervical tissue (both physiologic and pathologic) has characteristic electrical and optical properties. TruScan* scans the cervix using a combination of low level electrical impulses and light pulses at various frequencies. The measured response or tissue signature is compared algorithmically in real time to a databank of previously determined cervical tissue types. If a match is found the result is then classified into one of three categories; normal, low-grade squamous intraepithelial lesion (LSIL) and high-grade squamous intraepithelial lesion/invasive cancer.

The device is presently being evaluated in the Whittington Hospital, London, and consists of a 17 cm long handle with a 5 mm diameter tip into which is built the components necessary for the electrical/optical stimulation and detection of the cervix. This relays signals between the cervix and a portable console which houses the microprocessor responsible for the identification of tissue types (Fig. 5.62). A cusco's speculum is used to visualize the cervix and the probe is gently passed over the surface of the cervix. An instantaneous result is made available to the operator via a series of lights positioned on the handle of the device and a summary printout can be obtained showing the highest grade lesion identified during the course of the examination. The whole process generally takes between 1 and 2 minutes and can be performed by anyone who is competent at taking a smear test, with a minimum of instruction.

Studies at the author's unit show that the TruScan* system has a high degree of acceptability among women when compared with the pap smear. A total of 152 women were surveyed and the findings revealed that women experience less anxiety, pain, and after effects like bleeding with TruScan* than with the pap smear. In addition significantly more women preferred the system to the smear and felt reassured about the possibility of having an immediate result. Importantly, 82% (95% CI 75–88%) of women responded that the TruScan* system would encourage them to attend for screening, compared with 18% (95% CI 12–25%) for the pap smear (Quek *et al.*, 1998).

The TruScan* tissue classification is based on a reference diagnosis established primarily by review of colposcopic and histologic results. As a result they do not map directly to cytologic classification systems and could potentially

be used to resolve cytologically equivocal smear results (Quek *et al.*, 1998). Initial studies using an early prototype suggested that false-positive/negative rates in the order of 10% were achievable (Coppleson *et al.*, 1994). Ongoing clinical trials are underway to evaluate the efficacy of the system:

1 as an adjunct to the pap smear;
2 as a form of triage for women with minor cytologic abnormalities;
3 as a primary screening alternative to the pap smear.

Visual inspection-based techniques

Speculoscopy

Speculoscopy is a visual screening procedure that uses low power magnification and chemoluminescent light, which improves observer ability to detect acetowhite changes on the cervix (Lonky & Edwards, 1992). A chemoluminescent light is used to illuminate the cervix in a darkened room and a handheld optic with magnification is then used to examine the cervix for acetowhite areas after the application of 5% acetic acid. This technique has been proposed as a an adjunct to the cervical smear to improve the overall sensitivity for the detection of clinically signifiant CIN (pap plus Speculoscopy, The Trylon Corp, Torrance, CA) (Wertlake *et al.*, 1997).

Other techniques

The use of visual inspection techniques as a screening test is included here only for completeness. They are not proposed as adjunctive tests to the pap smear. These techniques have been proposed for use in developing countries where resources do not permit the establishment of cytologic screening. In fact the World Health Organization (1996) has recommended the evaluation of visual inspection techniques to identify early curable cancer in these countries.

The unaided naked-eye speculum examination of the cervix (also referred to as downstaging) which has been used in India has not been found to be satisfactory in the detection of cervical precancer, having very low positive predictive values (Sehgal *et al.*, 1991; Singh *et al.*, 1992; Nene *et al.*, 1996; Wesley *et al.*, 1997). However two other techniques using 3–4% acetic acid followed by inspection either with magnification (gynoscopy) or without (cervicoscopy) have shown initial promise (Sankaranarayanan *et al.*, 1997). A recent study in Zimbabwe compared cervicoscopy with pap smears in over 10000 women (University of Zimbabwe/JHPIEGO Cervical Cancer Project 1999). The result of this study was that cerviscoscopy was shown to have a high sensitivity for the detection of cervical precancer when compared with pap smears. However, the corresponding specificity was lower.

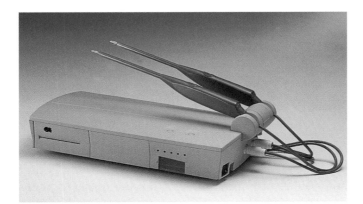

Fig. 5.62

New developments

Fluorescence spectroscopy

This technique has recently appeared as one of the new diagnostic techniques for CIN. It is a non-invasive real-time technique that measures the autofluorescence of tissue based on the amount of natural occurring fluorophores. It would seem as though there are possible differences in fluorophores between malignant and premalignant tissue, and this could account for differences in autofluorescence in the different grades of CIN. Diagnostic algorithms can be developed by using fluorescence spectroscopy that allow reasonable sensitivities and specificities to be developed for the diagnosis of CIN (Ramanujam *et al.*, 1994; Ramanuma *et al.*, 1996). Preliminary results compare favorably to sensitivities in respect of colposcopy when performed by an experienced observer (Mitchell *et al.*, 1999). In a recent review, Mitchell *et al.* (1999) compared fluorescence spectroscopy with other diagnostics techniques using colposcopic biopsy as the reference standard. They calculated receiver operator characteristic (ROC) curves for the different techniques. Fluorescence spectroscopy performed better than colposcopy and other techniques in the diagnosis of squamous intraepithelial lesions (SIL) and they suggested that this real-time technique had the potential of being employed for diagnosis especially by inexperienced operators. However, large-scale trials will be required to validate these findings.

5.12 Problems in cytologic screening in the postmenopausal era

Alterations in function

In the postmenopausal era, the estrogen stimulus is withdrawn, resulting in a general deterioration in the tissues of the lower genital tract. This is seen particularly in the cervix and vagina where the squamous epithelium, dependant on estrogens for maturity, becomes thin and atrophic. This results in the alteration of the structure of the exfoliative cells and leads to an increase in local vaginal infection. In turn, this will further distort the quality of the exfoliated cells (Fig. 5.63).

As the epithelium of the cervix becomes thin and atrophic, it decreases in height to only a few cells with the result that the nuclear:cytoplasmic ratio increases. It must be remembered that the cytoplasm is reduced in quantity, rather than the nucleus is increased, and this may lead to some difficulty in interpretation and differentiation from a CIN. In the case of a CIN, the opposite process occurs in that the cytoplasm remains static in quantity but the nucleus increases. One way to differentiate between the two is to look for mitotic figures that are not seen in the atrophic epithelium. It is also important for the pathologist to recognize that the nuclei are smaller than those found in a CIN. Compounding this problem is the fact that biopsies taken at this time are usually fragmented and of poor quality, owing to the thinness and fragility of the

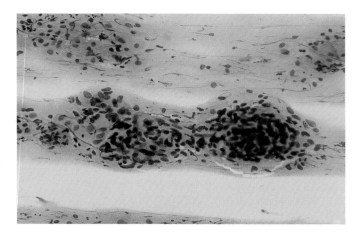

Fig. 5.63

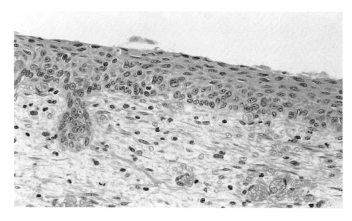

Fig. 5.64 A biopsy of postmenopausal squamous epithelium with the nuclei appearing slightly more prominent than normal due to the loss of cytoplasm. There is no increase in nuclear size, although some hyperchromasia is present. No mitotic activity is present in the epithelium (1). The stroma is inactive (2) but does show the presence of epithelial capillaries. Because of the lack of estrogenic stimulus, maturation and stratification are minimal or absent (as in this case). There is an increased likelihood of petechial hemorrhages occurring during the collection of a postmenopausal smear; this is apparent from the prominence of the capillaries beneath a very atrophic and thinned epithelium.

epithelium. An example of a biopsy taken in the postmenopausal period is shown in Fig. 5.64.

Exfoliated cells also present a classic picture in the postmenopausal era. The nuclei are usually very pale with a very fine chromatin pattern. However, the presence of superadded infection, resulting from the vulnerability of the unestrogenized vaginal mucosa, results in the presence of numerous polymorphous and other inflammatory cells. Degenerative changes, such as pyknosis and karyorrhexis, within the exfoliated cells also confuse the cellular pattern. The presence of infection may cause the nuclei to appear more active than they would normally be. This can result in an increase in false-positivity.

The frequent occurrence of false-negative smears in the postmenopausal period is also as a result of this inflammatory process, in that the normal parabasal cells may become swollen, show some nuclear distortion, and appear similar to dyskaryotic cells. This produces a similar picture to that seen in the postpartum period.

Screening in the postmenopausal era

The postmenopausal era is a time of increased incidence of invasive carcinoma, be it squamous or glandular. False-negative smears can arise not only because of the presence of increased cervicovaginal infection, as mentioned above, but also because of the retraction of the abnormal (atypical) epithelium within the endocervical canal as a result of tissue contraction. It has been shown by some authors (Hartman *et al.*, 1986) that small endocervical lesions could be missed by conventional cytologic sampling.

The size of the lesion and its influence on false-negative rates has already been discussed (Barton *et al.*, 1989) and it has been shown that the overall size of an underlying CIN lesion is more important in determining the cytologic grade than is the histologic grade itself. Therefore, if there is a small lesion situated high in the endocervical canal, then there is a very high risk of a false-negative smear being obtained. This is particularly important for the detection of CIN in women who present with a mildly dyskaryotic smear (Bethesda classification; low-grade squamous intraepithelial lesion) in whom a small CIN 3 endocervical lesion may exist in the presence of a low-grade (i.e. CIN 1) intraepithelial lesion of the ectocervix or lower endocervical canal region. This type of smear in a postmenopausal woman should not be ignored and a repeat smear should be obtained using an endocervical brush (Barton *et al.*, 1989; Jarmulowicz *et al.*, 1989).

Overcoming the problem of collection in the postmenopausal era

It is well known that sampling errors are the major cause of false-negative smears; this is particularly so in the postmenopausal era, as mentioned above in respect of the position and size of endocervical lesions. To overcome this problem in the postmenopausal era various devices have been used to increase the harvest of endocervical cells. There is a higher collection rate of abnormal cells when endocervical columnar cells are present (Vooijs *et al.*, 1985). It has also been shown that the detection of abnormalities in subsequent smears containing endocervical cells was higher when the first "negative" smear did not contain any endocervical cells. Vooijs *et al.* (1985) have shown that with proper instruction in sample taking, endocervical cells can be present in 96% of cervical smears.

The solution to the problem of harvesting endocervical cells lies with the spatulas used for collection. The Ayre's spatula, with its short and blunt endocervical tip, is unsuitable for use in the narrow external os and retracted squamocolumnar junction present in the postmenopausal female. Various plastic and wooden spatulas have been introduced through the years, and the English Aylesbury spatula offers an improvement (Wolfendale *et al.*, 1987). This device, with its narrow endocervical tip, has improved the quality of smears taken from the endocervix. However, it was not till the endocervical brushes were developed that dramatic improvements in cell collection from this area occurred. These brushes (Figs 5.65 & 5.66) are plastic and can be used in conjunction with a spatula device that cleans the ectocervix. The endocervical brush has been shown to increase the presence of endocervical cells so that they are found in 97–98% of samples; this doubles the detection rate of abnormalities in the canal (Boon *et al.*, 1986). These endocervical brushes sample not only the squamocolumnar junction within the endocervical canal but also any glandular lesions present in that area.

---

*Subsequently, Papnet® has ceased to trade and the patents and intellectual property have been purchased by other companies.

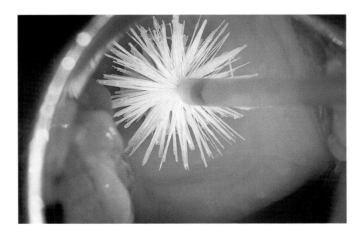

Fig. 5.65 An endocervical brush developed in the Department of Gynaecological Oncology, Queen Elizabeth Hospital, Gateshead, UK.

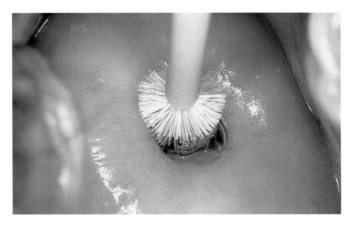

Fig. 5.66 An endocervical brush developed by the Mendscand Company, Malmö, Sweden.

5.13 References

Anderson, M.C. (1995) Glandular lesions of the cervix: diagnostic and therapeutic dilemmas. *Baillière Clin Obstet Gyn* **9**,105.

Anderson, M.C., Jordan, J., Morse, A. & Sharp, F. (1992) *A textbook and Atlas of Integrated Colposcopy*. Chapman and Hall Medical, London.

Autier, P., Coibion, M., De Sutter, P. & Wayemberg, M. (1999) Cytology alone versus cytology and cervicography for cervical cancer screening: a randomized study. *Obstet Gynecol* **93**(3),353.

Ayre, J.E. (1948) Cervical cytology in the diagnosis of early cancer. *JAMA* **136**,513.

Barton, S., Jenkins, D., Hollingsworth, A. & Singer, A. (1989) An exploration for the problems of the false negative cervical smear. *Br J Obstet Gynaecol* **96**,492.

Bavin, P.J., Giles, J.A., Deery, A., Crow, J., Griffiths, P.D., Emery, V.C. *et al.* (1993) Use of semi-quantitative PCR for human papillomavirus DNA type 16 to identify women with high grade cervical disease in a population presenting with a mildly dyskaryotic smear report. *Br J Cancer* **67**,602.

Beeby, A.R., Keating, P.J., Wagstaff, T.I. *et al.* (1993) The quality and accuracy of cervical cytology: a study of five sampling devices in a colposcopy clinic. *J Obstet Gynecol* **13**,276.

Boon, M.E., Alons-van-Cordelaar, J.J.M. & Rietveld-Scheffers, P.E.M. (1986) Consequences of the introduction of combined spatula and cytobrush sampling for cervical cytology. Improvements in smear quality and detection rates. *Acta Cytol* **30**,264.

Boon, M.E., Baak, J.P.A., Kurver, P.J.H., Overdiep, S.H. & Verdonk, G.W. (1981) Adenocarcinoma in situ of the cervix: an undiagnosed lesion. *Cancer* **48**,768.

Bousefield, L., Pacey, F., Young, Q., Krumins, I. & Osborn, R. (1980) Extended cytologic criteria for the diagnosis of adenocarcinoma-in-situ of the cervix and related lesions. *Acta Cytol* **24**,283.

Boyes, D.A. (1981) The value of a pap smear program and suggestions for its implementation. *Cancer* **48**,613.

British Society for Clinical Cytology (BSCC). (1994) Borderline nuclear changes in cervical smears: Guidelines on their recognition and management. *J Clin Pathol* **47**,92.

Campion, M.J., McCance, D.J., Cuzick, J. *et al.* (1986) Progressive potential of mild cervical atypia: Prospective cytological, colposcopic, and virological study. *Lancet* **2**,237.

Christophereson, W.M., Nealon, N., Gray, L.A. Snr. (1979) Noninvasive precursor lesions of adenocarcinoma and mixed adenosquamous carcinoma of the cervix uteri. *Cancer* **44**,975.

Coppleson, M., Reid, B.L., Skladnev, V. *et al.* (1994) An electronic approach to the detection of pre-cancer and cancer of the uterine cervix: a preliminary evaluation of the Polrprobe. *Int J Gynecol Cancer* **4**,79.

Corkhill, M., Knapp, D., Martin, J. & Hutchinson, M.L. (1997) Specimen adequacy of Thin Prep® sample preparations in a direct-to-vial study. *Acta Cytol* **41**,39.

Cox, T.J., Lorincz, A.T., Schiffman, M.H. *et al.* (1995) Human papillomavirus testing by hybrid capture appears to be useful in triaging women with a cytologic diagnosis of atypical squamous cells of undetermined significance. *Am J Obstet Gynecol* **172**,946.

Cuzick, J., Szarewski, A., Terry, G. *et al.* (1995) Human papillomavirus testing in primary cervical screening. *Lancet* **345**,1533.

Cuzick, J., Terry, G., Ho, L., Hollingsworth, T. & Anderson, M. (1992) Human papillomavirus type 16 DNA in cervical smears as a predictor of high grade intraepithelial neoplasia. *Lancet* **339**,959.

De Sutter, P.H., Coibion, M. & Vosse, M. (1998) A multicentre study comparing cervicography and cytology in the detection of cervical intraepithelial neoplasia. *Br J Obstet Gynaecol* **105**,613.

Duncan, I.D. (1997) Screening programmes: results and expectations. In: Franco, E. & Monsonego, J. (eds) *New Developments in Cervical Cancer Screening and Prevention*, p. 187. Blackwell Science, Oxford.

Eskridge, C., Begneaud, W.P. & Landwehr, C (1998) Cervicography combined with repeat Papanicolaou test as triage for low-grade cytologic abnormalities. *Obstet Gynecol* **92**,351.

Evans, D.M., Hudson, E.A., Brown, C.L. *et al.* (1986) Terminology in gynaecological cytopathology; report of the working party of the British Society for Clinical Cytology. *J Clin Pathol* **39**,933.

Ferenczy, A., Franco, E. & Arseneau, J. (1996) Diagnosic performance of hybrid capture human papillomavirus deoxyribonucleic acid assay combined with liquid-based cytologic study. *Am J Obstet Gynecol* **175**,651.

Ferenczy, A., Robitaille, J. & Franco, E. (1996) Conventional cervical cytologic smears vs. ThinPrep smears—a paired comparison study on cervical cytology. *Acta Cytol* **40**,1136.

Ferris, D.G., Payne, P. Frisch, L.E. *et al.* (1993) Cervicography: adjunctive cervical cancer screening by primary care physicians. *J Fam Pract* **37**,158.

Ferris, D.G., Wright, T.C., Litaker, M.S. *et al.* (1998) Triage of women with ASCUS and LSIL on pap smear reports: management by repeat pap smear, HPV testing or colposcopy? *J Fam Pract* **46**,125.

Giles, J.A. (1989) The accuracy of repeat cytology in woman with mildly dyskaryotic smears. *Br J Obstet Gynaecol* **96**(9),1067.

Hall, S., Lorincz, A., Shah, F. *et al.* (1996) Human papillomavirus DNA detection in cervical specimens by hybrid capture: correlation with cytologic and histologic diagnoses of squamous epithelial lesions of the cervix. *Gynec Oncol* **62**,353.

Hartman, B., Kaplan, B. & Dun, D. (1986) Morphometric analysis of dysplasia in cervical cone biopsy specimens in cases with false negative cytology. *Obstet Gynecol* **68**,832.

Hatch, K.D., Schneider, A. & Abdel-Nour, M.W. (1995) An evaluation of human papillomavirus testing for intermediate and high-risk types as triage before colposcopy. *Am J Obstet Gynecol* **172**,1150.

Herber, A. (ed.) (1995) *Achievable Standards, Benchmarks for Reporting and Criteria for Evaluating Cytopathology*. NHSCSP, Sheffield.

Hutchinson, M., Isenstein, L.M., Goodman, A. *et al.* (1994) Homogeneous sampling accounts for the increased diagnostic accuracy using the ThinPrep processor. *Am J Clin Pathol* **101**,215.

Jarmulowicz, M.R., Jenkins, D., Barton, S.E. & Singer, A. (1989) Cytological status and lesion size: a further dimension in cervical intraepithelial neoplasia. *Br J Obstet Gynaecol* **96**,1061.

Kesic, V.I., Soutter, W.P., Sulovic, V. (1993) A comparison of cytology and cervicography in cervical screening. *Int J Gynecol Cancer* **3**,395.

Kinney, W.K., Manos, M.M., Hurley, L.B. *et al.* (1998) Where's the high grade cervical neoplasia? The importance of minimally abnormal Papanicolaou diagnoses. *Am J Obstet Gynecol* **91**,973.

Koos, L.G. (1992) *Diagnostic Cytology and its Histopathologic Basis*, 4th edn. J.B. Lippincott, Philadelphia.

Korn, A.P., Judson, P.L. & Zaloudetz, C.J. (1998) Importance of atypical glandular cells of uncertain significance in cervical cytologic smears. *J Reprod Med* **43**,774.

Koss, L.G. (1989) The Papanicolaou test for cervical cancer detection: a triumph and a tragedy. *JAMA* **261**,737.

Koss, L.G., Lin, E., Schreiber, K., Elgert, P. & Mango, L. (1994) Evaluation of the Papnet Cytological Screening System for quality control of cervical smears. *Am J Clin Pathol* **101**(2),220.

Koss, L.G., Stewart, F.W., Foote, F.W. *et al.* Some histological aspects of behaviour of epidermoid carcinoma in situ and related lesions of the uterine cervix. *Cancer* **16**,1160.

Kreiger, P. & Bibbo, M. (1997) Our journey towards improved accuracy in cytology: the role of new technologies. *Acta Cytol* **41**,11.

Laara, E., Day, N.E. & Hakama, M. (1987) Trends in mortality from cervical cancer in the Nordic countries: association with organised screening programmes. *Lancet* **1**,1247.

Lee, K.R. (1997) Papanicolaou smear sensitivity for adeno-carcinoma in situ of the cervix. A study of 34 cases. *Am J Clin Pathol* **107**,30.

Lee, K.R., Ashfaq, R., Birdsong, G.G. *et al.* (1997) Comparison of conventional Papanicolaou smears and a fluid-based, thin-layer system for cervical cancer screening. *Obstet Gynecol* **90**,278.

Londsborough, P., Ho, L., Terry, G. *et al.* (1996) Human

papillomavirus genotype as a predictor of persistence and development of high grade lesions in women with minor cervical abnormalities. *Int J Cancer* **69**,364.

Lonky, N.M. & Edwards, G. (1992) Chemoluminescent light improves observer ability to visualize aceto-white epithelium. *Am J Gynecol Health* **6**,11.

Lonky, N.M., Navare, G.L., Saunders, S. *et al.* (1995) Low grade Papanicolaou smears and the Bethesda System: a prospective cytopathologic analysis. *Obstet Gynecol* **85**,716.

Lorincz, A. (1996) Hybrid capture method for detection of human papillomavirus DNA in clinical specimens. *Papillomavirus Rep* **7**,1.

Lorincz, A. (1999) Cervical cancer screening clinical trial results. Proceedings of the 17th International Papillomavirus Conference, January 1999, Charleston. *Lancet* **253**,1382.

McGoogan, E. & Reith, A. (1996) Would monolayers provide more representative samples and improved preparations for cervical screening? *Acta Cytol* **40**,107.

Maini, M., Lavie, O., Comeerci, G. (1998) The management and follow-up of patients with high-grade cervical glandular intraepithelial neoplasia. *Int J Gynecol Cancer* **8**,287.

Mango, L.J. (1994) Computer-assisted cervical cancer screening using neural networks. *Cancer Lett* **77**,155.

Manos, M.N., Kinney, W.K., Hurley, L.B. *et al.* (1999) Identifying women with cervical neoplasia—using human papillomavirus DNA testing for equivocal Papanicolaou results. *JAMA* **281**(17),1605.

Meisels, A. & Fortin, R. (1976) Condylomatous lesions of the cervix and vagina. I. Cytological patterns. *Acta Cytol* **20**,505.

Metcalf, K.S., Sutton, J., Moloney, M.D. *et al.* (1994) Which cervical sampler? A comparison of four methods. *Cytopathology* **5**,219.

Mitchell, H., Medley, G. & Giles, G. (1990) Cervical cancers diagnosed after negative results on cytology: perspective in the 1980s. *BMJ* **300**,1622.

Mitchell, M.F., Cantor, S.B., Ramanujam, N. *et al.* (1999) Fluorescence spectroscopy for diagnosis of squamous intraepithelial lesions of the cervix. *Obstet Gynecol* **93**(3),462.

Morell, N.D., Taylor, J.R., Snyder, R.N. *et al.* (1982) False negative cytology rates in patients in whom invasive cancer subsequently developed. *Obstet Gynecol* **60**,41.

National Audit Office (1998) *The Performance of the NHS Cervical Screening Programme in England.*

National Cancer Institute Workshop. (1988) The 1988 Bethesda system for reporting cervical/vaginal cytologic diagnoses. *J Am Med Assoc.* **262**,931.

National Cancer Institute Workshop. (1992a) The revised Bethesda system for reporting cervical/vaginal cytologic diagnoses: Report of the 1991 Bethesda Workshop. *Anal Quant Cytol Histol* **14**,161.

National Cancer Institute Workshop (1992b) The revised Bethesda System for reporting cervical/vaginal cytologic diagnoses: Report of the 1991 Bethesda Workshop. *Acta Cytol* **36**(3),273.

Nene, B.M., Deshpande, S., Jayoant, K. *et al.* (1996) Early detection of cervical cancer by visual inspection: a population-based study in rural India. *Int J Cancer* **68**,770.

Nobbenhuis, M., Walboomers, J.M., Helmerhorst, T.J., Rozendaal, L. *et al.* (1999) Relation of human papillomavirus status to cervical lesions and consequences for cervical cancer screening: a prospective study. *Lancet* **354**,20.

Nuovo, J., Melnikow, J., Hutchison, B. & Paliescheskey, M. (1997) *J Am Board Fam Pract* **10**(6),390.

Office for National Statistics. (1996) *Monitor; Population and Health.* MB1 96/2.

Papanicolaou, G.N. (1928) *New Cancer Diagnosis.* Proceedings Third Race Betterment Conference, Battle Creek, Michigan. Race Betterment Foundation.

Papanicolaou, G.N. (1954) *Atlas of Exfoliative Cytology.* The Commonwealth Fund, New York.

Papanicolaou, G.N. & Traul, H.F. (1999) Diagnosis of uterine cancer by the vaginal smear. The Commonwealth Fund, New York. Now published by Harvard University Press, Cambridge, Mass. (In press.)

Pisani, P., Parkin, D.M. & Ferlay, J. (1993) Estimates of the worldwide mortality from 18 major cancers in 1985. Implications for protection and projection of future burden. *Int J Cancer* **55**,891.

Pritchard, J. (ed.) (1996) *Quality Assurance Guidelines for the Cervical Screening Programme.* NHSCSP, Sheffield.

Purola, E. & Savia, E. (1977) Cytology of gynecologic condyloma acuminatum. *Acta Cytol* **21**,26.

Quek, S.C., Mould, T., Canfell, K. *et al.* (1998) The Polarprobe—emerging technology for cervical cancer screening. *Ann Acad Med Singapore* **27**,712.

Ramanujam, N., Mitchell, M.F., Mahadevan, A. *et al.* (1994) Fluorescence spectroscopy: a diagnostic tool for cervical intraepithelial neoplasia (CIN) *Gynecol Oncol* **52**,31.

Ramanujam, N., Mitchell, M.F., Mahadevan-Jansen, A. *et al.* (1996) Cervical precancer detection using a mutivariate statistical algorithm based on laser induced fluorescence spectra at multiple excitation wavelengths *Photochem Photobiol* **64**,720.

Reagan, J.W. & Harmonic, M.J. (1956) The cellular pathology in carcinoma in situ; a cytohistopathological correlation. *Cancer* **9**, 385.

Reagan, J.W., Ng, A.B.P. & Wentz, W.B. (1969) Concepts of genesis and development in early cervical neoplasia. *Obstet Gynecol Surv* **24**,860.

Reid, R., Greenburg, M.D., Lorincz, A. *et al.* (1991) Should cervical cytological testing be augmented by cervicography or human papillomavirus deoxyribonucleic acid detection? *Am J Obstet Gynecol* **164**,1461.

Richart, R.M. (1968) Natural history of cervical intraepithelial neoplasia. *Clin Obstet Gynecol* **10**,748.

Sankaranarayanan, R., Syamalakumari, B., Wesley, R. *et al.* (1997) Visual inspection as a screening test for cervical cancer control in developing countries. In: Franco, E. & Monsonego, J. (eds), *New Developments in Cervical Cancer Screening and Prevention*, Blackwell Science, Oxford. p. 411.

Sasieni, P. (1996) Cervical sampling devices. *BMJ* **313**,1275.

Sasieni, P., Cuzick, J. & Farmery, E. (1995) Accelerated decline in cervical cancer mortality in England and Wales. *Lancet* **346**, 1566.

Saurel, J. (1996) Adenocarcinoma in situ of the cervix uteri: cytologic and histologic aspects. *Ann Pathol* **16**(5),374.

Sehgal, A., Singh, V., Bhambhani, S. & Luthra, U.K. (1991) Screening for cervical cancer by direct inspection. *Lancet* **338**,282.

Selvaggi, S.M. & Haefner, H.K. (1997) Microglandular endocervical hyperplasia and tubal metaplasia: pitfalls in the diagnosis of adenocarcinoma on cervical smears. *Diagn Cytopathol* **16**,168.

Sigurdsson, K. (1995) Quality assurance in cervical cancer screening: the Icelandic experience 1964–1993. *Eur J Cancer* **31**,728.

Singer, A. (1995) Cervical cancer screening: state of the art. In: Jones III, H.W. (ed.) *Cervical Intraepithelial neoplasia*, p. 43. Ballière, London.

Singh, V., Sehgal, A. & Luthra, U.K. (1992) Screening for cervical cancer by direct inspection. *BMJ* **304**,534.

Siziopikou, K.P. (1997) Cytologic features of neoplastic lesions in endocervical glands. *Diagn Cytopathol* **17**,1.

Smith, P.A. & Turnbull, L.S. (1997) Small cell and "pale" dyskaryosis. *Cytopathology* **8**,3.

Soutter, P. (1986) Should patients with mild atypia in a cervical smear be referred for colposcopy? *Br J Obstet Gynaecol* **93**(1),70.

Stafl, A. (1985) Cervicography: a new method for cervical cancer detection. *Am J Obstet Gynecol* **152**,192.

Stewart, C.J.R. (1993) Borderline nuclear abnormality in cervical smears: a cytological review of 2000 cases with histological correlation. *Cytopathology* **4**(6),339.

University of Zimbabwe/JHPIEGO Cervical Cancer Project. (1999) Visual inspection with acetic acid for cervical-cancer screening: test qualities in a primary-care setting. *Lancet* **353**,869.

Usman, F. (1998) Cervical screening: management of patients referred for colposcopy with smear abnormalities less severe than dyskaryosis. *Cytopathology* **9**,100.

Van Wijngaarden, W.J., Duncan, I.D. & Hussain, K.A. (1995) Screening for cervical neoplasia in Dundee and Angus: 10 years on. *Br J Obst Gynaecol*, **102**,137.

Vooijs, P.G., Elias, A., van der Graf, Y. & Verling, S. (1985) Relationship between the diagnosis of epithelial abnormalities and the composition of cervical smears. *Acta Cytol* **29**,323.

Walker, E.M., Dodgson, J. & Duncan, I.D. (1986) Does mild atypia on a cervical smear warrent further investigation? *Lancet* **2**(8508),672.

Wertlake, P.T., Francus, K., Newkirk, G.R. *et al.* (1997) Effectiveness of the Papanicolaou smear and speculoscopy compared with the Papanicolaou smear alone: a community-based clinical trial. *Obstet Gynecol* **90**,421.

Wesley, R., Sankaranarayanan, R., Mathew, B. *et al.* (1997) Evaluation of visual inspection as a screening test for cervical cancer. *Br J Cancer* **75**,436.

Wilbur, D.C. (1995) Endocervical glandular atypia: A "new" problem for the cytologist. *Diagn Cytopathol* **13**(5),463.

Wilbur, D.C., Prey, M.U., Miller, W.M., Pawlick, G.F. & Colgan, T.J. (1998) The AutoPap system for primary screening in cervical cytology—comparing the results of a prospective, intended-use study with routine manual practice. *Acta Cytol* **42**,214.

Wolfendale, M.R., Howe-Guest, R., Usherwood, M.M. & Draper, G.J. (1987) Controlled trial of a new cervical spatula. *Br Med J* **294**,33.

Wright, T.C., Sun, X.W. & Kuolos, J. (1995) Comparison of management algorithms for the evaluation of women with low-grade cytologic abnormalities. *Obstet Gynecol* **85**,202.

Chapter 6
Diagnosis of Cervical Precancer
The use of colposcopy

6.1 Introduction

In the diagnosis of cervical precancer the three modalities, namely cytology, colposcopy and histopathology are interlinked and complementary. They must be used by the clinician, who should understand and be aware of the advantages and disadvantages of each technique. The realization that there is a variable malignant potential in many cervical epithelial lesions has been translated into a more realistic classification of these lesions by the use of the three modalities. Each has now rationalized the classification into lesions that are at high or low risk of progression to malignancy.

Histopathologists reserve the term high-grade cervical intraepithelial neoplasia (CIN) for those lesions that are reckoned to be true precursors of invasive cancer. Likewise, the experienced colposcopist is now able to differentiate lesions into those that are at either high or low risk of progression to malignancy, while cytologists using revised classifications also stress the cellular changes that suggest either low- or high-grade squamous intraepithelial lesions (LSIL or HSIL respectively).

The cytologic assessment of the cervix provides the important link between the gynecologist and the patient. In most screening programs, it is the cervical smear that provides a clue to the presence of abnormality within the cervix and lower genital tract. As a result of this information the clinician is able to select those patients who will need further diagnostic assessment, that is, by colposcopy.

6.2 Which cytologic abnormalities need further investigation?

The presence of an abnormal smear should alert the clinician to the fact that there may well be a precancerous lesion in the cervical epithelium. At present, a number of findings within a cervical smear should dictate either referral of a woman to a specialist clinic where colposcopy can be performed, or examination of the cervix by the practitioner. The indications for referral for colposcopic examination of the cervix are as follows:
1 Any smear suggestive of invasive cancer.
2 The presence of LSIL (The Bethesda System [TBS]) or mild dyskaryosis/borderline nuclear changes (British Society for Clinical Cytology [BSCC] classification); usually two such abnormal smears over a 6-month period as there is a high rate of spontaneous regression. However there is

an increasing argument for the referral of women with a single mildly abnormal smear as studies have shown that among women with minor cytologic abnormalities, up to 30% will have high-grade squamous intraepithelial lesion.
3 The presence of HSIL (TBS) or moderate to severe dyskaryosis.
4 Persistent unsatisfactory smears.
5 The presence of glandular lesions, especially of severe glandular atypia/adenocarcinoma-in-situ (AIS).

Obviously any clinial suspicion of invasive cancer on the cervix would qualify the patient for colposcopic assesment. The presence of contact bleeding of the cervix, of intermenstrual and irregular bloodstained vaginal discharge, or of a suspicious lesion of the cervix, such as a hypertrophied transformation zone, should immediately alert the clinician to the possible presence of cervical malignancy.

6.3 Colposcopy: the initial clinical examination

The types of abnormal smear that qualify the patient for a colposcopic examination were listed in the preceding section. Once the patient has been recommended for an examination there are a number of conditions that must be satisfied by the colposcopist before a satisfactory opinion can be given on the nature of the lesion. It is important that:
1 The clinician be familiar with the different morphologic features of the epithelium and its vasculature that may harbor precancerous lesions.
2 The clinician should have a knowledge of the extent of any lesion and, most importantly, any progression of this lesion within the endocervical canal.
3 The clinician employs accurate methods of biopsy to sample the epithelium of either the endo- or ectocervix; within the former, endocervical curettage may be used.
Figure 6.1 shows the varied topographic arrangements of the major pathologic lesions within the cervix and its epithelium that give rise to abnormal (atypical) colposcopic findings. The important features of these lesions that are noted on the colposcopic examination can be seen.

6.4 The rationale for the use of colposcopy in the diagnosis of cervical precancer

Colposcopy with associated biopsy is described as the "gold standard" for the diagnosis of cervical precancer. In

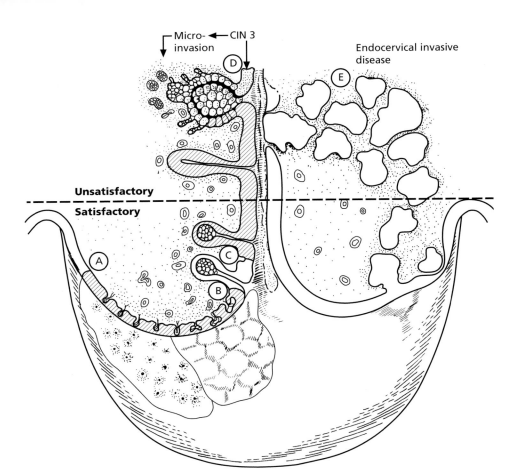

Micro- ◄── CIN 3
invasion

Endocervical invasive
disease

Unsatisfactory
Satisfactory

Fig. 6.1 A diagrammatic representation of the cervix showing the different topographic arrangement of the pathologic epithelia that may be examined by colposcopy. (A) and (B) An ectocervical area of epithelial abnormality with specific morphologic features and associated abnormal vascularity giving rise to the characteristic punctation and mosaic appearances that are visible colposcopically. (C) (shaded) A cervical intraepithelial neoplasia (CIN) lesion extends into the endocervix; the upper limit is not visible. Continuation of the lesion above a certain line (dashed horizontal line) signifies the border between a satisfactory and, in this case, unsatisfactory colposcopic examination (the upper extent of the lesion is not visible). (D) (stippled) An endocervical lesion such as the one shown here may be purely an extension of major intraepithelial disease, such as CIN 3, or may occur in conjunction with an early invasive cancer, i.e. microinvasive carcinoma. Special techniques are needed to determine the exact extent of this lesion within the endocervix. (E) Very occasionally, endocervical invasive carcinoma may present initially in this area within the endocervical canal. Examination is required to ensure that such lesions as this are not missed; the presentation would be that of an unsatisfactory colposcopic examination.

the USA approximately 50 million Papanicolaou smears are performed annually and of these approximately 2.5 million (5%) show evidence of low-grade abnormalities and the usual management of these low-grade lesions is a combination of both colposcopy and directed biopsy. The cost of these procedures has been estimated at approximately $6 billion annually.

There have been very few objective analyses of the efficacy or performance of colposcopy. Recently, however, a detailed study by Mitchell *et al.* (1998) has confirmed that colposcopy, when compared with other diagnostic techniques in medicine, has a very acceptable sensitivity, specificity and positive predictive value. This study is in the form of a meta-analysis of some 86 articles in which colposcopy had been used. They used a variety of statistical methods which compared colposcopy with other diagnostic techniques. They showed that the actual sensitivity of diagnostic colposcopy was high ranging between 87% and 99%, but its specificity was lower at between 23% to 87%. In the diagnosis of high-grade epithelial lesions there were characteristic distinguishing features that allowed them to be better separated from low-grade lesions and it appeared that this differentiation was easier to perform than on separating low-grade lesions from physiological cervical epithelium. This difference supported the validity of the Bethesda cytologic classification, which has been criticized as being arbitrary in its subdivisions. This study was important in that it presented statistical methods that could be used for the evaluation of other diagnostic and screening tests (like HPV testing, Cervicography, TruScan*, etc.) in comparison with colposcopy.

6.5 Colposcopic appearance of the abnormal (atypical) cervical epithelium

The colposcopic morphology of the abnormal (atypical) epithelium harboring the cervical precancerous lesion (or CIN) is dependent on a number of factors. These include:

1 Thickness of the epithelium—a result of a number of cells and their maturation.
2 Alterations in surface contour and any associated changes in the covering epithelium (keratinization).
3 Variations in blood vessel patterns.

When acetic acid is applied to this epithelium certain changes occur within the cellular proteins and, more especially, within the cytokeratin portion of the tissue (see p. 37). This biochemical change is seen through the colposcope as a whitening or opaqueness occurring within the visible epithelium. The change is transient and reversible. By comparison, the normal epithelium washed with acetic acid remains unchanged, retaining its translucent pink color. Also, a sharp line develops between the normal and abnormal (atypical) epithelium with the application of acetic acid.

When iodine solution is applied to normal tissue, a brownish stain develops due to the inherent glycogen content. This is the so-called iodine positive or Schiller's test. Other tissue types have variable staining reactions and these will be discussed below.

Morphology of the abnormal (atypical) epithelium

The effect of acetic acid and iodine

Before acetic acid is applied, the normal translucent squamous epithelium reflects the underlying vascular connective tissue. Once acetic acid has been applied and coagulation of the cellular proteins has occurred, the squamous epithelium becomes progressively opaque, initially developing a flat dull appearance that masks the reflection of the underlying connective tissue (see Figs 3.1 & 3.2, p. 34). If there is a thickened or extremely cellular epithelium, as is found in the major-grade CIN lesions (i.e. CIN 3), then the opacity is such that the lesion becomes progressively more white. Because there is a lack of glycogen in this tissue, the application of iodine will produce a relative whiteness within the epithelium; this forms the basis for the iodine or Schiller's test.

In normal epithelium there are minimal amounts of protein and large amounts of glycogen, especially within the cytoplasm, while in the abnormal (atypical) epithelium there is protein in the cell membrane, nuclei, and cytoplasm, but very little glycogen. In lesions where there are significant amounts of both protein and glycogen, as is found in the minor-grade CIN lesions, acetic acid will produce only a slight whitening and opacity of the epithelium. Likewise, the application of iodine will show a weak and unequal staining.

Acetowhite changes are the most important of all the colposcopic features because they are associated with the spectrum of change from normal epithelium (i.e. immature squamous metaplasia) to cancer. Therefore the epithelial changes that may be associated with acetowhiteness include:
1 Immature squamous metaplasia.
2 Healing—regenerating epithelium.

3 Congenital transformation zone.
4 Human papillomavirus infection.
5 CIN.
6 Adenocarcinoma-in-situ.
7 Adenocarcinoma.
8 Invasive squamous carcinoma.

It is therefore important that the physiological and minor pathologic changes are differentiated from more severe neoplastic alterations (i.e. CIN/cancer) within the epithelium. The degree of acetowhiteness is one of four specific colposcopic features that differentiate the normal from the abnormal (atypical) cervical epithelium. The three other features are:
1 Margins.
2 Surface contour.
3 Vascular patterns.

In a study by Kierkegaard *et al.* (1995) the relationship between specific colposcopic signs and histologic grade of cervical lesions was explored. Using logistic regression analysis, it was found that, among others, intensity of acetowhite change, distinct margins and pathology of vessels as single findings were highly statistically correlated to the histologic grade.

Margins

The margins of the abnormal (atypical) cervical epithelium are graded according to a number of features which include the sharpness, shape and thickness of the border and the presence of internal margins.

In more severe or high-grade epithelial abnormalities (CIN) as seen in Figs 6.2a and 6.16 (p. 110) the margins exhibit a distinct raised edge (3). These types of high-grade lesions may be located within a larger low-grade lesion and have an internal margin or demarcation. This is seen in relation to the area 1 and its surrounding tissues and in areas 2 and 3 in Fig. 6.2b. In low-grade or minor lesions the

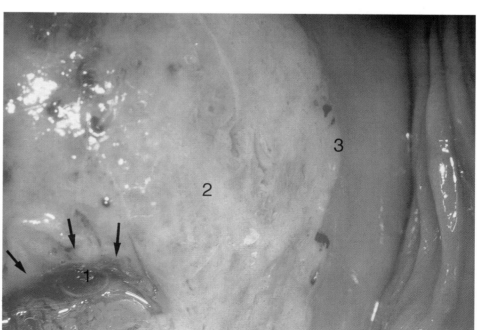

Fig. 6.2 (a) Acetowhite change within the transformation zone showing the upper limit of the process (arrow) within the endocervical canal (1). The thick, abnormal (atypical) epithelium at (2) has stained extremely white and a sharp border (3) indicates the original squamocolumnar junction. (*Continued.*)

Fig. 6.2(a)

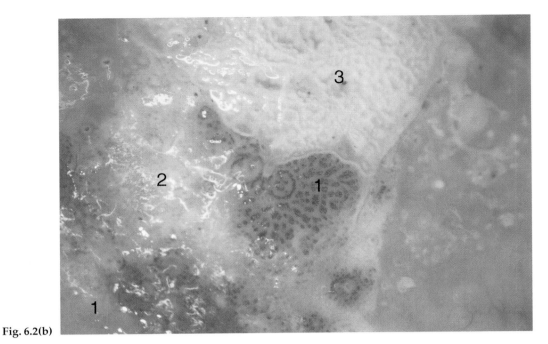

Fig. 6.2(b)

Fig. 6.2 (*Continued*) (b) Punctation (1) seen after the application of acetic acid with acetowhiteness at (2) and changes suggestive of the presence of human papillomavirus (HPV) at (3); this latter tissue also shows acetowhiteness. (*Continued.*)

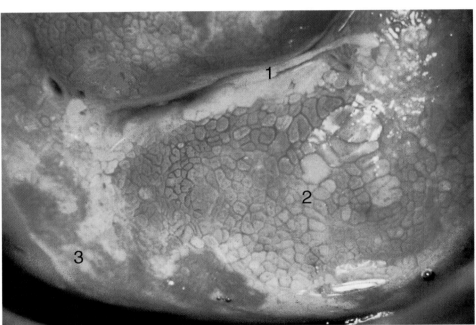

Fig. 6.2(c)

Fig. 6.2 (*Continued*) (c) A mosaic vascular pattern showing coarse mosaic epithelium within a wide field of acetowhiteness that extends into the endocervical canal at (1). The mosaic pattern is at (2) and the sharp squamocolumnar junction is outlined at (3). Note the variation in intercapillary distance within the mosaic field; this indicates different grades of precancerous change. (*Continued.*)

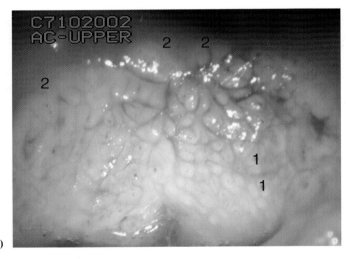

Fig. 6.2(d)

Fig. 6.2 (*Continued*) (d) dense acetowhite epithelium with a coarse mosaic pattern is obvious. Wide intercapillary distances exist as well as the presence of tufted glands at (1). The original squamocolumnar junction is at (2) and the new squamocolumnar junction within the canal cannot be seen.

margins are usually described as irregular, feathered, angular or geographic and indistinct. "Satellite" lesions or exophytic micropapilliferous condyloma-like lesions are similarly low-grade. The contour of these edges or margins is clearly seen in Figs 6.59–6.62 and 6.101 (pp. 129–30, 140).

The effect of surface contour

The stereoscopic magnification produced by colposcopy enables the surface contour to be visualized and can be described as smooth, papillary, nodular, uneven or even ulcerated. For instance, native squamous epithelium has a smooth surface, while columnar epithelium is recognized as grape-like and papillary (see p. 46). High-grade CIN (p. 110), and particularly CIN 3 and early invasion, give an uneven, slightly elevated surface (Fig. 6.16); while the frankly invasive lesions have a nodular or polypoid surface (see p. 145) that finally develops to an ulcerated or exophytic growth pattern (see p. 147).

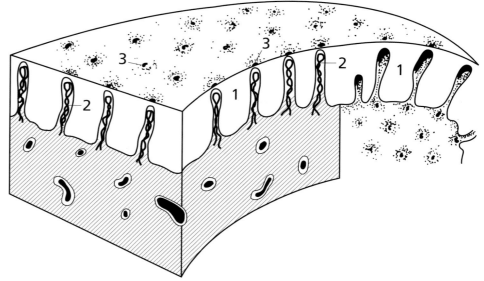

Fig. 6.3(a)

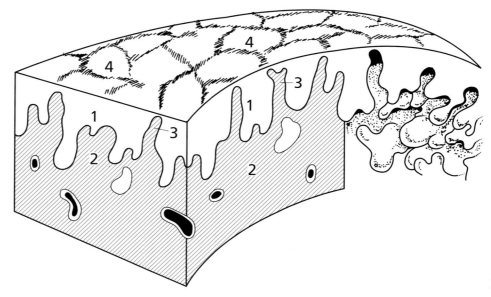

Fig. 6.3 (a) Representation of the punctate areas seen colposcopically. Between the epithelial buds (1), there is a vascular bundle (2) that nearly reaches the surface where the squamous epithelium is very thin. This allows the vessels to be seen through the surface (3). Vessels within the stromal connective tissue can be easily seen. (b) Representation of the mosaic pattern with the epithelial buds (1) protruding into and ramifying within the stromal connective tissue (2). The capillaries between these epithelial buds (3) come close to the surface and where the epithelium is thin the mosaic pattern is easily seen (4).

Fig. 6.3(b)

The colposcopic signs in relation to degrees of aceto-whiteness, margins, vessel formation, and iodine staining, have been used by a number of authors (Reid *et al.*, 1984; Reid, 1990) to differentiate low- and high-grade epithelial lesions and thereby to establish a colposcopic index grading system. This will be described later.

Vascular patterns

Punctation and mosaic

Often in epithelium stained with acetic acid intraepithelial vessels will be absent, but sometimes the appearance of these vascular elements is sufficiently characteristic to warrant names being given to the abnormal appearance. There are two vascular patterns found within the abnormal epithelium: punctation and mosaic. Combinations of these two patterns may also exist. When the capillaries are studded throughout the epithelium and are seen end-on as red points, the term *punctation* is used. Equally common is the appearance of capillaries in a wall-like structure which subdivides blocks of tissues in a honeycomb fashion; this is the so-called *mosaic* pattern.

Punctation is easily recognized by dilated, often twisted, and irregular terminating vessels that are of a hairpin type and can be elongated and arranged in a prominent punctate pattern (Figs 6.2b, 6.3a & 6.5). The area is usually well-defined so that a sharp line separates the normal from the abnormal epithelium (Fig. 6.2b). This pattern of punctation is also seen when there is an inflammation of the tissue, especially in relation to trichomonal infection and cervicitis. The dilated hairpin capillaries are usually diffuse across the ectocervix, with the actual capillaries lying close together with no sharp separation line between normal and abnormal tissue.

In the mosaic pattern the capillaries are arranged parallel to the surface, forming a quasi pavement-like appearance (Figs 6.2c,d & 6.3b). The vessels enclose a vascular field that ranges from small to large and may be regular or irregular in shape (Fig. 6.2c). The vessels themselves may have a complex outline. Histologically, the abnormal (atypical) epithelium forms buds that push, and sometimes ramify, into the connective tissues but are held in place by the basement membrane. When acetic acid is applied to the tissue, a pattern of small white cobblestones is produced, each corresponding to an epithelial bud and surrounded by a red margin that corresponds to the above-described blood vessels. If iodine is applied to the tissue, the abnormal (atypical) squamous epithelium becomes straw-colored and the mosaic pattern disappears.

Formation of punctation and mosaic

One of the mechanisms that has been proposed for the formation of punctation and mosaic epithelium is that during the development of squamous metaplasia within the exposed columnar epithelium, exposure to a mutagenic agent results in the production of an atypical metaplastic process. Kolstad and Stafl (1982) have described the development of punctation and mosaic structures in relation to this atypical metaplasia. They demonstrated that in atypical metaplasia the individual stromal papillae did not coalesce or fuse but the metaplastic squamous epithelium completely filled the clefts and folds of the ectocervical

columnar epithelium (Fig. 6.4a–f). The central vascular networks of the previously grape-like papillae (6.4a) of the columnar epithelium remained as thick stromal papillae (6.4b) surrounded by metaplastic epithelium. At a later stage of development the blood supply of the surface epithelium is probably greater than that found in the normal transformation zone. Any application of acetic acid will show the stromal papillae as red fields surrounded by "white strands" of metaplastic epithelium (6.4c). As atypical metaplastic development proceeds, it is characterized by increased proliferative activity of the epithelium within the clefts, with the resulting compression of the stromal papillae (6.4d–f). Kolstad and Stafl showed that the vessels within these papillae undergo dilatation and proliferation near the surface (6.4d & e) or tend to form a basket-like vascular network around buds of abnormal (atypical) epithelium (6.4d). As seen in Fig. 6.4, a lesion derived from these changes would appear colposcopically as puncta-

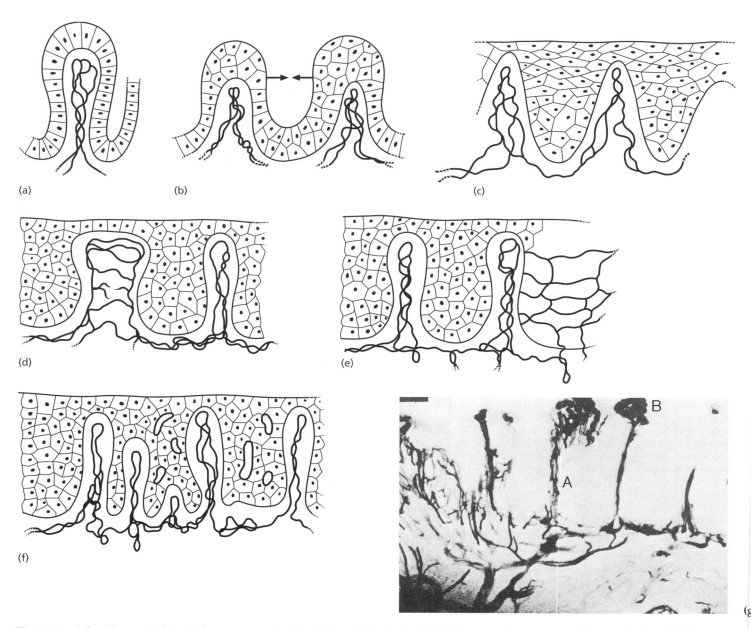

(a)   (b)   (c)

(d)   (e)

(f)   (g)

Fig. 6.4 (a–g) Development of atypical squamous metaplasia (after Kolstad & Stafl, 1982). For an unknown reason the metaplastic epithelium starts to grow in buds or blocks, while the central vascular network, for example the villi of the columnar epithelium, remains as punctate or mosaic vessels that extend close to the surface of the epithelium. The mosaic vessel form basketlike structures around the blocks of neoplastic cells. (g) is a photomicrograph (angiography using alkaline phosphatase 125 μm section) demonstrating this effect. It shows coiled intraepithelial capillaries at A with numerous subepithelial vessels ending in a capillary network beneath the epithelium at B.

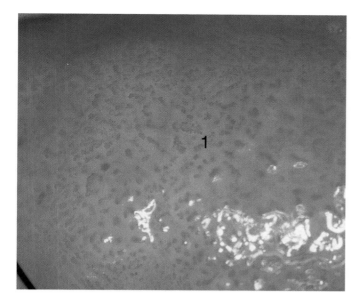

Fig. 6.5 Punctation (1) within a field of intraepithelial neoplasia. This widespread and variable field of punctuated vessels indicates the presence of various degrees of high- and low-grade cervical intraepithelial neoplasia (CIN). Capillaries toward the center of the field are more spaced, indicating a higher degree of CIN compared with the capillaries at the periphery, which are more closely spaced and indicate a lesser degree of abnormality.

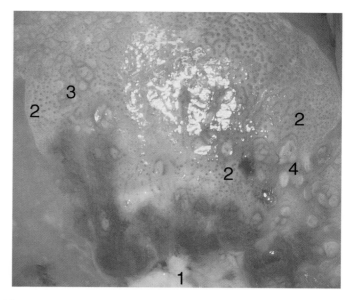

Fig. 6.6 Punctation and mosaic patterns exist in this field of cervical intraepithelial neoplasia (CIN). The endocervical canal is at (1) and areas of punctation exist at (2), but these vary and the more widely spaced capillaries indicate a higher grade of CIN. The same applies in area (3) where there is variation in the intercapillary distance within the mosaic epithelium. In area (4) thick, white epithelium surrounds some gland openings. This lesion comprised essentially low-grade CIN [around (2)] with small areas [around (3) and (4)] of high-grade CIN.

tions and/or a mosaic structure (6.4d). The reason why the epithelium sometimes grows more symmetrically and forms punctations (Fig. 6.5) and at other times grows in larger blocks and forms a mosaic (Fig. 6.6) was not known by Kolstad and Stafl. The development of both mosaic and punctation patterns within the transformation zone is basically similar and so it is not surprising that both can be found in the same lesion, as shown in Fig. 6.6.

Another important feature when assessing an area of mosaic or punctation is intercapillary distance. This refers to the distance between the corresponding parts of two adjacent vessels or to the diameter of fields delineated by network or mosaic-like vessels. In native squamous epithelium the intercapillary distance averages about 100 µm but in preinvasive, and certainly invasive cancer this increases as the malign nature of the lesion increases.

However not all punctation and mosaic patterns are abnormal. This emphasis on abnormal vascular patterns has often led to inexperienced colposcopists overlooking a more severely atypical area, as the majority of squamous intraepithelial lesions do not have colposcopically atypical vessels. Punctation and mosaic may also be found in normal epithelium. In fact Bajardi *et al.* (1959) showed that only 18% of cervices in which mosaic and punctation were present had an underlying neoplastic change. Mosaicism and punctation can also be found in association with acanthotic epithelium (Burghardt *et al.*, 1998), which is a characteristic of the congenital transformation zone (see Section 4.11). In this situation there is extensive budding and branching of the dermal papillae and the interdigitating epithelial pegs (Figs 4.48b,c [p. 67], Fig. 4.50 [p. 68]). The intercapillary distances are variable but are usually not excessive which helps its distinction from a neoplastic

lesion. In the latter the epithelial pegs (i.e. of CIN) are wider, thicker and more irregular.

Burghardt *et al.* (1998) believe that mosaic and punctation appear to be more common outside the transformation zone than within it. He believes that 70% are associated with benign acanthotic epithelium and 30% with CIN. In contrast, within the transformation zone, these patterns correspond to CIN in 80% and with benign acanthotic epithelium in 20% of cases. However most authors would contend that CIN is restricted to the transformation zone, bounded by the original squamocolumnar junction and the new squamocolumnar junction.

Atypical vessels

Atypical vessels have a characteristic appearance and are associated with significant major pathologic changes within the epithelium (Fig. 6.7a–c). They are described as terminal vessels and are characterized by irregularities in shape, course, density, caliber, and spatial arrangement, where the intercapillary distance is larger than that seen between the vessels of the original squamous epithelium. In many cases the vascular pattern may be so irregular that it is indeed impossible to determine whether the pattern is either punctation or mosaic. The atypical vessels may be found in areas where typical punctation and/or mosaic patterns exist. It would seem that by proliferation of these vessels the areas of ordinary mosaic and punctated changes will eventually develop into areas of atypical vessels (Burghardt, 1991). When an irregular pattern such as this develops within fields of punctation and mosaic it may represent the first signs of early invasion, and usually involves the most superficial parts of the basketlike atypical mosaic

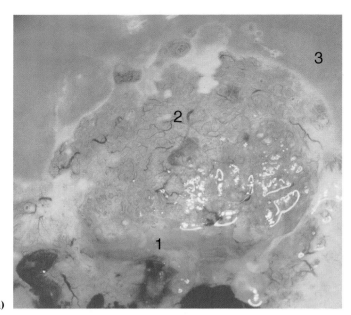

Fig. 6.7(a)

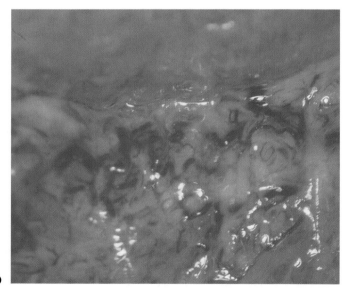

Fig. 6.7(b)

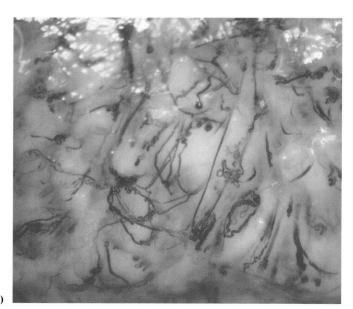

Fig. 6.7(c)

vessels starting to proliferate into the adjacent mosaic fields. Meanwhile, the punctation vessels can be seen with the tops of their loops running parallel with the surface, covered by only a few cell layers. Kolstad and Stafl (1982) believed these horizontal and superficial vessels to be distinctive and indicative of early stromal invasion.

Initially, it seems as though the intercapillary distance within the precancerous tissue is reduced, but as the lesion becomes more malign relatively larger avascular areas are formed. The malign cells are nourished by atypical branches or networklike vessels which, in turn, endow the surface tissue with a coarse meshwork appearance. Kolstad and Stafl (1982) report that they have never seen this type of vessel configuration in a CIN lesion. The atypical vessels branching into these avascular areas show great variation in size, shape, and course; it would seem that the vascular growth has to keep pace with the rapid growth of the malignant cells (Fig. 6.7b & c). Sometimes the growth of these latter cells is so rapid that the blood supply cannot keep up and necrosis develops.

Atypical branch vessels never form the fine network seen in the branch vessels of the transformation zone (Figs 6.8 & 6.9). They do not have the regular treelike pattern with subsequent decrease in the diameter of single branches as is found in physiologic tissues.

Epithelial vascularity is best demonstrated using the technique of saline colposcopy, in which the cervical surface is painted with physiologic saline and viewed at 16× magnification and with a green filter. The blood vessels become obvious and easier to see after the saline has been applied. However, when 3–5% acetic acid is used there is an immediate acetowhitening of the squamous component of the epithelium with a dramatic reduction in the clarity of the vascular pattern. With the green filter *in situ*, and following the application of saline, the red blood vessels appear as dark objects and become much more readily visible. A number of major grade CIN and early invasive lesions are featured in Figs 6.10–6.13.

Fig. 6.7 (a) Atypical vessels seen in a very invasive squamous carcinoma involving both endo- (1) and ectocervix (2). There is a combination of networklike and branched atypical vessels (2). The networklike vessels have an irregular course with sharp bends and show color variation. Branched vessels also have an irregular pattern, and such branches show a characteristic decrease in diameter. Original squamous epithelium is at (3).

(b) Very atypical branching of vessels within the endocervix in an early invasive squamous carcinoma. The gross variation in caliber and irregularity is easily seen by comparison with the physiologic branched vessels in Figs 6.8 and 6.9.

(c) Very irregular and atypical vessels with a corkscrew appearance based on an original branching or network pattern and present in an early invasive carcinoma. Before acetic acid is applied these atypical vessels are visible through the translucent gel formed by the epithelial buds; formation of such gel is characteristic of early invasive carcinoma. The vascular network varies in density in different parts of the tumor and sometimes large vascular loops can be seen to have emerged from the stroma, run over the surface, and then descended into the deeper parts. These large vessels often project considerably above the surface, while the smaller ones are narrow and have a corkscrew configuration.

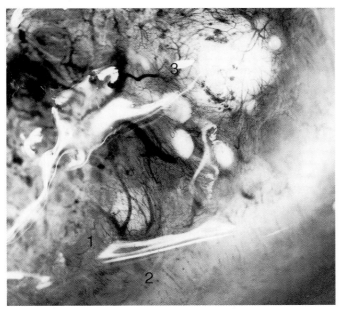

Fig. 6.8

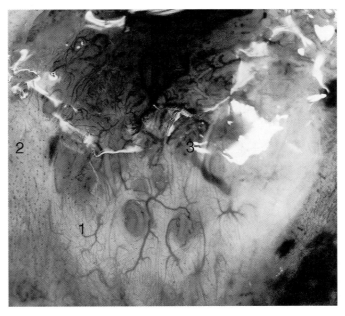

Fig. 6.9

Figs. 6.8 and 6.9 Saline colposcopy has been used to highlight the three types of vessel seen in the normal cervix. A dense and fairly regular meshwork of very fine capillaries, described as *coiled network capillaries*, is seen at (1) in both photographs.

The second type, the so-called *hairpin capillaries*, are characterized by one ascending and one descending branch of a very-fine-caliber vessel; these course together and form a small loop. They sometimes give the appearance of a fine and regular

punctate pattern, as seen at (2) in Figs 6.8 and 6.9.

The third type, occurring predominantly in the transformation zone, is composed of terminal vessels that are seen running parallel with the surface and branching in a treelike manner. These are called *branched vessels* and are shown at (3) in both photographs. Branched vessels divide dichotomously and ultimately lead into a fine network of capillaries with normal intercapillary distances.

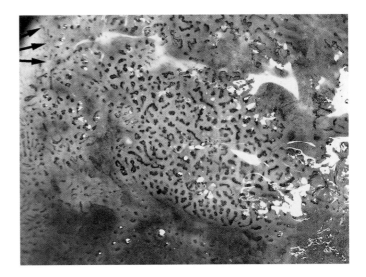

Fig. 6.10 This lesion was shown histologically to be a cervical intraepithelial neoplasia (CIN) 3 with early microinvasion. It has three features that are characteristic of major-grade lesions. First, there is a large intercapillary distance associated with a regular and coarse punctation pattern, with the dilated terminal vessels having a forked or antler-type appearance; this has been referred to as a double capillary pattern. Second, there is an irregular surface contour, seen by reference to the uneven response of the photographic flash; and third, a sharp border exists (arrowed).

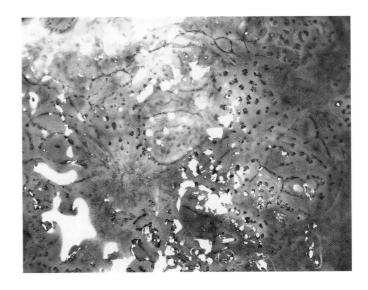

Fig. 6.11 Wide intercapillary distances exist between the hairpinlike punctated vessels and there is a large basketlike dilated vessel in the center, adopting a classic mosaic pattern. The underlying lesion is a cervical intraepithelial neoplasia (CIN) 3.

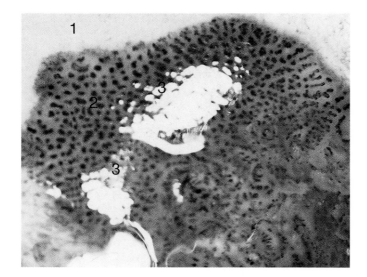

Fig. 6.12 This small focal lesion shows many of the features described for a high-grade precancerous lesion. First, there is a sharp line of demarkation between the native squamous epithelium (1) and the punctated area (2). Second, the lesion is darker than the surrounding tissue; and third, the irregularity (3) on the surface can be clearly seen by the irregular flash reflection. The fourth abnormal sign is that of the hairpinlike and atypical punctated vessels that are coarse; in some places these terminal vessels extend into small papillomatous excrescences (papillary punctation).

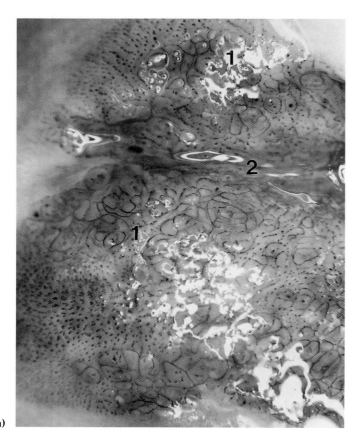

Fig. 6.13(a)

Fig. 6.13 (a) This large lesion, which covers most of the ectocervix (1) and extends into the endocervix at (2), shows five major features characteristic of a high-grade precancerous lesion. First, the vascular pattern is a combination of mosaic and punctation. Clearly demarkated punctation vessels are seen toward the periphery of the lesion, while in the area extending into the endocervix (2) mosaic-type terminal vessels are seen (1). There is a combination of circular, polygonal, hairpin, and occasionally irregular vessels. Some are smoothly curved while others curve irregularly and occasionally there are intertwining strands of dilated capillaries of varying caliber. Like the punctation vessels, these mosaic vessels are observed in relatively distinct areas. Second, the intercapillary distance is increased and variable, signifying variation in the severity of the cervical intraepithelial neoplasia (CIN). Third, there is irregularity in the surface contour: the stereoscopic nature of colposcopy and the magnification have accentuated this feature. The native squamous epithelium at the periphery has a smooth surface, while the CIN lesion, which occupies the whole of the transformation zone, has an uneven surface and is sightly raised compared with the surrounding epithelium. The variation in the flash reflection further accentuates this irregularity. Fourth, there is variation in color tone; this is obvious between the native squamous epithelium and the darker central CIN lesion. Fifth, there is a clear line of demarkation between the native squamous epithelium and the CIN lesion.

(b) A combination of mosaic and punctation patterns exist in this high-grade CIN lesion. However, there is also some leukoplakia (1) present and one area has small plaques that occasionally coalesce to form larger ones. The outline of the area is irregular. Leukoplakia may hide the true nature of the underlying epithelium, although in this lesion the punctation, mosaic pattern, and atypical branching of the surrounding vessels make the lesion an obvious high-grade CIN or early invasive lesion. A sharp line of demarkation associated with the irregular surface contour and the obvious difference in color tone in relation to the native squamous epithelium at (2) are other obvious features of the high-grade lesion.

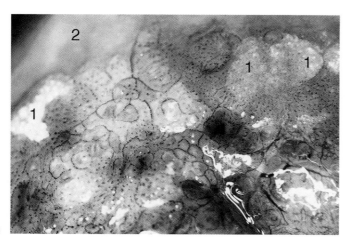

Fig. 6.13(b)

The vascular pattern of early invasion

As has already been discussed, atypical vessels usually indicate invasive cancer (Fig. 6.7a–c). In the earlier stages of invasion it may be difficult for the colposcopist to note a clear distinction between the vascular patterns of CIN, namely punctation and mosaic, and these atypical vessels. In most instances high-grade CIN and early invasion are found together in the cervix, and only a small focus of slightly atypical vessels is seen in a more extensive area of an otherwise typical punctation and mosaic pattern. This is shown in Fig. 6.14a. In this lesion not only is there a difference in color tone and a clear line of demarkation between the native squamous epithelium and the actual precancerous lesion (arrowed), but also there are variations within the vessel characteristics. At (1) there is a typical punctated appearance, signifying a high-grade lesion, but at (2) the mosaic pattern has changed to one of a coarse and irregular structure with extremely large intercapillary distances between the vessels. There is also an avascular-type whiteness appearing within the epithelium. All these features indicate early invasion. In area (3) the smoother mosaic pattern still exists and there is a reduction in the intercapillary distance compared with the area of early invasion at (2).

During the initial development of atypical vessels in areas of typical mosaic and punctation patterns there may be a reduction in the intercapillary distance (Kolstad, 1965; Kolstad & Stafl, 1982). However, as the malignant cells proliferate, so large avascular areas, signified by an increased intercapillary distance, develop. This is clearly seen in Fig. 6.14b, where the typical punctate pattern has been disrupted by the developing atypical capillary loops, which run parallel with the surface into the field of punctation, and where there has been an initial reduction in the intercapillary distance.

When an adenocarcinoma or an anaplastic carcinoma develops it frequently demonstrates a vascular pattern that differs from that of the squamous lesions described so far. The vascular pattern of an adenocarcinoma is consistent with the concept, expounded by Kolstad (1965), that the atypical vessels originate from the central capillary network of the papillary columnar epithelium. The adenocarcinomas seem to derive their nutrition through the central capillary system; this is in contrast to the well-differentiated squamous cell cancers that seem to have a microcirculation characterized by peripheral vessels that surround the epithelial buds but do not seem to have any penetrating vessels. The undifferentiated lesions tend to have fine capillaries penetrating between the epithelial buds of malignant cells. Therefore, the intercapillary distance in these undifferentiated malignancies may be quite normal in many areas. An example of such an early adenomatous malignancy is seen in Fig. 6.14c, where the papillary nature of the columnar epithelium can still be seen with atypical vessels present. The sharp demarkation (arrowed) between the native squamous and the abnormal capillary structures is obvious.

There would seem to be a correlation between definite vascular patterns and the early stages of adenocarcinoma.

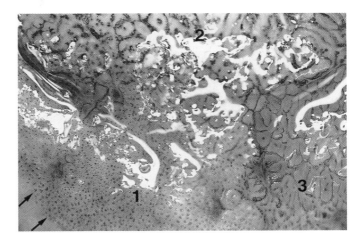

Fig. 6.14(a)

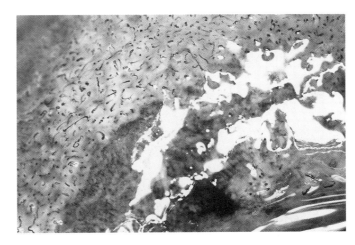

Fig. 6.14(b)

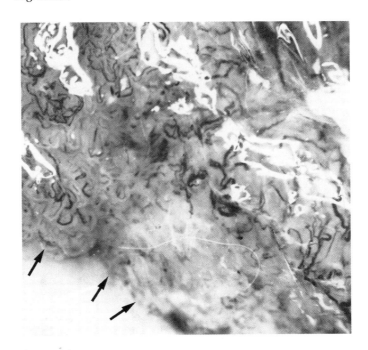

Fig. 6.14(c)

Ueki (1985) and Ueki and Sano (1987) have proposed that there exist specific vascular patterns that are representative of these early stages. These are seen diagrammatically in Fig. 6.15a (adapted from Ueki, 1985). The upper six vessels

Non-malignant

Network-like (NV-1)	Red dotted (NV-2)	Red spotted (NV-3)	Branch-like (NV-4)	Linear (NV-5)	Loop-like (NV-6)

Malignant

Glomeruloid hairpin-like (AV-1)	Corkscrew-like (AV-2)	Mosaic (AV-3)	Tendril-like (AV-4)	Waste-thread-like (AV-5)	Willow-branch-like (AV-6)	Root-like (AV-7)

Fig. 6.15(a)

outlined are present in non-malignant squamous lesions, while the lower seven (including Fig. 6.15b) exist in squamous malignancy. However, in the case of adenocarcinoma, there may be a mixture of both types. As will be seen later in this chapter, there would seem to be specific types associated with the corresponding colposcopically recognized adenocarcinomatous change. It would likewise appear that while mosaic and punctation changes are found in squamous epithelium, they would seem never to be present in adenocarcinomas. However, they are found in some adenosquamous lesions.

Ueki believes that the most common vascular pattern in cases of adenocarcinoma is that of the root-like vessels. In these early stages only one or two such vessels are noted, but in the more advanced stages they are more numerous. Thread-like vessels, described by Ueki (1985) (Fig. 6.15a & b), may also be seen, while in advanced cases tendril-like vessels increase in conjunction with willow-branch vessels. Corkscrew vessels seem never to be present in adenocarcinomatous lesions. Further description of adenocarcinomas is given in Section 6.14 (p. 153).

6.6 The classification of colposcopically abnormal (atypical) cervical epithelium

In the preceding section all the colposcopic features of precancerous and cancerous change within the cervical epithelium were described. A universally agreed classification of these features was formulated at the International Federation of Cervical Pathology and Colposcopy (IFCPC) meeting in Rome (May 1990) (as quoted by Burghardt, 1991; Coppleson & Pixley, 1992b). Previous attempts at classification were hampered by the varied and perplexing terminology that has existed among various national societies.

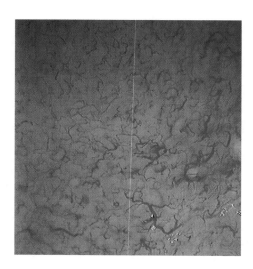

Fig. 6.15 (b) This shows a combination of root and waste thread-like atypical vessels.

The classification is based on the fact that most cervical intraepithelial lesions arise within the transformation zone. The classification also recognizes that there are frequently abnormal colposcopic appearances, most notably attributed to HPV, that occur within the original squamous epithelium. These lesions have little or no neoplastic potential and generally represent the subclinical papillomavirus infection (SPI) that will be described below. However, it was felt that it was no longer appropriate to describe all abnormal (atypical) colposcopic appearances as representing images present within the broad category of the atypical transformation zone. This had not previously been recognized by IFCPC terminology.

Table 6.1 International colposcopic terminology.

Normal colposcopic findings
Original squamous epithelium
Columnar epithelium
Normal transformation zone

Abnormal colposcopic findings
(within the transformation zone)
Acetowhite epithelium*
   Flat
   Micropapillary or microconvoluted
Punctation*
Mosaic*
Leukoplakia*
Iodine negative
Atypical vessels

Colposcopically suspect invasive carcinoma

Unsatisfactory colposcopy
Squamocolumnar junction not visible
Severe inflammation or severe atrophy
Cervix not visible

Miscellaneous findings
Non-acetowhite micropapillary surface
Exophytic condyloma
Inflammation
Atrophy
Ulcer
Other

* Indicates minor or major changes. Minor changes: acetowhite epithelium, fine mosaic, fine punctation, thin leukoplakia. Major changes: dense acetowhite epithelium, coarse mosaic, coarse punctation, thick leukoplakia, atypical vessels, erosion. (Ratified by the International Federation of Cervical Pathology and Colposcopy, at Rome, Italy, May 1990.)

There has been recent criticism of this classification by many authors, particularly Burghardt (1991) who believes that "there are many colposcopic images which show all the attributes of physiological epithelium within the transformation zone but whose native colour and reaction with acetic acid or iodine show them to be abnormal." He calls the previously defined atypical transformation zone, the unusual transformation zone.

The words "atypical" and "abnormal" have been used in many classifications over the last 30 years. Indeed, "abnormal" is used in the new IFCPC classification. In Spanish, and to a lesser extent in German, the word "atypical" has serious connotations, while the word "abnormal" in these languages is too close to "normal." Coppleson and Pixley (1992b) have proposed a compromise that would use both "atypical" and "abnormal." The authors agree with this and these terms will be used synonymously throughout this text. The IFCPC classification is presented in Table 6.1.

6.7 Colposcopic examination of the precancerous/cancerous cervix

The most important part of the examination of the abnormal (atypical) colposcopic epithelium is to obtain a clear view of the full topography and morphology of the lesion (Fig. 6.1). The topography involves determining the outer and inner limits of the abnormal (atypical) region, while the morphology involves making a precise examination of all the features detailed in the previous section, such as vascular pattern, intercapillary distance, surface contour, color tone, and clarity of demarkation. The assessment of the inner limit is one of the most important parts of the examination because it will allow distinction to be made between a satisfactory and an unsatisfactory colposcopy.

A satisfactory or an unsatisfactory colposcopy

A satisfactory colposcopic examination is defined as one in which the new squamocolumnar junction and the full extent of abnormal (atypical) epithelium are visible. An unsatisfactory examination is one in which the new squamocolumnar junction is not visible (Figs 6.16–6.19), or where severe inflammation or severe atrophy make it impossible for the examiner to determine the upper limits of the lesions. The limits are clearly defined by the new squamocolumnar junction and it signifies the upper extent of the abnormal (atypical) epithelium within the endocervical canal. An example of this can be seen in the histologic specimen in Fig. 6.20; this specimen has resulted from a loop excision of an ecto- and endocervical lesion. The ectocervical part of the lesion is present between points (1) and (2), while the endocervical limits extend from (2) to (3) with the new squamocolumnar junction in the region of (3). The lesion itself is a high-grade intraepithelial lesion (CIN 3) and extends deep into the glands of the endocervix at (4). The area between (2) and (3), situated high in the endocervical canal, would most likely have been associated with an unsatisfactory colposcopic picture.

Grading of the abnormal (atypical) colposcopic findings

The great variability shown in precancerous and cancerous changes is such that no single appearance can be called characteristic. The admixture of the variable blood vessel patterns with varying degrees of epithelial maturity associated with alterations in surface contour, color, and demarkation all determine the great variability in the resulting image. A number of grading systems have been devised to increase the objectivity of colposcopic grading and reduce the inter- and intraobserver variability. This provides a less subjective approach to the differentiation between low and high grade colposcopic changes. One such system, is suggested by Coppleson and Pixley (1992b). The scheme employs a practical subdivision of the appearances into those that are insignificant (grade 1), significant (grade 2), and highly significant (grade 3). In grade 1, the lesions show minimal neoplastic potential and invasion is likely to be years away, if it ever occurs; grade 2 comprises lesions that have a neoplastic potential but where invasion is not imminent; and grade 3 covers those lesions that have a high neoplastic potential and where invasion is imminent. The Coppleson and Pixley (1992b) subdivision allows some diagnostic and prognostic

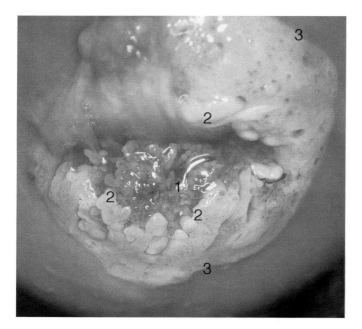

Fig. 6.16 A satisfactory colposcopic picture has been obtained for the posterior lip with the original columnar epithelium at (1), the new squamocolumnar junction at (2), and the original squamocolumnar junction at (3). On the anterior lip, the upper limit of the lesion is not so clearly seen as on the posterior lip, and it seems to be hidden behind some mucus. Until this mucus is removed, the nature of the epithelium on the anterior lip cannot be determined, and this constitutes an unsatisfactory picture.

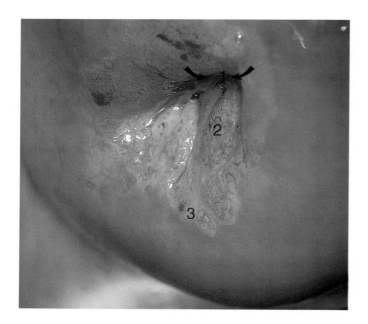

Fig. 6.17 An unsatisfactory colposcopic image is shown with the abnormal (atypical) and high-grade epithelial lesion (2) extending into the endocervix (1, arrowed). The upper limit cannot be seen. The original squamocolumnar junction is at (3).

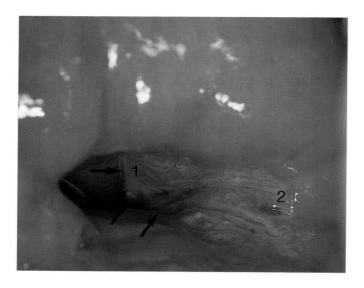

Fig. 6.18 An example of an unsatisfactory colposcopic image of the abnormal (atypical) epithelium (1) that extends high into the endocervix with only one part of its upper limit visible and arrowed. The lateral extent of the lesion is in area (2). However, the anterior, posterior and medial margins cannot be seen.

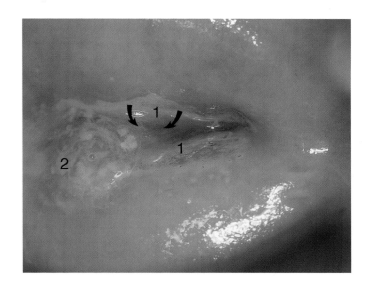

Fig. 6.19 Dense acetowhite epithelium (1), the upper limit of which cannot be seen within the endocervical canal (arrowed). This constitutes an unsatisfactory colposcopic picture. The lateral limit of the lesion is at (2).

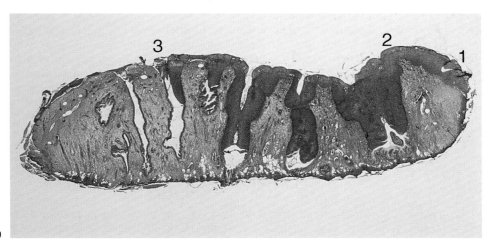

Fig. 6.20

Fig. 6.21 A grade-1 insignificant lesion with acetowhite shiny epithelium (2) extending into the endocervix (1). The upper limit of the lesion is arrowed. The indistinct borders at (3), the shiny acetowhite epithelium, and the fine-caliber vessels with a small intercapillary distance (4) are characteristic of these minor lesions.

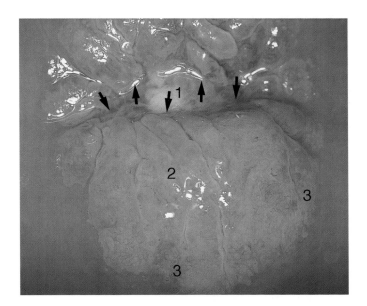

correlations to be made. Definitions of the grades are as follows.

Grade 1 (insignificant, not suspicious)—acetowhite epithelium, usually shiny or semitransparent, borders not necessarily sharp; with or without fine-caliber vessels, often with ill-defined patterns; absence of atypical vessels; small intercapillary distance (Fig. 6.21).

Grade 2 (significant, suspicious)—acetowhite epithelium of greater opacity with sharp borders; with or without dilated-caliber, regularly shaped vessels; defined patterns; absence of atypical vessels; usually increased intercapillary distance (Figs 6.22 & 6.23).

Grade 3 (highly significant, highly suspicious)—very white or gray opaque epithelium with sharp borders;

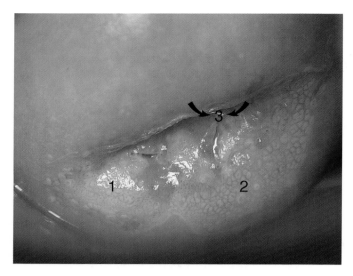

Fig. 6.22 A mixture of grade-1 (insignificant) and grade-2 (significant) lesions. The area at (1) is a grade-1 area with shiny acetowhite epithelium, indistinct borders, and very-fine-caliber vessels. In comparison area (2) shows a grade-2 area with sharper borders, regularly shaped vessels, and an increased intercapillary distance. This abnormal (atypical) epithelium extends into the endocervical canal (3) and is arrowed. The overall colposcopic image is unsatisfactory.

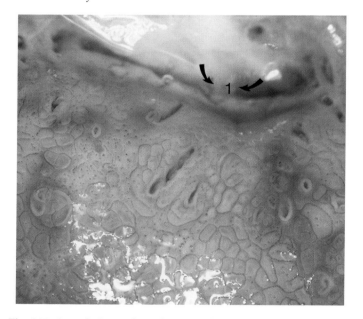

Fig. 6.23 A grade-2 significant lesion with the acetowhite epithelium showing greater opacity, dilated-caliber, regularly shaped vessels, and an increased intercapillary distance. There are gland openings with a thickened white epithelium. The overall colposcopic image is unsatisfactory and the abnormal (atypical) epithelium (arrowed) extends out of view into the endocervix (1).

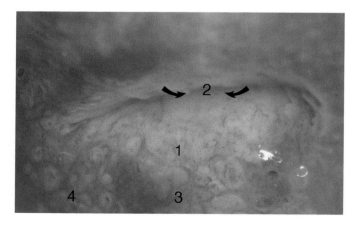

Fig. 6.25 (*Opposite*) (a) A grade 3 (highly significant, highly suspicious) lesion with very white or gray opaque epithelium (2) extending out of view into the endocervix (1, and arrowed). The sharp original squamocolumnar junction is at (3). This is an unsatisfactory colposcopic image.

(b) A grade 3 (highly significant, highly suspicious) lesion with very white or gray opaque epithelium (2) extending out of view into the endocervix (1, and arrowed). There is a sharp border (3) with atypical vessels present at (4); these give a distinctive color-tone difference between the atypical transformation zone and the original squamous epithelium. On the posterior lip (5) there is an outer area with an indistinct border and no atypical vessels are present.

(c) A grade 2 (significant, suspicious) lesion extending across the ectocervix. The acetowhite epithelium has variable degrees of opacity. The area surrounding (1) is of a translucent acetowhite epithelium with irregular feathery margins consistent with a diagnosis of HPV/low-grade epithelial atypia. The area surrounding (2) on the posterior lip has an obvious sharper, well-defined margin (arrowed) and the acetowhiteness is of a greater opacity than that seen on the anterior lip. There are no obvious vascular changes. These changes at (2) are consistent with a high-grade epithelial lesion (grade 2). When grading is undertaken using the Reid–Coppelson Colposcopic Index, a score of 5 is obtained, made up as follows: 2 points are given for color, 2 for margins and surface configuration (there is an area of internal demarcation), 1 point for vessels (absent vascular patterns). Note that further points would have been given but no iodine staining is available. However, the final score of 5 puts the lesion into the high grade SIL category.

(d) A lesion showing both low and high grades of abnormality. On the anterior lip, the predominant epithelium around (1) is of a low intensity acetowhitening which is not completely opaque. The lesion margins are feathered or finely scalloped at (2) and a poorly formed mosaic pattern predominates through the outer half of the acetowhite epithelium (3). The arrows mark an internal margin enclosing a raised higher intensity acetowhite area. This is seen at (4) on the anterior lip and a similar area is present at (5) on the posterior lip. Using the Reid–Coppelson Colposcopic Index, the color of the lesion (at the denser central acetowhite area) scores one point. The margins and surface configuration scores 2 in view the presence of an internal margin. One point is given in the central area where there are absent vessels. It was not possible to iodine stain but it is most likely that it would have scored at least 1 or possibly 2, giving a total of 5 or 6, making it a high grade lesion. Loop excision showed this area to be composed of CIN 1 and CIN 2.

(e) This photograph shows a wide area of low intensity acetowhitening, not completely opaque at (1) with irregular margins and a central "raised" area (2) on the anterior lip.

The color is accentuated by the flash photography but a higher power view in Fig. 6.25f reveals this area as having a micropapillary surface configuration (1). Peripheral to this in Fig. 6.25f there is an area of poorly defined fine mosaic consistent with SPI. Using the Reid–Coppelson colposcopic index, 0 points would be allocated for color, 0 points for the lesion margin and the surface configuration, and 0 points for vessels. Iodine staining was not available but even so, the lesion is unlikely to score more than one point in total, making it LSIL or HPV/atypia. This lesion, although spectacular in appearance, was associated with a very benign epithelial change. This shows the utility of the Reid–Coppelson Colposcopic Index.

Fig. 6.24 (*Left*) A grade 3 (highly significant, highly suspicious) lesion with very white or gray opaque epithelium (1) extending into the endocervical canal (2, arrowed). Occasional atypical vessels are present on the posterior lip (3) and there are gland openings with thickened white epithelium at (4). This latter appearance is referred to as gland cuffing and represents an extension of the cervical intraepithelial neoplasia (CIN) process into the subepithelial glandular crypts.

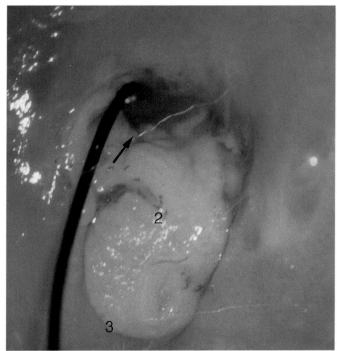

ig. 6.25(a)

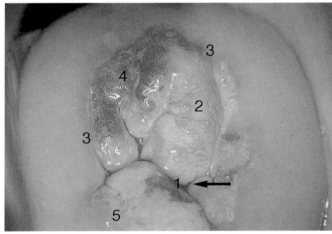

ig. 6.25(b)

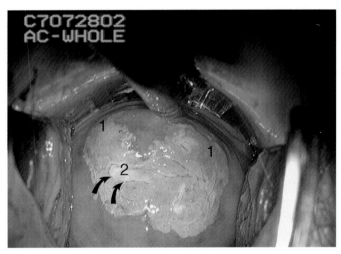

ig. 6.25(c)

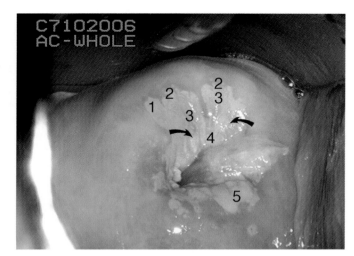

Fig. 6.25(d)

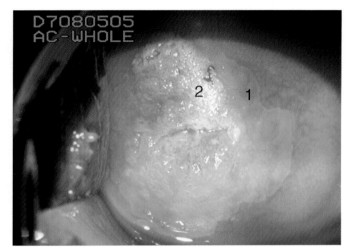

Fig. 6.25(e)

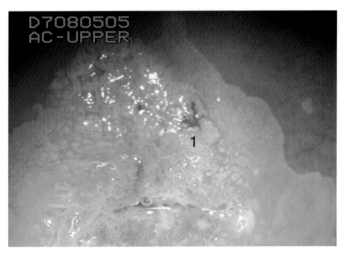

Fig. 6.25(f)

dilated-caliber, irregularly shaped, often coiled, occasional atypical vessels; increased but variable intercapillary distance; sometimes irregular surface contour—microexophytic epithelium (Figs 6.24 & 6.25).

In grade 1 the histologic features can be: (i) those of meta-plastic epithelium (immature, mature, or acanthotic epithelium); (ii) an SPI; or (iii) CIN 1. In grade 2 the lesions usually correspond to those of CIN 2 to 3. In grade 3, CIN 3 or early invasion can be anticipated. Examples of the various grades of lesion can be seen in Figs 6.21–6.25.

In other classifications it would be assumed that the grade 1 of Coppleson and Pixley's classification corresponds to the so-called minor- or low-grade lesions, while grades 2 and 3 correspond to major- or high-grade lesion.

Another grading system is the Reid Colposcopic Index (RCI) (Reid, 1993). The following description has been modified from Reid's original description by Professor Malcolm Coppleson in collaboration with Dr Richard Reid. This takes into account four colposcopic appearances: (i) color; (ii) lesion margin and surface configuration; (iii) vessels; and (iv) iodine staining. These four colposcopic signs are assigned points ranging from 0–2 (see Table 6.2). The results are then added to derive an overall colposcopic index which predicts the histologic diagnosis as shown in Table 6.3. Examples of the useage of this classification in practice are shown in Figs 6.25c–e.

The effect of patient age on colposcopic detection of CIN

A study by Zahm *et al.* 1998, on a cohort of 967 women found that patient age affects the colposcopic detection of CIN lesions. In that study, women under 35 years with CIN had more pronounced colposcopic changes than in the over 35 age group. The colposcopic parameters used included degree of acetowhiteness, surface configuration, intercapillary distances, and the distinctness of borders between acetowhite and normal epithelium. They also measured the relative epithelial thickness and number of cell layers between the two age groups and postulated that the decreased epithelial thickness and cell proliferation in the over 35 age group resulted in less prominent colposcopic features, suggests that in this age group women with trivial colposcopic changes should undergo biopsy so as to ensure complete histologic evaluation.

Unsatisfactory colposcopy: examination of the endocervical canal

Abnormal (atypical) epithelium extending high into the endocervix presents a problem to the clinician. Very often the upper limit can be clearly defined by using simple examination methods. Once the upper limit has been found, the clinician can be satisfied that no further areas of precancerous or cancerous tissue exist above that line. This applies only to squamous lesions because abnormal glandular changes may well exist higher. The clinician will be alerted to the fact that such glandular changes exist by finding abnormal (glandular) cytology.

The simplest method of defining the upper limit of the lesion is to use a small cotton-tip bud. In Fig. 6.26 such an examination is under way. An area of grade-2 abnormal (atypical) epithelium (3) extends into the endocervix (1). The upper limit (2) can be clearly seen and has been brought into view by pressure of the cotton-tip bud (4) on the posterior lip of the cervix. In Figs 6.27 and 6.28 a previous laceration in the cervix has produced an unsatisfactory colposcopic picture. An area of very mild acetowhite epithelium (grade 1) (2), whose outer limit is at (3), seems to extend into the endocervix. This patient presented with mild dyskaryotic smears (Bethesda LSIL). In Fig. 6.28, two cotton-tip swabs have been used to separate the lateral lips of the deformed cervix, and the upper limit within the endocervix can be clearly seen at (1).

In Figs 6.29–6.31 the area of grade-2 abnormal (atypical) epithelium is seen at (2) and its extension into the

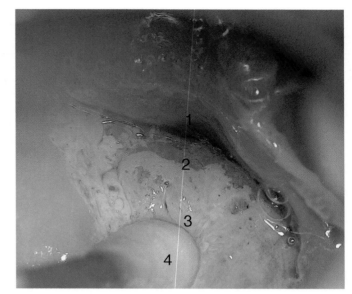

Fig. 6.26

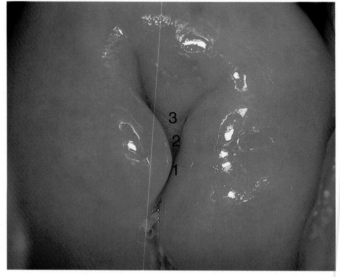

Fig. 6.27

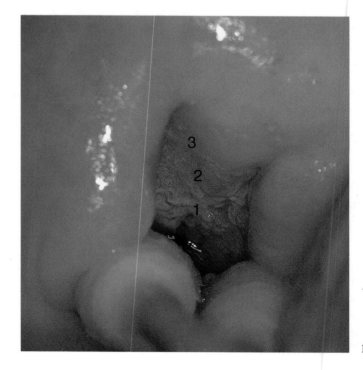

Fig. 6.28

Table 6.2 The modified Reid Colposcopic Index (RCI)*.

Colposcopic signs	Zero points	One point	Two points
Color	Low intensity acetowhitening (not completely opaque); indistinct acetowhitening; transparent acetowhitening Acetowhitening beyond the margin of the transformation zone Pure snow-white color with intense surface shine (rare)	Intermediate shade— gray-white color and shiny surface (most lesions should be scored in this category)	Dull, oyster-white Gray
Lesion margin and surface configuration	Microcondylomatous or micropapillary contour† Flat lesions with indistinct borders Feathered or finely scalloped margins Angular, jagged lesions§ Satellite lesions beyond the margin of the transformation zone	Regularly shaped symmetrical lesions with smooth, straight outlines	Rolled, peeling edges‡ Internal demarcations between areas of differing colposcopic appearance; a central area of high-grade change and peripheral area of low-grade
Vessels	Fine/uniform caliber vessels¶ Poorly formed patterns of fine punctation and/or mosaic Vessels beyond the margin of the transformation zone Fine vessels within microcondylomatous or micropapillary lesions††	Absent vessels	Well-defined coarse punctation or mosaic, sharply demarcated**
Iodine staining	Positive iodine uptake giving mahogany brown color Negative uptake of insignificant lesion, i.e. yellow staining by a lesion scoring three points or less on the first three criteria Areas beyond the margin of the transformation zone, conspicuous on colposcopy, evident as iodine negative areas, such areas are frequently due to parakeratosis‡‡	Partial iodine uptake —variegated, speckled appearance	Negative iodine uptake of significant lesion, i.e. yellow staining by a lesion already scoring four points or more on the first three criteria

*Colposcopic grading performed with 5% aqueous acetic acid and 1% iodine solution. (Crystalline iodine 0.5 g/potassium chloride/g/distilled water 100 ml.)

†Microexophytic surface contour indicative of colposcopically overt cancer is not included in the scheme.

‡Epithelial edges tend to detach from underlying stroma and curl back on themselves. Note: prominent minor grade lesions are often overinterpreted and subtle avascular patches of HSIL can easily be overlooked.

§Score zero even if part of the peripheral margin does have a straight course.

¶At times, mosaic patterns containing central vessels are characteristic of low-grade histologic abnormalities. These minor grade lesion capillary patterns can be quite pronounced. Until the physician can differentiate these fine from coarse vascular patterns, overdiagnosis is the rule.

**Branching atypical vessels indicative of colposcopically overt cancer are not included in the scheme.

††Generally, the more microcondylomatous the lesion, the lower the score. However, cancer can also present as a condyloma although this is a rare occurrence.

‡‡Parakeratosis: a superficial zone of cornified cells with retained nuclei.

Table 6.3 Colposcopic prediction of histologic diagnosis using the Reid Colposcopic Index (RCI).

RCI (overall score)	Histology
0–2	LSIL–HPV/atypia
3–4	Overlap*
5–8	HSIL

*3 points likely to equate with LSIL; 4 points with HSIL.

endocervix is at (1). In Fig. 6.29 it is also marked with an arrow. The outer limit of the lesion is at (3). In Fig. 6.30 the cervix has been opened with a pair of Desjardin's (gallbladder) forceps. The upper limit, represented by the new squamocolumnar junction, comes into view on the anterior lip at (1), but is not completely visible on the posterior lip until the forceps have been further opened (Fig. 6.31). At this stage a small area of acetowhite epithelium is visible at the 6-o'clock position, just inside the endocervix.

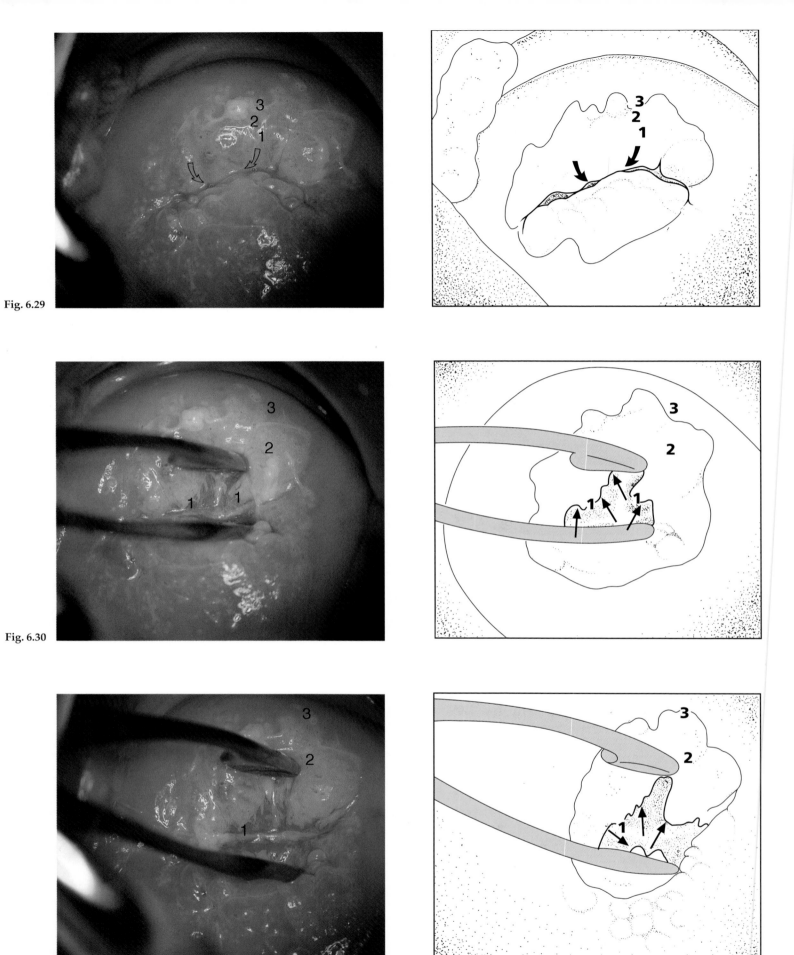

Fig. 6.29

Fig. 6.30

Fig. 6.31

This view in Fig. 6.31 represents a satisfactory colposcopic image. However, the lesion does extend into the lower endocervical canal and this must be taken into consideration when treatment is given. The lesion is of a major-grade consistency, and histologic sampling (cone biopsy) showed it to be composed of CIN 3. There was no evidence of invasion.

The diagrams opposite Figs 6.29–6.31 more clearly demonstrate, by virtue of using the Desjardin's forceps, the upper limits (arrowed) of the abnormal (atypical) epithelium as delineated by the new squamocolumnar junction within the endocervical canal. The usefulness of the Desjardin's forceps is further seen in Figs 6.32–6.35a and the accompanying traces.

In Fig. 6.35b–d a cervicoscope has been employed to determine the extent of abnormal epithelium and lesions within the endocervix. This device and the microcolpohysteroscope (of Hamou) are accessory diagnostic aids and will be discussed in more detail later.

Further examination of the endocervical canal: after treatment of cervical precancer

The follow-up of patients treated for precancerous cervical disease is most important (Figs 6.36–6.40). With all the techniques employed, be they excisional or local destructive, there is always the risk of some constriction of the ecto- and endocervix. This constriction may range from complete

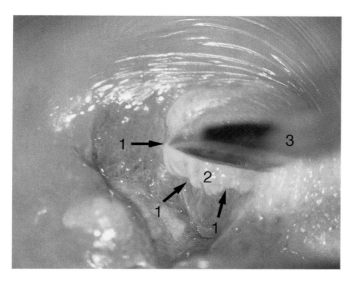
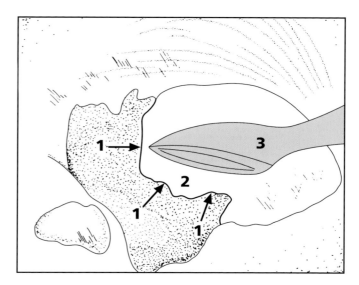

Fig. 6.32 The upper blade of the Desjardin's forceps (3) has been used to outline clearly the upper extent (new squamocolumnar junction) of the abnormal (atypical) epithelium (2) within the endocervical canal; this can be seen as a sharp line (1) and is arrowed. The lesion is of grade 1, and biopsy revealed the presence of cervical intraepithelial neoplasia (CIN) 1 with human papillomavirus (HPV) changes.

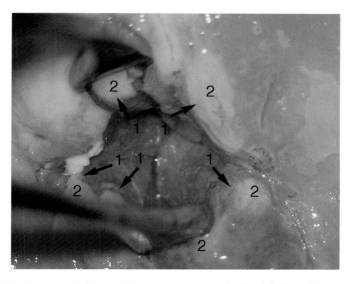
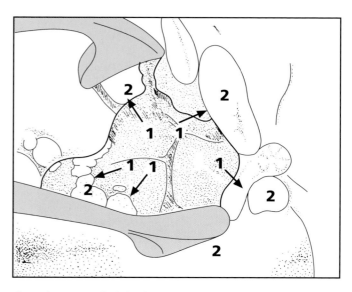

Fig. 6.33 Grade-2 acetowhite abnormal (atypical) epithelium (2) extends into the endocervix, which has been opened with Desjardin's forceps. The upper limit, the new squamocolumnar junction, is seen at (1) and is arrowed just within the endocervical margins.

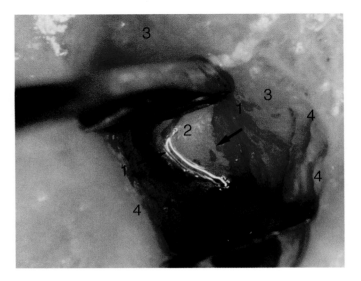

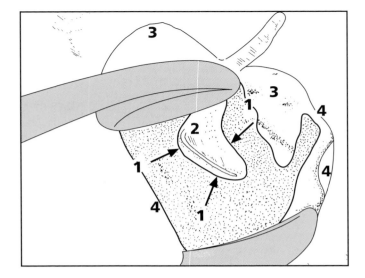

Fig. 6.34

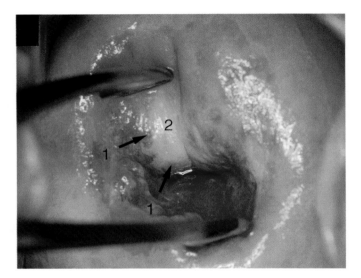

Fig. 6.35(a)

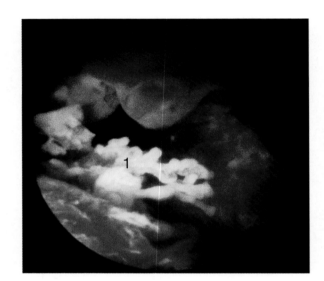

Fig. 6.35(b)

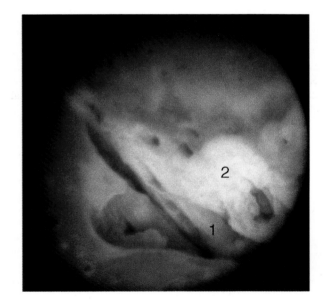

Fig. 6.35(c)

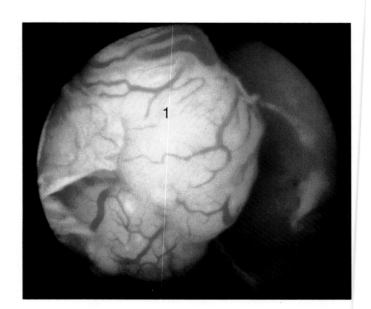

Fig. 6.35(d)

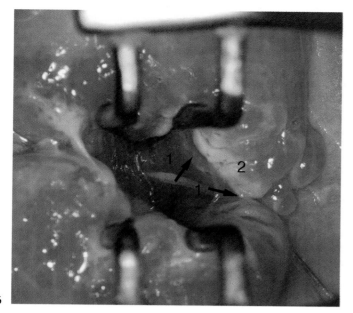

Fig. 6.36

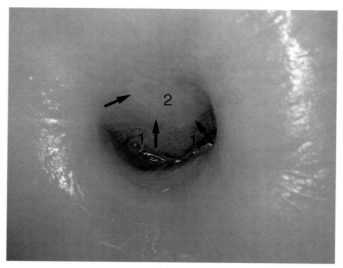

Fig. 6.37

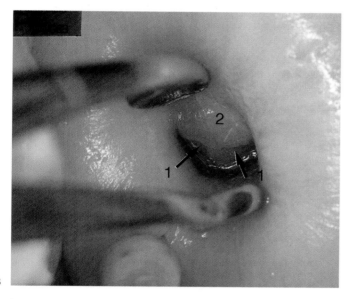

Fig. 6.38

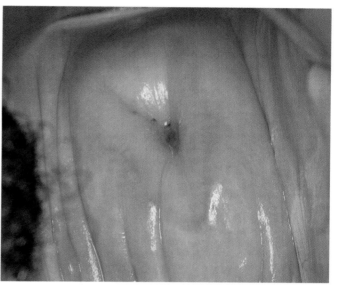

Fig. 6.39

Fig. 6.34 (*Opposite above*) An area of abnormal (atypical) epithelium (2) extends high into the endocervix. Its upper limit can be clearly seen at (1, arrowed) once the Desjardin's forceps have been inserted. Metaplastic squamous epithelium exists at (3) and the original squamocolumnar junction is at (4).

Fig. 6.35 (*Opposite below*) (a) Endocervical acetowhite epithelium (minor grade) (2), histologically composed of immature metaplastic epithelium, whose upper limit is at (1) (arrowed). Cervical smears on three occasions showed mild dyskaryosis (Bethesda LSIL). (b) A cervicoscope inserted within the endocervical canal, with saline irrigation at 20–30°C, showed altered white papillae (1) that, when stained with acetic acid, appeared very white and suspect, and in conjunction with abnormal glandular cytology demanded biopsy which revealed early papillary adenocarcinoma. (c) Cervicoscopy revealed a small focal patch of endocervical (2) acetowhite epithelium (grade 3) with an area of low-grade epithelium (1) that extends from the ectocervix. (d) Cervicoscopy shows an endocervical yellow nodular growth with atypical vessels (rootlike and willow-branch capillaries, Ueki (1985)) which histologically revealed a poorly differentiated tubular adenocarcinoma. This case demonstrates the value of endocervical cerviscopy in patients with abnormal glandular cytology with no obvious ectocervical lesion.

Fig. 6.36 (*Left above*) A small area of abnormal (atypical) grade-1 epithelium exists at (2), and the upper limit, the new squamocolumnar junction, is seen at (1, arrow) after the introduction

of Kogan's endocervical forceps. This residual epithelium is all that remains from a previous high-grade lesion that had been treated with cryotherapy some 9 months earlier.

Fig. 6.37 (*Right above*) A minor-grade lesion is shown at (2), the upper limit of which is seen within the endocervical canal (1, and arrowed); this cervix had been subjected to laser evaporation therapy some 12 months earlier. The initial lesion had been a cervical intraepithelial neoplasia (CIN) 3, that extended into the endocervix.

Fig. 6.38 (*Left above*) An endocervical low-grade lesion exists at (2) and its upper limit is at (1, arrow). Desjardin's forceps are needed to visualize the full extent of this completely endocervical lesion. Laser vaporization therapy had been used to destroy a major-grade lesion 2 years previously.

Fig. 6.39 (*Right above*) The cervix of a woman treated some 12 months earlier with laser cone biopsy for a cervical intraepithelial neoplasia (CIN) 3. The external os is constricted and will just about allow the passage of an endocervical brush appliance for cytologic purposes. Local anesthetic may need to be inserted around the external os, and tenaculum forceps applied to the anterior lip to provide countertraction when the device is gently but firmly inserted into the endocervical canal. It is important to insert the anesthetic needle into the posterior part of the cervix and also well lateral to the external os. If this is not done, then blood from the injection site may flow back into the endocervix and thereby contaminate the cytologic specimen.

stenosis to the inability to allow passage of the normal devices used to harvest endocervical cells in follow-up surveillance.

The projection of the abnormal (atypical) epithelium within the endocervix can be followed using the devices previously mentioned, such as the cotton-tip swab or Desjardin's (gall-bladder) forceps. Kogan's endocervical forceps, used extensively in the USA, may also be used and these are shown in Fig. 6.36. Other techniques that may be used to ensure opening of the constricted endocervix to obtain an adequate smear include the insertion of a hydroscopic device which can be removed after 24 hours. The only problem with this device is that its removal may well cause abrasion of the endocervical epithelium and so produce bleeding; this leads to difficulty not only in obtaining but also in interpreting the endocervical smear. The administration of estrogens, especially to postmenopausal females, will ensure some softening and possibly dilatation of the constricted endocervical canal (Cartier, 1984). However, if an excessive amount of scar tissue exists, then it may be difficult for exogenous estrogens to produce any effective dilatation.

In some instances it may be necessary to insert a local anesthetic into the cervix so that an endocervical cytologic brush appliance can be forcibly introduced into a very stenosed external cervical os. The cervixes seen in Figs 6.39 and 6.40 would represent such a case.

Colposcopic biopsy

A biopsy of the abnormal (atypical) epithelium of the cervix is imperative if local destructive treatment of CIN is contemplated. Such treatment usually consists of either cryotherapy, deep radial diathermy, laser evaporation or cold coagulation and should be confined to cases where there is no suggestion of invasion either colposcopically or histologically. The colposcopic biopsy and its assessment by an experienced pathologist is an important procedure to be carried out before any further treatment is undertaken. It should be noted, however, that colposcopic punch biopsy does not always resolve the subjective difficulties with colposcopy. It has a false-negative rate of between 41% and 54% (Byrne *et al.*, 1988; Skehan *et al.*, 1990; Howe & Vincenti, 1991) and in addition may miss glandular abnormalities (see p. 150).

There is an increasing move towards using the diathermy loop excision as both a diagnostic and therapeutic modality. Indeed the "see and treat" technique relies on this. However the contention that the diathermy loop should replace punch biopsy is not completely proven. Ang *et al.* (1995) in a comparison between directed punch biopsy and loop excision showed a satisfactory correlation between both techniques in respect of histologic detection of low-grade lesions; but the punch biopsy missed two cases (0.8%) of microinvasive lesions which were predicted as high-grade SIL on both punch biopsy and smear.

The biopsy site is selected from the area with the most severe degree of abnormality. It is the authors' policy to take multiple biopsies under a suitable local anesthetic block administered with a dental syringe. The forceps used

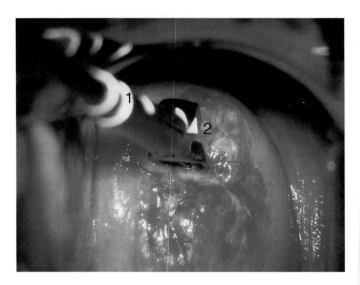

Fig. 6.41 Eppendorfer forceps with a rotating 25-cm shaft (1) are being used to biopsy an area of abnormal (atypical) epithelium (2) on the anterior cervical lip.

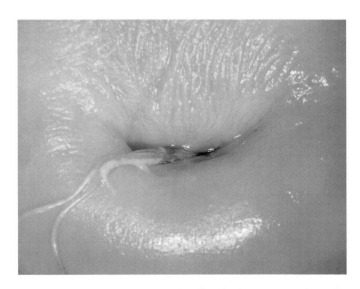

Fig. 6.40 The cervix some 18 months after diathermy coagulation for a major-grade lesion. This cervix has constricted to a narrow transverse opening. It could not be dilated with either Desjardin's or Kogan's forceps when cervical dilatation was necessary to procure an endocervical sample. The tail of an intrauterine device can be clearly seen. The use of an endocervical dilator (as shown in Fig. 7.72b) will be helpful.

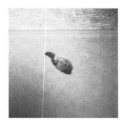

Fig. 6.42 Photograph of a 5 mm forceps biopsy (from the case shown in Fig. 6.41) orientated on filter paper with the epithial surface uppermost.

vary in shape and efficiency, but with some it is very difficult to obtain a biopsy from a site where the epithelium is on a particularly curved surface of one of the cervical lips (Figs 6.41 & 6.42). It may be necessary to use an Iris hook or teneculum to steady the tissue while the biopsy is being taken. Some of the modern biopsy forceps have a toothed jaw which facilitates better application to the tissue.

After the biopsy has been taken, the bleeding can be stopped by the use of astringent agents. Monsell's solution (ferric subsulfate) can be placed immediately on the area, or a more simple procedure is to apply a silver nitrate stick immediately. The stick should be left in place for at least 1–2 minutes and can then be removed.

A small diathermy loop has been developed to obtain samples of abnormal tissue. This was popularized in Paris by Dr Rene Cartier nearly 20 years ago and is shown in Figs 6.43 & 6.44. As will be discussed later (Chapter 7), the trend for complete removal of the transformation zone using a large diathermy loop has reduced the indications for its use.

Handling of the biopsy specimen

Once the biopsy specimen has been obtained, it must be handled correctly so that the maximum amount of information can be obtained from it. The biopsy should include at least 3–4 mm of underlying stroma and encompass about 5 mm in length of the cervical epithelium (Fig. 6.42). The authors prefer to place the biopsies in buffered formalin. The biopsy should be orientated so that sections can be cut at right angles to the surface mucosa. The biopsy may be still present in the biopsy forceps when they have been removed from the vagina. The specimen in Figs 6.41 and 6.42 will

need to be gently removed from the jaws of the forceps and then oriented on the chosen material. When it arrives in the laboratory, it will be described, measured and embedded in wax for later sectioning as a single block. Initially three superficial levels will be sectioned by microtome with shallow steps in between. Leveling will begin at the first representative full face section of the block. Routine staining is with hematoxylin and eosin. Perhaps 5–10% of one face of the block will be examined microscopically.

Microcolpohysteroscopic examination of the endocervical canal

With a microcolpohysteroscopic examination further evidence can be obtained as to the nature of the epithelium within the endocervix. The tissue can be stained with Waterman's blue ink, which will be taken up *in vivo* by squamous cells. The blue-stained epithelium can then be visualized with a microcolpohysteroscope in direct contact with the epithelium. The device has a 60× magnification and a resolution of 2 μm.

The microcolpohysteroscope is an original instrument with multiple uses; it can be used for diagnosis and also for therapeutic hysteroscopy. Cells can be viewed both microscopically and macroscopically (Hamou, 1991). In the latter case, a panoramic view of the cervical canal can be obtained. In Fig. 6.45 (a) the device is shown with a focusing screw, allowing both a direct and a second ocular view. The direct ocular view extends from 1× (Fig. 6.45b) to 20× magnification, and in the contact mode, wherein the microcolpohysteroscopic lens is in contact with the tissue stained with a supravical stain, the magnification can be extended up to 60×. In the second ocular position

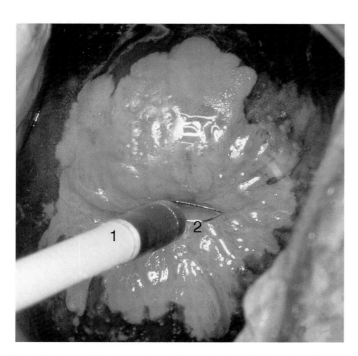

Fig. 6.43 A small diathermy loop biopsy device (1), developed by Dr Rene Cartier, is used to take a biopsy from minor-grade abnormal (atypical) epithelium at (2).

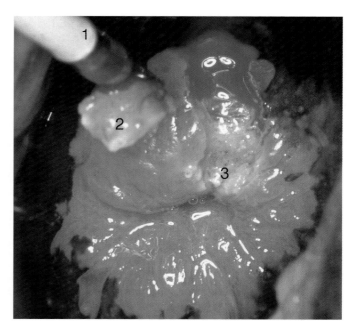

Fig. 6.44 The biopsy loop (1) shown in Fig. 6.43 has now taken a small area of tissue (2). The defect that extends from the endocervical canal to the outer limit of the lesion can be seen at (3). Small gland openings are visible in the depth of the defect toward the endocervical margin. An extremely satisfactory sample can be obtained by this method.

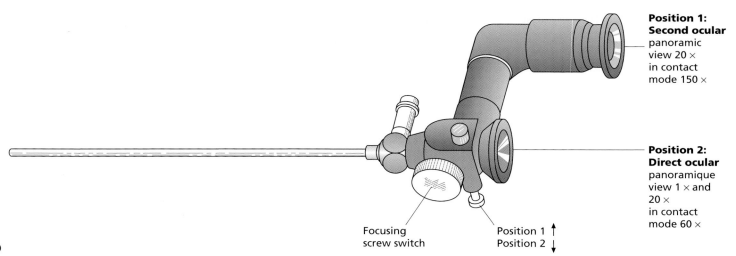

Position 1:
Second ocular
panoramic
view 20 ×
in contact
mode 150 ×

Position 2:
Direct ocular
panoramique
view 1 × and
20 ×
in contact
mode 60 ×

Focusing
screw switch

Position 1 ↑
Position 2 ↓

Fig. 6.45(a)

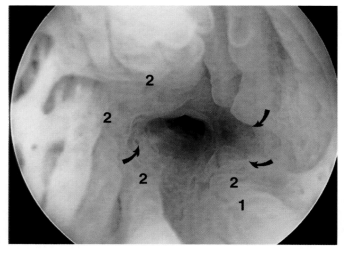

Fig. 6.45(b)

Fig. 6.45 (b) shows a panoramic view of the endocervical canal. Physiological epithelium is present with squamous metaplastic epithelium at (1) with the new squamocolumnar junction at (2).

the panoramic view is at 20× magnification, and in the contact mode is at 150× magnification. There is a wide viewing angle of 90° and a depth of field ranging from infinity to millimeters from the distal end of the instrument.

When to perform an examination

An examination is optimally performed in the preovulatory phase, when the cervical orifice is open and the mucus is clear. Desquamation and slight adhesiveness of the cells of the cervix in the luteal phase tend to hinder visualization. For the postmenopausal female it is recommended that ethanyl estradiol be given for 8 days prior to the examination (as described above for viewing the unsatisfactory cervix) to facilitate the passage of the device. With experience the technique can be performed during a bleeding episode. The distal lens makes contact with the epithelium and so a plasma film develops between it and the mucosa; this film acts like the oil of an immersion microscope and leads to improved resolution.

The examination

The equipment necessary for the examination is shown in Fig. 6.46. The microcolpohysteroscope is at (1), (2) is a 25-cm-long pointed dissection forceps, (3) a stabilizing

tenaculum, (4) a vaginal speculum, (5) a container with Waterman's blue ink, and (6) a container with 2% Lugol's iodine. The third container is a bowl of sterile water.

Once the cervix has been exposed, it must be cleaned with a cotton pledget soaked in saline to eliminate secretions, mucus, and cellular debris. If there is copious cervical

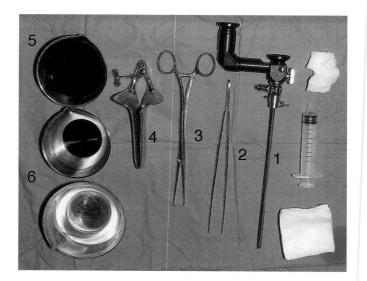

Fig. 6.46

mucus, the cervix can be compressed between the blades of the speculum; this will expel the mucus, which can then be removed using a cotton pledget.

Staining procedure

Lugol's iodine solution, used to determine the extent of abnormal epithelium, is generously applied across the ectocervix. The tissue can then be examined at 20× magnification and has an appearance comparable with that seen during the initial steps of colposcopy. Once the areas have been evaluated, the Waterman's blue ink should be applied. It is preferable to apply small quantities directly to the external os and endocervix. To stain the endocervix effectively, pledgets are soaked in the ink, held with the 25-cm forceps, and gently inserted into the endocervical canal.

Passage of the microcolpohysteroscope

The microcolpohysteroscope is used with a high magnification of 60× or 150×. Any tremor made by the user will consequently be magnified and will hinder observation. It is suggested that the left hand holds the middle of the telescope between the thumb and index finger with the other fingers supporting the edge of the posterior blade of the speculum. The right hand holds the proximal lenses and the right elbow should be placed on a firm surface. The examiner should be seated. In this manner very precise movements can be made with the distal end and any tremors are minimized.

The first step is to observe the cells of the cervix at 60× magnification. This permits overall observation of the cellular topography and determination of the distribution of the glandular structures. It is recommended that scanning is carried out by exerting slight pressure with the tip of the endoscope on the mucosa and progressing in a circular fashion. This preliminary evaluation at 60× magnification permits a rapid scan of the cervix and localization of any suspect areas. The new squamocolumnar junction is examined in its entirety, and once any suspicious areas have been examined the index finger is moved gently to change the magnification to 150×. At this magnification it is possible to evaluate the nuclear:cytoplasmic ratio and any nuclear abnormalities.

Grading of endocervical abnormalities

Hamou (1991) has defined three grades of abnormality within the endocervix that may be visualized with the microhysteroscopic system. Grade 1 defines normal cervical epithelium in a narrow transformation zone without nuclear abnormality (Fig. 6.47). Grade 2 describes what Hamou refers to as dystrophies (these include all benign lesions, such as colpitis, metaplasia, leukoplakia, mosaicism, and condyloma, but exclude neoplasia). Grade 3 describes neoplasia and this epithelium is found in a high concentration in the same optic field which shows nuclei with diameters greater than 15 µm (Figs 6.48–6.50). These changes can only be seen using 150× magnification. Hamou believes that the success of this technique depends

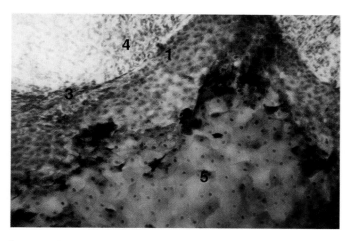

Fig. 6.47 The transformation zone at a magnification of 150×. In approximately 90% of cases this transformation zone is narrow, entirely contained within the optic field, and shows intermediate (1) and deep (2) layers of squamous epithelium where all the metaplastic and dysplastic processes may be seen. The blue line of the squamocolumnar junction is seen at (3), separating the glandular (columnar) (4) from the squamous epithelium (1,2). Pyknotic and superficial squamous cells are present at (5).

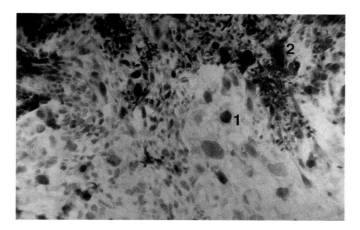

Fig. 6.48 The view, seen through the microcolpohysteroscope, of a neoplastic area in which there are severe nuclear abnormalities [(1) and (2)]. In particular, the greatly enlarged nuclei (greater than 15 µm) are associated with hyperchromasia, anisokaryosis, and a reduced nuclear:cytoplasmic ratio. There is excessive dyschromasia (measure of the chromatin (DNA) concentration) and polymorphism of nuclear abnormalities; the appearance is suggestive in this case of "moderate dysplasia with condyloma" (Hamou, 1991).

on the experience of the examiner and meticulous attention to detail during the procedure.

Other cervicoscopic appearances and pathologic findings

Using the cervicoscope, Ueki (1985) and Ueki and Sano (1987) have studied endocervical precancerous lesions. They have defined two types of endocervical lesion; in the first the lesion occurs in conjunction with an ectocervical abnormality, and in the second there is purely an endocervical neoplastic lesion. These two types will be described in more detail later.

For the first type, Ueki found that the abnormal ectocervical CIN-containing epithelium was acetowhite in 55% of

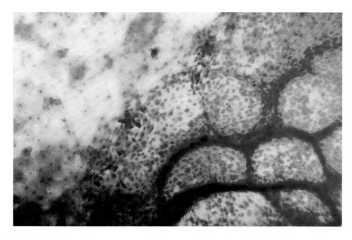

Fig. 6.49 Mosaicism seen at 150× magnification. Residual papillae are covered by an immature epithelium. The squamous thickening separating the pseudopapillae, described by Hamou (1991), is identified by the darker blue coloration. These papillae appear as simple arches centered above the vascular axis that appears between the immature epithelium composed of a few parabasal layers. The lack of obliteration of the interpapillary furrows that lie deep within the epithelium allows the characteristic "mosaic" appearance to be easily identified by the colposcopist.

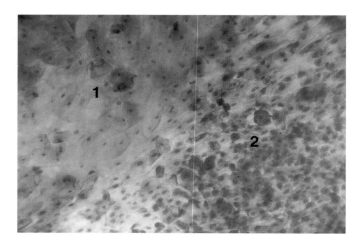

Fig. 6.50 Microcolpohysteroscopic view of a major-grade lesion. The external limits of the lesion can be seen with the mature squamous epithelium to the left and labeled (1); the beginning of the lesion with major-grade features is at (2).

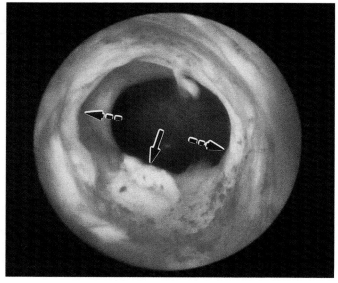

Fig. 6.51(ai)

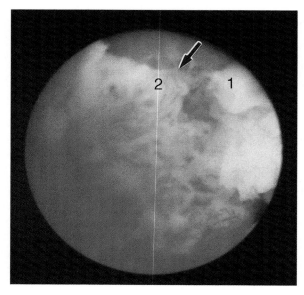

Fig. 6.51(aii)

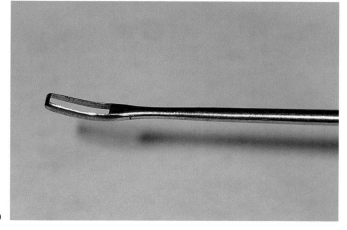

Fig. 6.51(b)

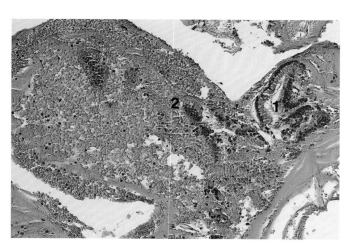

Fig. 6.51(c)

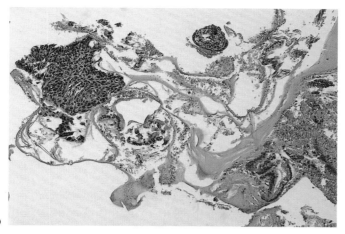

Fig. 6.51(d)

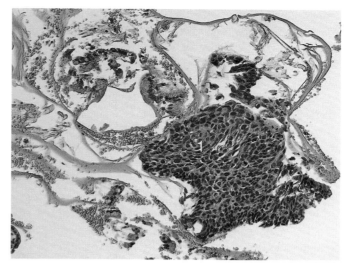

Fig. 6.51(e)

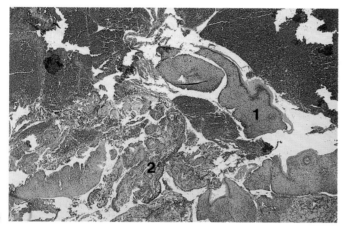

Fig. 6.51(f)

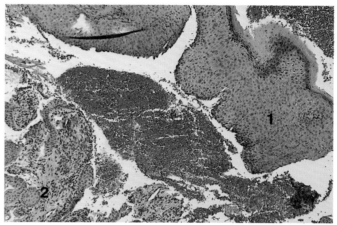

Fig. 6.51(g)

Fig. 6.51 (a) Endocervical adenocarcinoma in a 61-year-old parous patient who presented with an abnormal glandular cytology.

(i) Cervicoscopy shows a lesion limited to the endocervix at some distance from the external os. Keratosis (arrowed) and ring-like white epithelium (broken arrows) with some root and hairpin-like capillaries can be seen in the 11 o'clock position. (ii) A higher magnification of the view in (i) shows a small papillary lesion (2) containing the glomerular, hairpin, and corkscrew fine blood vessels described by Ueki (1985). An area of keratosis is at (1). Pathology of this lesion showed it to be a very early but well-differentiated papillary adenocarcinoma.

(b) The sharp endocervical curette.

(c) Photomicrograph of tissue removed by endocervical curettage; there are fragments of endocervical epithelium at (1) and an amorphous blood clot at (2).

(d) and (e) Low- and high-power views of endocervical curettings; strips of neoplastic squamous epithelium of high-grade disease can be seen at (1).

(f) and (g) Endocervical curettings seen with (f) low-power and (g) high-power magnification. The tissue contains strips of squamous epithelium. Because there is no stroma available it is difficult to preclude the presence of invasion. In (g), detached fragments of "abnormal" epithelium (1) can be seen with columnar epithelium associated with immature squamous metaplasia (2).

cases, punctated in 25%, and mosaic in 15%. Keratosis with atypical vessels occurred infrequently. However, he showed that punctation and mosaicism were very unusual in the endocervical extension of these lesions, but the frequency of leukoplakia and atypical vessels was increased in this site. The reason for these specific changes within the endocervix is not known.

Ueki classified in the second group those endocervical lesions that were suspect, because the cytology was positive or suspicious, but in which there was no obvious ecto-cervical abnormality. However, the endocervical findings were mainly those of leukoplakia followed by atypical vessels and punctation; sometimes an unexpected transformation zone was found wholly within the endocervix. If such a transformation zone exists within the endocervix, it should be carefully examined because any hypertrophy of

the surface or "white rings", which signify endocervical gland openings containing CIN, will necessitate curettage or biopsy. These lesions seem to be of a limited extent.

Ueki and Sano (1987) believe that lesions of invasive cancer in the endocervix are characterized by surface elevation, ulceration, and altered papillae, as shown in Fig. 6.51a. Lesions that suggest alteration from a precancerous to a cancerous state in this area are usually associated with leukoplakia and atypical vessels with punctation.

Endocervical curettage

A biopsy of the endocervical canal can be obtained using an endocervical curette (Fig. 6.51b). Although this is used extensively in the United States (Talebian *et al.*, 1977; Drescher *et al.*, 1983; Hatch *et al.*, 1985; Krebs *et al.*, 1987), it is less popular in Europe (Burghardt, 1991; Anderson *et al.*, 1992). It is reserved for those cases in which there is uncertainty as to the existence of an unsuspected abnormality within the endocervical canal above the new squamo-columnar junction. It is also useful after treatment of a precancerous lesion in cases where the cervical canal is partly stenosed and where it is difficult to see the new squamo-columnar junction. However, with the advent of the endocervical brush to harvest cells from the endocervix, use of endocervical curettage would seem to be limited (Anderson *et al.*, 1988).

One of the major objections to endocervical curettage is the fact that only fragments of tissue are obtained (Fig. 6.51c–g). It is difficult to judge the relationship of the epithelium to the stroma, especially when this has been disrupted. No indication as to the depth of involvement of the neoplastic tissue within the stroma, namely the occurrence of microinvasive cancer, can be given. A second objection is that it is a painful procedure when carried out without anesthetic.

The procedure itself is performed with a sharp spoon-shaped or curved curette (Fig. 6.51b), which can be inserted through a narrow os. Once the curette has been positioned inside the canal, a circumferential scraping technique is used; the curette is then withdrawn and any tissue that remains within the jaws of the instrument is washed into the fixative solution. Residual tissue, such as fragments on the ecto- or endocervix, can be picked out with forceps and placed in the fixative.

While carrying out the actual procedure, the clinician should pay attention to the consistency of the cervical wall. If the endocervix has a firm and regular feel, then it is unlikely to possess within its depths invasive cancer. However, if the tissue removed is friable, and bleeding is excessive, then invasive disease is more likely.

The use of cervicoscopy or microcolpohysteroscopy, as described above, would seem to be much more logical diagnostic techniques than the blind endocervical curettage that is still employed in many countries.

How accurate is endocervical sampling?

It has been very difficult to answer the question as to how sensitive and specific is endocervical sampling, regardless of whether it is being carried out by use of a cytologic brush smear or curettage. Most studies have either examined too few subjects (Sesti *et al.*, 1990) or been retrospective, in that women who have had both satisfactory and unsatisfactory colposcopy have had the final histology determined by either punch biopsy or cone biopsy. In others the diagnosis of CIN was made on punch biopsy material before local destructive therapy was given (Drescher *et al.*, 1983; Hatch *et al.*, 1985; Krebs *et al.*, 1987). In many of these studies, no significant pathology was available. There has been no information on the value of a negative endocervical sampling, or on whether a negative result would, indeed, influence treatment when colposcopy is unsatisfactory.

In a recent study by Anderson *et al.* (1992), 100 females, who had abnormal cervical smears and were selected for cone biopsy according to the current colposcopic criteria (see Chapter 7) randomly underwent endocervical sampling with either the Kevorkian curette or the endocervical brush. The latter group comprised 47 females. The cytology and histology results from the endocervical sampling were compared with the results of the cone-biopsy histology, and it was found that the overall sensitivity of endocervical sampling was 56% with a false-negative rate of 44% and a negative predictive rate of 26%. Breakdown of these figures showed that the sensitivities of curettage and brush cytology samples were 57 and 53% respectively; the specificity was 69% but the small number of cases listed means that the accuracy of this latter figure is doubtful. Although the overall false-negative rate was 43%, this rate for curettage was 46% and for brush sampling was 45%.

Anderson *et al.* concluded that the two recognized sampling methods have high false-negative rates and a correspondingly low ability to predict freedom from disease (26% negative predictive value). These sampling methods certainly missed significant CIN and invasive lesions, and their value in, for instance, avoiding negative cone biopsy when the endocervical sample is negative is seriously questioned by Lopez *et al.* (1989). It would seem from his study that endocervical sampling should not influence the management when the colposcopy is unsatisfactory.

Identification of the abnormal (atypical) epithelium: Schiller's iodine test

Schiller's iodine test, originally described by Schiller in 1929, is used to delineate areas that are likely to contain a cervical precancer. Glycogen-containing squamous epithelium is usually fully differentiated and will stain strongly with iodine, giving rise to the so-called iodine-positive state. Other epithelia that fail to take up the stain are called iodine negative; such tissues include columnar epithelium, immature metaplastic squamous epithelium, SPI, and some invasive cancers.

The Lugol's iodine solution that is applied to the cervix and forms the basis of the Schiller's iodine test, is a 1% iodine solution consisting of 2g iodine, 4g potassium iodide, and 200g distilled water. The basic test depends on the interaction between iodine and glycogen. Glycogen-containing vaginal epithelium of premenopausal females takes up the iodine and stains an intense mahogany brown. This contrasts with the areas that do not contain glycogen, and consequently will not stain with iodine; these are the iodine-negative or Schiller-positive areas.

Abnormal (atypical) epithelium, or epithelium that contains an excessive amount of keratin (acanthotic epithelia), is glycogen free and reacts with the iodine solution to stain a characteristic yellow. The area of abnormality are clearly outlined, at (2) in Figs 6.52–6.55. After the menopause, and coincident with a decline in estrogen production, application of iodine solution to the vagina will produce a stippled brown appearance, whereas the cervix may stain light brown or yellow (Figs 6.56 before Schiller's & 6.57 after Schiller's).

There are a number of false-positive results of Schiller's test that are not uncommon; these are particularly likely to

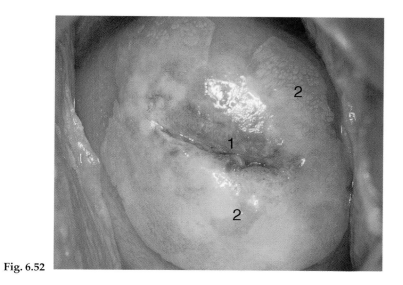

Fig. 6.52

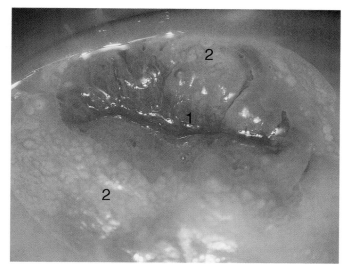

Fig. 6.54

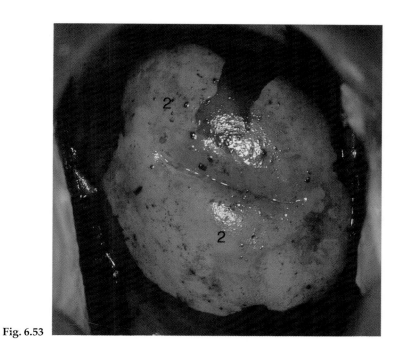

Fig. 6.53

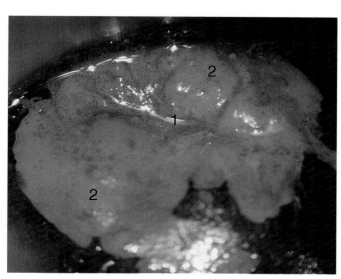

Fig. 6.55

Figs 6.54 and 6.55 Iodine solution reacting with a minor-grade colposcopic lesion to produce a typical yellow shade of iodine negativity. The cervical canal is at (1) and abnormal (atypical) epithelium at (2) (Figs 6.52, 6.54; before application).

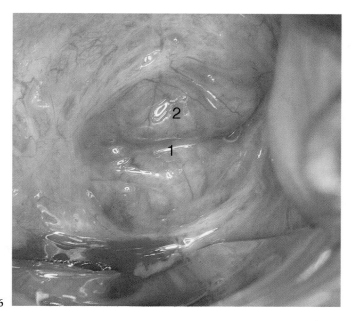

Fig. 6.56

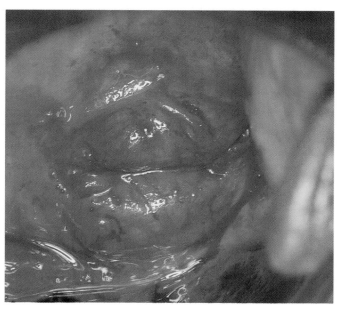

Fig. 6.57

be produced when there is much immature metaplasia in the cervix, as is found after a recent pregnancy. Likewise, large areas of acanthotic epithelium, such as are found in the congenital transformation zone, will also be Schiller positive and iodine negative. These conditions may cover large areas of the cervix and extend into the vagina.

6.8 The concept of human papillomavirus infection and cervical precancer

As has been discussed in Chapter 2, it would seem that very few precancerous lesions of the cervix are not in some way associated with human papillomavirus infection (HPVI) (Richart *et al.*, 1992; Schiffman *et al.*, 1993; Bosch *et al.*, 1995). The virus causes many morphologic changes within the transformation zone and beyond, and these may be difficult to interpret. Much controversy surrounds their diagnosis and natural history. In the following sections, their varied presentations will be considered.

HPV produces two types of lesion on the cervix. These are: (i) clinical condylomata of various forms; and (ii) a sub-clinical non-condylomatous type that is only obvious after the application of acetic acid.

The condylomatous lesions have been described histologically by Burghardt (1991) and their colposcopic representations are as follows.

The so-called *papillary condyloma* is the most common type and is composed of thickened epithelium that forms excrescences; these are supported by a scaffold of elongated and delicate stromal stalks that are rich in blood vessels (Fig. 6.58a). There is a variable degree of surface

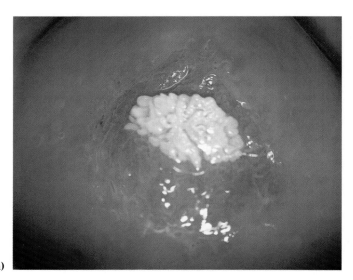

Fig. 6.58(a)

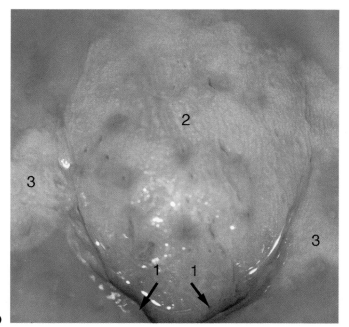

Fig. 6.58(c)

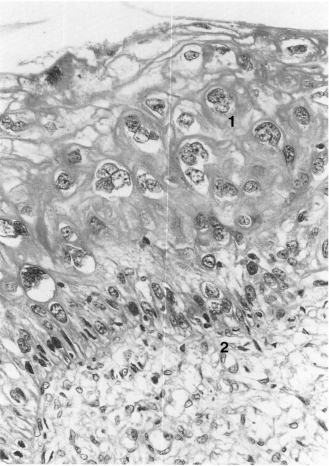

Fig. 6.58(b)

Fig. 6.58 (b) Biopsy from a lesion that showed signs of subclinical papillomavirus infection (SPI); the classic features of koilocytosis and multinucleation (1) are present, especially within the middle and superficial layers. There is pleomorphism and hyperchromasia in the basal layers, and an increase in cellular proliferation. The stroma can be seen at (2).

(c) SPI showing a multifocal acetowhite area (2) with irregular indistinct margins and obvious satellite lesions (3). The lesion extends into the endocervical canal (1, arrow) and presents an unsatisfactory colposcopic picture in that the upper limits of this change cannot be seen. Close observation of the pattern in the main area of abnormality at (2) shows it to be of a micropapillary character. There is a distinct change in color between the area extending into the endocervical canal and the main area at (2). The latter is a pearly white, whereas the central area is a darker gray; excision biopsy of this endocervical area showed it to be a cervical intraepithelial neoplasia (CIN) 2. The tissue at (2) contained lesions of HPV/CIN 1.

keratinization. The epithelium is squamous with a prominent basal layer as well as a thick layer of prickle cells that, in turn, are overlain by a zone of cells with clear cytoplasm and reminiscent of normal cervical squamous epithelium. The clear cytoplasm is due to a large perinuclear halo that is offset by rather dense cytoplasm. These cells are often binucleated or multinucleated and are referred to as koilocytes (Fig. 6.58c). They are characteristic of viral condylomata and occasionally show nuclear abnormalities.

The *spiked condyloma* forms the second type and is characterized by numerous fine, fingerlike epithelial projections. The cellular glycogen content is variable and koilocytes are present.

The third type, *flat condyloma* (Figs 6.59 & 6.60), is characterized by the presence of the HPV antigen and koilocytes. Not only are perinuclear halos present but there is nuclear pleomorphism with dense cytoplasm in the cells of the middle and superficial zones of the epithelium. For a diagnosis of an HPV-related lesion to be made, nuclear atypia must be present. Pronounced atypia and atypical mitoses are lacking. The stromal papillae are elongated. Some of

these flat condylomata can be found outside the original squamocolumnar junction on the original squamous epithelium itself. The authors consider this type to be synonymous with SPI.

A fourth, and uncommon, type of condyloma is the so-called *inverted condyloma* that is characteristically present within the area of endocervical crypts. Surface projections are distinctly keratinized.

It is impossible to distinguish histologically between a flat condyloma and low-grade CIN. Lesions such as that shown in Fig. 6.58c must be regarded as HPV related, but no inference can be made regarding the HPV type or the natural history of the lesion.

The *subclinical papillomavirus infections* (SPIs) have been described in detail by Coppleson and Pixley (1992a) (Figs 6.58b & 6.61–6.64). They are referred to as clinically unapparent, minor-grade lesions and show a number of features that differentiate them from more significant CIN or high-grade lesions. These subclinical lesions contain many of the histologic features of the condylomatous types described above. The proposed grading system of Reid

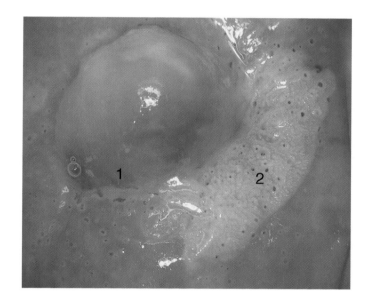

Fig. 6.59 The micropapillary nature of a localized flat condylomatous area is shown at (2). The gland openings are obvious within this area. The very shiny snow-white color is typical of a clinical papillomavirus infection. Punch biopsy of this focal lesion showed it to be a flat condyloma with hyperkeratosis and slight epithelial basal changes, consistent with cervical intraepithelial neoplasia (CIN) 1. The endocervical canal is at (1).

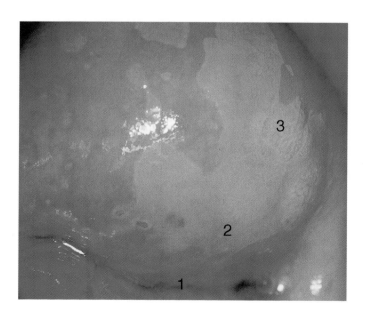

Fig. 6.60 This minor grade of subclinical papillomavirus infection (SPI) shows a characteristic geographic shape. The cervical canal is at (1). The shiny snow-white color and indistinct acetowhitening are typical of a flat condyloma, and an obvious micropapilliferous change is present at (3). Punch biopsy of the area (2) showed it to be a flat condylomatous wart with very minor atypical changes.

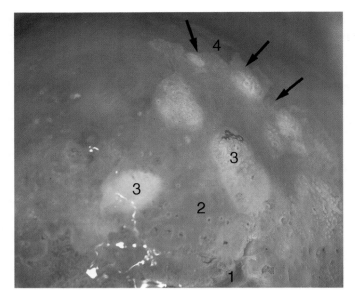

Fig. 6.61 An area of subclinical papillomavirus infection (SPI) indicated by the semitransparent acetowhitening at (2) with more obvious lesions of a condylomatous nature at (3). Close inspection will show them to be composed of small micropapilliferous lesions (3), although some have a grayish white acetoepithelial covering that is suggestive of hyperkeratinization. The border to the lesion is angular and jagged (arrowed), and a satellite lesion (4) can be seen outside the boundary in the 1-o'clock position. The endocervix is at (1).

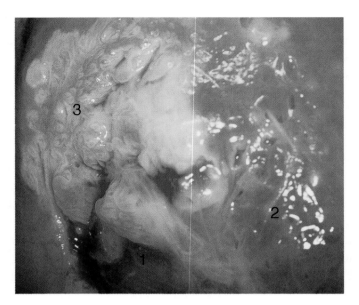

Fig. 6.62 An area of subclinical papillomavirus infection (SPI) at (3) showing the gray shiny acetowhite epithelium that is characteristic of these lesions. The lesion is within the transformation zone and some parts of it can be seen to contain a distinct capillary pattern. These vessels have a uniform capillary loop with a very fine mosaic pattern. The boundary of the lesion appears irregular with an angular configuration. At (2), an area of columnar epithelium exists in association with some metaplastic epithelium. The endocervical canal is at (1).

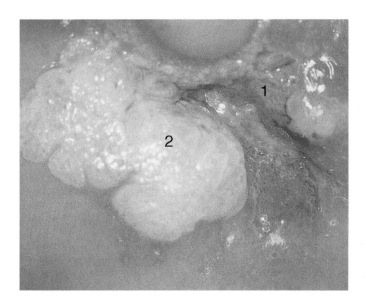

Fig. 6.63 An extremely hyperkeratotic subclinical papillomavirus infection (SPI) (2) with a less pronounced but micropapillary lesion at (1) extending a short distance into the endocervical canal, but remaining within the transformation zone. The micropapillary nature of the hyperkeratotic area at (2) can be clearly seen with its irregular and slightly fissured borders. Biopsy of this area showed it to be a flat condyloma with marked keratosis and some minor epithelial basal changes (cervical intraepithelial neoplasia (CIN) 1).

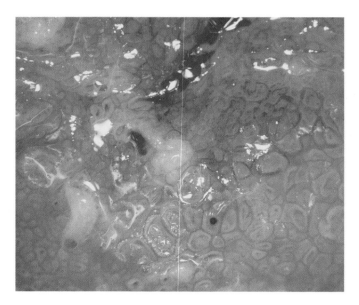

Fig. 6.64 A subclinical papillomavirus infection (SPI) lesion with a pronounced mosaic capillary pattern. The mosaic pattern consists of uniform fine vessels that are rather loosely and randomly arranged as a form of horizontal mesh. These vessels are vertically and horizontally oriented. The vascular pattern in these lesions is usually more ill-defined with less complete boundaries than is the true mosaic angioarchitecture of the high-grade lesions. Close inspection of this pattern shows that there are irregular mosaic-type patterns with a large central vessel; these are characteristic of the low-grade histologic atypia. This lesion was shown to be composed of HPV/CIN 1 epithelium.

et al. (1984), which distinguishes between condylomatous and noncondylomatous lesions of similar appearance, has been found by many authors (Burghardt, 1991) to be cumbersome and unsatisfactory. This system, however, of relevance and some of its criteria will be used here to classify various HPV lesions.

Colposcopic appearance of condylomatous and subclinical papillomavirus lesions

The condylomatous lesions that were described above are sometimes difficult to distinguish from lesions of a more malignant nature, yet many of them are reversible and benign. Colposcopically, they have a typical appearance with a vascular micropapilliferous or frondlike surface. Their pathology is described and represented later. After the application of acetic acid, the surface becomes blanched and usually there is a definitive acetowhite change that may persist for some time (Figs 6.65 & 6.66).

Lesions can be single or multiple, and may even occur outside the lateral limits of the transformation zone. With increasing keratinization, the surface may appear to be walled or heaped up, resembling the surface of the cerebral cortex. This brainlike appearance has been called encephaloid or microconvoluted (Figs 6.67–6.69). Such a presentation may be difficult to distinguish from that seen in an early verrucous-type carcinoma because these warty excrescences occur in both types of lesion. The types of condyloma that have been described may intermingle and also occur in association with SPI. It may be extremely difficult to distinguish between the subclinical lesions and CIN. Consequently, biopsy may be the only method of procuring a final diagnosis.

The difficulty in distinguishing between subclinical HPV infections and high-grade CIN lesions is due to the fact that although SPI lesions are characterized colposcopically by a micropapillary and fine vascular arrangement analogous to a miniature condyloma, they may also present as a flat plaque of acetowhite epithelium that broadly resembles a high-grade CIN lesion. Biopsy is necessary in these cases. It is not surprising that there is a wide variety of morphologic patterns; these have been described by Reid *et al.* (1984) and Reid (1990), whose classification has been referred to above.

Some of the possibly confusing features of such lesions are shown in Figs 6.67–6.70. In Fig. 6.70, an extensive area of

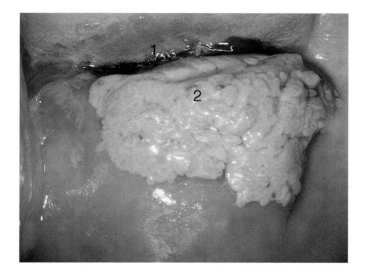

Fig. 6.65 After the application of acetic acid, the papillae whiten and are more easily recognized (2). The majority of the blood vessels, that are visible, for example in the condyloma featured in Fig. 6.71, are now masked. The acetic acid has caused the papillae to retract and separate. They have become shortened and rounded, and the isolated papillae can be seen more clearly. The lesion extends into the endocervical canal at (1).

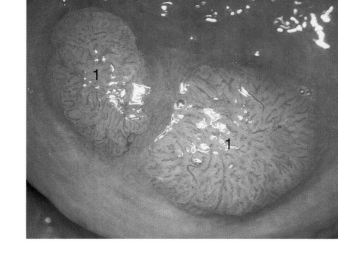

Fig. 6.66 A very abnormal vascular pattern exists on the surface of two condylomatous lesions (1) on the posterior cervical lip. Indeed, bizarre and atypical vessels of markedly variable caliber are present. Some show a staghorn-like appearance that is sometimes also seen in inflammatory lesions. Although there is a sharp edge to the lesions, they may be confused with an early invasive carcinoma. The appearance of these condylomata, once acetic acid has been applied, is seen in Fig. 6.74.

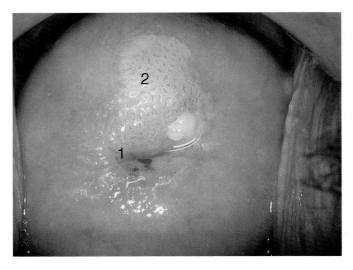

Fig. 6.67

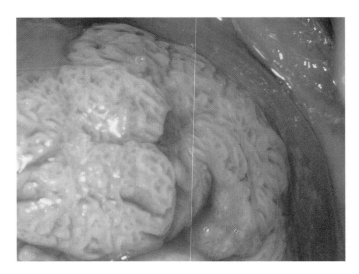

Fig. 6.68

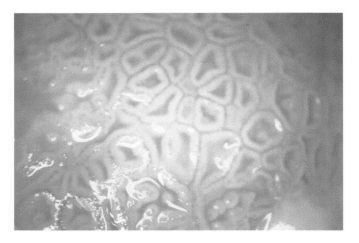

Fig. 6.69

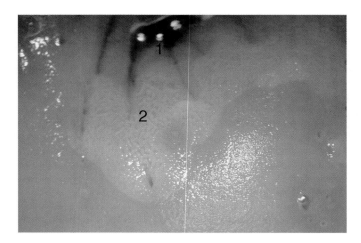

Fig. 6.70

the ectocervix is covered by a snow-white lesion (2) that appears indistinct when acetic acid is applied. It projects into the endocervix at (1). There is an obvious micropapillary surface arrangement. It also has an indistinct, angular, and rather jagged edge. The whole lesion would seem to have arisen just proximal to the squamocolumnar junction within the transformation zone. The lesion does extend into the endocervix and may present the colposcopist with a problem in diagnosis. Biopsies will be needed to differentiate this lesion from a high-grade lesion. Indeed, excision biopsy of this area showed it to be composed of a flat condyloma with minor basal changes that were consistent with CIN 1.

Figures 6.67–6.69 show the typical brainlike microconvoluted epithelial derangements that are associated with SPI. The pattern seen at (2) in Fig. 6.67, and in more detail in Figs 6.68 & 6.69 [the endocervix is at (1)], is caused by the nondilated but uniform-caliber capillaries underlying the surface, and with hyperkeratosis between the vessels. Histologically, markedly elongated papillae are seen, each containing a blood vessel, or several vessels, of varying caliber. Because of the thickness of the epithelium and the height of the stromal papillae, the resulting surface configuration of many of these subclinical HPV lesions is coarser than that seen in similar colposcopic lesions that

occur as a result of abnormal (atypical) epithelia. As has been mentioned, it may be impossible to distinguish between a flat SPI-type condyloma and abnormal (atypical) epithelium.

Colposcopic appearances of condylomata and their differentiation from malignant lesions

The colposcope allows one to differentiate between a condyloma and possible invasive lesions. Before the application of acetic acid, condylomata appear as soft, very poorly defined tumorous lesions that are dark reddish. The papillae are poorly individualized but the vessels are clearly visible (Figs 6.66 & 6.71–6.73). These vessels are described as sinuous and irregular, sometimes varicose, and may be comma-shaped, resemble a stag's horn, or even adopt a corkscrew appearance. These latter appearances are very similar to those seen in invasive carcinoma, especially of the papillary or verrucous form. It is not surprising that there are similarities because in both types new capillaries develop within the connective tissue to provide increased nourishment for the growth of the benign or malignant epithelial proliferations.

Prior to the application of acetic acid, the irregular vessels are visible through the translucent squamous

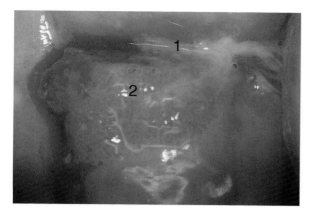

Fig. 6.71

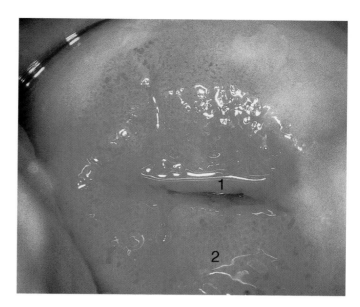

Fig. 6.72

epithelium. Once the acetic acid has been applied, the squamous epithelium becomes coagulated and masks the outline of the vessels (Figs 6.65, 6.74 & 6.75). However, the individual papillae can then be seen more clearly.

Further pathologic appearances of HPV and HPV/CIN-associated lesions

The varied pathologic features of HPV infection have been described already. Before embarking on a correlation of the diagnostic methods used to detect cervical precancer and the problems entailed, it would seem appropriate to further examine a number of features in the pathology of both HPV and HPV/CIN associated lesions (Figs 6.76–6.81).

6.9 Correlation of diagnostic methods in the detection of cervical squamous precancer

Cytology and colposcopy are the major diagnostic techniques used in the detection of cervical squamous precancer. Unfortunately, each involves a certain margin of error. However, by using colposcopy, it has been possible to iden-

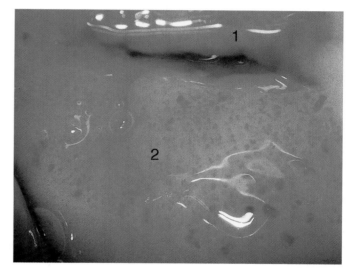

Fig. 6.73

Fig. 6.71 (*Above*) Condyloma characterized by comma-shaped and staghorn-like blood vessels (2) before the application of acetic acid. With this appearance an early papillary endocervical carcinoma cannot be excluded. The endocervical canal is at (1).

Figs 6.72 and 6.73 (*Above right*) Before the application of acetic acid, a generalized vascular pattern is obvious through the translucent squamous epithelium (2). At the higher magnification shown in Fig. 6.73, the fingerlike projections of these vessels with central capillary loops can be seen. Before the application of acetic acid (as seen in Fig. 6.75), this vascular pattern would be regarded as suspicious because some of the vessels, especially those seen in Fig. 6.72, have an atypical appearance. The endocervical canal is at (1).

Fig. 6.74 (*Below right*) Acetic acid, applied to the lesions seen in Fig. 4.66, has caused the whitening of the two condylomatous lesions (1), and the papillae can now be clearly seen toward the margins of the lesion. The vessels are completely masked, as the acetic acid has caused them to retract. On the anterior lip, there is an irregular-edged acetowhite epithelium (2). This is typical of subclinical human papillomavirus (HPV) disease. There is no neoplasia present within the cervix.

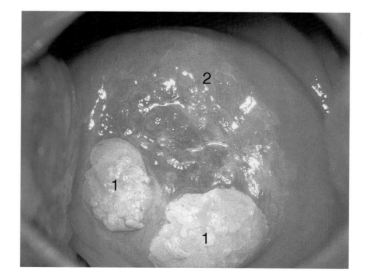

Fig. 6.74

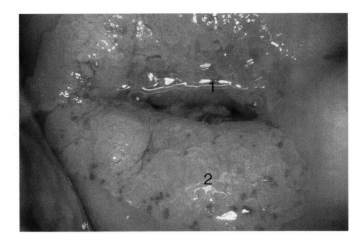

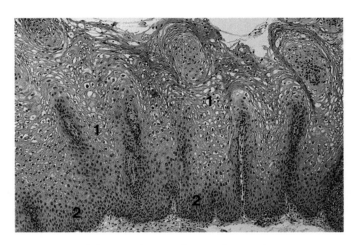

Fig. 6.75 The application of acetic acid to the cervix shown in Fig. 6.72 and 6.73 reveals a distinct flat condylomatous appearance. Some of the vessels can still be seen as punctated dark lesions within the flat condyloma at (2). The individual papillae now appear short and rounded, and are clearly visible. The endocervix is at (1).

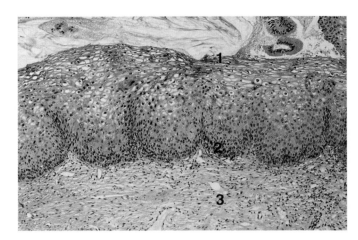

Fig. 6.76 Squamous epithelium showing features of wart virus infection; the surface (1) displays prominent koilocytic changes in the cells immediately beneath the surface. The basal cells (2) show some nuclear atypia and the lesion is classified as a flat condyloma (subclinical papillomavirus infection). There is a mild inflammatory infiltrate in the stroma at (3).

Fig. 6.78 A condyloma with a papillary surface configuration. There are widespread areas of koilocytosis at (1); normal stroma is present at (2).

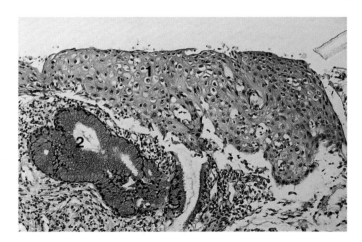

Fig. 6.77 Metaplastic-type squamous epithelium with human papillomavirus (HPV) changes at (1) overlying columnar epithelium in a gland crypt (2).

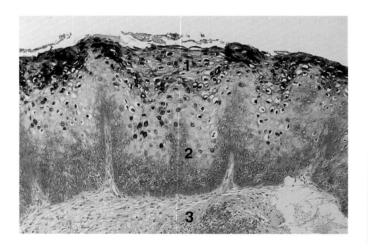

Fig. 6.79 Viral antigen staining (in-situ hybridization) shows intense staining of the nuclei of the koilocytes (1). There is slight atypia of the basal layers at (2) and normal stroma at (3). This is a low-grade epithelial lesion.

tify some of the reasons for the failings of cytology, especially in respect of its false-negative rate (Jarmulowicz *et al.*, 1989; Al-Nafussi *et al.*, 1993). It would seem that the higher the grade of lesion, that is CIN, the larger is the area of cervix occupied by the abnormal (atypical) squamous

epithelium, and the more likely it is for the process also to involve the glandular crypts. Furthermore, it would seem that the size, both area and depth, of the lesion increases with age for the same grade of CIN (Barton *et al.*, 1989; Jenkins, 1990). It has also been shown that the different

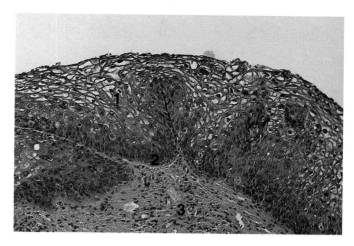

Fig. 6.80 Epithelium, showing wart viral infection, with prominent koilocytic changes and the occasional abnormal mitotic figure.

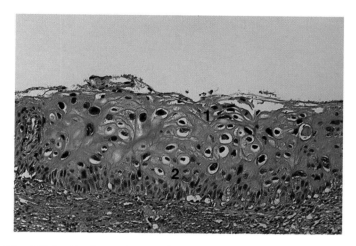

Fig. 6.81 In this photomicrograph, wart virus infection with striking koilocytic change exists within the very flattened epithelium (1). The nuclei of the koilocytes are enlarged and hyperchromatic. The basal nuclei (2) are atypical. In the absence of abnormal mitotic figures this lesion should be classified as a low-grade cervical intraepithelial neoplasia (CIN).

grades of CIN may occur simultaneously within the same cervix and present with just one cellular type in the cervical smear (Tidbury & Singer, 1992). In such conditions, it is the CIN with the largest area that would seem to dictate the type of smear that results. This can be shown by reference to Fig. 6.82, from the study by Jarmulowicz *et al.* (1989); a correlation was made between the grades of repeat smears and the area occupied by each lesion, as determined from excised material. Figure 6.83 shows the correlation between the most advanced grade of CIN and the size of the particular CIN lesion. It can be seen that the more severe (high grade) the lesion, the larger the area occupied. This will obviously have an effect on the smear taken from such an area. Indeed a study by Kierkegaard *et al.* (1995) comparing specific colposcopic findings with histology found that lesion size larger than 50% of the visible cervix as a single finding was highly statistically correlated to the histologic grade (odds ratio of 3.6; 95% CI, 2.1–6.3 for high-grade SIL).

This strong relationship between the cytologic grade and the extent of CIN is most important. About two-thirds of females with severe dyskaryosis HSIL will have CIN 3, another 20% will have CIN 2, and 10% will have CIN 1 or HPVI; less than 5% will have no detectable lesion (Singer *et al.*, 1984). Likewise, one-third of females with moderate dyskaryosis will have CIN 3 and a similar proportion will have CIN 2. These results indicate that moderate and severe dyskaryosis HSIL are good indicators of high-grade CIN, even if they do not always predict the exact histologic grade; in any case, this is subject to observer error. The risk of invasive cancer associated with a severe dyskaryosis HSIL is high, even when those smears that are thought to be suggestive of invasion are excluded. Several studies (Kohan *et al.*, 1985; Soutter *et al.*, 1986; Walker *et al.*, 1986) have shown that 20–40% of females with mild dyskaryosis LSIL turn out, following a colposcopic or excisional biopsy, to have high-grade CIN and up to 25% will have CIN 3 (Fig. 6.82).

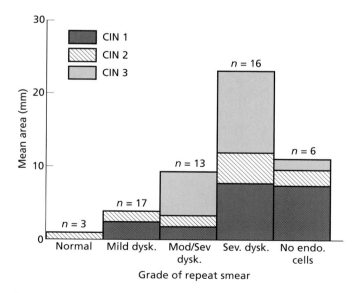

Fig. 6.82 Correlation between smear grade and the area (mm²) of cervical intraepithelial neoplasia (CIN) in excision biopsy material. (From Jarmulowicz *et al.*, 1989. With kind permission of *Br J Obstet Gynaecol.*)

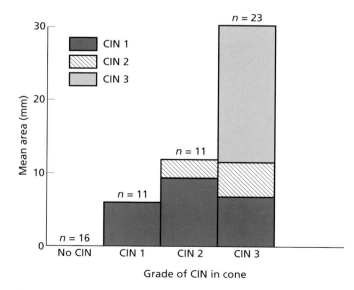

Fig. 6.83 Correlation between the most advanced grade of cervical intraepithelial neoplasia (CIN) and the size of the individual CIN lesion. (From Jarmulowicz *et al.*, 1989. With kind permission of *Br J Obstet Gynaecol.*)

The precancerous potential of small CIN 3 lesions is difficult to ascertain because they are usually associated with large areas of CIN 1 that are more likely to be sampled and yield the mildly dyskaryotic (LSIL) smears. In many cases, the CIN 3 lesion will eventually be identified by a major-grade cellular abnormality if cytology is repeated (Barton *et al.*, 1989).

It seems that a correlation can be made between the cytology, colposcopy, and pathology of the lesion and the risk of it being associated with invasive cancer. The low-grade precancer is typified by subclinical HPV infection and CIN 1. Such lesions are generally judged colposcopically to be small, and are associated with low-grade smear abnormalities (LSIL, such as borderline or mild dyskaryosis). As was pointed out in Chapter 2 these lesions are associated with viral types HPV 6 or 11 in the cervix. A substantial minority will regress and there is a very small risk of invasive disease. The high-grade lesions, on the other hand, are typified by the large CIN 3 lesion, which is diagnosed by high grade cytology, histology and colposcopy, and have a high risk of invasion and recurrence after treatment (Shafi *et al.*, 1993). This risk is most likely related to the size of the CIN 3 component and the associated HSIL cytology (moderate or severe dyskaryosis) (Jenkins, 1990).

There would also seem to exist an interface between the high- and low-grade precancers, which include the CIN 2 and small CIN 3 lesions. These are lesions that may progress to become larger but at this stage probably do not represent a high-risk group for the presence of invasion. They may be associated with any grade of smear abnormality and account for the vast majority of high-grade histologic CIN 3 lesions that are associated with low-grade cytology. There is a further interface at the opposite end of the spectrum in respect of high-grade precancer and the development of invasion.

Combination of the three diagnostic modalities forms the basis for efficient management of cervical precancer. In the following, this combination will be examined and correlations will be made between cytology, colposcopy, and pathology for individual CIN lesions.

Examples of the correlation of diagnostic methods

In HPV/CIN 1/LSIL

Case 1

Figure 6.84 shows a low-grade (LSIL) smear from a 22-year-old including occasional dyskeratotic and binucleated koilocytotic squamous cells with no other features (central cells in field). The nuclear changes include a relatively increased nuclear diameter.

The transformation zone (Fig. 6.85a) is seen to contain an area on the posterior lip of acetowhite epithelium that is shiny and semitranslucent with indistinct borders in relation to the original squamocolumnar junction (dashed line). The acetowhite epithelium extends to the new squamocolumnar junction (arrowed). A high-power view as seen in Fig. 6.85b shows the epithelium to have sur-

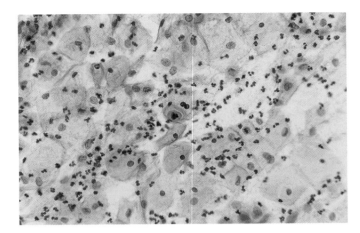

Fig. 6.84

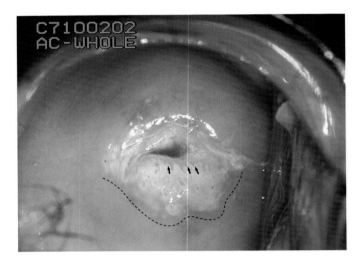

Fig. 6.85(a)

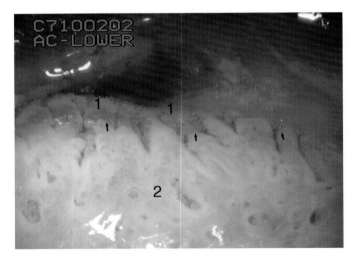

Fig. 6.85(b)

rounded areas of original columnar epithelium which are seen as (1). A sample taken by punch biopsy (2) shows an epithelium with evidence of HPV infection and superbasal cell proliferation representing either basal cell hyperplasia or CIN 1 (Fig. 6.86).

The overall impression from cytology, colposcopy and histology is of a lesion with HPV/CIN 1/LSIL.

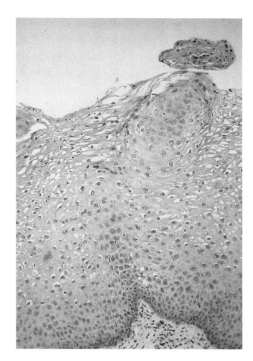

Fig. 6.86

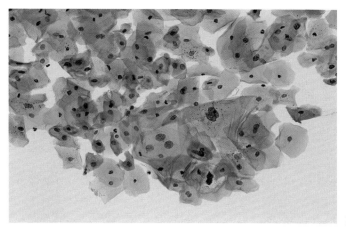

Fig. 6.87

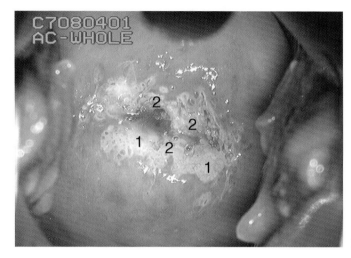

Fig. 6.88

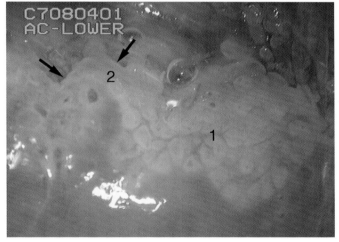

Fig. 6.89

Case 2

A 24-year-old female presented with a smear that was highly suggestive of HPV infection with typical koilocytes and mild dyskaryosis (LSIL) as in Fig. 6.87. When the cervix was examined (Fig. 6.88), it was found that there was an area of atypical (abnormal) epithelium on the posterior lip (1) associated with changes of immature metaplasia in the rest of the cervix (2). A high power view of the atypical (abnormal) epithelium, as seen in Fig. 6.89 shows an area of regular mosaic epithelium (1) adjacent to tissue representing immature metaplasia at (2) with the new squamo-columnar just seen and arrowed. A punch biopsy taken from (1) shows the typical features of HPV infection with or without CIN 1 (LSIL) (Fig. 6.90). At (1) in the superficial layer, koilocytes are present whereas at (2) there is some basal cell proliferation. There is very mild nuclear atypia and multinucleation is prominent. The stroma (3) is normal.

Case 3

Another example involving a low-grade lesion is shown in Fig. 6.91; here, cytology in a 26-year-old woman revealed the presence of koilocytotic and dyskaryotic cells suggesting CIN 1 and wart virus infection (LSIL). The colposcopy (Fig. 6.92) also shows features suggestive of a low-grade lesion; these include a shiny white acetowhite epithelium (1) and a margin of indistinct irregular edges (2). Satellite lesions are present on the left of the photograph at (3). Punch biopsy (Fig. 6.93), taken from point (1), reveals an area with a flat condyloma and abundant koilocytosis. The atypical cells extend through the epithelium with some differentiation in the middle and upper thirds, and atypical basal changes. This type of epithelial change is consistent with a CIN 1/LSIL lesion.

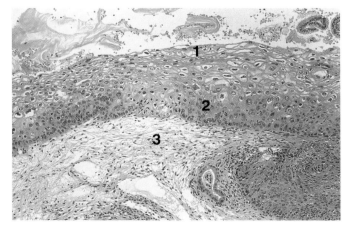

Fig. 6.90

In moderate-grade epithelial lesions

Figure 6.94 shows a smear from a 29 year-old female; this smear is suggestive of CIN 2. The cells are intermediate cells with dyskaryotic nuclei, some binucleation and koilocytosis. Colposcopy (Fig. 6.95) shows a lesion consistent with high-grade disease. Following the application of acetic acid, there is a general acetowhitening of the transformation zone and mild accentuation of the surface contour. The acetowhitening is not as pronounced as it has been in previous low-grade lesions, but has a dull-white character. The lower border of the lesion at (3) is sharp and this is an important sign in the differentiation of high- and low-grade colposcopic lesions. There is also variation in the color tone between the original squamous epithelium and the abnormal (atypical) epithelium; this is more pronounced in the high-grade than in the low-grade lesions. The abnormal (atypical) epithelium (2) extends toward the canal (1) and the upper extent of this epithelium is highlighted by the arrows. This is a grade 2 (Coppleson & Pixley, 1992a) colposcopic lesion.

A punch biopsy (Fig. 6.96), taken from point (3) on the posterior lip, shows CIN 2 in the superficial layers (1), and an increase in atypical suprabasal cells (2) that extend through about half the epithelial thickness. Nuclear atypia and hyperchromasia are present. Multinucleate cells are common and mitotic figures can be seen extending into the middle part of the epithelium. A histologic diagnosis of CIN 2 is made.

In high-grade epithelial lesions

A 31-year-old woman has presented with a severely dyskaryotic (HSIL) smear (Fig. 6.97). There are abnormalities within both the nucleus and cytoplasm, and the former shows enlargement, variation in size and shape, and hyperchromasia. There is also an irregular nuclear outline. The cytoplasm is variable and the smear is typical of a high-grade lesion.

The colposcopy (Fig. 6.98) shows an area within the transformation zone especially on the anterior lip of very dense acetowhite epithelium (1). An internal margin is present at (2) and an area of less dense acetowhite epithelium is present at (3). Other areas on the lateral margins of the ectocervix show features of both insignificant and non-suspicious epithelium (grade 1) at (4) and also of significant, suspicious grade 2 epithelium (5). The sharp upper border of the new squamocolumnar junction can be clearly seen (arrowed) on both on the anterior and posterior lips although in the real colposcopic view (when the speculum is removed into the vagina) the atypical (abnormal) epithelium retracts high into the endocervix. At (6), there is an area of loss of superficial epithelium which is characteristic of high grade disease; in this case, as a result of trauma from the examination. Excisional biopsy showed a central CIN 3 lesion, surrounded by peripheral CIN 1 and CIN 2. The excisional biopsy (Fig. 6.99) shows an area of CIN 3.

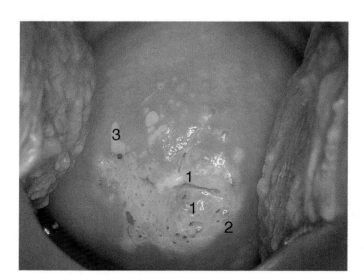

Fig. 6.91

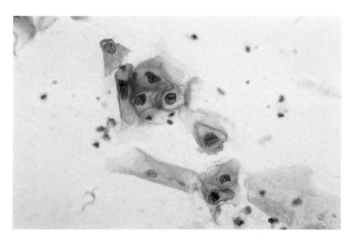

Fig. 6.92

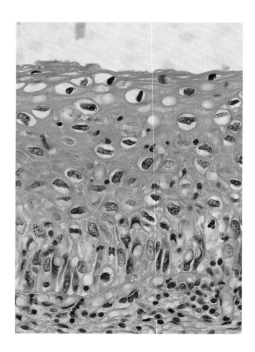

Fig. 6.93

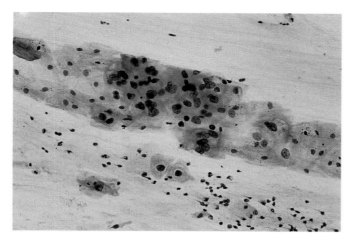

Fig. 6.94

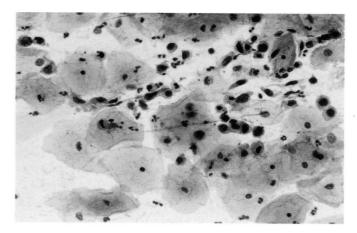

Fig. 6.97

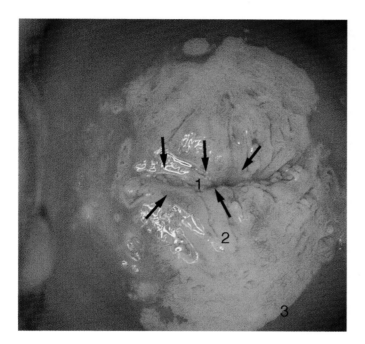

Fig. 6.95

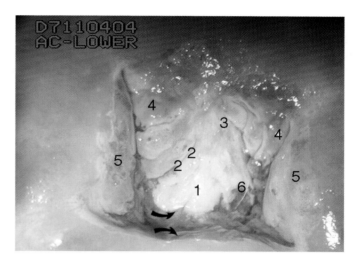

Fig. 6.98

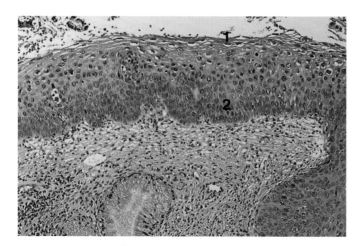

Fig. 6.96

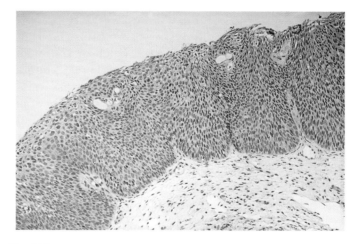

Fig. 6.99

6.10 Lack of correlation between diagnostic methods

In the previous section, examples were given of correlation between the diagnostic methods. In many cases, however, there is a lack of correlation. Four such cases will now be presented and the reasons for this lack will be discussed. In each, the lack of correlation was principally because there was a small CIN 3 lesion and in three of the cases this was found to exist in association with a larger area of CIN 1. In all cases, the smear yielded mildly dyskaryotic cells (LSIL). It was only by meticulous colposcopy with directed punch biopsy that the major-grade lesion, albeit small, was found.

The biologic potential of the small CIN 3 lesions is unknown (Jenkins, 1990; Shafi *et al.*, 1991, 1993). It may represent an earlier stage of progression or a lesion progressing slowly to invasion. Much of the evidence for the high rate of progression of CIN 3 to invasion comes from older studies of women who were initially diagnosed cytologically as having severe dyskaryosis (HSIL) strongly associated with a large CIN 3 lesion.

As has been discussed previously, the size of the CIN lesion is also important in determining the risk of false-negative smears (Barton *et al.*, 1989). It has been shown that colposcopically large lesions, those involving more than two quadrants of the cervix, are unlikely to produce a false-negative smear, whereas the false-negative cytology rate for lesions smaller than this is greater than 50%. In a recent study (Barton *et al.*, 1989), one-third of the cases of false-negative cytology occurred with lesions that occupied less than 10% of the area of the transformation zone. These lesions were almost entirely CIN 1. The importance of the proportion of the transformation zone that is occupied by different-sized lesions, and their effect on the resultant cytology (as discussed above) suggests that small lesions may escape cytologic sampling by eluding inclusion in the cell sample. It would seem that a certain threshold concentration of abnormal cells, in proportion to normal cells, may also be required for detection. This probably explains the following four cases.

Figure 6.100 is a colpophotograph from a 34-year-old female who had shown a negative cytology at regular yearly intervals. The smear that prompted this colposcopic examination was of a mild dyskaryosis (LSIL). The colposcopic examination revealed a small patch of acetowhite epithelium at (2) on the edge of the endocervix (1). The area has a relatively sharp border but there was no associated vascular change. The color tone is different from that of the surrounding epithelium, and the surface contour is slightly elevated. However, punch biopsy revealed the presence of CIN 3 (high-grade disease). It could be speculated that a larger area of abnormal (atypical) epithelium of a high grade nature existed on the anterior lip but that this had been destroyed during parturition when a physiologic erosion occurred.

Figure 6.101 is a colpophotograph from a 27-year-old woman who presented with mild dyskaryosis (LSIL). Colposcopy revealed an extensive area of acetowhiteness on the anterior lip between areas (2) and (3). This abnormal (atypical) epithelium is suggestive of SPI. A shiny white epithelium associated with the irregular indistinct border at (3) supports this diagnosis. The upper extent of the acetowhite epithelium is arrowed within the endocervical canal (1).

The colposcopist noted some abnormal vessels within

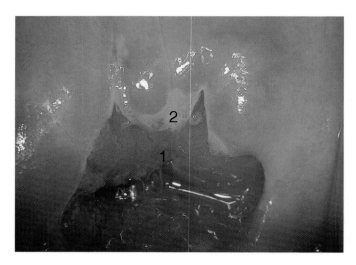

Fig. 6.100

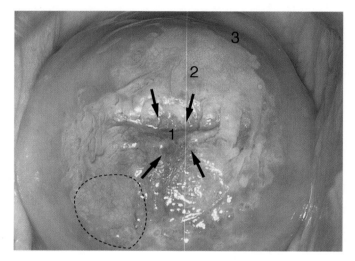

Fig. 6.101

the area (circled). These atypical vessels have an irregular branched pattern, and, on close examination, can be seen to have variable-diameter branches. Although this did not represent an extreme example of atypical vascularity, a punch biopsy was taken and revealed the presence of CIN 3 (high-grade disease). This is another example of a small area of CIN 3 occurring within the transformation zone that was predominantly occupied by a minor-grade lesion.

Figure 6.102 is a colpophotograph from a 29-year-old woman with a mildly dyskaryotic smear. At colposcopy, an area of acetowhite change was noted surrounding the cervical os which consists in the main of low-grade CIN changes as evidenced by the faint irregular acetowhite margins at (1). However, on the posterior lip there is an internal border surrounding an area of denser acetowhite

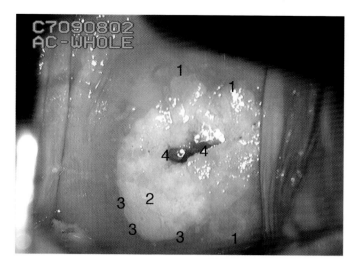

Fig. 6.102

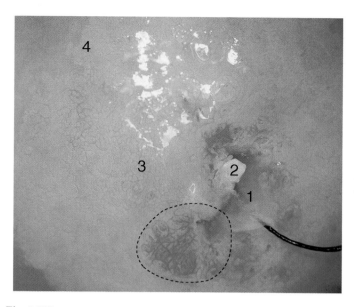

Fig. 6.103

change (2), which is in association with a sharp and raised external border (3). The new squamocolumnar junction is seen at (4) and the examination is thus deemed satisfactory. Multiple punch biopsies were taken which were reported as showing CIN 1 in relation to (1) and CIN 2 to 3 at (2). This case portrays another example where a small area of major-grade disease, surrounded by a lager of minor-grade disease, is discovered only by precise colposcopically directed biopsy.

The woman whose cervix is represented in Fig. 6.103 presented with a mildly dyskaryotic (LSIL) smear. A small condyloma is present at (2) and obtrudes into the endocervix (1), from which is projecting an intrauterine device (IUD) cord. A very fine mosaic pattern is present at (3) and involves most of the ectocervix. An irregular indistinct border is present at (4). These features are characteristic of a subclinical papillomavirus infection and indicate a low-grade lesion. However, the colposcopist noted that in the area that has been circled, there were vessels of a coarse mosaic nature. Patterns like this can also be associated with papillomavirus, but in this case a punch biopsy revealed the presence of CIN 3 (high-grade disease). It is suggested that the major portion of the cytologic sample constituted cells from the large area of minor-grade disease; the small area of major-grade disease yielded a small cellular sample compared with that produced from the rest of the cervical epithelium.

6.11 The diagnosis of early invasion

Early invasive squamous cell carcinoma: colposcopic diagnosis

The colposcopic detection of early invasive carcinoma depends on a number of features. Besides those defined (by Coppleson, 1992) previously in association with high-grade epithelial lesions, there are a number that must be added. These are:
1 Size of lesion.
2 Presence of different epithelial types within the lesion.

3 Increased vascularity.
4 Ulceration.

It is very difficult to diagnose by colposcopy any early stromal invasion that extends only a fraction of a millimeter into the stroma. Many of these foci arise from glands that are involved with CIN 3 and the colposcopic appearance is essentially that of the parent surface epithelium with the invasive foci protruding from the base. Burghardt (1991) recognized the importance of the size of the lesion as an indicator of early invasive disease. He showed that the larger the area of abnormal (atypical) epithelium, the more likely was the occurrence of an early invasive lesion. Other authors have confirmed these findings (Tidbury & Singer, 1992) (Tables 6.4 & 6.5) and showed that an area of CIN 3 from which invasion develops was some seven times larger than an area of CIN 3 that had no associated invasion.

Burghardt (1991) has also shown that where early stromal invasion has occurred, it is more common to find different epithelial types of the CIN spectrum associated with the invasion.

Increased epithelial and stromal vascularity is also suggestive of invasion, and as has been described above, a wide intercapillary distance, the presence of atypical vessels, and an irregular surface are all features of a high-grade lesion. However, there are many reports in the literature where "not all early invasive lesions were associated with atypical vessels" (Kolstad & Stafl, 1982). In these cases, a more complex pattern of epithelial abnormality such as a combination of acetowhiteness, punctation, mosaic, a raised irregular punctate surface, and a large lesion, were more common than abnormal vascularity.

Ulceration, which masks the surface epithelium, is likewise a not uncommon feature of early invasive disease.

The diagnosis of early invasion therefore requires a combination of both colposcopic and pathologic indicators. The colposcopic features have already been described, and for the pathology, the recent International Federation of

Table 6.4 Comparison of total length of cervical intraepithelial neoplasia (CIN) 3 in cone biopsies containing microinvasive squamous carcinoma (diagnosed following abnormal cytology).

		Length of CIN 3 (mm)			
	n	Mean	(SD)	(SEM)	Range
*Previous study**					
Smears					
Mild	22	0.6	(1.7)	(0.4)	0.0–7.9
Moderate	15	5.3	(15.7)	(4.1)	0.0–60.7
Severe	21	9.5	(15.5)	(3.4)	0.0–53.7
Present study†					
Microinvasive carcinoma	39	63.5	(37.2)	(6.0)	11.4–162.4

*Jarmulowicz *et al.* (1989).

†From Tidbury and Singer (1992). Reproduced by kind permission of *Br J Obstet Gynaecol.*

Table 6.5 Relation (in terms of the number of biopsies) between cytologic grade/microinvasive cancer and total length of CIN 3 present in cone biopsies.

	Length of CIN 3 (mm)			
	<1	1–9.9	10.0–19.9	>20
*Previous study**				
Smears				
Mild	20	2	0	0
Moderate	11	2	1	1
Severe	11	5	1	4
Present study†				
Microinvasive carcinoma	0	0	3	36

*Jarmulowicz *et al.* (1989).

†From Tidbury and Singer (1992). Reproduced by kind permission of *Br J Obstet Gynaecol.*

Gynecology and Obstetrics (FIGO) statement concerning morphological parameters (1995) has placed objective limits on the extent of early invasion (see Table 1.1a, p. 10). Under this classification stage Ia is defined as early invasive carcinoma of the cervix; this stage can only be diagnosed by microscopy and is further subdivided into stages Ia1 and Ia2. Stage Ia1 describes microscopic stromal invasion to a depth of 3 mm. The more important Ia2 stage describes a lesion with a depth of invasion of no more than 5 mm from the base of either the surface or glandular epithelium from which the disease originates. For stage Ia, the second dimension of measure, the horizontal spread, must not exceed 7 mm (Burghardt, 1992a). Other features, such as capillary-like (endothelial) space-involvement and specific growth patterns, must also be examined. The latter involve those that may be confluent, sprayed, or fingerlike. More advanced lesions of early invasion are sometimes referred to as colposcopically suspect/overt invasive carcinomas. Many of these show an extension of invasion beyond the 5-mm limit.

In the examples presented here, an early invasive lesion is suspected colposcopically. Both the acetic acid and saline techniques of colposcopy have been used to illustrate various features of the lesion. In Fig. 6.104a, the application of acetic acid has removed the very pronounced vascular pattern that existed at (2) and that was seen when the saline technique was used (Fig. 6.105a). In Fig. 6.104a, the epithelium is extremely white and has a matted opaque color in areas (2) and (3). The surface is irregular (3) and the area has sharp borders (4). There is an obvious color-tone difference between the native and the abnormal (atypical) epithelium. The large extent of the lesion, which occupies most of the ectocervix, would raise suspicion of early invasion. The upper extent, as signified by the new squamocolumnar junction, of the lesion in the endocervical canal (1, and arrowed) cannot be seen.

In Fig. 6.105a, the marked and abnormal vascularity can be seen. Areas of coarse punctation and mosaicism are visible, especially on the anterior lip in area (2). A hemorrhage has already been induced within the endocervix (1,

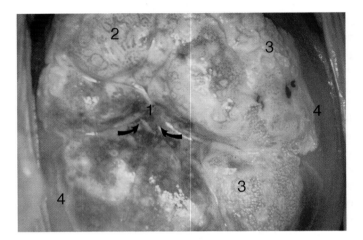

Fig. 6.104(a)

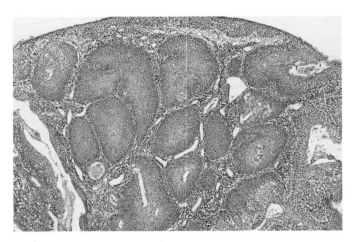

Fig. 6.104(b)

and arrowed) when saline was gently applied. This contact bleeding is another suspicious feature indicating the presence of high-grade epithelial disease.

Various epithelial types exist within this lesion. A punch biopsy (Fig. 6.104b), taken from point (2), reveals the presence of CIN 3 (1) but with no extension into the underlying

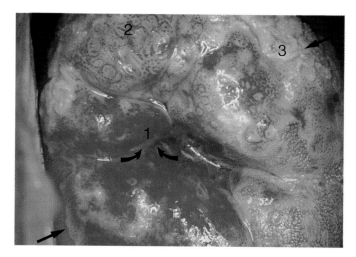

Fig. 6.105(a)

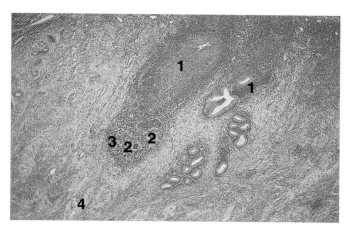

Fig. 6.105(b)

stroma (2). There is, however, advancement of this high-grade lesion into the crypts (3). Excision biopsy of this whole area revealed the presence of early stromal invasion. A section of this biopsy specimen is shown in Fig. 6.105b; the CIN 3 lesion is seen at (1), areas of early invasion to a depth of about 2 mm are present at (2), and there is a surrounding intense inflammatory cell infiltration (3) within the stroma at (4).

There is a further colposcopic feature that is characteristic of a major-grade lesion and may be associated with early invasion. This is the presence of tufted glands within an area of abnormal (atypical) epithelium. In such cases the abnormal (atypical) epithelium occupies the gland and forms a cuff that surrounds the secretory duct of the gland and penetrates to a variable depth. Following the application of acetic acid, it is recognized as a spot that is whiter than the rest of the lesion, is depressed, and has at its center a hole or slit. Occasionally, it has the appearance of a raised rim surrounding the gland orifice. A prominent entrance to a gland crypt can sometimes be found in benign situations as, for example, when the epithelium is normal and acanthotic, and in these cases the ring around the gland entrance will be less pronounced and thinner than in the corresponding major-grade lesion. In Fig. 6.106a a number of these gland clefts have been indicated (arrowed). They are associated with an area (2) of coarse mosaicism that is demarkated from an outer area of fine mosaicism by a sharp border. The upper limit of the lesion can be easily seen projecting into the endocervix at (1). Excision biopsy of this large lesion revealed the presence of early stromal invasion (stage Ia1) in relation to area (2); CIN 2/3 was present in the area between (3) and (4).

In some lesions gland crypts may be present beneath the epithelium and may have no obvious surface opening. Such a situation exists in Fig. 6.107, where a very extensive area of abnormal (atypical) epithelium (3), from which a punch biopsy has been taken and which is indicative of a high-grade lesion, extends across the ectocervical anterior lip and into the endocervical canal (1). Removal of the biopsy tissue reveals the presence of a glandular crypt from which yellow mucus exudes (2). No other signs of gland openings exist on this abnormal epithelial surface. It is most

important to appreciate this, as the abnormal (atypical) epithelium may extend deep into the stroma via the gland cleft. The histology of the punch biopsy taken from the area around (2) is shown in Fig. 6.108 where the epithelium is of a CIN 3 (1) and extends into the glands (2). Excision biopsy of the abnormal (atypical) epithelium revealed the presence of early invasive carcinoma (stage Ia2).

Further examples of the colposcopic appearance of early invasion are seen in Figs 6.106b, 6.107, 6.109–10, 6.111b. In all these examples no obvious clinical evidence of invasion existed. However, these subclinical appearances of early invasion were immediately recognized when colposcopy was used.

Importance of pathology in diagnosis

As mentioned earlier, it is extremely difficult to judge the extent of early invasion from a colposcopic assessment and only histology can make the objective diagnosis (Burghardt, 1992a). The early stages of invasion can be recognized as tiny buds of invasive cells (1) penetrating beneath the basement membrane (2) into the underlying stroma (3) (Fig. 6.111ai). These cells have the appearance of those of the CIN 3 tissue from which they have usually arisen. As invasion occurs, the cells become more differentiated than those of the overlying CIN 3. There is usually a stromal reaction involving localized lymphocytes. Edema also accompanies this infiltration as the neoplastic tissue gives rise to a loosening of the stroma.

With further invasion, there is involvement of the lymphatic channel, after which generalized growth into the surrounding stroma and tissues of the cervix occurs (Fig. 6.111(aii)). Unless detailed sections are made, it is possible to miss early invasion that has extended beyond the defined limits. It is necessary to take between 25 and 40 sections to make an accurate diagnosis. If fewer sections are taken, as is usual in clinical practice, small areas of invasion may be missed. For example, in Fig. 6.111c the smear from the cervix of a 47-year-old female suggests squamous cell carcinoma. The endocervix is at (1) (arrowed). However, on the ectocervix (2) there is a depressed whitish lesion with an irregular base. The groove surrounding the lesion, which has a very irregular surface contour, suggests that invasive

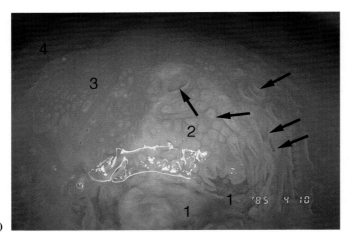

Fig. 6.106(a)

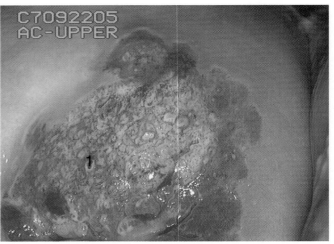

Fig. 6.106(b)

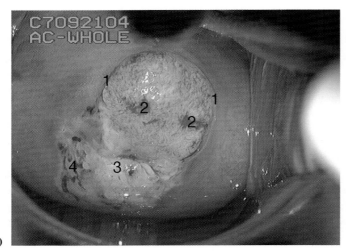

Fig. 6.106(c)

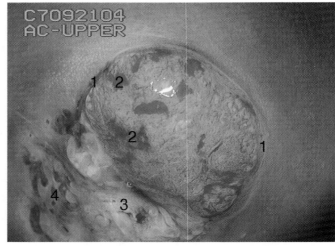

Fig. 6.106(d)

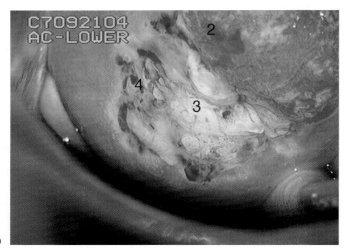

Fig. 6.106(e)

Fig. 6.106 (a) A 25-year-old woman with severe dyskaryosis on colposcopy. (b) The abnormal (atypical) epithelium extends well into the endocervix making it an unsatisfactory colposcopy. There is coarse punctation and mosaic on the anterior lip. There is a distinct color tone difference between atypical (abnormal) epithelium and the surrounding tissue. There are tufted glands at (1) and the atypical (abnormal) epithelium occupies the whole of the transformation zone that can be seen. Excision biopsy of the cervix showed the presence of early microinvasive disease.

(b–d) Large atypical (abnormal) transformation zone shows features that are highly suggestive of early invasive carcinoma. The rolled edges at (1) encompass an area on the anterior lip of marked vessel irregularity and contact bleeding with disruption of the superficial epithelium surrounding the area marked at (2). On the posterior lip (Fig. 6.106e) at (3), there is dense acetowhite epithelium with a papilliferous surface configuration. There is further disruption of the epithelium at (4). Excisional biopsy showed an invasive carcinoma with a depth of penetration of 5.6 mm below the basement membrane with marked vascular lymphatic permeation. This is an example of a stage Ib1 cancer which will be described in Section 6.12 on p. 147.

disease is present. There is also a difference in color tone between this area and the surrounding tissue, and abnormal vessels can be seen in the base of the depressed area. The area above and surrounding the internal os (1) is also very abnormal and indicative of a high-grade lesion.

Pathologic specimens were taken from multiple areas of this cervix and they showed that the medial part of the lesion possessed cancerous tissue that had in-

vaded to a depth of 3 mm. However, sections of the lateral area (in the area of the depressed whitish lesion) showed gross lymphatic involvement with malignant cells. This diagnosis was most important in determining the appropriate treatment. Unless multiple sections had been taken, the very small area of highly invasive disease (i.e. the lymphatic permeation) would have been overlooked.

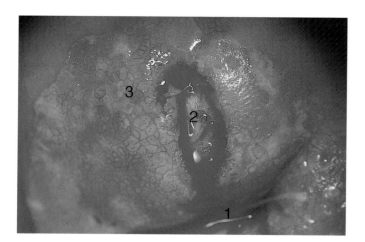

Fig. 6.107

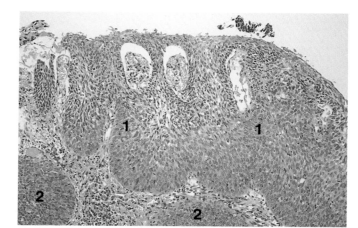

Fig. 6.108

Fig. 6.109 The raised papilliferous appearance (2) within the transformation zone was highly suggestive of early invasive disease. Contact bleeding occurred just above the endocervix (1). The outlines of atypical vessels are just visible at the edge of the transformation zone (3). Although the appearance of the cervix could be mistaken for an ectopy, the presence of a severely dyskaryotic (high-grade squamous intraepithelial lesion) smear in conjunction with the atypical vascularity indicates the possible presence of early invasion. Excision biopsy revealed the presence of early invasion (stage Ia2).

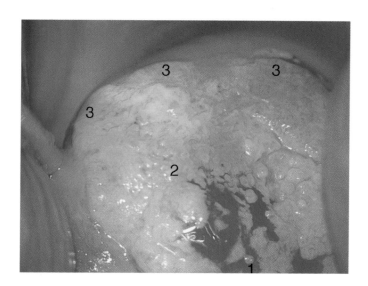

Fig. 6.110 The abnormal (atypical) epithelium extends well into the endocervix (1, arrow), giving an appearance of an unsatisfactory colposcopy. Coarse punctation exists at area (2), but abnormal vessels exist around the upper and outer left margins of the cervix (3). There is a distinct color-tone difference between this area and the surrounding tissue. Large dilated vessels are highly suggestive of early invasion. A small ulcerated area also exists on the posterior lip at the entrance to the endocervix. Excision biopsy of this lesion showed it to be an early invasive carcinoma of stage Ia2.

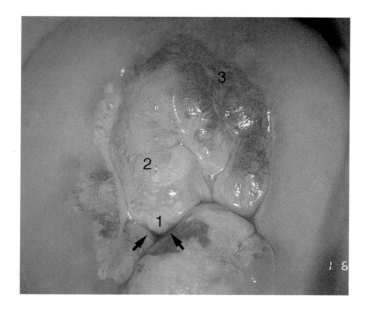

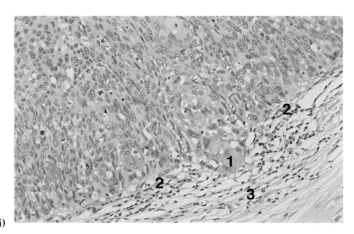

Fig. 6.111(ai)

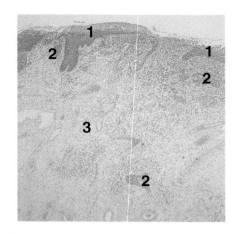

Fig. 6.111(aii)

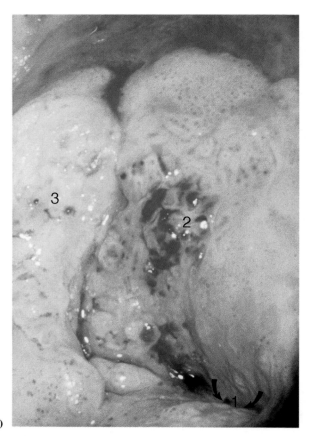

Fig. 6.111(b)

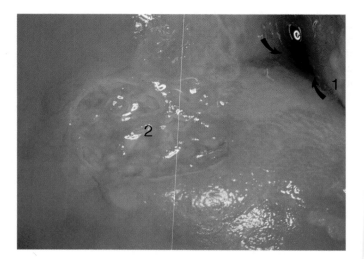

Fig. 6.111(c)

Fig. 6.111 (aii) This shows CIN 3 (1) with tongues of invasive squamous carcinoma (2) infiltrating the stroma (3) to a depth of 3.3 mm (FIGO Stage Ia2)

(b) The color-tone difference between this exceedingly white lesion and the surrounding epithelium is obvious; it extends high into the endocervix (1, and arrowed). Abnormal vessels are present in a leash at (2) and show coarse punctation; there are further abnormal vessels in the area (3). Excision biopsy showed this to be early invasive carcinoma of stage Ia2.

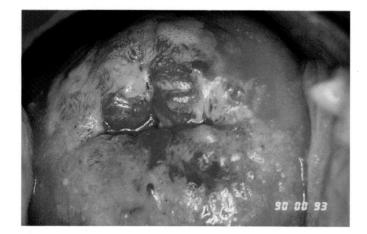

Fig. 6.112

Figure 6.112 shows a large and major-grade lesion. The central reddish area suggested the presence of invasive carcinoma. A cone biopsy was performed, and even though 34 multiple sections were taken, only a very small area of invasive disease (invasion to a depth of 3.5 mm) was found in three sections. The remainder showed the presence of CINs 2 and 3. It had been expected that the pathology would show large areas of early invasion.

The case presented in Fig. 6.113 shows the variation in depth of invasion that can occur between different areas of the same cervix. A wide excision biopsy showed between 2 and 5 mm of invasion (Fig. 6.114) that could not have been predicted colposcopically.

Fig. 6.113(a)

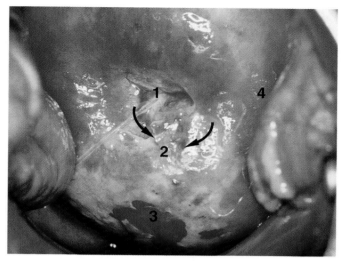

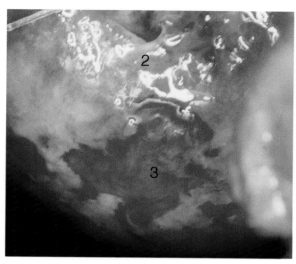

Fig. 6.113(b)

Fig. 6.113 (a) and (b) The cervix of a 42-year-old female who presented with a severe dyskaryotic smear (high-grade squamous intraepithelial lesion). An area of hyperemia extends across the anterior cervix and projects into the left vaginal fornix at (4). In (a) there is an irregular contour to the tissues surrounding the endocervix (1, and arrowed). Very abnormal (atypical) epithelium exists at (2) and an ulcerated area (3) is also visible. This can be seen more clearly in the high-power view of the posterior cervical lip shown in (b). In early invasive lesions, the abnormal (atypical) epithelium is particularly vulnerable as it lacks cohesiveness and is easily detached. This can occur not only during an examination but also from normal vaginal trauma. Its appearance is highly suggestive of early invasive disease. The pathology of an excision biopsy taken from this cervix is shown in Fig. 6.114.

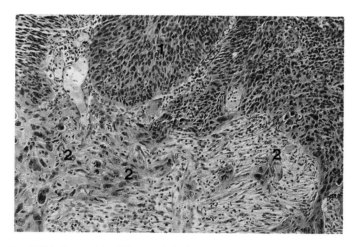

Fig. 6.114 An excision biopsy of the lesion shown in Fig. 6.113 reveals the pathology seen here. There is a cervical intraepithelial neoplasia (CIN) 3 lesion at (1), and within the stroma there are infiltrating malignant cells (2). They have penetrated to a depth of 5 mm and have involved the endothelial lined lymphatic spaces. A section of tissue from around area (4) in Fig. 6.113a showed invasion to a depth of 2 mm.

6.12 Preclinical invasive carcinoma (colposcopically overt/suspect): colposcopy and pathology

There are a number of instances where early invasive carcinoma is not recognized by the traditional methods of inspection; palpation, probing, and endocervical curettage. These lesions are called preclinical invasive carcinomas, and most become obvious when the illuminated magnification of colposcopy is used. This entity is also referred to as the colposcopically suspect/overt carcinoma (Coppleson, 1992). Previously, these lesions were referred to as stage Ib occult carcinomas. This term was used for those lesions where a single invasive focus, or confluent foci in invasion, showed more than 5-mm penetration into the stroma. However, in contradistinction to the overt carcinomas, they cannot be detected by the usual clinical examination techniques described above. These lesions have very marked morphologic features that become evident colposcopically after the application of acetic acid; these features include, marked raised edges, the so-called mountain range appearance that is representative of an irregular surface contour, and very obvious and bizarre blood vessels of altered caliber, size, shape, direction, and arrangement (see Fig. 6.10b–e, p. 144).

Coppleson (1992) believes that colposcopy should play the predominant role in determining the mode of treatment for these preclinical invasive carcinomas. It must be emphasized that the microinvasive carcinomas (stages Ia1 and Ia2), described above, are also defined as preclinical invasive; early invasive cancer as stage Ib1 (see Table 1.1a, p. 10).

Three pathologic specimens are presented (Figs 6.115–6.117) from women who showed no obvious clinical signs of overt carcinoma, although colposcopy and subsequent pathology diagnosed the presence of early invasive carcinoma. In Fig. 6.115 strands of invasive cells (1) and (2) have permeated the stroma (3) to a depth of 7 mm. The lesion was designated a stage Ib1 squamous carcinoma. In Fig. 6.116 a CIN 3 lesion (1) extends into a gland (2); the gland itself (3) projects to a depth of 5.5 mm. A focus of

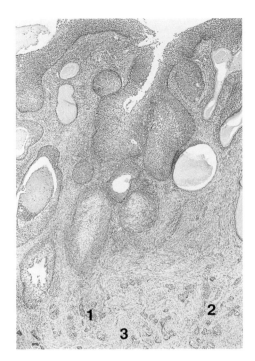

Fig. 6.115

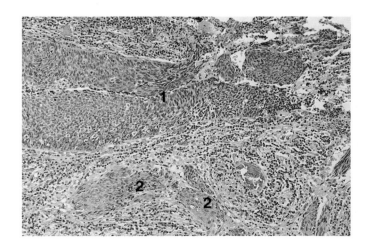

Fig. 6.116

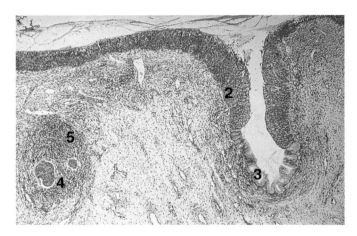

Fig. 6.117

microinvasion is seen at (4) and there is intense round cell infiltration at (5). Accurate measurement placed the depth of invasion at 4.5 mm from the surface. However, the extent of the lesion was approximately 9 mm along the surface, and other areas of invasion projected to a depth of up to 6 mm. In Fig. 6.117, a CIN 3 lesion exists at (1) and there are nests of malignant cells in the stroma (2). These cells penetrate to a depth of 7 mm; in this figure, however, invasion is to a depth of 1.5 mm. The lesion is classified as a stage Ib1 (a clinical lesion no greater than 4 cm in size) carcinoma.

In the following three cases the lesions were, again, not immediately identified as invasion until a colposcopic examination had been performed. They are classed as stage IB which includes clinical lesions confined to the cervix or as in these cases preclinical lesions greater than stage IA which were assessed and measured with the aid of colposcopy. In the case shown in Fig. 6.118, a major-grade cytologic smear indicated the need for colposcopy, but it

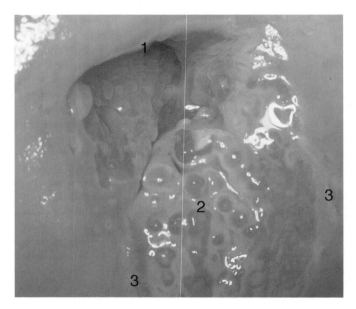

Fig. 6.118

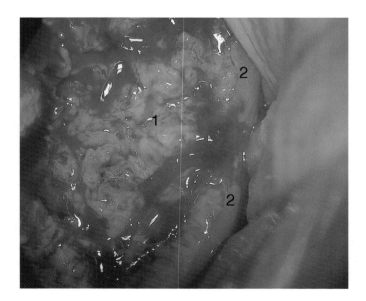

Fig. 6.119

was only when this examination was performed that the severe nature of the lesion was diagnosed. Very atypical vessels are seen at (2) within this small tumor, whose sharp borders can be seen at (3). The endocervix is at (1). This lesion was an endophytic early invasive cancer of stage Ib1. However, the cervix had appeared essentially normal until colposcopy was employed; there had been no clinical symptoms or signs.

The exophytic lesion shown in Fig. 6.119 was classified as an "ectopy with contact bleeding" until colposcopy was used to display the true malignant nature of this lesion; atypical vessels exist in the region of the endocervix at (1). The lateral margin is seen at (2). Unfortunately, there were no clinical symptoms until the lesion had expanded to occupy most of the cervix. This was a clinical cancer of stage Ib2 (clinical lesions greater than 4 cm in size) and exfoliative cytology had given unsatisfactory results on two occasions.

In the case shown in Fig. 6.120, a "benign polyp with contact bleeding" was said to exist on the cervix. However, the use of colposcopy revealed atypical vessels (2) that extended from the region of the endocervix (1). The vaginal fornix is seen at (3). As in the previous case, cytology had been unsatisfactory.

The use of colposcopy is indicated in situations not only where an abnormal cytology dictates but also where a suspicious appearance of the cervix requires further detailed visual examination. Likewise, the finding of an abnormal sign, such as contact bleeding, is a definite indication for colposcopy.

6.13 Precancerous glandular lesions of the cervix

Epidemiology

Cervical adenocarcinoma and its precursor lesions have been only recently included in the list of HPV-associated genital lesions (Griffin & Wells, 1995; Hörding et al., 1997). The evidence linking HPV with cervical adenocarcinoma is derived from a number of studies demonstrating the presence of oncogenic HPV types in a substantial proportion of both invasive and preinvasive glandular lesions of the uterine cervix (Leminen et al., 1991; Duggan et al., 1994; Hörding et al., 1997). Adenocarcinoma of the cervix is a complex lesion, with several different histologic types being recognized. Similarly, adenocarcinoma-in-situ (AIS) is an unknown quantity, whose diagnostic criteria are not yet universally agreed (Jaworski et al., 1988; Lee et al., 1991; Saurel, 1996). Even more debatable are the existence of less severe forms of glandular precancer lesions (Wilbur, 1995).

By comparison with squamous cell carcinoma, adenocarcinoma and adenosquamous carcinoma of the cervix are significantly more uncommon lesions, representing some 10% of all malignant primary tumors of the uterine cervix (Leminen et al., 1991; Griffin & Wells, 1995). However, a large number of studies from different countries show that the incidence of cervical adenocarcinomas has increased during the past two decades (Shingleton et al., 1981; Tamimi

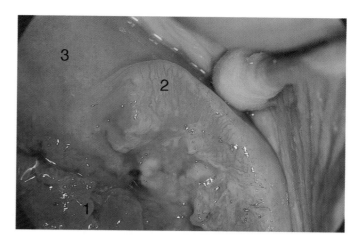

Fig. 6.120

& Figge, 1982; Duk et al., 1989; Shroyer, 1993; Griffin & Wells 1995). Unfortunately, much of the increase in cervical adenocarcinoma is in young women, namely, those under 35 years of age (Griffin & Wells 1995; Quinn, 1997). The median age, reported in several series, is between 33 and 42 years, with the youngest ranging from 22 to 24 years (Luesley et al., 1987).

The evolution of invasive adenocarcinoma of the cervix appears to follow a similar pattern as for squamous carcinoma (Anderson, 1995). However, the precursor lesions of cervical adenocarcinoma are currently less well-defined, and continue to pose serious diagnostic problems for colposcopists and pathologists alike (Wilbur, 1995; Saurel, 1996). An indication of these diagnostic difficulties is that many studies have found a higher rate of previous false-negative, previous cervical smears among patients with adenocarcinomas as compared with squamous cell carcinomas (Wilbur, 1995). Still more worrying is the fact that most cervical adenocarcinoma or high-grade CGIN (AIS) is either discovered incidentally after biopsy for squamous intraepithelial lesions or else after a variable period of time in a "holding" category of "borderline glandular cells" (BSCC classification) or "atypical glandular cells of uncertain significance" (AGCUS–The Bethesda System; Korn et al., 1998; Maini et al., 1998).

Colposcopic diagnosis

It has been stated by many authors (Brown & Wells, 1986; Fu et al., 1987; Luesley et al., 1987; Laverty et al., 1988) that there are no obvious colposcopic features that allow clear prediction of AIS. In many series, it is rare to find that the lesion has been diagnosed on colposcopy alone. Coppleson (1992) believes that most lesions originate within the transformation zone or its immediate environs, and that the stark acetowhiteness of either the individual or fused villi in discrete patches are a sign of AIS (Fig. 6.121a–d). This author further believes that the surrounding villi may appear normal. When the lesion is mixed, the surrounding tissue has an appearance characteristic of CIN. Ueki (1985) insists that with use of the cervicoscope, an endoscopic technique using either saline or acetic acid, it is possible to

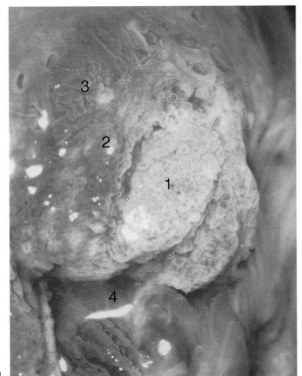

Fig. 6.121(a)

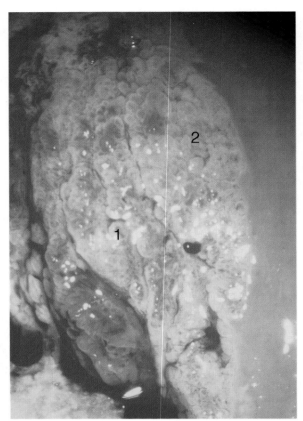

Fig. 6.121(b)

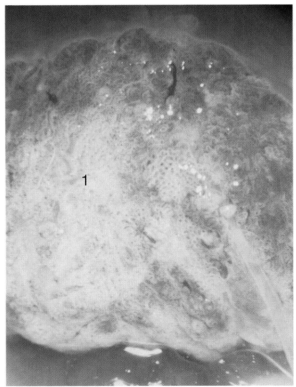

Fig. 6.121(c)

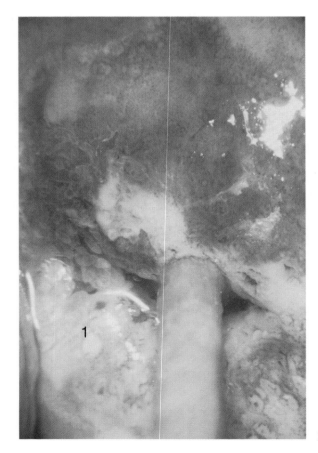

Fig. 6.121(d)

view the endocervix and observe various morphologic features that indicate the presence of glandular neoplasia. The presence of gland openings without white tufts, a surface elevation with irregularity and, in advanced cases, necrosis associated with a variety of vessel patterns make up the morphologic features of AIS and early adenocarcinoma.

Ueki believes that cervicoscopy offers an accuracy of 90% for the diagnosis of AIS.

Wright *et al.* (1995) believe that at present most colposcopists do not easily recognize AIS because of its rarity and

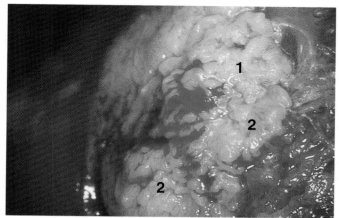

Fig. 6.121(e)

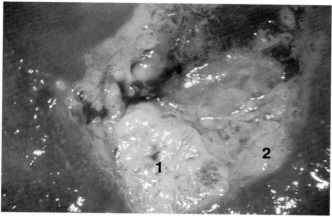

Fig. 6.121(i)

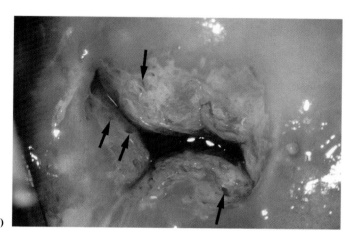

Fig. 6.121(f)

Fig. 6.121 (a) Acetowhite papillary epithelium (1) within an area of metaplastic epithelium (2); some native columnar epithelium is present at (3). Abnormal glandular cells were seen in the smear, and histologic examination with a punch biopsy taken at (1) confirmed the diagnosis. A subsequent excision biopsy confirmed the presence of adenocarcinoma-in-situ (AIS). The endocervical canal is at (4).

(b) A dense acetowhite papillary pattern is shown at (1) and some metaplastic squamous epithelium is developing at (2). AIS is present in an excision biopsy taken at (1).

(c) In this AIS at (1), the villi appear irregular, unequal, and stain intense white with the application of acetic acid. There seems to be an excess of mucus exuding from the surface. Enlarged gland openings can also be seen within the transformation zone.

(d) An area of AIS showing classic intense acetowhite staining at (1); this extends to the endocervical canal, in which a small swab stick can be seen. A similar area of intense white staining is present on the anterior lip.

(e) A dense acetowhite papillary lesion overlying normal columnar epithelium is seen at (1). Papillary configuration is also noted at (2). Biopsy of this lesion showed it to be an early stage invasive adenocarcinoma.

(f) Large gland openings are seen and arrowed in association with a variegated patchy red and white color to the lesion which appears after acetic acid application. The AIS lesion occupies the endocervical canal (1) and its linear length measured 15 mm.

(g) Small papillary excrescences (1), in association with epithelial budding (2), are seen after the application of acetic acid in a lesion that was AIS.

(h) Characteristic blood vessels are seen in the AIS lesion which also has fusion of the villus structures. Blood vessels are described as "waste-thread-like" occurring centrally with "character-writing-like" blood vessels seen at the 11-o'clock and 1-o'clock area. These vessels are also found in adenocarcinoma. (i) A mixed lesion is seen with the AIS portion located between the 6 and 10-o'clock position (1) with the less pronounced CIN 3 lesion (2) seen between 2- and 5-o'clock. (After acetic acid application.)

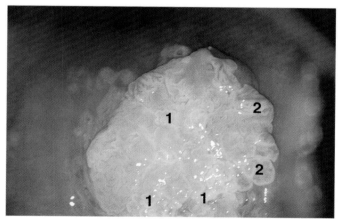

ig. 6.121(g)

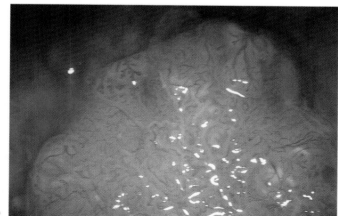

g. 6.121(h)

lack of prescribed distinguishing features. The latter may be due to the fact that AIS often produces only minor alterations of the surface contour as well as the fact that neoplastic glands are buried beneath the surface. Notwithstanding these characteristics, Wright *et al.* (1995) described detailed colposcopic findings of suspected glandular (AIS) lesions which are in relation to eight surface patterns or blood vessel structure. They described the *surface* patterns as:

1 Elevated lesions with an irregular acetowhite surface, usually overlying columnar epithelium but not contiguous with the squamocolumnar junction. These lesions may develop as a single elevated and demarcated lesion with an

irregular surface (Fig. 6.121e) or alternatively after the application of acetic acid the lesion demonstrates fused acetowhite villi in discrete patches, which resemble immature squamous metaplasia. These patches may not be associated with a squamous border in contrast to the high-grade squamous intraepithelial lesions which are usually contiguous with this border.

2 Large gland crypt openings in association with other abnormal (colposcopic) features producing excessive mucus (Fig. 6.121f).

3 Papillary lesions occasionally seen in association with fused villi resembling the early stages of squamous metaplasia. They are also seen in association with epithelial budding (Fig. 6.121g).

4 Epithelial budding (Fig. 6.121g) appears as tissue proliferation wherein the resultant projections look swollen and rounded. These appearances have to be differentiated from the early stages of immature squamous metaplastic epithelium. There is a broad base to them and they can coexist with finger-like papillary projections.

5 Variegated red and white lesions which appear similar to areas of immature metaplastic epithelium after acetic acid application. Their surface epithelium however is friable and frequently contains large gland openings (Fig. 6.121f & g).

The *blood vessel* structure of both AIS and invasive adenocarcinoma (Fig. 6.121h) can coexist and are described

on p. 108 (Fig. 6.15a). The most common variety are those vessels that are described as "waste-thread-like", "tendril-like", and where there exist either single or multiple dots in association with other very vascular patterns (Fig. 6.121h).

At one end of the spectrum of precancerous glandular changes, colposcopic appearances may be like those described above for AIS. However, at the other extreme, changes may be minimal (Fig. 6.122a). Even when a high-grade intraepithelial glandular lesion (Fig. 6.122b) is present, there may be very little colposcopic evidence. In some cases, where the AIS has changed to early invasion, a similar situation may prevail, in that there may be limited or no obvious change. Such an example is shown in Fig. 6.122b; a 32-year-old female presented with an abnormal glandular cytology, but excision biopsy of the cervix (Fig. 6.122c) revealed the presence of intraepithelial squamous disease with early glandular invasive disease.

Topographic studies of precancerous lesions have shown that glands with an associated lesion may penetrate as deep as 5 mm into the stroma (Bertrand *et al.*, 1987). The linear extent along the canal has been estimated by Ostor *et al.* (1984) as between 0.5 and 25 mm, with a mean of 12 mm. If measured from the external os, a few lesions extend to up to 30 mm. The frequency of multi-focality is about 15%. These findings have important implications with regard to treatment by excision biopsy.

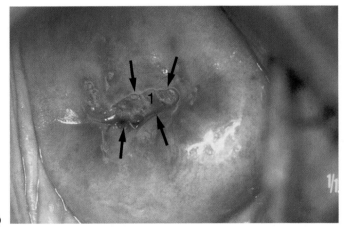

Fig. 6.122(a)

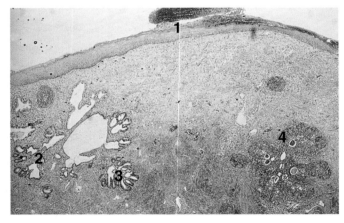

Fig. 6.122(c)

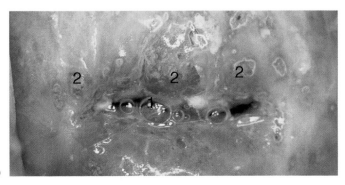

Fig. 6.122(b)

Fig. 6.122 (a) An unsuspected glandular atypia was found in this cervix of a 42-year-old woman who presented with an abnormal glandular smear. Excision biopsy after a cervicoscopic examination revealed glandular atypia with adenocarcinoma-in-situ (AIS). The endocervix is at (1). The new squamocolumnar junction is arrowed. (b) The transformation zone of this 32-year-old woman is completely normal but cytology suggested the presence of both squamous and glanular neoplasia. The endocervix is at (1) and small islands of columnar epithelium exist at (2). Excision biopsy confirmed the presence of squamous carcinoma-in-situ [cervical intraepithelial neoplasia (CIN) 3] with an early glandular invasive lesion (c). (c) The excision biopsy of the cervix seen in (b). There is normal squamous epithelium at (1), and underlying this covering epithelium there are a few normal gland crypts (2) with areas of AIS at (3). A focus of early invasive adenocarcinoma is present at (4).

Relevance to management

In mixed cases where AIS coexists with a squamous intraepithelial neoplasia (Fig. 6.121i) (i.e. CIN) the AIS component may be destroyed during ablative treatment (i.e. with cryosurgery or CO_2 laser vaporization) along with the more distal squamous lesion, without ever being recognized. Despite this problem, studies of consecutive patients (Bertrand *et al.*, 1987) submitted to routine electrosurgical loop excision for squamous cellular abnormalities reported a prevalence of AIS cases of 2%. Approximately one half of AIS cases have an accompanying squamous (i.e. CIN) component which is often of a high-grade nature and usually colposcopically visible whereas the AIS component may lie proximal and involve the cervical canal or be found beneath the metaplastic epithelium or in an atypical (abnormal) transformation zone out of colposcopic view (Fig. 6.121f). As a result the cytology may only represent the abnormal squamous component, thus influencing the colposcopist to manage the squamous lesion at the expense of the glandular. Indeed, the colposcopic punch biopsy may confirm only the presence of the squamous lesion with the AIS component only being detected either in the excisional biopsy or at later hysterectomy.

6.14 Colposcopic diagnosis of early adenocarcinoma of the cervix

In some cervixes in which AIS is found, the characteristic findings are as shown in Fig. 6.121a–i; there is dense acetowhiteness of the individual or fused villi that exist as discrete patches within the transformation zone. However, there are a number of instances in which adenocarcinoma is associated with minimal colposcopic findings, as has been shown in the two cases discussed above (Fig. 6.122a–c). In another similar case (shown in Figs 6.123 and 6.124), evidence of early invasive adenocarcinoma was also found. It seems that when early glandular invasion develops, there maybe few distinctive features within the glandular epithelium to alert the clinician to this possibility.

Ueki (1985) and Ueki and Sano (1987) have, however, described five colposcopic appearances that they believe are associated with early adenocarcinoma. In the first type, there is a papillary structure that develops within the columnar epithelium; before the application of acetic acid, this has a pale yellow and sometimes hemorrhagic color. Acetic acid turns these lesions milky white. Each papilla is large, but there is no uniformity of size, and large-diameter openings are found within the epithelium. Such lesions are shown in Figs 6.125–6.129, 6.139, 6.141–6.144. These are similar to the gland openings described in the colposcopic description of AIS.

In the second type of early adenocarcinoma the transformation zone is composed of epithelium that is thick, dull, pale orange, and shows specific vascular patterns (Ueki, 1985). The third type of colposcopic appearance is composed of atypical vessels (Figs 6.131–6.134, 6.138–6.140).

The fourth and fifth types, which are uncommon, may either be composed of a granulated surface tissue in conjunction with abnormal vessels, or adopt the appearance of a mucus-secreting lesion. In this latter case the cervix is enlarged, rubbery, and covered with copious amounts of exudate. These lesions are shown in Figs 6.137 and 6.138.

Notwithstanding the above morphologic features, there are instances in which other presentations of early

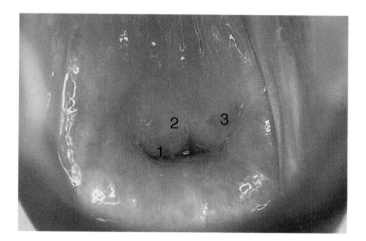

Fig. 6.123 Abnormal glandular cells were found in the cervical smear from this 54-year-old parous female. Examination of the cervix showed essentially normal findings with some whitening of the endocervical squamous epithelium (1) with a few gland openings present at the external os (2). In the 2-o'clock position there is a small area of true erosion (3) that results from wiping with a cotton swab. Excision biopsy revealed an early invasive glandular lesion (as shown in Fig. 6.124).

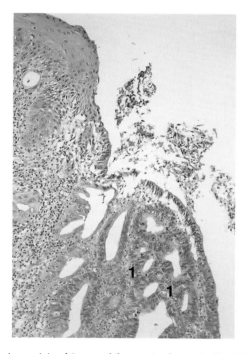

Fig. 6.124 An excision biopsy of the cervix shown in Fig. 6.123; a small lesion is present with glands containing increased amounts of chromatin. Some glandular buds have a back-to-back configuration (1). The pattern is highly suggestive of adenocarcinoma-in-situ. In another area of the specimen there was evidence of early invasion.

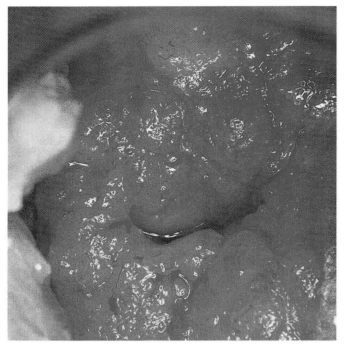

Fig. 6.125

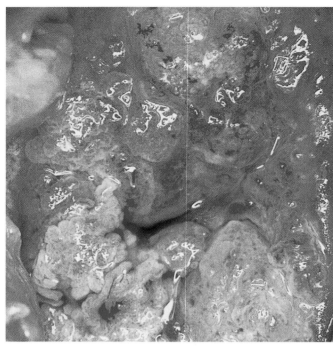

Fig. 6.126

Figs 6.125 and 6.126 A well-differentiated but early papillary adenocarcinoma is visible, which could be mistaken for a large cervical ectopy. Closer examination shows that the cervix is swollen and has a cauliflower-like appearance. The surface is eroded, irregular, and yellowish, and on the right lateral posterior lip

papillary excrescences become more visible after the application of acetic acid. The other areas have a granulated appearance. There is also an abnormal vascular pattern, as described by Ueki (1985). In Fig. 6.126, acetic acid has been applied and the papillae now appear white and of various sizes and shapes.

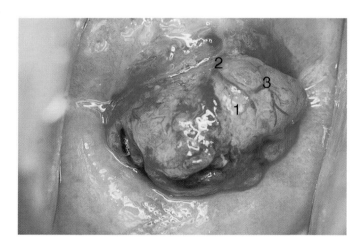

Fig. 6.127 A large endocervical polyp showing branchlike vessels which, on closer inspection, can be seen to develop into a leash of small atypical vessels that have a branching and network-type configuration. There are also small vessels of the willow-branch and waste-thread configurations described by Ueki (1985). Biopsy shows an early adenocarcinoma. Acetic acid has been applied to the cervix and this has produced a reduction of the previously very obvious abnormal vasculature (2 and 3), and a very white stained epithelium (1) has developed.

adenocarcinoma may occur. For example, in Fig. 6.127, the large endocervical polyp is shown to be of an early adeno-carcinoma. Likewise, the papillary type of early adeno-carcinoma shown in Figs 6.125 and 6.126, could well be

mistaken for a large cervical ectopy. The same applies to the more extreme lesions portrayed in Figs 6.128 and 6.130 and the accompanying pathology in Fig. 6.129. A close colposcopic examination is essential whenever cytological (Ng, 1988) or clinical suspicion exists for adenocarcinoma; excision biopsy of any suspicious area should be undertaken.

The examples presented clearly show the preclinical presentation and essentially nonsuspicious appearance of many early and advanced adenocarcinomas. Three further cases are shown in Figs 6.131–6.134, wherein a seemingly benign cervical lesion harbored an invasive lesion. Figure 6.131 is a colpophotograph of a 44-year-old female who presented with minor glandular abnormalities. There is a color-tone difference between the transformation zone (2) and the normal original squamous epithelium at (3). The endocervical canal is at (1). A close-up of the posterior lip (Fig. 6.132) shows abnormal vessels (2) and some ulceration. The vessels are branched and have an atypical pattern, especially on the right of the photograph. Further views (Fig. 6.133) into the endocervix show a very white papillary epithelium at (1); contact bleeding is already occurring from the abnormal vessels at (2). Following this highly suspicious finding an excision biopsy (stained with Van Gieson's stain) was taken, the pathology of which (Fig. 6.134) is indicative of an adenocarcinoma (1) invading into stroma (2). Ueki (1985) has classified lesions with this mor-phology as of a transformation-zone type. In his series, they

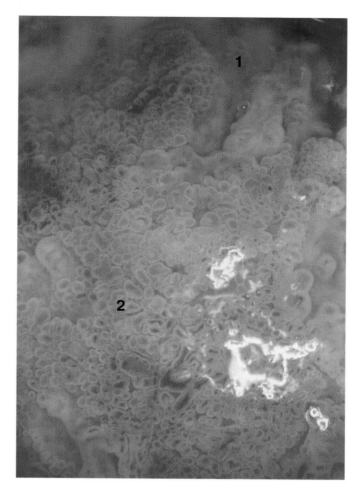

Fig. 6.128

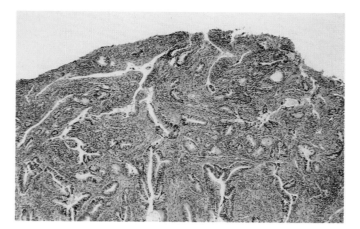

Fig. 6.129

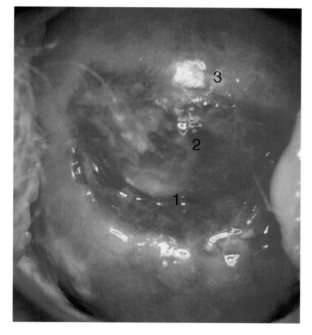

Fig. 6.131

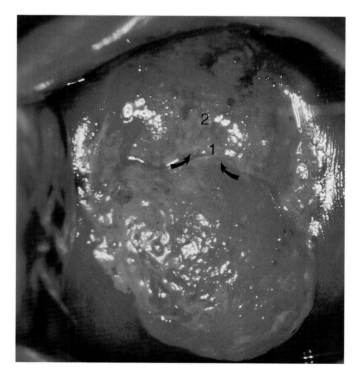

Fig. 6.130

Fig. 6.128 (*Left above*) A papillary adenocarcinoma that could be mistaken for a cervical ectopy. There were no clinical features to indicate the presence of early adenocarcinoma in this 34-year-old woman who had contact bleeding. Close examination shows that there are numerous irregular and large papillae. The endocervical canal is at (1) and the adenocarcinoma with its distinctive villi is at (2). A biopsy of this lesion can be seen in Fig. 6.129.

Fig. 6.129 (*Right above*) This photomicrograph of the lesion seen in Fig. 6.134 shows an invasive adenocarcinoma stained with Van Gieson's stain.

Fig. 6.130 (*Left below*) A papillary lesion occupies the posterior cervical lip and has irregular and distorted papillae. Iodine has been applied to the cervix but there has been very little uptake. However, on the anterior lip there has been partial uptake and this indicates the squamous nature of the tissue at (2). The abnormal (atypical) epithelium in that area and on the posterior lip extends into the endocervix (1, and arrowed). Excision biopsy of this suspicious papillary lesion showed it to be an early adenocarcinoma.

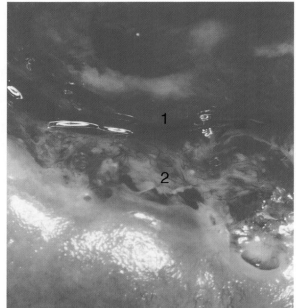

Fig. 6.132

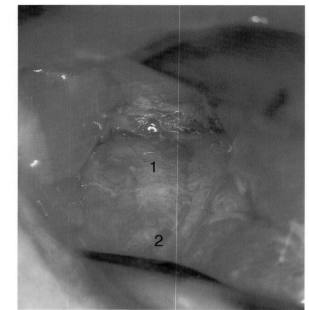

Fig. 6.133

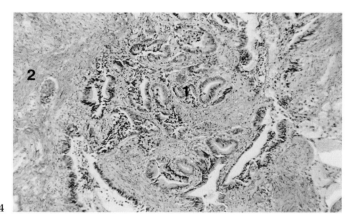

Fig. 6.134

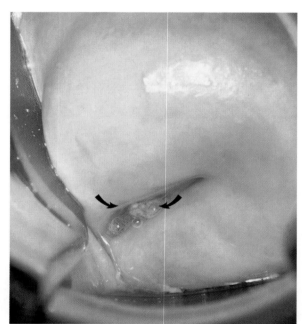

Fig. 6.135

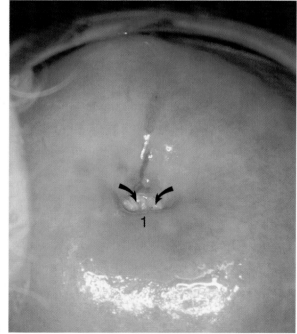

Fig. 6.136(a)

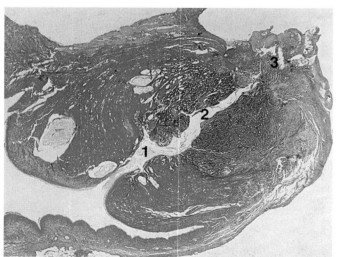

Fig. 6.136(b)

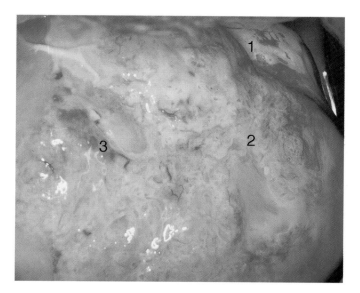

Fig. 6.137 A large, mixed, granulated and smooth epithelial-type lesion is present across the endo- and ectocervix and has very atypical vessels. Thick white epithelium is present on the anterior ectocervix at (1), and at (2) there are distended villi that are irregular and unequal. The vessels (3) are of the type described by Ueki (1985) as root-, tendril- and corkscrew-like. These can also be seen in the high-power view of the central part of the posterior lip shown in Fig. 6.144. Acetic acid application has caused a slight whitening and pale yellow appearance.

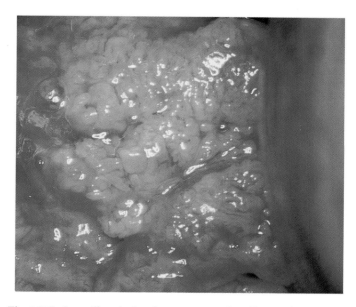

Fig. 6.139 A papillary lesion that appears pale yellow and is clearly demarkated; there is also a hemorrhagic surface that is typical of an adenocarcinoma. This appearance can easily be confused with that of a benign "ectopy".

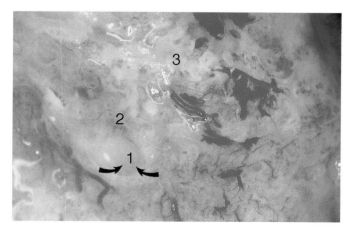

Fig. 6.138 A high-power view of the area between points (2) and (3) in Fig. 6.143. It shows grossly atypical vessels (as described in Fig. 6.143) and some contact bleeding. Excision biopsies from this area and its surrounds revealed the presence of adenosquamous carcinoma.

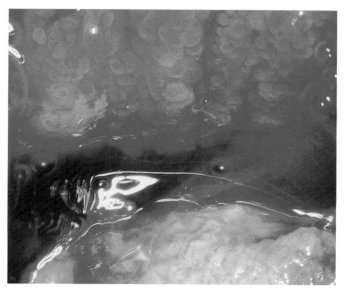

Fig. 6.140 This view within the endocervix shows individual villi that are large and nonuniform. The generalized hemorrhagic appearance forms a background to the tissue on the anterior cervical lip. Closer inspection would reveal that each papilla has abnormal vessels within it, especially of the so-called glomeruloid or hairpin types described by Ueki (1985) and Ueki and Sano (1987).

accounted for 9% of all early adenocarcinomas. In one-third of cases an adenosquamous carcinoma existed.

The other two cases demonstrated in Figs 6.135 and 6.136a and b show how small endocervical polyps can also masquerade as endocervical adenocarcinoma. In Fig. 6.135, small buds can be seen to emerge through the external os (arrowed); these are associated with glandular abnormality in a cervical smear. An excision biopsy of the cervix revealed the presence of early adenocarcinoma. In the second patient (Fig. 6.136a), who was 60 years old, a subtotal hysterectomy had been performed 15 years earlier. The

patient had been treated with 5 mg dienestrol daily, and a routine cervical smear from the residual cervix had suggested the presence of squamous carcinoma. After the application of acetic acid, colposcopy showed a small white area at the external os (1, and arrowed). An excision biopsy (Fig. 6.136b) of the cervix showed a zone of CIN 3 just inside the endocervix (1), but in position (2) there is an obvious adenocarcinoma within the canal. The upper margin of the

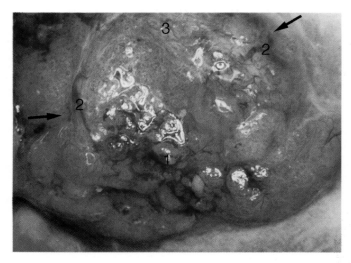

Fig. 6.141 This cervix is that of a 45-year-old parous female who has a large area of ectropion on the posterior cervix. Close inspection shows that the tissue is raised and papillary (1), has an irregular surface, and is a pale yellow–red. The arrows point to large rootlike vessels (2), and some willow-branch, fine waste-thread, and glomeruloid vessels (3) are also present (as described by Ueki, 1985). No acetic acid has been applied.

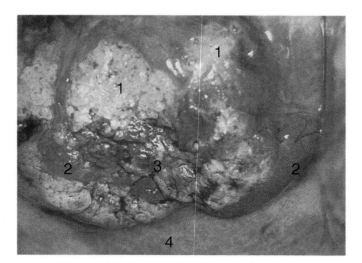

Fig. 6.142 Acetic acid has now been applied to the cervix shown in Fig. 6.141. There is partial whitening of the papillary structures (1), which appear larger and whiter than those of the normal columnar epithelium (2). There is more irregularity within the adjacent columnar epithelium (3) than would be seen in areas of physiologic columnar epithelium. The posterior vaginal fornix is at (4). Biopsy of this lesion showed it to be a well-differentiated adenocarcinoma.

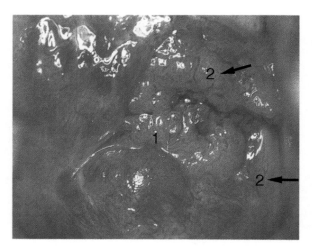

Fig. 6.143 This cervix is that of a 48-year-old parous woman who presented with postcoital bleeding; on colposcopic examination a yellowish papillary area could be seen at (1). Contact bleeding was produced from this area. Close inspection of each papilla will show that there are linear, waste-thread, or glomeruloid vessels. Arrows at (2) signify further areas where there are other abnormal vessel types. This view is before the application of acetic acid.

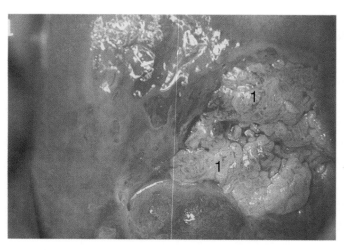

Fig. 6.144 After the application of acetic acid to the cervix shown in Fig. 6.143, the papillary area around the cervical os (1) becomes white. The papillae are of various sizes and are confluent in one area. There is a granular appearance to the white epithelium around the endocervix. Excision biopsy of this central area revealed the presence of a poorly differentiated tubular adenocarcinoma in conjunction with a moderately differentiated squamous cell carcinoma.

excision is at (3). Unfortunately, in this patient metastases were already present within the iliac lymph nodes. Both these cases show the value of surveillance by endocervical smears in those patients where the transformation zone has receded to within the canal. In the second case it also shows the benefit of cytologic surveillance in any female who retains a residual cervix after a subtotal hysterectomy.

In Figs 6.137–6.144 various examples of invasive glandular and, in some cases, squamous cancers are seen. They reinforce comments previously made above concerning the difficulty that may sometimes arise in diagnosis; especially in respect of their differentiation from benign disease such as cervical "ectopy".

6.15 References

Al-Nafussi, A.I., Colquhoun, M.K. & Williams, A.R.W. (1993) Accuracy of cervical smears in predicting the grades of cervical intraepithelial neoplasia. *Int J Gynecol Cancer* **3**,89.

Anderson, D.J.M., Strachan, F. & Parkin, D.E. (1992) Cone biopsy: has endocervical sampling a role? *Br J Obstet Gynaecol* **99**,668.

Anderson, M.C. (1995) Glandular lesions of the cervix: diagnostic and therapeutic dilemmas. *Baillières Clin Obstet Gynecol*, **9**(1),105.

Anderson, W., Fiersen, H., Barber, S. & Tabbraah, S. (1988) Sensitivity and specificity of endocervical curettage and the endocervical brush for the evaluation of the endocervical canal. *Am J Obstet Gynecol* **159**,702.

Ang, M.S., Kaufman, R.H., Adam, E. *et al.* (1995) Colposcopically directed biopsy and loop excision of the transformation zone. Comparison of histologic findings. *J Reprod Med* **40**(3),167.

Ayer, B., Pacey, F. & Greenberg, M. (1988) The cytologic diagnosis of adenocarcinoma in situ of the cervix uteri and related lesions. II. Microinvasive carcinoma. *Acta Cytol* **32**,318.

Bajardi, F., Burghardt, E., Kern, H. & Kroemer, H. (1959) Nouveaux resultats de la cytologie et de la colposcopie systematiques dans le diagnostique precoce du cancer du col del'uterus. *Gynecol Prst* **5**,315.

Barton, S.E., Jenkins, D., Hollingworth, A. & Singer, A. (1989) An explanation for the problem of the false negative cervical smear. *Br J Obstet Gynaecol* **96**,482.

Bertrand, M., Lickrish, G.M. & Colgan, T.J. (1987) The anatomic distribution of cervical adenocarcinoma in situ: implications for treatment. *Am J Obstet Gynecol* **157**,21.

Bosch, F.X., Manos, M.M., Munoz, N. *et al.* (1995) Prevalence of human papillomavirus in cervical cancer: a worldwide perspective. International biological study on cervical cancer (IBSCC) Study Group. *J Natl Cancer Inst* **87**,796.

Brown, L.J.R. & Wells, M. (1986) Cervical glandular atypia associated with squamous intraepithelial neoplasia—a premalignant lesion? *J Clin Pathol* **39**,22.

Burghardt, E. (1991) *Colposcopy, Cervical Pathology, Textbook and Atlas*, 2nd edn. Georg Thieme Verlag, Stuttgard.

Burghardt, E. (1992a) Pathology of early invasive squamous and glandular carcinoma of the cervix (FIGO stage Ia). In: Coppleson, M. (ed.) *Gynaecological Oncology*, Vol. 1, 2nd edn, p. 609. Churchill Livingstone, Edinburgh.

Burghardt, E., Pickel, H. & Girardi, F. (eds) (1998) In: *Colposcopy Cervical Pathology*, 3rd edn, p. 78. Thieme, Stuttgart, New York.

Byrne, P., Jordan, J., Williams, D. *et al.* (1988) Importance of negative result of cervical biopsy directed by colposcopy. *Br J Med* **296**,172.

Cartier, R. (1984) *Practical Colposcopy*, p. 30. Laboratoire Cartier, Paris.

Coppleson, M. (1992) Early invasive squamous and adenocarcinoma of the cervix (FIGO stage 1a): clinical features and management. In: Coppleson, M. (ed.) *Gynaecological Oncology*, Vol. 1, 2nd edn, p. 631. Churchill Livingstone, Edinburgh.

Coppleson, M. & Pixley, E. (1992a) Effects of human papillomavirus infections. In: Coppleson, M. (ed.) *Gynaecological Oncology*, Vol. 1, 2nd edn, p. 303. Churchill Livingstone, Edinburgh.

Coppleson, M. & Pixley, E. (1992b) International colposcopic terminology. In: Coppleson, M. (ed.) *Gynaecological Oncology*, Vol. 1, 2nd edn, p. 309. Churchill Livingstone, Edinburgh.

Cox, J.T., Schiffman, M.H. & Winzelberg, A.J. (1992) An evaluation of human papilloma testing as part of referral to colposcopy clinic. *Obstet Gynaecol* **80**,389.

Drescher, C., Peters, C. & Roberts, J. (1983) Contribution of endocervical curettage in evaluation of abnormal cervical cytology. *Obstet Gynecol* **62**,343.

Duggan, M.A., Benoit, J.L., McGregor, S.E. *et al.* (1994) Adenocarcinoma in situ of the endocervix: human papillomavirus determination by dot blot hybridization and polymerase chain reaction amplification. *Int J Gynecol Pathol* **13**,143.

Duk, J.M., Aalders, J.G., Fleuren, G.J., Krans, M. & de Bruijn, H.W.A. (1989) Tumor markers CA 125, squamous cell carcinoma antigen, and carcinoembryonic antigen in patients with adenocarcinoma of the uterine cervix. *Obstet Gynecol* **73**,661.

Evans, D.M., Hudson, E.A., Brown, C.L. *et al.* (1986) Terminology in gynaecological cytopathology; report of the working party of the British Society for Clinical Cytology. *J Clin Pathol* **39**,933.

Fu, Y.S., Berek, J.S. & Hilborne, L.H. (1987) Diagnostic problems of in situ and invasive adenocarcinomas of the uterine cervix. *Appl Pathol* **5**,47.

Griffin, N.R. & Wells, M. (1995) Premalignant and malignant glandular lesions of the cervix. In: Fox, H. & Wells, M. (eds) *Haines and Taylor Obstetrical and Gynaecological Pathology*, 4th edn, p. 323. Churchill Livingstone, New York.

Hamou, J. (1991) Hysteroscopy and microcolpohysteroscopy—text and atlas. Appleton and Lange, Norwalk, CA.

Hatch, K., Shingleton, H., Orr, J., Gore, H. & Soong, S. (1985) Role of endocervical curettage in colposcopy. *Obstet Gynecol* **63**,403.

Hörding, U., Daugaard, S. & Visfeldt, J. (1997) Adenocarcinoma of the cervix and adenocarcinoma of the endometrium: distinction with PCR-mediated detection of HPV DNA. *APMIS* **105**,313.

Howe, D.T. & Vincenti, A.C. (1991) Is large loop excision of the transformation zone (LLATZ) more accurate than colposcopically directed punch biopsy in the diagnosis of cervical intraepthelial neoplasia? *Br J Obstet Gynaecol* **98**,588.

Jarmulowicz, M.R., Jenkins, D., Barton, S.E. & Singer, A. (1989) Cytological status and lesion size: a further dimension in cervical intraepithelial neoplasia. *Br J Obstet Gynaecol* **96**,1061.

Jaworski, R.C., Pacey, N., Greenberg, M.L. & Osborne, R.A. (1988) The histological diagnosis of adenocarcinoma in situ and related lesions of the cervix uteri. *Cancer* **61**,1171.

Jenkins, D. (1990) Pathology of lower genital tract premalignancy. In: Singer, A. (ed.) *Clinical Practice of Gynaecology*, Vol. 2, p. 70. Elsevier, New York.

Kierkegaard, O., Byralsen, C., Hansen, K.C., Frandsen, K.H. & Frydenberg, M. (1995) Association between colposcopic findings and histology in cervical lesions: the significance of the size of the lesion. *Gynecol Oncol* **57**(1),66.

Kohan, S., Noumoff, J. & Beckman, E.M. (1985) Colposcopic screening of women and atypical Papanicolaou smears. *J Reprod Med* **30**,383.

Kolstad, P. (1965) The development of the vascular bed in tumours, as seen in squamous cell carcinoma of the cervix uteri. *Br J Radiol* **38**,216.

Kolstad, P. & Stafl, A. (1982) *Atlas of Colposcopy*, 3rd edn, p. 84. Churchill Livingstone, Edinburgh.

Korn, A.P., Judson, P.L. & Zaloudetz, C.J. (1998) Importance of atypical glandular cells of uncertain significance in cervical cytologic smears. *J Reprod Med* **43**,774.

Krebs, H., Wheelock, J. & Hert, G. (1987) Positive endocervical curettage in patients with satisfactory and unsatisfactory colposcopy; clinical implications. *Obstet Gynecol* **69**,601.

Laverty, C.R., Farnsworth, A., Thurloe, J. & Bowditch, R. (1988) The reliability of a cytological prediction of cervical adenocarcinoma in situ. *Aust NZ J Obstet Gynaecol* **28**,307.

Lee, K.R., Manna, E.A. & Jones, M.A. (1991) Comparative cytological features of adenocarcinoma in situ of the uterine cervix. *Acta Cytol* **35**,117.

Leminen, A., Paavonen, J., Vesterinen, E. *et al.* (1991) Human papillomavirus types 16 and 18 in adenocarcinoma of the uterine cervix. *Am J Clin Pathol* **95**,647.

Lopez, A., Pearson, S., Mo, R. *et al.* (1989) Is it time for a reconsideration of the criteria for cone biopsy? *Br J Obstet Gynaecol* **96**,1345.

Luesley, D.M., Jordan, J.A., Woodman, C.B., Watson, N. & Williams, D.R. (1987) A retrospective review of adenocarcinoma in situ and glandular atypia of the uterine cervix. *Br J Obstet Gynaecol* **94**,699.

Maini, M., Lavie, O., Comeerci, G. *et al.* (1988) The management and follow-up of patients with high-grade cervical glandular intraepithelial neoplasia. *Int J Gynecol Cancer* **8**,287.

Mitchell, M.F., Schottenfeld, D., Zortolero-Luna, G. *et al.* (1998) Colposcopy for the diagnosis of squamous intraepitherial lesions: a meta-analysis. *Obstet Gynecol* **91**,626.

Ng, A.B.P. (1988) Microinvasive adenocarcinoma and precursors of adenocarcinoma of the uterine cervix. In: Wied, G.L., Koss, L.G. & Reagan, J.W. (eds) *Compendium on Diagnostic Cytology*, 6th edn, *Tutorials in Gynecology series*. University of Chicago Press, Chicago.

Ostor, A.G., Pagano, R., Davoren, R.A.M. *et al.* (1984) Adenocarcinoma in situ of the cervix. *Int J Gynecol Pathol* **3**,179.

Quinn, M.A. (1997) Adenocarcinoma of the cervix. Are there arguments for a different treatment policy? *Curr Opin Obstet Gynecol* **9**,21.

Reid, R. (1990) Colposcopy of cervical pre-invasive neoplasia. In: Singer, A. (ed.) *Clinical Practice of Gynaecology*, Vol. 2, p. 117. Elsevier, New York.

Reid, R. (1993) Biology and colposcopic features of human papillomavirus associated cervical lesions. *Obstet Gynecol Nth America* **20**,123.

Reid, R., Stanhope, C.R., Herschman, B.R., Crum, C.P. & Agronow, S.J. (1984) Genital warts and cervical cancer. IV. A colposcopic index for differentiating subclinical papillomaviral infection from cervical intraepithelial neoplasia. *Am J Obstet Gynecol* **149**,815.

Richart, R.M., Foux, J.F. & Winkler, B. (1992) Pathology of cervical squamous and glandular intraepithelial neoplasia. In: Coppleson, M. (ed.) *Gynaecological Oncology*, Vol. 1, 2nd edn, p. 557. Churchill Livingstone, Edinburgh.

Saurel, J. (1996) Adenocarcinoma in situ du col uterin. Aspects cytologiques et histologiques. *Ann Pathol* **16**,374.

Schiffman, M.H., Bauer, H.M., Hoover, R.N. *et al.* (1993) Epidemiologic evidence showing that human papillomavirus infection causes most cervical intraepithelial neoplasia. *J Natl Cancer Inst* **85**,958.

Schiller, J. (1929) Jodpinselung und Abschabung des Portioepithels. *Zentralbl Gynäkol* **53**,1056.

Sesti, J., Farne, C., Mattei, M. & Piccione, E. (1990) Role of endocervical curettage in the diagnostic work-up of pre-invasive cervical lesions. *Int J Gynaecol Obstet* **31**,153.

Shafi, M.I., Dunn, J.A., Buxton, E.J. *et al.* (1993) Abnormal cervical cytology following large loop excision of the transformation zone: a case controlled study. *Br J Obstet Gynaecol* **100**,145.

Shafi, M.I., Dunn, J., Finn, C.B., Kettoe, S., Buxton, E. & Jordan, J. (1993) Characterization of high and low grade intraepithelial neoplasia. *Int J Gynecol Cancer* **3**,203.

Shafi, M.I., Finn, C.B. & Luesley, D.M. (1991) Lesion size and histology of atypical cervical transformation zone. *Br J Obstet Gynaecol* **98**,490.

Shingleton, H.M., Gore, H., Bradley, D.H. & Soong, S.J. (1981) Adenocarcinoma of the cervix I. Clinical evaluation and pathologic features. *Am J Obstet Gynecol* **139**,799.

Shroyer, K.R. (1993) Human papillomavirus and endocervical adenocarcinoma. *Hum Pathol* **24**,119.

Singer, A., Walker, P., Tay, S.K. & Dyson, J. (1984) Impact of introduction of colposcopy to a district general hospital. *Br Med J* **289**,1049.

Skehan, M., Soutter, W.P., Lim, K. *et al.* (1990) Reliability of colposcopy and directed punch biopsy. *Br J Obstet Gynaecol* **97**,811.

Soutter, W.P., Wisdom, S., Brough, A.K. & Monaghan, J.M. (1986) Should patients with mild atypia in a cervical smear be referred for colposcopy? *Br J Obstet Gynaecol* **93**,70.

Talebian, F., Shayan, A., Krumhoz, A., Palladino, V. & Mann, L. (1977) Colposcopic evaluation of patients with abnormal cervical cytology. *Obstet Gynecol* **49**,670.

Tamimi, H.K. & Figge, D.C. (1982) Adenocarcinoma of the uterine cervix. *Gynecol Oncol* **13**,335.

Tidbury, P. & Singer, A. (1992) CIN III; the role of lesion size in invasion. *Br J Obstet Gynaecol* **99**,583.

Ueki, M. (1985) In: Ueki, M. (ed.) *Cervical Adenocarcinoma — A Colposcopic Atlas*, p. 18. Ishiyaku Euro-America Inc., St. Louis.

Ueki, M. & Sano, T. (1987) In: Ueki, M. & Sano, T. (eds) *Endocervical Carcinoma — A Cervicoscopic Atlas*, p. 9. Ishiyaku Euro-America Inc., St. Louis.

Walker, E.M., Dodgson, J. & Duncan, I.D. (1986) Does mild atypia on a cervical smear warrant further investigation? *Lancet* **2**,672.

Wilbur, D.C. (1995) Endocervical glandular atypia: A "new" problem for the cytologist. *Diagn Cytopathol* **13**,463.

Wright, V.C., Lickrish, G.M. & Shier, R.M. (1995) In: *Basic and Advanced Colposcopy — A Practical Handbook for Diagnosis*, 2nd edn, Chapter 12, p. 12. Biomedical Communications, Houston.

Zahm, D.M., Nindl, I., Greinke, C., Hoyer, H. & Schneider, A. (1998) Colposcopic appearance of cervical intraepithelial neoplasia is age dependant. *Am J Obstet Gynecol* **179**(5),1298.

Chapter 7
Management of Cervical Precancer

7.1 Introduction

In the last three decades, management of the patient with an abnormal smear has undergone a series of significant changes. The standard therapy in the late 1960s for any patient with a "positive" cervical smear was excision, utilizing either a cone biopsy of the cervix or, for the older patient who was no longer likely to bear children, some form of hysterectomy. Often these procedures resulted in considerable morbidity, such as the increased risk of miscarriage following cone biopsy, or even mortality following the more extensive hysterectomy techniques (Way et al., 1968; Jones et al., 1979).

When the colposcope was reintroduced to Europe and North America in the early 1970s, more appropriate, less aggressive, and more accurate techniques of therapy appeared. Initially these involved applications of the existing technology, refined by use, with the guidance of colposcopy following initial punch biopsy of any cervical lesion. This use of the colposcope as a biopsy director and treatment guide versus its use as a primary diagnostic and screening tool, continues to be the fundamental difference between Anglo–American–Australian and continental European practice.

7.2 Rationale behind treatment

The precancerous nature of cervical intraepithelial neoplasia (CIN) has been discussed in Chapters 1 and 6. In recent years, there has developed a body of opinion that has questioned the treatment of all such CIN lesions and, as will be discussed in this chapter, recent evidence suggests that possibly all major-grade (CIN 2, CIN 3, HSIL) lesions should be treated, whereas minor-grade (CIN 1, LSIL) lesions should be managed more conservatively, albeit with the aid of new methods of viral testing to determine the presence of high-risk HPV types, thereby identifying an increased risk of progression of minor-grade lesions as well as indicating the presence of high-grade lesions when minor-grade cytology exists (Cuzick et al., 1992; Terry et al., 1992; Mansell et al., 1994; Cox, 1995; Hatch, 1996; Ferris et al., 1998; Manos et al., 1999).

Over the last decade the trend has been directed toward more conservative methods of managing CIN, with special emphasis being placed on techniques of local destruction. However, over the last 3 to 4 years, reservations have been expressed about the suitability of these modalities, espe-

cially with the development of invasive cancer in a number of women who had been treated conservatively, and also with reference to the accuracy of colposcopically directed biopsies (McIndoe et al., 1989; Partington et al., 1989; Vergote et al., 1992; Wright et al., 1992a; Shafi et al., 1997). This has coincided with the recent introduction of the large loop diathermy excision technique. A large multicenter study covering over 13 000 treatments has recorded the continuing small risk of patients treated with conservative modalities to develop invasive cancer many years after their initial therapy. The risk in this series was still present up to 14 years following treatment (Soutter et al., 1997).

Notwithstanding these reservations, there is still a great demand for conservative management in treating CIN lesions and, indeed, success rates for both conservative and excisional methods are similar. In this chapter, the topics of whom to treat, the methods available for treatment, the mechanisms for follow-up after treatment, and the reasons for failure will be considered. Initially, a detailed description will be given of the colposcopic and pathologic characteristics of CIN lesions that are a prerequisite to determining what, if any, treatment should be undertaken.

7.3 Colposcopic and pathologic characteristics of CIN lesion: a prerequisite to treatment

Colposcopy plays a major role in the decision of what particular treatment should be given for any individual CIN lesion. As has been pointed out in Chapters 4 and 6, the cervical transformation zone contains the CIN lesion within the colposcopically recognizable abnormal (atypical) epithelium. Before considering treatment, the colposcopist must examine three essential characteristics of the lesion. These are: (i) the limits and nature of the abnormal (atypical) epithelium; (ii) the risk and extent of glandular involvement; and (iii) the extent of the CIN within the endocervix.

The limits and nature of the abnormal (atypical) epithelium

After carrying out an initial visual examination, the colposcopist will be able to determine the outer limits of the lesion at the original squamocolumnar junction, and the internal limits at the new squamocolumnar junction. The lesion will be contained within the boundaries of these two junctions. If the new squamocolumnar junction cannot be adequately visualized because of its position within the endocervical canal, then the colposcopic examination must be deemed unsatisfactory.

Once these limits have been determined, the nature of the lesion must be considered. As has been described in Chapters 4 and 6, it is now accepted that in colposcopic terms there are minor- and major-grade lesions. The minor-grade lesions are usually smaller than their major-grade counterparts, and are essentially ectocervical. As a CIN/SIL lesion becomes more severe, its size increases (Holzer & Pickel, 1975; Giles *et al.*, 1987; Jarmulowicz *et al.*, 1989). Also, the larger the extent of the surface lesion, the more likely it is to involve the glandular crypts of the cervix (Abdul-Karim *et al.*, 1982; Jarmulowicz *et al.*, 1989; Kierkegaard, 1995); Boonstra *et al.* (1990) have also suggested that CIN 3 increases in extent, depth, and endocervical involvement with age.

Glandular involvement

Extension of CIN into the endocervical crypts or glands occurs frequently and to a variable extent, as can be seen in Fig. 7.1a. Colposcopically, the finding of gland cuffing (see Fig. 6.106 on p. 144), the appearance of a rim of acetowhite epithelium around the gland or crypt entrance, suggests involvement of the crypt with CIN (Fig. 7.1a). However, the depth of such gland extensions is impossible to determine colposcopically. A number of studies have shown the range of depth of glandular involvement in association with CIN 3 lesions. Anderson and Hartley (1980) found that 88.6% of the 343 conization specimens with CIN 3 had some crypt involvement by CIN. The mean depth of this involvement was 1.24 min, the maximum was 5.22 min, and the maximum +3 SD (includes 99.7% of the population) was 3.80 min. Boonstra *et al.* (1990) found that the mean depth of CIN 3 crypt involvement was 1.6 min in the 66 cone specimens they examined.

A full histologic assessment of the depth of glandular involvement requires an excision biopsy, that is, cone biopsy. However, the colposcopic punch biopsy taken by the colposcopist allows the extent and depth of crypt involvement to be determined, and provides an important prognostic sign. Jarmulowicz *et al.* (1989), in a study of local treatment of CIN 3, showed that recurrence was highly likely when there was extensive crypt involvement (depth greater than 1.7 min) or a mitotic count greater than 34 metaphase mitoses per 10 high-power fields in the pretreatment biopsy.

The importance of a pathology examination to assess the extent of crypt penetration by CIN can be seen in Fig. 7.1b, which shows a longitudinal section through a cone biopsy specimen where the lesion is predominantly in the endocervical canal (1). The endocervical glands extend for a few millimeters into the stroma (2). Although the lesion has been completely removed at the ectocervical (3) and stromal (2) margins, the endocervical margin (4) cannot with confidence be said to be clear. The difficulties of determining the exact depth of glandular involvement by CIN has, to some extent, limited confidence in the conservative techniques, such as laser vaporization or cryotherapy. As "conservative" treatment methods have developed, it has become generally accepted that treatment, by either excision or tissue destruction, to a depth of approximately 6–7 mm should be achieved to produce an optimal clearance rate.

It is now felt that expansion of the gland and central degeneration or necrosis of the gland involved is an ominous sign of either impending or associated invasion. These changes should be noted particularly when the excision is reported as incomplete.

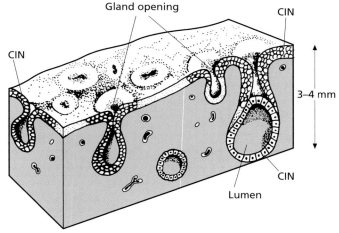

Fig. 7.1(a)

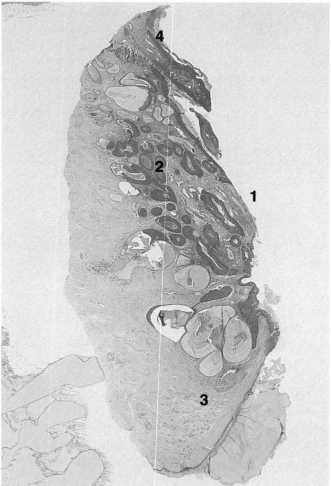

Fig. 7.1(b)

Fig. 7.1 (a) Diagrammatic representation of a cervical intraepithelial neoplasia (CIN) lesion involving the glands and crypts. Around the gland openings there is the colposcopic sign of gland cuffing (1); this indicates the presence of CIN involving the glandular elements. (b) Longitudinal section through a cone biopsy specimen.

Endocervical extension

The extension of any CIN lesion into the endocervix means that its upper limit is situated there. However, it may be difficult to determine the height of the disease within the endocervix, and various techniques, such as microcolpohysteroscopy (p. 121), must be employed to examine the endocervical canal and evaluate any extension of the CIN. It is only by defining the lesion limits that the appropriate treatment can be selected. Figure 7.2 shows how various treatment techniques can be tailored to deal with the wide and variable extent of a CIN lesion within the ectocervix, and especially within the endocervix. On the left, where the entire limits of the abnormal (atypical) epithelium (shaded) are readily visible to the colposcopist, a conservative (ablative) technique can be used, removing tissue in a dome-shaped configuration to a depth of 6–10 mm. Where the lesion extends into the endocervical canal and the upper limits cannot be confidently seen (central diagram), an excisional technique must be used (i.e. cone biopsy, excision using either a cold knife, laser, or loop), producing a cylindric defect. Where there is a combination of a wide ectocervical and an extended endocervical lesion (right-hand diagram), a combination of peripheral tissue destruction (1) vaporization and central excision (2), the so-called top hat procedure, will optimize treatment without the need to remove large volumes of the cervix.

7.4 Colposcopically directed biopsy

As the role of conservative techniques of treatment developed, it was accepted as mandatory that the histologic nature of the cervical lesion would be known prior to treatment. An initial colposcopic assessment of the cervix (p. 120) is performed, and the most significant area of abnormality is biopsied. The skill in determining this area has to be acquired through a thorough understanding of all the morphologic manifestations of epithelial abnormality.

The inexperienced colposcopist is advised to seek confirmation of any suspect epithelial type by carrying out a biopsy. Sometimes, when a variety of colposcopic appearances are present, multiple biopsies are appropriate. These must be carefully directed and documented. It is pointless to take a large number of apparently random biopsies in the hope that a significant lesion may be found. A careful audit of the results of colposcopically directed biopsy must also be made to reduce to an absolute minimum the number of "geographic misses."

It has been found even in the best centers, that when conservative treatment systems with pretreatment punch biopsy have been changed from ablative (cryosurgery, electrodiathermy, cold coagulation, and laser) to excisional (loop diathermy and laser cone biopsy), the rate of diagnosis of microinvasive and early invasive cancers of the cervix has risen markedly (Buxton et al., 1991; Vergote et al., 1992). This has cast doubt on the accuracy of punch biopsy. It is obvious that the expertise of the colposcopist determines the accuracy of this type of biopsy. Three major studies have examined the efficacy of colposcopically directed punch biopsies.

McIndoe et al. (1989) examined 196 patients who were considered suitable to undergo local destructive treatment with laser vaporization and who had a prior punch biopsy taken from the most abnormal area within the transformation zone. Each patient was then treated with small laser excision cone biopsy. They found that two patients had microinvasive carcinoma and one had adenocarcinoma-in-situ (AIS); all these were diagnosed by cone biopsy and missed by punch biopsy. Sixteen patients were found to have lesions that were categorized as two or three grades worse by laser excision biopsy than by punch biopsy. McIndoe et al. surmised that because of the apparent inaccuracy of the colposcopic biopsy, small laser excision cone biopsies should be recommended as the treatment of choice in CIN. However, Sze et al. (1989) reviewed 15 studies involving over 1000 patients; the accuracy of diagnosis of colposcopically directed biopsy was compared with ultimate cone biopsy or hysterectomy. The percentage of patients with lesions that were more severe than initially diagnosed by punch biopsy ranged from 1% to 10%. In a total of 1975 patients, only 16 invasive cancers were missed by colposcopically directed biopsy.

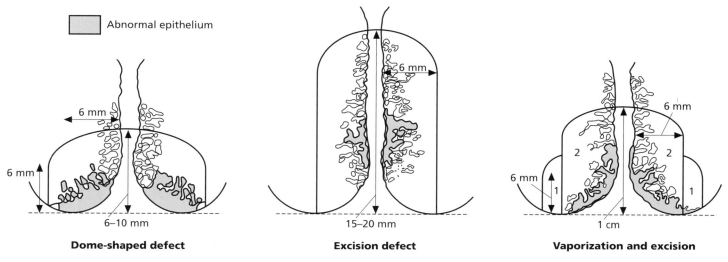

Dome-shaped defect   **Excision defect**   **Vaporization and excision**

Fig. 7.2

The third study, by Buxton *et al.* (1991), where the newly introduced diathermy loop excision biopsy of the transformation zone was employed, was a prospective study of 243 women who had been examined by colposcopy with directed punch biopsy of the most severe lesion. The histology of the punch biopsy and the excised transformation zone, and the size of the abnormal lesion were all measured; it was found that in 132 (54%) of the 243 women there was discordance between the results of the punch biopsy specimen and the loop excision specimen. In 62 (47%) of these 132 females, a more severe lesion was found in the excised transformation zone; these lesions included three unsuspected cases of AIS and one very early microinvasive carcinoma. In 39 (41%) of the 96 women in whom a lesion of CIN 3 or more severe was found in the loop excision specimen, the paired punch biopsy had suggested a lesion of lesser severity. In small-area lesions, a punch biopsy was more likely than the large excision specimen to have shown more severe disease. Buxton *et al.* (1991), concluded that direct punch biopsy was an inadequate endpoint technique by which to judge the severity of an epithelial lesion. They felt that it had important implications for patient management and the design of trials in which punch biopsy was used as an end-point method for assessing CIN could lead to incorrect conclusions.

The authors feel that colposcopically directed biopsy can still be employed safely, but it is essential to perform multiple biopsies to reduce the risk of missing an early invasive lesion. However, the reservations expressed above about biopsy must be taken into consideration.

7.5 Which lesions to treat

The introduction by Richart (1990) of the concept of low and high-grade lesions has formalized the view, held by pathologists and clinicians for some time, that there seems to be a spectrum of epithelial change, from mild epithelial lesions at one end to undifferentiated lesions at the other extreme. The move for a more simplified approach using this grading system has been supported by others from studies showing that lesser grade lesions (CIN 1) have a low rate of progression (Campion *et al.*, 1986; Rome *et al.*, 1987; Syrjanen *et al.*, 1987). In one such study, Robertson *et al.* (1988) showed that of 1781 patients who exhibited mild dyskaryosis in cervical smears taken between 1965 and 1984, only 10 developed invasive cancer. Four of these were diagnosed soon after presentation and three developed many years later after default from follow-up. Only one occurred during cytologic surveillance and a further two after referral for colposcopy. They also found, during an initial surveillance, that cervical smears reverted to normal in 46% of patients within 2 years, and during a longer term follow-up none of these patients developed invasive cancer. Indeed, three-quarters of those followed in a life analysis table had not relapsed after 14 years. It is on the understanding that many, or most, low-grade lesions will undergo regression, compared with the potential for high-grade lesions to proceed to invasive cancer, that it is possible to make the following recommendations concerning which CIN lesions to treat.

Östör (1993) in a critical review of the natural history of CIN has confirmed the spectrum of regression and progression in CIN 1, 2 and 3. This ranges from a regression rate of 60% in CIN 1 to a progression of 12% from CIN 3 to invasive cancer. He emphasized the need to use factors other than morphologic to determine the prognosis in individual patients.

High-grade lesions: CIN 2 to 3/HSIL

On the basis of the discussion in Chapter 6, it would seem wise to treat all lesions in this category of severity. It is unclear how urgent therapy is but, at present, no technique exists to tell the clinician when a lesion is likely to become invasive.

Low-grade lesions: CIN 1/LSIL

The available evidence suggests that this group is not associated with a high risk of progression with time (Östör, 1993). In addition, significant regression may occur. Two options concerning the management of these low-grade lesions are obvious.

1 Observation only

Observation with serial monitoring by cytology, with or without colposcopy, has been shown to be highly effective in detecting the development of major-grade lesions (Jones *et al.*, 1992). Regression will reveal itself, and progression to a higher grade should be identifiable so that appropriate treatment can be instituted. The role of viral testing to determine the presence of high-risk DNA types is quickly becoming an accepted part of the management protocol (Nobbenhuis *et al.*, 1999). The confirmation of such types and their semiquantitative measurement by polymerase chain reaction techniques (Cuzick *et al.*, 1992; Terry *et al.*, 1992) will greatly assist in the triage of these low-grade lesions (Schiffman, 1993). More recently, hybrid capture techniques have been widely used with satisfactory results (Ferenczy *et al.*, 1996; Hall *et al.*, 1996; Lorincz, 1996). This has been discussed in detail in Chapter 2 (p. 29).

2 Proceed to treatment as soon as is practical

Both options have their advantages and disadvantages, but clearly the more conservative approach reduces unnecessary intervention for lesions that will regress. Long-term follow-up without treatment may not only induce a level of anxiety in the patient but also increase the follow-up workload for the individual clinic.

Protagonists of immediate treatment argue strongly in its favor against the background of an anticipated cure rate of more than 90% with one treatment and the availability of therapy in an outpatient department or office environment.

Both approaches have the problem that they must somehow address a remarkable increase over the last 5 years in the prevalence of low-grade lesions. This has resulted in an increased load on clinical facilities. It would seem to the authors that a CIN lesion, especially a small one involving less than one quadrant of the cervix, that is diagnosed histologically with an accompanying mild dyskaryotic smear, can be left untreated if there is adequate cytologic follow-up.

The role of HPV testing has recently been defined in the exceptionally well screened Icelandic population by Sigurdsson *et al.* (1997). They defined the role of HPV testing by either hybrid capture or PCR assays as limited to "identifying women with low grade smears and koilocytosis or low grade colposcopic biopsies that are at risk of concealing or developing high grade histologic lesions." A recent study by Manos *et al.* (1999) showed that the use of hybrid capture (HCII, Digene Corp.) to detect high risk oncogenic HPV types on women with low-grade smear abnormalities could accurately identify those who had high-grade SIL.

7.6 Prerequisites for treatment

Having assessed the cervix, the colposcopist is now in a position to determine whether the lesion may be treated by one of two methods, namely excision, or local destruction with preoperative biopsy. The choice as to which to use depends on certain criteria that must be considered by the colposcopist. These are as follows.

1 Is there any suspicion, within the atypical transformation zone, of the presence of invasive cancer? If there is evidence, then the procedure must be excision. Any extensive (large area) major-grade lesion must also be regarded as an indication for excision, as it has been shown (Tidbury *et al.*, 1992) that invasive cancer is most likely to arise from a large CIN 3 lesion.

2 Is the colposcopy satisfactory or unsatisfactory? Any significant extension of a lesion within the endocervix must be viewed with suspicion and is usually a contraindication to local destruction.

3 Is there correlation between the cytology and the colposcopy? For example, the colposcopic finding of a supposedly low-grade lesion and the cytologic report of the presence of a high-grade lesion would indicate that the lesion should be excised.

It is important for the colposcopist to be aware of the referral cytology, and also whether within that cytology report there is mention of any atypical glandular cells indicating the possibility of glandular intraepithelial neoplasia (GIN) or adenocarcinoma. The issue of endocervical curettage and its effect on the choice of treatment has already been discussed (p. 125). In recent years, there has been a very significant move towards excisional therapies obviating many of the dilemmas mentioned above.

7.7 Methods of treatment

Once the prerequisites for treatment have been confirmed, then a choice can be made between excision and local destruction. Each will be discussed below.

Local destructive techniques

The following conservative methods all depend on eradication of the localized lesion by its physical destruction. It is imperative that any such method destroys the CIN contained within the cervical glands or, more correctly, the crypts, as discussed above. Therefore, to be totally effective, these methods must destroy the tissue to a depth of at least 6–7 mm, especially if the CIN is situated in the crypts. There are four local destructive techniques:

1 Cryotherapy, or freezing of the area by the application of probes; anesthesia is not usually required.

2 Cold coagulation, usually without, or with some local, anesthesia.

3 Electrodiathermy, under either local or general anesthesia.

4 Carbon dioxide (CO_2) laser evaporation, usually with local anesthesia.

A. Cryosurgery

Principle

The principle of cryosurgery is that when a liquid vaporizes, or a gas expands, heat is drawn from the surrounding environment. Some of the earlier devices used for cryosurgery involved liquid nitrogen or freon gases, but now almost all machines use nitrous oxide, which is readily available in all hospitals and clinics (Creasman *et al.*, 1984).

Equipment

The equipment (Fig. 7.3) consists of a hand-held probe (1) that terminates in a hollow tip (2); this can be changed to suit the size and contour of the cervix. The gas is channeled through a narrow tube (3) into the tip, from which it is removed by a wider bore tube and exhausted to the outside air. The cryoprobe tip, which is placed against the area to be treated (Fig. 7.4) is cooled by this gaseous expansion and the cervix is superficially frozen, resulting in cell death.

Technique

The patient will already have had an initial colposcopic assessment, during which preliminary biopsies will have been made and reported on. Upon returning to the clinic, the patient is informed of the results and proposed treat-

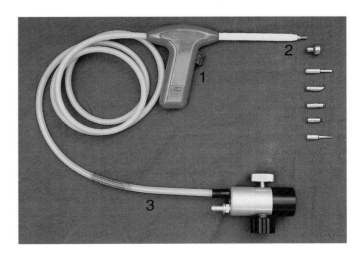

Fig. 7.3

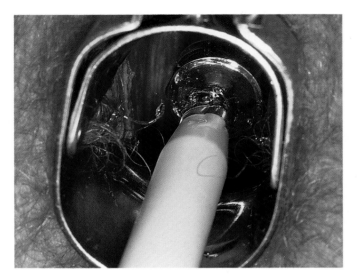

Fig. 7.4

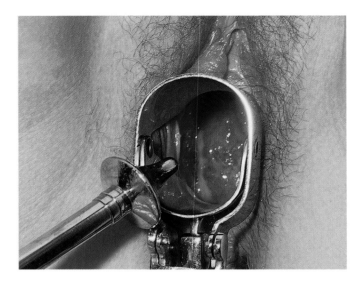

Fig. 7.5

ment and should be allowed to ask questions and receive a full explanation of the procedure, its complications, and sequelae.

The patient is then placed in the lithotomy position and the largest comfortable Cusco's speculum is inserted into the vagina to expose the cervix, in order to keep the cervix and probe tip clear of the vagina. Colposcopy then determines the size of the lesion. A suitable probe tip is then chosen and screwed into the cryoprobe, which is then inserted into the vagina under direct vision (Fig. 7.5).

The most effective, and now standard, technique is to use a freeze–thaw–refreeze process (Creasman *et al.*, 1984). Each element of the freeze cycle lasts for 120 seconds; the aim is to achieve a peripheral "iceball" of approximately 4 mm (Fig. 7.6). This infers that the depth of freeze will also be approximately 4 mm, meeting to a large extent the depth-of-treatment recommendations mentioned above. At the end of the treatment cycle the probe is defrosted and gently removed from the cervix. The freeze crater (1) has completely covered the lesion with a small (3 mm) margin of normal tissue around (2). In Fig. 7.7 an application (1) of antibiotic cream is being placed in the cervical crater; however, its use is controversial.

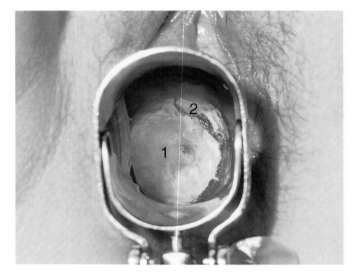

Fig. 7.6

Healing

Following treatment, the cervix will go through the usual repair process that occurs when tissue has been destroyed. The area will become demarcated and a slough will develop. In Fig. 7.8, such a slough (1) can be seen; this will usually separate at around 10 days. At this time there may be some slight bleeding or increase in discharge, usually of a clear mucous consistency. Thereafter, new squamous epithelium will migrate inward from the periphery and cover the defect with a firm strong epithelium.

Post-treatment patient information and instructions

The patient is given a series of written recommendations that, if followed, will aid rapid and full healing of the cervix.

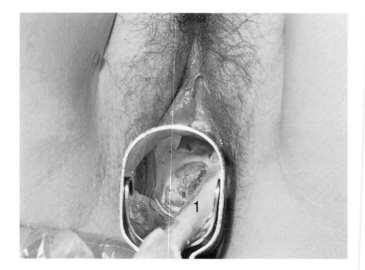

Fig. 7.7

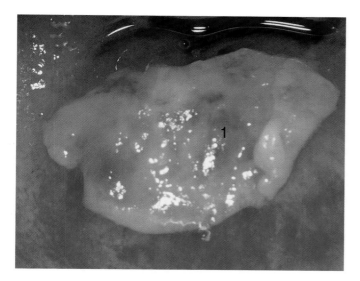

Fig. 7.8

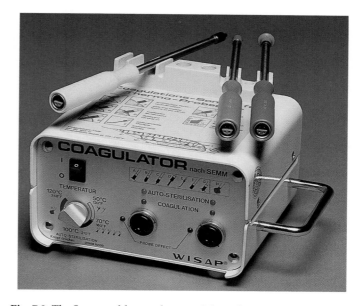

Fig. 7.9 The Semm cold coagulator and three thermoprobes.

1 The patient should avoid sexual intercourse for 4 weeks.
2 The use of tampons should be avoided for the first menstrual period after treatment.
3 Heavy and prolonged exercise should be avoided for 4 weeks.
4 Patients will experience a series of reactions, of which they should be forewarned:

(a) A profuse watery discharge will develop and may persist for 2–3 weeks. The discharge may be so heavy as to require the wearing of sanitary protection.

(b) A small amount of spotting may occur as the slough separates. This is normal. Bleeding that is significantly heavier than that which occurs during a menstrual period is not normal and is usually a sign of infection; medical advice should be sought.

(c) An offensive discharge indicates infection and should be actively treated with local vaginal cleansing and use of an antibiotic, if appropriate.

Complications

Among patients, cryosurgery is the most acceptable of all the conservative techniques as it can be performed in an outpatient department and there is virtually no pain. At worst, a mild menstrual-type cramp will be felt.

The most frequently reported sequela of cryosurgery is a profuse watery discharge that may persist for 2–3 weeks. Bleeding is relatively rare. If it does occur, it is usually slight, mixed with discharge, and most commonly occurs at the time of the separation of the slough. The cervix heals well, leaving a characteristic appearance of radial ridging. The squamocolumnar junction is often found to lie just within the endocervical canal. Some authorities feel that this is advantageous as it reduces the risk of new lesions occurring. Others consider it to be a disadvantage as it renders access and colposcopic monitoring rather more difficult.

Infection of the sloughing area may occur but responds well to a short course of antibiotics and local cleansing.

Results of treatment

Although patient acceptability is very high, cryosurgery has a lower clearance rate than other conservative techniques. Some authors have claimed clearance rates of about 95% (Benedet *et al.*, 1992). However, the general experience appears to be that a rate of 85% is more frequently seen (Monaghan *et al.*, 1982; Anderson *et al.*, 1988). Success in treating some CIN 3 lesions was shown to be lower in two studies (Ostergard, 1980; Walton *et al.*, 1980); these gave rates of clearance of only 61 and 68%, respectively. Like other local destructive methods, the size of the lesion and not the biologic stage of the CIN seems to influence the chances of success and of complete clearance.

B. Cold coagulation

The Semm cold coagulator was introduced into gynecologic practice in 1966. It was primarily used for the local destruction of benign cervical lesions. Many authors have confirmed its wide applicability in the treatment of precancerous conditions of the cervix (Gordon & Duncan, 1991; Loobuyck & Duncan, 1993). The equipment (Fig. 7.9) consists of a series of varying sized Teflon-coated thermoprobes that are rapidly heated electrically. The equipment is relatively cheap and has proved remarkably popular within Europe and the UK.

Technique

The patient is given a colposcopic examination in the standard manner, and the site and extent of the lesion are confirmed. A biopsy is taken and the patient returns to the clinic for definitive treatment if the conditions for safe usage of local destructive techniques have been satisfied. Gordon and Duncan (1991) have reported a "see and treat" policy involving immediate treatment following biopsy.

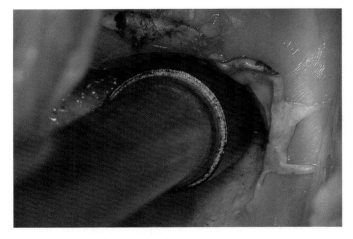

Fig. 7.10 The thermoprobe is applied to the cervix and activated. Sloughing of the skin can be seen alongside the probe head.

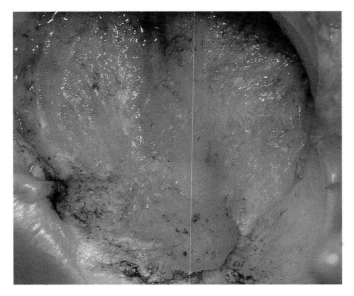

Fig. 7.11 The treated cervix is dry with a central pale area of destroyed tissue.

This technique, however, relies on very-high-quality colposcopy and is not generally recommended. They only use this technique when the entire limits of the lesion are fully visible and when there is no suggestion of an invasive lesion. Two to four biopsies are taken at this time.

The thermoprobe is applied to the lesion, and two to five overlapping applications are required to cover adequately the abnormality (Fig. 7.10). The thermoprobe heats the tissues to 120°C, thereby literally boiling the tissues. De Cristofana *et al.* (1988) showed that cold coagulation at 120°C for 30 seconds achieves a depth of destruction of at least 4 mm within the cervix. Hemostasis is automatic (Fig. 7.11). The whole procedure takes less than 2 minutes. Local analgesia is often used; in a recent study, Goodman and Sumner (1991) showed that compared with laser vaporization, 155 women requiring treatment for CIN found the cold coagulation treatment to be less painful and quicker. Patients are given a prescription of triple sulfonamide cream to insert into the vagina throughout the next week.

Follow-up

As with other conservative techniques, primary follow-up is with cytology (in some units cervicography is employed purely to monitor the appearance of the ectocervix). Colposcopy is used only when there is persistent or recurrent cytologic abnormality.

Results of treatment

In a review by Gordon and Duncan (1991) of 1661 patients treated over a 14-year period, 1628 patients were successfully reviewed. There were excellent clearance rates of 98% at 4 months and 87% at 5 and 10 years. The primary clearance rate was 93% (1518/1628). As with other ablative conservative techniques, there was a significant post-treatment carcinoma rate of 4/1628; this is a slightly higher rate than that reported by Paraskevaidis *et al.* (1991) for laser ablation.

In the study by Gordon and Duncan (1991), the practice was to offer cold coagulation when the patient presented for the first visit, at which time the colposcopist expected that the diagnosis would be no worse than CIN 3. Overall, 97% of women were treated at this first visit, but only in 30 women (2%) was the histology more minor than expected, or contained glandular epithelium. However, 22 females showed no persistent cervical disease at a later date and follow-up for up to 10 years was achieved in 87% of cases. Repeat cold coagulation was used for persistent and recurrent CIN 3 lesions, but this technique was less successful under these conditions and was not advised.

Pregnancy post-treatment

The evidence shows that cold coagulation, like other conservative techniques, does not adversely affect pregnancy. The major advantage of cold coagulation is its relative cheapness and wide applicability. The major disadvantages, as with other ablative techniques, are that the tissue destroyed is not available for analysis, the depth of treatment is difficult to determine, and its efficacy depends on high quality colposcopy.

The outcome of 226 pregnancies reported in the Gordon and Duncan (1991) study showed surprisingly low rates of preterm miscarriage or the need for operative delivery.

C. Radical electrocoagulation diathermy

This simple and effective technique has been extensively used worldwide in the treatment of CIN. The equipment is readily available in all operating theaters and is relatively inexpensive. Chanen (1989) feels that the technique is more effective than either cryosurgery or the CO_2 laser for destroying larger areas of abnormality; he also uses this method where *"anatomic limits of the lesion can be exposed to the colposcope."* This extension of the role of a conservative technique has proved extremely successful in practice. As an added safeguard, Chanen advocates the use of further biopsies and/or endocervical curettage to make a better assessment of lesions that extend into the endocervical canal. The technique is, however, more limited in its application to lesions that extend onto the vagina. The greater accuracy and control over the depth of treatment achieved with laser surgery make this modality superior in these circumstances. The technique works by coagulating and destroying the epithelium and epithelium within glands. However, the latter may impair an adequate depth of destruction because it will stimulate the exudation of mucus, which, in turn, has a pronounced insulating effect; consequently, to achieve the required depth of destruction, application of heat must be continued until no more mucus is produced. The varied arrangement in number and topography of the clefts and glands within the cervix requires corresponding variation in the duration and depth of application of the heat source. Healing is usually complete within 4 weeks. Chanen and Rome (1983) in Australia have documented the excellent results of a large series of patients treated with this method. Its major disadvantage is that its application causes pain, and usually a short general anesthetic is required, although some series have reported the successful use of local analgesia (Chanen, 1989).

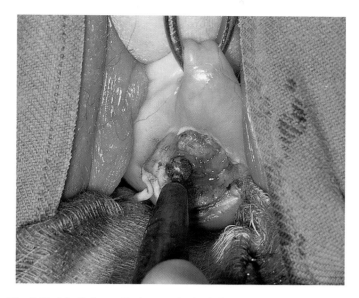

Fig. 7.12 A ball electrodiathermy device is being used to coagulate the abnormal (atypical) epithelium. The endocervix and part of the ectocervix have been obliterated to a depth of at least 10 mm beyond the lateral extent of the lesion. Pressure must be maintained on the diathermy probe because mucus exudation will insulate the tissue from the heat.

Technique

All patients should be given a preliminary assessment, in which the cervix is examined with the colposcope and appropriate biopsies are taken. The results of these biopsies must be available before radical electrodiathermy treatment is begun. Either local or sedo-analgesia can be used, and colposcopy is performed to confirm the initial findings. Chanen and Rome (1983) have recommended that the cervix be first dilated to counter the risk of postoperative stenosis. The cervix is then painted with Lugol's iodine solution. The equipment consists of a standard diathermy delivery unit producing 40–45 W; the needle electrode is used to perform a series of radial cuts to 2–3 mm beyond the iodine-negative areas. This segmentation of the cervix is carried down to approximately 5–7 mm. The needle is used to slice radial cuts into the cervix to open any Nabothian follicles and deal with any CIN that may extend into the gland crypts. The segments are then removed using a ball electrode (Fig. 7.12); this leaves a conical crater that is at least 7 mm deep (Fig. 7.13).

The clinician should take care not to touch the vagina with the diathermy unit during the procedure, as this would cause electrical burns. Postoperative cold-water douching of the area has been recommended, but has not been found by the authors to be necessary.

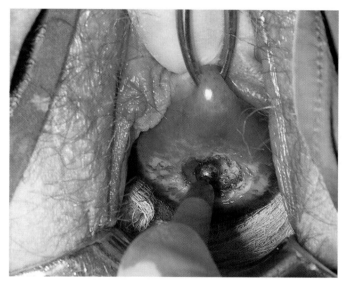

Fig. 7.13 A conical crater can be seen within the cervix.

has been no significant alteration in pregnancy performance subsequent to radical electrodiathermy. He noted that there was a slight increase in cervical dystocia; this resulted in a lengthening of labor for some patients.

Postoperative course

Following radical electrodiathermy, the patient will experience the same problems as those found after laser treatment. Secondary hemorrhage may occur and is usually associated with infection. Scarring and stenosis are more common after electrodiathermy, but there are no recorded series showing difficulties with future pregnancies. Most cervixes heal with an accessible squamocolumnar junction; there is often peripheral ridging and wrinkling, as found after cryosurgery (Fig. 7.14.). In Chanen's experience there

Results of treatment

Chanen and colleagues in Melbourne, Australia, have one of the largest series to date using this method (Chanen & Hollyock, 1974; Chanen & Rome, 1983). In their 1983 report, they described 1864 patients with histologically proven CIN; about two-thirds of cases were CIN 3. CIN was eradicated by one treatment in 97% of these patients, and 93% of all patients were under 30 years of age. There were 62 patients with either persistent or recurrent disease, but 44 of these were cured by either directed biopsy or further diathermy. Progression to invasive cancer during follow-

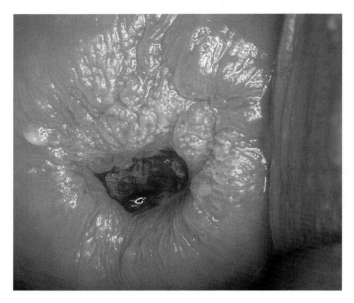

Fig. 7.14 The washed-leather appearance after electrodiathermy. The squamocolumnar junction is clearly visible just inside the endocervical canal.

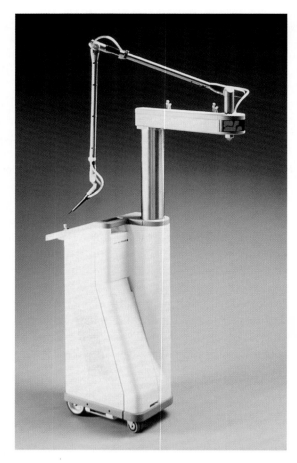

Fig. 7.15 A free-standing CO_2 laser machine with an articulated arm that connects to a micromanipulator which is attached to the colposcope. In this figure, a handpiece is at the terminal end of the articulated arm.

up has not been reported. The experience of Chanen *et al.* is similar to that of proponents of laser and cryosurgery, in that failures seem to be related more to the extent of the lesion or to a lack of firmness in the application of the heating current. Other smaller series have quoted success rates that range from 85% to 94% (Seshadri & Cope, 1985; Woodman *et al.*, 1985; Giles *et al.*, 1987). In a further publication from Australia, where electrocoagulation diathermy was used to obliterate a clinical human papillomavirus infection (HPV), and so possibly influence the later development of CIN, it was shown that no advantage was gained, as the rate of recurrence or persistence of HPV was exactly the same in a control group who were not given diathermy (Mitchell & Medley, 1989).

D. Carbon dioxide laser vaporization

The use of the CO_2 laser is now widely accepted as one of the most effective forms of treatment of CIN. Although at present the loop electrosurgical excision procedure has become more popular, there is no evidence to suggest that the results between CO_2 laser vaporization and loop excision will vary significantly. The advantages and disadvantages of the two techniques will be described later (Ali *et al.*, 1986; Benedet *et al.*, 1992; Volante *et al.*, 1992).

The term "laser" is an acronym for light amplification by stimulated emission of radiation. The laser converts energy, such as heat, light, or electricity, into a radiant form of energy that is produced at a specific wavelength, determined by the type of laser. CO_2 lasers, for example, produce energy at a wavelength of 10.6 µm; this is in the infrared portion of the spectrum and invisible to the human eye. This energy can be focused on a specific spot, 1.5 to 2 mm in diameter, by a system of mirrors and lenses, and at its focal point the laser releases an enormous amount of energy. Any tissue at this focal point is vaporized at the speed of light. The laser itself is attached to the colposcope and at all times

the area to be destroyed is under the direct vision of the person performing the laser surgery. Manipulation of the beam is extremely simple.

Equipment

Most modern lasers (Fig. 7.15) are free-standing and have a cabinet that contains the helium and nitrogen gas mixtures and the tubes for developing the coherent light beam. The beam is transferred via a series of articulated arms, each with a surface-reflecting mirror at the junction. A column, to which the articulating arm is attached, is capable of movement both up and down; the control (microprocessor) panel allows for a multiplicity of power and time selection. The arm terminates either in a handpiece, which is used for free lasering in exposed areas such as the vulva, or, more commonly, in a micromanipulator that can be attached to a colposcope head. This latter arrangement allows the light to be reflected from the terminal mirror, which can be angled by the micromanipulator, which is coupled (1) to the front piece of the colposcope (Fig. 7.16). A manipulator (2) at its upper part allows precision control over the emanating laser beam by free movement through a 360° arc. The lasers are arranged so that the light is "focused" at a focal length that maximizes the power density, and thus the cutting and vaporization potential of the device. Modern lasers have a variable spot-size facility, (determined by adjusting the circular ring (3)),

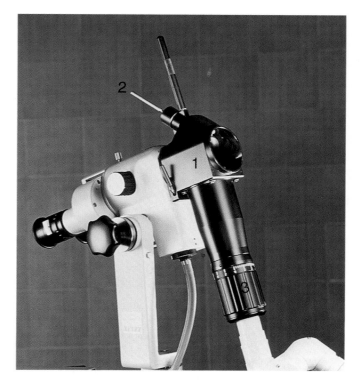

Fig. 7.16

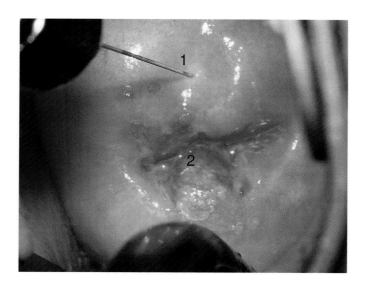

Fig. 7.17

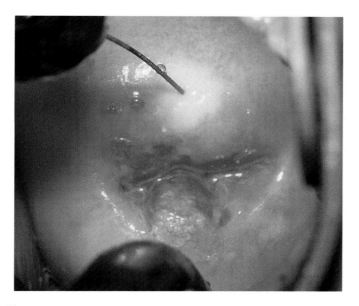

Fig. 7.18

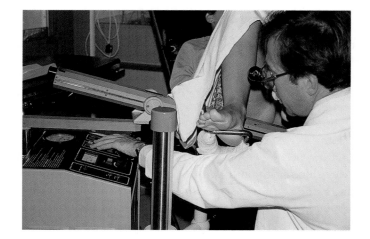

Fig. 7.19

varying from 0.2 to 2 mm, to allow the laser to be used in various modes, such as cutting, vaporization, or coagulation.

Procedure

The CIN lesion within the atypical transformation zone will have already been outlined using acetic acid. Its lateral borders can be easily defined by using Lugol's iodine solution; this contrasts the normal area with the abnormal area and gives the operator an accurate indication as to where the most atypical lateral parts of the transformation zone exist. This procedure is adopted prior to all local destructive techniques. The lesion can also be outlined by the laser beam (see Fig. 7.21 on p. 172).

Although the laser can be used without analgesia, and was used thus in the early days, it is now accepted that a combined analgesic and vasopressor agent will give a higher degree of patient compliance and acceptability. In Fig. 7.17, a fine dental syringe and needle (1) is being used to inject at one of four sites (i.e. 12-, 3-, 6-, and 9-o'clock positions) around the ectocervix immediately peripheral to the lesion site (2). Approximately 4 ml solution is injected. In Fig. 7.18, blanching is clearly seen when the fluid is injected to a depth of about 5 mm. Once the local analgesic has been injected, the appropriate setting is chosen on the laser machine (Fig. 7.19). Many lasers have a super pulse mode that, because of the configuration of the beam geometry, produces less tissue damage. However, the authors do not feel that this mode has advantages over the normal mode of delivery.

The aim of laser vaporization is to remove a block of tissue approximately 8–10 mm deep; this produces a dome-shaped defect that will incorporate any involved glands within the ecto- or endocervix (Fig. 7.20). Although the

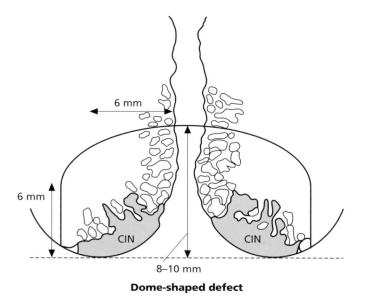

Fig. 7.20

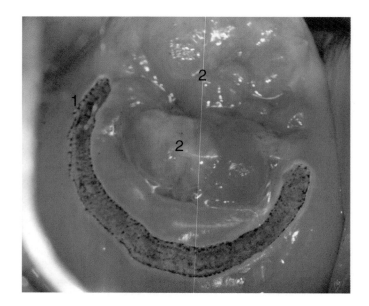

Fig. 7.21

edges of this defect are 6–7 mm deep, it is commonly found that the center will be up to 8–10 mm deep. This does not, however, produce any adverse effect for the patient.

The procedure commences some 3–4 mm beyond the edge of the atypical transformation zone at the 6-o'clock position, and the laser beam is moved rapidly over the tissues. This rapid movement reduces thermal tissue conductivity and minimizes potential scarring. It also reduces the heat build-up within the tissues, thereby reducing uterine contractions, which may otherwise distress the patient. The operator should use the highest possible power density, because the longer the beam is in contact with the tissues, the more the surrounding normal tissues will be damaged and the slower will be the healing process.

After the area has been outlined, the actual vaporization can be performed using one of two techniques. In the first, the procedure commences in the posterior area (1), the lesion (2) having already been visualized (Fig. 7.21).

The laser beam initially vaporizes a posterior area, thereby preventing blood from running down into the operative field. The beam is moved in multiple directions, either diagonally, horizontally, or vertically to prevent furrowing. The second technique, and the one used by the authors, involves a vertical movement whereby, commencing posteriorly, the beam is moved onto the endocervix and then down again, with each furrow of destruction overlapping the previous one, very similar to the effect of mowing a lawn.

The operator's right hand works the micromanipulator, and the left holds a small cotton bud or swab. As soon as bleeding occurs, the cotton bud is placed on that point to reduce blood contamination, because any blood will immediately take up a laser beam and so reduce the beam's efficiency. Using this vertical approach, it is easy to recognize bleeding points as soon as they develop. Once the posterior lip has been destroyed, the anterior lip can be similarly dealt with. The vertical technique is methodic and also allows an even depth of destruction to be achieved. Penetration is usually to a depth of at least 6 mm and this

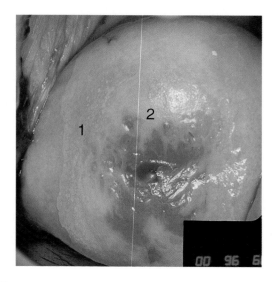

Fig. 7.22

should adequately deal with any CIN lesion within the cervical crypts. It is sometimes necessary to perform superficial laser vaporization to destroy subclinical wart viral lesions that may be associated with the CIN.

This technique is shown in Figs 7.22–7.25; punch biopsy had revealed not only the presence of subclinical papillomavirus infection (SPI) but also CIN 2/3. In Fig. 7.22, the sharp lateral (outer) outline of the atypical transformation is seen; multiple biopsies in the peripheral area (1) showed the presence of subclinical viral infection, while biopsies taken at point (2), toward the endocervix, showed the presence of CIN 2 to 3. The upper limit of the lesion can be clearly seen. Vaporization of the peripheral area to a depth of only 2–3 mm is shown in Fig. 7.23, while in Fig. 7.24 the central area has been ablated to a depth of about 8 mm. Some 6 months later the area appears as seen in Fig. 7.25; the outer limit of the vaporization is at (1) and some metaplastic regenerating epithelium is at (2). The upper limit, the new squamocolumnar junction, can be clearly seen.

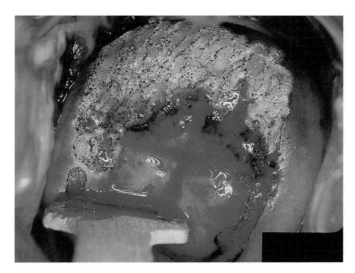

Fig. 7.23

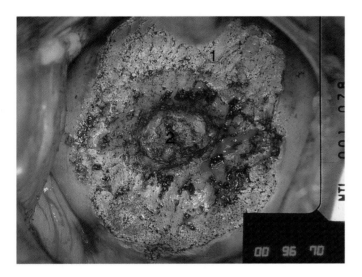

Fig. 7.24

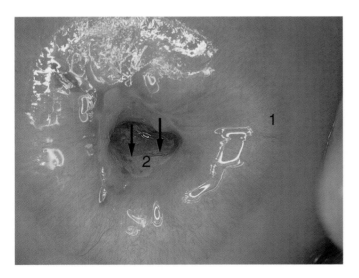

Fig. 7.25

Results

The results for laser vaporization have been extremely satisfactory. At present, most large series quote success rates of over 90%. A recent study by Benedet *et al.* (1992) of some

1811 women showed a cure rate for CIN of all grades approaching 96%. Volante *et al.* (1992), in a recent study of 334 patients, reported a similar cure rate with no invasive disease developing. In a study of 2130 women treated between 1980 and 1989, Paraskevaidis *et al.* (1991) had a failure rate of 5.6%, of which 71% developed during the 1st year of follow-up, 24% in the 2nd year, and 3% in the 3rd year. Disquietingly, they found two cases of microinvasion and one frankly invasive lesion following laser treatment; all these cases were diagnosed during the 2nd year of follow-up. Other studies (Rasbridge *et al.*, 1990) also showed high cure rates; Ali *et al.* (1986), in a study of 1157 women, noted a cure rate of 96% after one treatment.

7.8 Excision techniques for treating CIN

The use of excision techniques was the mainstay of the management of cervical dysplasia and carcinoma-in-situ (previous nomenclature) for many years; these involved hysterectomy and then cone biopsy, the latter being the less radical technique. However, the use of cone biopsy in large numbers of young women caused much disquiet because of the attendant morbidity (Jones *et al.*, 1979), and so it was not surprising that the locally destructive techniques, as described above, became popular. These methods are the treatment of choice for selected cases in which the entire abnormality is visible on the ectocervix, and in which there is no suggestion of invasion; this has been described under the prerequisites for treatment in Section 7.3. The principal disadvantage of local destructive treatment, however, is that a histologic examination of the entire lesion is not possible, and early invasive cancer may remain undetected (Paraskevaidis *et al.*, 1991).

Critics of the local destructive methods maintain that cytology, colposcopy, and biopsy together cannot exclude invasion with sufficient certainty to allow cone biopsy to be avoided. To test this premise, McIndoe *et al.* (1989) examined over a 12-year period women who had CIN and who were suitable for laser vaporization. During the initial part of the study all patients were treated by knife biopsy but in the second part, over some 6 years, laser vaporization was used in all those who had a satisfactory colposcopy and met other criteria that made them suitable for local destructive treatment. The rate of diagnosis of microinvasion, expressed as a percentage of all cases of CIN, fell from 3.45% when cone biopsy was used as the only treatment to 1.04% after the introduction of vaporization. McIndoe *et al.* concluded that a number of women, who were not recognized as having microinvasion may have been inappropriately treated using laser vaporization. With the advent of the laser (CO_2) cone biopsy technique, described below, McIndoe *et al.* (1989) found that a number of very early invasive cancers did indeed exist within another group of women who were eligible for laser vaporization. It would appear that these early lesions would have been missed had local destruction by laser vaporization been performed. In another study, by Vergote *et al.* (1992), 123 patients with histologically confirmed CIN, and who had had a satisfactory colposcopy, were treated by laser excision removal of the transformation zone. All these women would normally have been suitable for laser vaporization treatment. In three cases, histology of the laser excision specimen showed microinvasive lesions to be present. It was concluded that laser excision of the transformation zone was a suitable alternative to vaporization in patients with a satisfactory colposcopy.

These studies have led many authors to advocate the use of excision rather than local destruction techniques. At the moment, it must be left to the individual clinician to choose which technique gives the best results.

The techniques used for excision are as follows:
1 Cold knife biopsy.
2 Laser cone biopsy.
3 Large loop diathermy.
4 Hysterectomy: abdominal or vaginal.
However, before discussing these individually, it is important to consider the special problem of CIN extension to within the endocervix.

Special problems of endocervical extension

It has already been mentioned that lesions extending into the endocervix prove difficult to remove completely. Various techniques, such as microcolpohysteroscopy and cervicoscopy, have been used to assess the endocervical involvement of CIN. When CIN extends into the endocervical canal beyond the limits of detection with the colposcope, some excisional procedure that removes the entire length of the endocervical canal must be performed. In Fig. 7.26, an endocervical lesion (shaded area) and the excisional defect produced by its removal are diagrammatically represented. Figure 7.27 shows a further, similar case; the abnormal (atypical) epithelium (high-grade) is at (1) in the endocervix and the upper limits of its extent are arrowed.

This epithelium is in a cervix that was treated some 2 years previously by local destruction of a CIN 3 lesion. It is only with a "tailored" cone biopsy that this area can be effectively removed without the need to remove large amounts of the ectocervix. Indeed, in Fig. 7.26, the length of the excisional defect is 15–20 mm and the depth 6 mm; these are the dimensions that would be required to eradicate the residual CIN 3 lesion seen in Fig. 7.27.

Complete removal can be achieved where prior endocervical assessment has been made before a tailored excisional procedure. Soutter *et al.* (1984) reported their experience with tailoring cone (excision) biopsies to provide measurements of the endocervical involvement of CIN; they used microcolpohysteroscopy. In all 63 cone biopsies tailored in this way, the CIN was completely excised at the apex of the cone; this contrasted with 87 cone biopsies in which no visual control was used, and in which there were nine cases where the apex of the cone was involved with disease. Interestingly, in this series, no difference was noted between the length of the hysteroscopically controlled and uncontrolled cones. Other simple measures may sometimes be employed to determine the extent of endocervical involvement. In Figs 7.28 and 7.29, a major-grade lesion is seen to extend across the ectocervix (2); even with the insertion of Desjardin's forceps its upper limits cannot be determined (1). However, in this case microcolpohysteroscopy or cervicoscopy (after Ueki, 1985) would be needed to determine the upper limits of the lesion.

The cold knife cone biopsy

For years, the standard therapy for treating CIN and conserving the cervix was cold knife cone biopsy. This valuable technique has been somewhat superseded in recent years by the laser (CO_2) cone and, latterly, by the loop diathermy cone biopsy. Prior to the widespread availability of colposcopy, many cone biopsies were performed "blind" using this cold knife technique. Consequently, there was

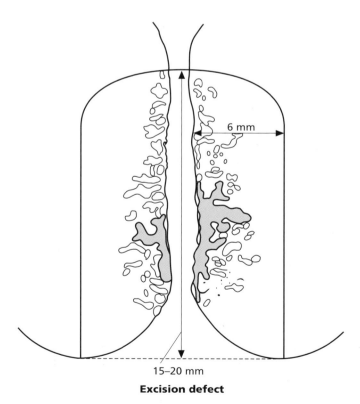

Excision defect

Fig. 7.26

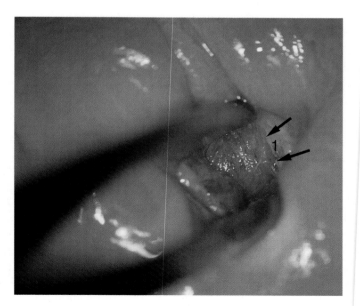

Fig. 7.27

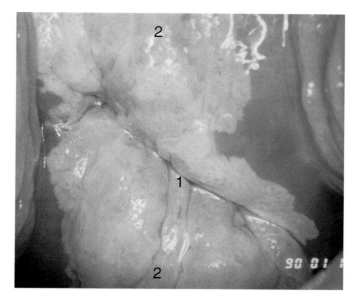

Fig. 7.28

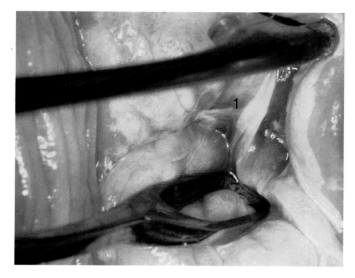

Fig. 7.29

tremendous variation in the amount of cervical tissue removed, and subsequent trauma to the cervix was significant. Large cone biopsies tended to be effective in dealing with the CIN at a "price," but there was a higher risk of pregnancy complications; smaller cone biopsies were less traumatic but tended not to remove the fundamental CIN problem. Colposcopy allows an accurate assessment to be made of the size of the lesion and, consequently, the clinician can more accurately determine and tailor the size of cone (excision) biopsy required.

No patient should receive treatment for an abnormal smear without first being given a colposcopic examination.

The aim of a cone biopsy is to achieve a combination of diagnostic and curative management. The tissue to be removed is the entire transformation zone with an extension into the endocervical canal to encompass the entire lesion. How deep this extension should be remains difficult to assess and the various methods employed to overcome this problem have been discussed above. There are a number of indications for cone biopsy.

Indications

The indications for cone (excision) biopsy (using either cold knife, CO_2 laser, or loop diathermy) are as follows:
1 The lesion extends into the endocervical canal to such an extent that a satisfactory assessment cannot be made colposcopically or by biopsy (unsatisfactory colposcopy).
2 The cytology gives repeated suggestion of an invasive lesion without there being colposcopic evidence.
3 There is suggestion of an invasive lesion on cytology, colposcopy, or biopsy.
4 An abnormal glandular lesion is suggested on cytology or colposcopy.
5 The cytology suggests a much more serious condition than do colposcopy or punch biopsy.
6 Endocervical curettage suggests a precancerous or cancerous lesion.

It must be recognized that in many parts of the world, where the newer excisional techniques, namely CO_2 laser and loop diathermy, are not available, there remains an important place for cold knife cone biopsy.

Technique

With the introduction of many reversible short-acting analgesics, such as Midazolam, it has been possible to perform extensive surgical procedures with the patient semiconscious and free from pain. With the subsequent use of reversal agents (e.g. Flumazenil), the patient can be fully conscious on leaving the operating room. Patients can therefore be given a choice of anesthesia for this procedure.

The patient should be placed in the lithotomy position. A Simm's or Auvard's speculum is placed in the vagina, exposing the cervix. The patient is recolposcoped and the site of the lesion confirmed. It is usual to utilize a technique for reducing blood loss during the procedure. A variety of methods, some extremely ingenious, have been tried; one is cryosurgery to freeze the cervix, with subsequent conization of the frozen cervical transformation zone. However, the most frequently used hemostatic techniques are either to insert lateral sutures to encompass the descending branches of the cervical arteries or to use a vasopressor agent that is injected directly into the substance of the cervix. The most popular agents are dilute adrenalin in local anesthetic, felypressin in local anesthetic, or bupivacaine and octapressin. Injections of these agents should surround the periphery of the ectocervical margin of the lesion and not be injected directly into the lesion because of the theoretic risk of implantation of CIN deep into the cervix.

Some clinicians recommend use of Lugol's iodine solution to assist in locating the ectocervical margins of the lesion; it is of no help in outlining the new squamocolumnar junction.

With a tissue forceps the cervix is grasped peripheral to the lesion and drawn down; the ectocervical incision is made with a pointed knife blade (a wedge), completely circumscribing the transformation zone and the lesion (Fig. 7.30). It is often easier to begin the incision posteriorly and then carry it on anteriorly, so that any bleeding runs away from the incision. Manipulating the cone with a tissue

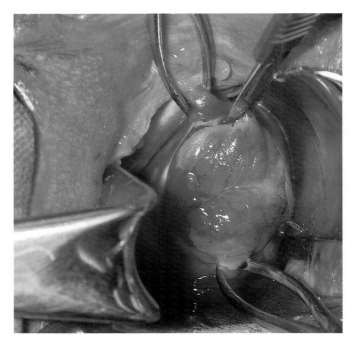

Fig. 7.30

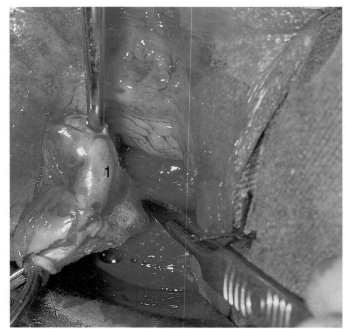

Fig. 7.32(a

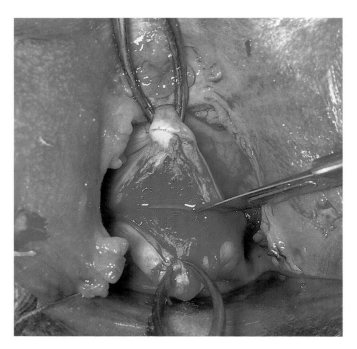

Fig. 7.31

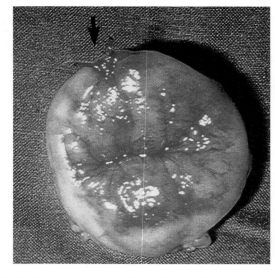

Fig. 7.32(b)

Fig. 7.32 (b) Gross photograph of a knife cone biopsy specimen, "os up," prior to fixation. There is a suture at 12 o'clock for orientation.

forceps, a vertical incision is then made into the cervix, angled toward the upper part of the endocervical canal (Fig. 7.31) so as to remove a conical block of tissue (1) (Fig. 7.32). The necessary depth of this cut is the great imponderable. It would appear that a depth of between 15 and 20 mm will clear most endocervical extensions. If the lesion extends for a large distance across the ectocervix and up into the endocervical canal, the upper limit of which can be clearly seen, then it will be necessary to perform a shallower cone excision. However, if there is little to be seen on the ectocervix and the lesion disappears out of sight into the endocervical canal, as in Fig. 7.29, then a proportionately longer cone will be needed. Fortunately, the latter situation rarely occurs in younger women, so that the risk of future

pregnancy complications, resulting from damage to the cervical sphincteric mechanism, does not apply.

Repairing the defect in the cervix

Traditionally, considerable efforts have been made to repair the cut surface of the cervix following cone biopsy. Figure 7.33 shows the use of one such previously popular technique (Sturmdorf) in which sutures were inserted to draw over the raw surface flaps of cervical epithelium that had been previously developed. The result at the time of surgery is commendably neat (Fig. 7.34). However, the scarring and disfigurement that can occur during the healing process plus the risk of covering over any residual precancerous lesion, thereby rendering satisfactory follow-up difficult or impossible to achieve, must first be considered. So long as local haemostasis can be achieved, it is better to simply freeze or cauterize the base of the cone cavity and allow spontaneous healing to occur. This results in the new squamocolumnar junction being accessible to

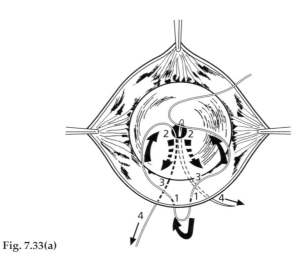

Fig. 7.33(a)

Fig. 7.33(b)

Fig. 7.33 (a & b) Scheme showing the technique for developing cervical skin flaps and inserting Sturmdorf sutures. The purpose of the Sturmdorf suture is to cover the posterior aspect of the bare cervical stump with a loose skin flap. The basic procedure is to draw the midpoint of the edge of the skin flap into the cervical canal on a double thread. The needles mounted on these two threads secure the flaps to the stump. It is initially anchored at the posterior cut end of the canal by transfixing the posterior wall of the stump with the two ends of the thread; one on the left side, in the 5-o'clock position, and one on the right side, in the 7-o'clock position. (a) The route taken by each end of the suture after it has been picked up at the midpoint of the edge of the posterior skin flap. The stitch commences by transversing the skin edge at 1A, and some surgeons prefer to use a double hitch or knot at this point. In any case, this is the midpoint of the suture length and each half will be inserted separately on each side with one end taken and inserted in the progression marked on the diagram 1 to 4; the other free end is then likewise inserted. (b) The effect when the stitch has been pulled tight and tied. Since the stitch embraces a major part of the cervical stump between its two halves or ends, it has value as a hemostatic agent and there is no need to worry about vessels bleeding from the ends of the stump.

cytological and colposcopic follow-up. Often, simple tamponade with a roll pack or large tampon will suffice.

Results of excision techniques

Excision techniques have been regarded as the "gold standard" for treatment of CIN. Almost all assessments of the results of treatment have revolved around the occurrence of invasive cancer following treatment. One of the difficulties in comparing the results of cone biopsy with more modern conservative therapies is that many of the cone biopsy series were carried out at a time when pretreatment colposcopic assessment was either not available or not used (Kolstad & Klem, 1976; Coppleson *et al.*, 1992).

There is broad agreement that the reporting of tumor-free margins on the cone biopsy specimen is a reliable indicator of clearance of the lesion, although some experts have reported residual CIN in subsequent hysterectomy specimens, obtained after apparently clear cone biopsies, to be between 12% and 60%. These figures were quoted by Coppleson *et al.* (1992) after an assessment of 13 studies. Latterly, the trend has been for most clinicians to adopt a policy of expectancy following cone biopsy in those cases where the margins are reported to be involved with disease. If a survey is made of the literature examining the results of treatment by local excision, then the number of subsequent overt invasive cancers is surprisingly limited. Coppleson *et al.* (1992), in reviewing some 19 series encompassing some 5480 women, described only 18 invasive lesions. It would therefore seem prudent, and indeed justified, in cases where the margins of the cone are affected with CIN to rely on follow-up cytology rather than move directly to hys-

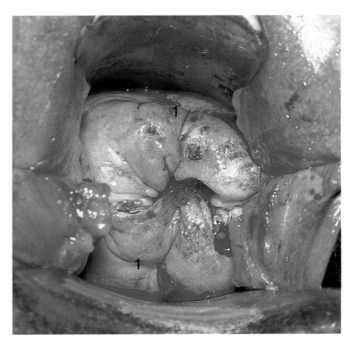

Fig. 7.34 The cervix has been fully reconstituted with the Sturmdorf stitches tied both anteriorly at the 12-o'clock position (1) and posteriorly at the 6-o'clock position (1). The cervix is covered by skin, except for a narrow band on each side; these disappeared when the anterior elevating stitch was cut.

terectomy. This policy of expectancy is reviewed immediately abnormalities are detected in surveillance cytology. Flannelly *et al.* (1997), have recently reviewed the long-term results of the treatment of 3500 women with LLETZ (large loop excision of the transformation zone) and have identified the patient with an incompletely cleared endo-cervical CIN lesion as being at highest risk of both recurrent CIN and for the older patient, invasive cancer. However the risk of recurrent CIN falls to that of the normal population after 5 years of negative cytology. The authors confirm an expectant management policy for all ages of women.

A possible reason why this form of treatment is so successful is that most excisional techniques also involve simultaneous treatment (once the cone has been removed) of the cone "bed" by either cryosurgery, cautery, or laser treatment; this effectively extends the limits of treatment beyond excision. If the specimen taken at the excisional procedure is reported to be incompletely excised or a cytological abnormality is reported at the review visit, resorting immediately to hysterectomy is now felt to be inappropriate for two reasons:

1 A true invasive lesion further in the cervix may be inadequately treated.

2 A second limited excisional procedure will usually deal with any further lesion or allow a diagnosis of an invasive area.

Laser cone biopsy

The CO_2 laser is excellent not only as a vaporizing instrument but also, when the spot size is reduced to 1 mm or less, as a slow cutting device. The facility to reduce the spot size, and thus increase the power (power density) of the beam, gives the surgeon a very accurate instrument with which to remove lesions from the cervix, vulva, etc. In many centers, laser cone biopsy has effectively replaced the cold knife conization procedure because of its accuracy, relatively small blood loss, low complication rate, and the potential to remodel the cervix; this results in an easily assessed squamocolumnar junction in the majority of cases.

The procedure can be performed either freehand or using the micromanipulator with the colposcope. The latter is the most frequently used.

Equipment

It is important to have a laser with a variable spot-size facility, and a suitable smoke-extraction device. It is essential that the speculum be light enough to allow maneuvering of the laser cone tissue and that the laser beam has access to the cervical surface.

Although the authors have used instruments such as fine Allis forceps for grasping the cone, currently the most popular instrument is the skin hook. These may be single or multiple [devised by one of the authors (AS)], as shown in Fig. 7.35.

Technique

In many centers the procedure is performed under local anesthetic in an outpatient clinic, although obviously general anesthetic or local anesthetic can be employed.

The cervix is exposed using a Cusco or Graves' speculum fitted with a smoke-extraction facility. The patient is colpo-

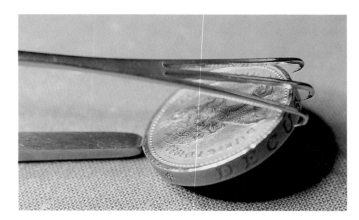

Fig. 7.35 The multiple skin hook (Singer claw; manufactured by Rocket, of London).

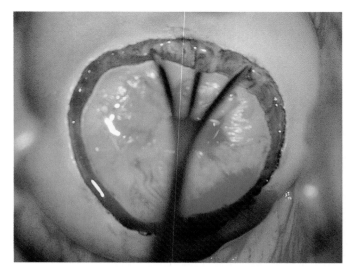

Fig. 7.36 A cone biopsy being grasped by a skin hook and drawn down. As this happens, tension is applied to the tissues, which can be easily divided by playing the laser beam over the surface. By moving the hooks around the periphery of the cone and steadily deepening the vertical cut, a cylindrical block of tissue is developed to an appropriate depth, usually 20 mm.

scoped and the extent of the lesion identified. A vasopressor agent is then injected to reduce blood loss during the procedure. As with the standard laser ablation, the transformation zone and the lesion are first circumscribed, leaving a margin of 3 mm around any lesion. This cut is deepened to approximately 3 mm, and the edge of the cone block is grasped with the skin hooks and retracted downward and sideways (Figs 7.36–7.39).

It is advantageous to biopsy the base of the cone defect to determine whether there is any residual lesion within the endocervical canal after the cone has been removed (Fig. 7.40). At the end of the procedure, the cylindrical defect remains; this can be easily measured using any simple measuring device (Fig. 7.41). Sometimes it may be necessary to extend treatment at the base. Others have recommended cutting a small dimple in the base, by undercutting with the laser the area just distal to the endocervical cut edge. This results in eversion of the endocervical epithelium, and it is believed that this simple procedure minimizes the risk of cervical stenosis.

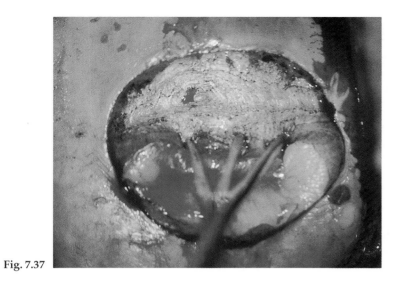

Fig. 7.37

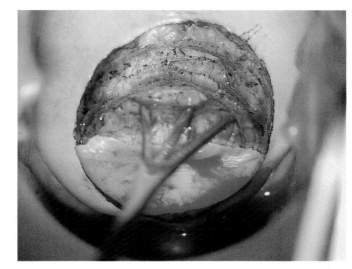

Fig. 7.38

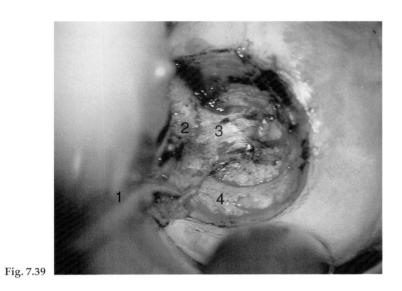

Fig. 7.39

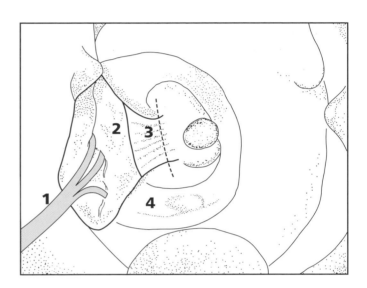

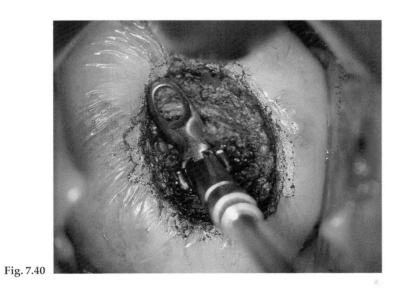

Fig. 7.40

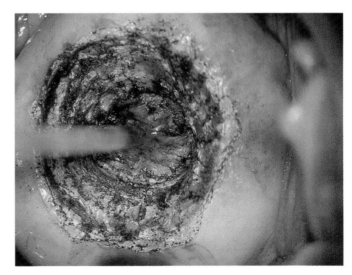

Fig. 7.41

Handling of the excised cone specimen

The excised cone specimen should be immersed intact in neutral buffered formalin for up to 24 hours fixation depending on its size. The recommended method of blocking the specimen is to take bread-kinfe cuts at 3 mm intervals to include both lips, and place each block with the same directional face down for sectioning. A sharp surgical skin blade is best for this purpose. After processing, longitudinal sections are examined and both endocervical and ectocervical margins are assessed. Where the disease extends to the first block taken, the block may be dewaxed and reversed. In this way the true resection edge can be examined. This should be necessary mainly where it is critical to measure an invasive lesion accurately.

Radial blocks are sometimes taken if the os is circular or open, but this technique has disadvantages in that the blocks end up being wedge-shaped, thereby causing problems with embedding and sectioning. With a long cone, as used in Fig. 7.27 (on p. 174), the endocervical part of the specimen can be cut transversely to obtain several circular blocks and, if necessary, the blocks from the tip of the cone may be cut at levels to assess the endocervical extreme (Anderson, 1992). The ectocervical part of the cone section is dissected using parallel anteroposterior cuts.

The edges of the cone may prove difficult to interpret. It is not unusual to find two zones of thermal injury. The zone at the margin of resection, which is approximately 50 μm thick, is characterized by extensive carbonization and charring. The other zone is much more variable in thickness and is characterized by tissue coagulation but lacks charring (Wright *et al.*, 1992b). In a study by Wright *et al.* (1992b) of 11 specimens obtained with the CO_2 laser, the coagulated zone ranged from 130 to 750 μm thick; the mean thickness was 411 μm. The extent of these zones will depend purely on the time taken by the operator to cut through the specimen. Figure 7.42 shows an example of these zones of injury at the edge of a cone biopsy (1).

Results

Although excision cone biopsy using either the cold knife or laser would seem to offer essentially similar success rates, there have been very few studies to confirm this contention. Tabor and Berget (1990), in a 5-year study of 425 women who were treated with either cold knife or laser conization, showed that the former gave a success rate of 92% and the latter a marginally higher rate of 95%. Incomplete excision at the margins warrant conservative review rather than immediate hysterectomy (Lopes *et al.*, 1993).

Complications of laser cone biopsy

The immediate postoperative problems seen after laser cone biopsy are essentially the same as those found after other excisional or local destructive procedures have been performed on the cervix. While the procedure is being carried out, hemorrhage may occur due to incomplete division of the vessels, or it may be associated with secondary infection of the defect site. Treatment is usually conservative, although occasionally surgical management may be required and, more rarely, supportive blood transfusion may be necessary.

Discharge is a common accompaniment to the healing process, and often lasts for a few weeks. So long as significant infection does not occur, no special treatment is needed. Pain is rarely felt following the procedure, even in the immediate postoperative period.

Longer term problems may arise as a result of variability in healing of the cervix. Most patients will be left with a cervix that has an accessible squamocolumnar junction with a small area of columnar epithelium visible (Figs 7.43 & 7.44). However, it is not uncommon for the cervix to appear as shown in Fig. 7.45, where there is a large area of

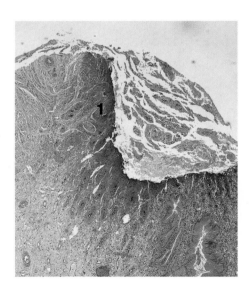

Fig. 7.42

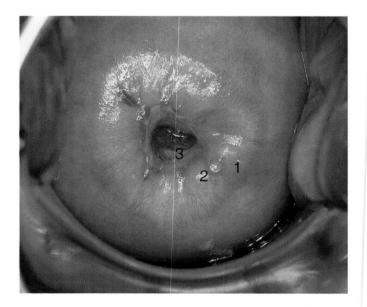

Fig. 7.43 A normal cervix after laser cone biopsy; this shows the result some 6 months after treatment. The edge of the treated area is at (1), the regenerating epithelium at (2), and the new squamocolumnar junction at (3).

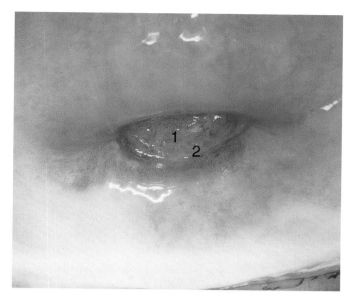

Fig. 7.44 A frequent finding after both laser conization and laser ablation is the appearance of a prominent "button" of columnar epithelium (1). This tends to appear after the removal of large volumes of tissue, leaving a wide defect. The edge of the regenerating area is at (2).

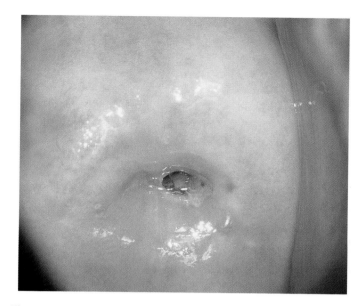

Fig. 7.46 A partially stenosed os after laser cone biopsy; the squamocolumnar junction is not accessible. The use of brush cytology or endocervical curettage is mandatory for proper follow-up assessment in such a case.

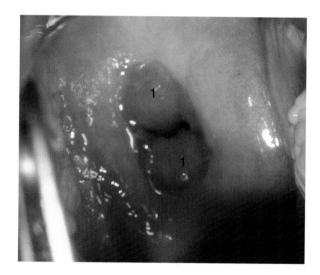

Fig. 7.45 An area of "ectopy" (columnar epithelium exposed on the ectocervix) developed 6 months after laser vaporization of a cervical intraepithelial neoplasia (CIN) lesion.

exposed columnar epithelium. Such situations may result in complaints of postcoital and intermenstrual bleeding or discharge. It may be necessary to stimulate metaplasia of this area by applying cryosurgery, cautery, or even laser vaporization to the columnar epithelium. For most patients, however, active treatment is not necessary. Nevertheless, it is possible for this exposed transformation zone to become infected yet again with the mutagenic agent that resulted in the development of the original CIN.

Rarely, the cervix may scar, producing a partial (Fig. 7.46) or complete stenosis of the os. This may be identified as an incidental finding at the time of cytologic review. Occasionally, the patient notices an alteration to the menstrual pattern with prolonged or reduced flow, and dysmenorrhea may develop. Mechanical dilatation of the cervix or cutting back the scar with a laser usually deals effectively with the problem.

Loop diathermy excision and cone biopsy

Wire diathermy loops have been used for many years to remove large and small lesions from the cervix. Cartier (1984) has used such small loops extensively to obtain biopsies from lesions on the cervix. Latterly, Prendiville et al. (1989) has shown that by using large diathermy loops a useful biopsy can be obtained with simultaneous and complete treatment being achieved. This has all the advantages of other minimally invasive conservative therapies and the added bonus that a large block of material can be obtained for pathologic assessment. The technique, when used in conjunction with the well-developed colposcopic assessment described above, has proved to be extremely popular for the majority of patients with abnormal cervical cytology.

Patient assessment and the development of treatment protocols

Patients are referred for colposcopy in the usual way, following the finding of a cytologic abnormality. Colposcopy is carried out in the usual manner, and any lesion is identified and its topography charted. Whereas with other conservative techniques the recommendation has been to make carefully representative biopsies and then bring the patient back to the clinic when a decision as to treatment has been made, with loop diathermy the possibility to combine the biopsy with treatment has led to the development of a "see and treat" policy for selected patients. It must be stressed that the patient must be effectively counseled and the procedure carefully explained. There is the risk of considerable psychological trauma if this is not done.

Loop diathermy excision was being developed in the UK at the same time as a radical reappraisal of the indications for treatment was taking place. Early experience with loop diathermy showed it to be a very effective method for removing the entire transformation zone; it had high patient acceptability and a small morbidity rate. In the initial enthusiasm for this technique, many patients had their lesions treated at the first visit only to find that the abnormality had been very minor or that no CIN existed in the removed tissue (Luesley *et al.*, 1990). Murdoch *et al.* (1991), also reported that 32.8% of patients had negative, metaplastic or inflammatory changes if loop diathermy was used to treat all cytologic abnormalities, increasing the pressure toward triaging patients into a higher risk high-grade cytologic abnormality group and a lower risk low-grade cytologic abnormality group. As pointed out above, considerable concern has been expressed about the mental anguish undergone by patients in whom there is the finding of an abnormal smear result; there is also an increase in anxiety associated with a visit to the colposcopy clinic (Brown *et al.*, 1988). Clearly, the development of a rapid "see and treat" policy was advantageous in reducing unnecessary and traumatic clinic visits, but this enthusiasm had to be tempered with a desire not to over-treat patients with minor abnormalities.

One of the consequences of the enhanced screening program that was successfully promoted in the UK, was that a considerable proportion of the smear tests reported showed minor abnormality, that is, mild dyskaryosis (Bethesda low-grade squamous intraepithelial lesions, LSIL) or less. Considerable attention has been paid to this problem, culminating in the general recommendation that the "see and treat" policy should be reserved for those patients with smears showing moderate or severe dyskaryosis (Bethesda high-grade squamous intraepithelial lesions, HSIL) or where there is a significant colposcopic lesion entering the endocervical canal; in these cases a loop diathermy cone biopsy (described below) should be carried out.

For patients with lesser cytologic or colposcopic abnormalities, the standard management of preliminary biopsy followed by a return visit to the clinic is to be recommended.

Patient consent

It is now generally felt that a simple form of consent should be utilized prior to the use of outpatient local anesthetic procedures. This is particularly important in the context of "see and treat." A simple document outlining the procedure which can be countersigned by the clinician is adequate.

Terminology

The original description by Prendiville *et al.* (1989) used the acronym LLETZ, which represented large loop excision transformation zone. In the USA, the acronym LEEP (loop electrical excision procedure) has been coined. The criteria for use are identical with those for LLETZ. In this text, we have differentiated between loop excision and loop cone biopsy, the former being used when the entire limits of the colposcopic abnormality an be seen, and the latter when the lesion enters the endocervical canal. This distinction has allowed comparison of loop excision with the equivalent conservative techniques of laser ablation, radical electro-diathermy, cryosurgery, and cold coagulation. Also, loop cone biopsy can be compared with cold knife and laser cone biopsy.

Equipment

The systems that are available consist of a combined cutting and coagulating facility (Fig. 7.47); this can be blended to be used with a single device, the loop (Figs 7.48 & 7.49). A wide variety of designs and sizes of loop are available. The device consists of an insulated barrel that can be inserted into a handpiece, very similar to that used in the standard operating-theater diathermy systems. The barrel terminates in a wire loop that is insulated to a variable extent, depending on the individual manufacturer and the clinician's desires. The stainless steel wire is made in either a thin flexible form or a thicker more rigid form. The rigid form is rather easier to use but does produce more thermal damage to the specimen produced. The fine flexible wire (Fig. 7.48) requires a delicate touch and an understanding of the three-dimensional nature of the block to be removed.

Following removal of the large loop specimen, a defect remains (Fig. 7.50); this must be carefully cauterized with the ball-headed cautery (Fig. 7.49), thereby sealing the entire defect.

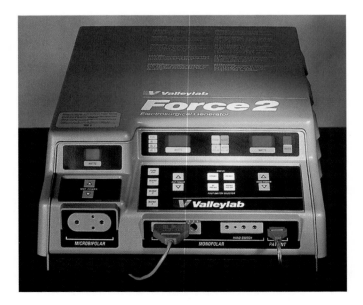

Fig. 7.47 A Valley Lab Force 2 electrodiathermy machine. These machines provide variable power for cutting and coagulation; the required power can be blended using a simple hand switch. The patient is "earthed" using an adhesive disposable jelly pad attached to the thigh. Use of the machine provides a high-quality cut resulting in minimal tissue damage through coagulation or thermal artifact. Hemostasis is easily and rapidly achieved. When the equipment is used in a modern colposcopy service it is important that there is no television interference.

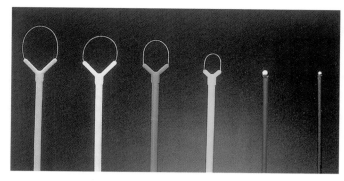

Fig. 7.48 Four fine wire loops of various dimensions with two diathermy ball devices (Utah Medical Products, Inc). (Courtesy of Professor W. Prendiville, Dublin.)

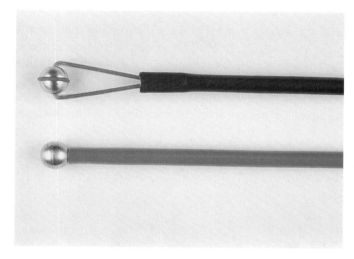

Fig. 7.49 Two diathermy devices, fixed ball (upper) and moveable-ball/roller-ball (lower) (Utah Medical Products, Inc). (Courtesy of Professor W. Prendiville, Dublin.)

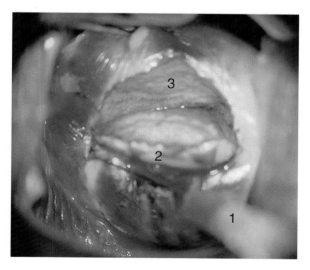

Fig. 7.50 The defect after large loop excision; the base may require careful cauterization to seal the surface. The lack of bleeding is entirely due to the injected vasopressor agent. The lack of thermal damage results from the use of the high-frequency electrosurgical unit. It is, however, essential to "seal" fully the surface using the ball electrode; otherwise, when the vasopressor agent wears off, profuse hemorrhage will occur. In this figure, the loop diathermy handle (1) with the loop attached has removed a small cone-shaped block of tissue (2) from the anterior lip of the cervix. The cone base is at (3).

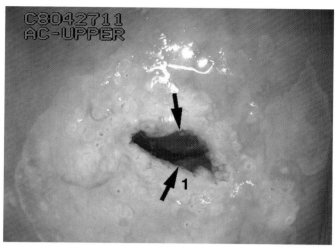

Fig. 7.51(a)

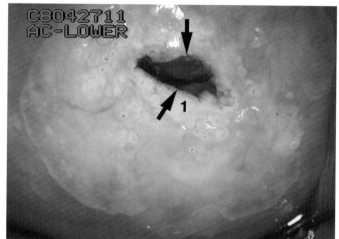

Fig. 7.51(b)

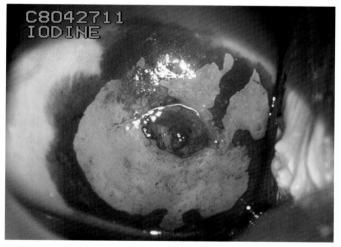

Fig. 7.51(c)

Fig. 7.51 (a) and (b) show a high grade lesion with well defined outer and inner limits (the new squamocolumnar junction is arrowed).

Technique

As with other conservative techniques, the patient is first told about the intended colposcopic assessment and possible treatment. With the patient in the lithotomy position, and a Cusco or Graves' speculum with a smoke-extraction facility in the vagina, the cervix is exposed and the patient colposcoped in the standard manner; the limits of the lesion are identified as shown in Fig. 7.51a–c, which depicts an area of abnormal (atypical) epithelium (high-grade) (1) whose outer and inner (new squamocolumnar junction) limits can be seen. The application of Lugol's iodine (Fig. 7.51c) has the added advantage of delineating the limits of the lesion more clearly, especially after the injection of local anesthetic which sometimes causes bleeding and can obscure the acetowhite margins. Where the circumstances meet the protocol described above for the safe employment of a "see and treat" policy, the patient (as in the case in Fig. 7.51) is informed of the treatment procedure to be followed.

An insulating diathermy pad is attached to the patient's thigh, the smoke-extraction facility is attached to the speculum, and a local anesthetic is injected into the cervix (Fig. 7.52). The preferred agent is Citanest 3% with octapressin (prilocaine hydrochloride 30 mg/ml, felypressin 0.03 iu/ml), a combination of a local anesthetic agent and a vasopressor. Using a fine dental syringe, the injection is delivered into the anterior and posterior lips of the cervix, taking care to inject peripherally to the lesion. If the cervix is broad or the lesion large, injection at the four cardinal points is recommended. The injection should be made gently and superficially, at first causing blanching of the cervix; thereafter, the needle may be injected slightly more deeply, but not in the manner used for a paracervical block.

An appropriately sized loop is chosen to encompass the entire lesion for removal in one block. In the author's (JM) experience, it is rarely necessary to use more than one "sweep" of the loop. In an early series (Murdoch et al., 1991), almost 70% of treatments were made with one sweep of the loop. That same series has recently been reviewed and in a 10-year period from 1989 to 1999, a total of 4944 loop cone biopsies were performed, of which 80% were made with a single sweep, 15% required two sweeps and only 5% required more than two sweeps of the loop. The loop is then laid over the transformation zone so as to encompass the lesion comfortably; if the fine wire loop is being used slight pressure is put on it so that it adopts a curved attitude to the cervix. The "cut" button on the handpiece is pressed and after a few seconds the wire begins to enter the cervix (Fig. 7.53). Some authors suggest pressing the "cut" button before touching the cervix. The wire is then followed, rather than pushed, through the cervix so that it exits beyond the lateral limit of the lesion (arrowed on Fig. 7.53). This movement can be made top-to-bottom or bottom-to-top, or even side-to-side, as the clinician prefers. Often the block sits on the cervix and can be lifted off with a small stick or a forceps (Fig. 7.54). Minimal bleeding should be experienced if the vasopressor agent has been injected correctly.

Once the loop cone has been removed, the defect is carefully diathermied using the ball electrode; special attention should be paid to the skin edges where bleeding frequently occurs (Fig. 7.55). The completed treatment leaves a shallow scoop defect in the cervix with a completely sealed surface (Fig. 7.56). For additional hemostasis, Monsel's solution (ferric subsulfate) may be applied to the base of the defect (Fig. 7.57). The speculum should then be closed slightly to release the pressure from the speculum blades on the anterior and posterior vaginal fornices while maintaining colposcopic vision (Fig. 7.58). This procedure often unmasks additional bleeding points which may then be further diathermied. Healing following loop diathermy excision or cone biopsy is similar to that following other conservative procedures; it leaves a cervix with an accessible squamo-

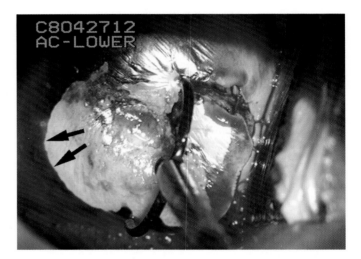

Fig. 7.53

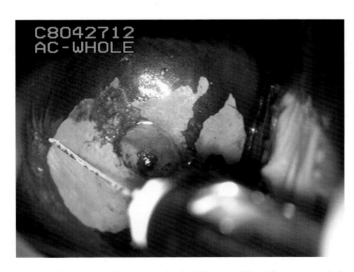

Fig. 7.52 Injection of local anesthetic (Citanest 3% with octapressin) using a dental syringe.

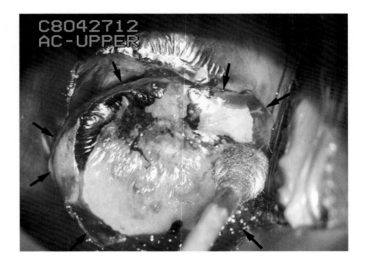

Fig. 7.54 The excised block of tissue in situ (arrowed) after a loop cone biopsy has been performed.

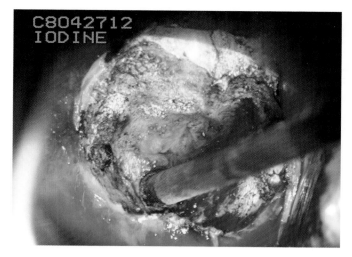

Fig. 7.55 Cauterization of the base using a diathermy ball electrode.

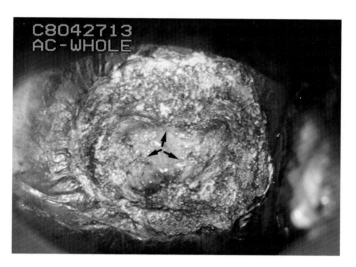

Fig. 7.56 This shows the completed treatment with the base of the treatment site having been sealed with ball diathermy. The endocervical tissue is arrowed.

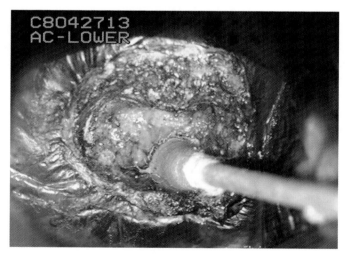

Fig. 7.57 Application of Monsel's solution (ferric subsulphate) to aid hemostasis.

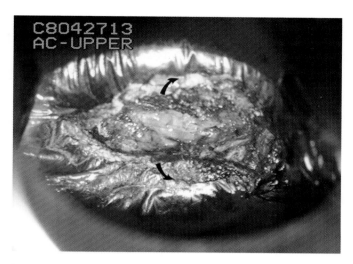

Fig. 7.58 View of the cervix after partial release of the speculum. This maneuver shows the "real" view of the cervix with the excised edges (arrowed) tending to approximate.

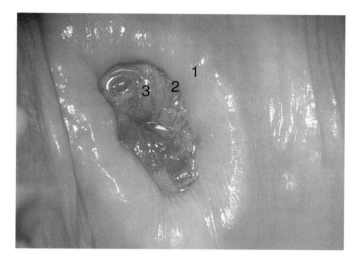

Fig. 7.59

columnar junction (2) surrounded by a narrow rim of scar (1) (Fig. 7.59). Figure 7.59 shows the cervix seen in Figs 7.53–7.58 some 3 months later, after healing. The large central area of columnar epithelium (3) is common following loop diathermy, as it is following laser surgery. Why there should be so much variability from patient to patient is not known. The large areas of ectopy commonly occur when a very wide lesion has been removed. The natural remodeling of the cervix does not appear to occur as frequently as it does following the removal of a smaller lesion.

Results

Histologic specimens

The high quality of the specimens produced by loop diathermy procedures, especially when fine wire loops are used, has impressed many pathologists. Figures 7.60–7.63 show how minimal is the thermal artifact on the cut edges of the specimens, and how easy it is to interpret the histologic changes on the ectocervical and endocervical ends of the specimen.

A study by Wright *et al.* (1992b) presented interesting

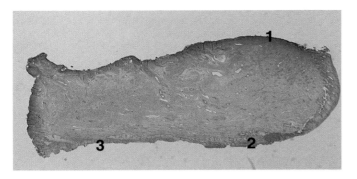

Fig. 7.60

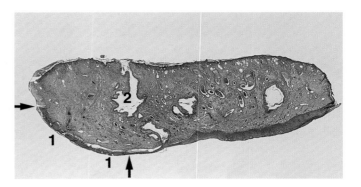

Fig. 7.62

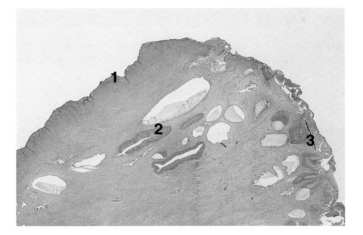

Fig. 7.61

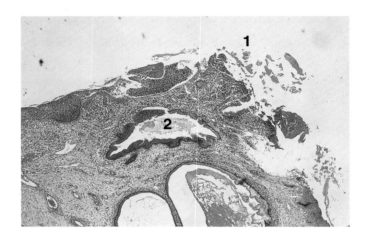

Fig. 7.63

information by comparing the histologic changes in the cervical epithelium and stroma following CO_2 laser conization with changes after excision biopsy using the loop electrosurgical excision procedure. Two zones of thermal injury were detected using either device (see Fig. 7.42 on p. 180), but there was no significant difference in the biocharacteristics or extent of thermal damage between the two methods. In 11 specimens from the CO_2 laser material the coagulated zone ranged from 130 to 750 μm in graded thickness with a mean thickness of 411 μm. When 40 specimens obtained using the loop were examined, the range of thickness of the coagulated zone was 150–830 μm with a mean difference of 396 μm. The difference in mean value of the thermal injury, measured in micrometers, between the laser and the loop was not significant. It was pointed out that extensive areas of carbonization and epithelial distortion of the margins of the excision were only occasionally present in specimens obtained by the electrosurgical excision but were almost invariably present in CO_2 laser specimens. However, in all cases, it was possible to evaluate, both histologically and cytologically, the epithelium in the stroma. Again, it must be pointed out that the extent of "damage" is directly related to the experience of the clinician.

In Fig. 7.60 a long loop cone biopsy is presented with minimal thermal damage (1); the excellent quality of the material over the lesion (2) with progression into the endocervical canal (3) can be seen. A high-power view of this in Fig. 7.61 shows the thermal damage (1), gland infilling (2), and the surface lesion at (3). In Fig. 7.62 another excellent specimen (stained with Van Gieson's stain) shows a CIN 3 lesion (1), whose ectocervical limits are seen between the arrows, with "clear" glands (2) and margins both ecto- and endocervical.

In Fig. 7.63 there has been incomplete excision at (1) and the excellent quality of the material facilitated the making of this important diagnosis. Indeed, Murdoch *et al*. (1992b) attempted to quantify and analyze the influence of a histologic report such as this (of incomplete excision of CIN after LLETZ) on the frequency of detection of residual CIN. They studied 721 woman who were diagnosed histologically on LLETZ specimens as having CIN and, in spite of the first-time treatment success rate, as assessed by cytology, of 95% at 3 months, only 56% of the women were reported to have had a complete histologic excision of CIN. A report suggesting incomplete excision was more likely with more severe CIN and extensive lesions, and where there was involvement of the endocervical canal. Furthermore, 21% with residual CIN had had an apparently complete excision of CIN by LLETZ.

It was concluded by the authors that a histologic report of incomplete excision of CIN by LLETZ does not equate with residual disease. The high treatment-success rate of LLETZ means that a report of incomplete excision should stimulate close colposcopic and cytologic follow-up to identify the small number of females with residual CIN after therapy.

Success rates

Many studies have already attested to the high success rate (95–96%) of this technique (Prendiville *et al*., 1989; Luesley *et al.*, 1990; Murdoch *et al.*, 1991). In a recent study by Bigrigg *et al.* (1994), 1000 women treated by LLETZ in 1990 were followed for at least 22 months. The rate of recurrence and residual lesions was 5.0% and 0.6% in the first and second years respectively. LLETZ was also effective when used as a repeat procedure; the negative histology rate was much higher (4.7% for initial procedures and 20% for repeat).

Probably one of the most interesting findings is the remarkable increase in diagnosis of early invasive cancer of the cervix following loop diathermy (Murdoch *et al.*, 1992a). Turner *et al.* (1992) described 33 consecutive patients with major-grade cytology who were subjected to loop diathermy conization. One case of unsuspected invasive cancer and two of microinvasion were diagnosed. Buxton *et al.* (1991) managed 243 women by colposcopy and directed punch biopsy and loop diathermy excision. There were three unsuspected cases of AIS and one early microinvasive carcinoma found.

Morbidity

The morbidity for this procedure is 2–4% (Murdoch *et al.*, 1991) with immediate discomfort and bleeding, or subsequent cervical stenosis leading to dysmenorrhea. However, in the study by Bigrigg *et al.* (1994), 250 out of the 1000 women who had a LLETZ procedure in 1990 answered a questionnaire concerning menstrual and fertility problems. No differences between them and a matched control group who had negative smears, was found. LLETZ would seem to have no effect on menstruation and fertility.

7.9 Management of extension of the abnormal (atypical) transformation zone

Uncommonly, the area of the atypical transformation zone is extensive, reaching to the periphery of the cervic and onto the vagina. It may extend well within the endocervix (Figs 7.64–7.66) giving rise to an unsatisfactory colposcopy. Previously, such an extensive lesion would have been treated by surgery, with removal of a large part of the cervix and vaginal fornices. A combination of wide peripheral laser vaporization and a deeper central vaporization or laser/loop diathermy excision allows the clinician nowadays to deal effectively with the entire area without removing large volumes of the cervix and causing serious surgical damage (Fig. 7.67a).

Technique

The procedure may be performed under local or general anesthetic. Biopsies will have been taken of the peripheral area of the transformation zone. In Fig. 7.66, for example, a colposcopically unsatisfactory central area (1) exists with an obvious minor- or "intermediate"-grade tissue present at (2) and (3). Biopsies taken at positions (2) and (3) showed CIN 3. The central area (1) was removed by excision biopsy and revealed very early microinvasive carcinoma; the peripheral areas that showed CIN 3 were subjected to laser vaporization.

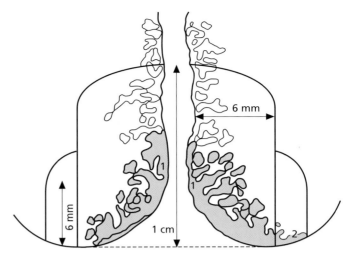

Vaporization and excision

Fig. 7.64 A diagrammatic representation of the wide extension of abnormal (atypical) epithelium onto the ectocervix; such a combination requires both vaporization and excision. This epithelium extends high into the endocervical canal (shaded) (1) and an excisional procedure will be needed for its complete removal. The abnormal (atypical) epithelium on the ectocervix (2) had already been biopsied and shown to be cervical intraepithelial neoplasia (CIN); this will require vaporization. The arrows point to the outer limits of the vaporization procedure.

When lesions extend onto the vaginal fornices (Figs 7.65 & 7.66), it is often prudent to perform the procedure under general anesthetic on a day-case basis, because the vaginal skin is extremely sensitive and it may not be easy to achieve complete analgesia using local anesthetic agents.

With the patient in the lithotomy position, a colposcopic examination maps out the lesion. It is useful to circumscribe the outer limits of the atypical transformation zone by laser. Cone biopsy is performed first using either laser or loop diathermy. Once the central area has been removed, the periphery can then be vaporized to a depth of 5 mm (Fig. 7.67). The fibers of the cervical stroma can be seen at the base of the treated area with minimal attendant bleeding. In Fig. 7.67a, the CIN lesion extended to the vaginal fornix (arrowed); this contrasts with the lesion seen in Fig. 7.66, where it extended to the vaginal mucosa (3).

In the cases pictured in Figs 7.65–7.67a, the peripheral area had already been sampled by punch biopsy, performed in the colposcopy clinic; this had revealed CIN 3. If there is any colposcopic or histologic suggestion of invasion, then undercutting, using the laser in the super pulse mode, of the abnormal (atypical) epithelium in the vaginal fornix or vagina will be necessary. This technique is described on p. 229.

The end results of the laser "top hat" procedures, involving excision of the endocervical extension of CIN, are also employed when using laser vaporization, loop diathermy excision, and loop diathermy cone biopsy. Fig. 7.67a is a good example.

7.10 Follow-up after treatment

Normal cytologic review 4–6 months after treatment is required. If the squamocolumnar junction is visible, as it

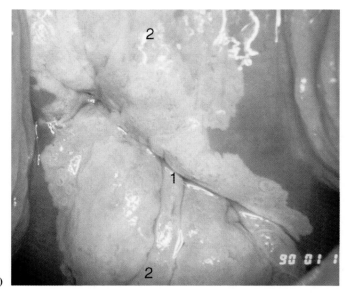

Fig. 7.65(a)

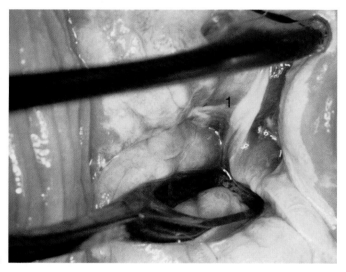

Fig. 7.65(b)

Fig. 7.65 (a) A large area of abnormal (atypical) epithelium (dense staining acetowhite) extends high into the endocervix (1) and onto the ectocervix (2) requiring excision, for the central area (1), and vaporization, of the peripheral area (2). (b) Shows the difficulty in finding the upper limit of the lesion.

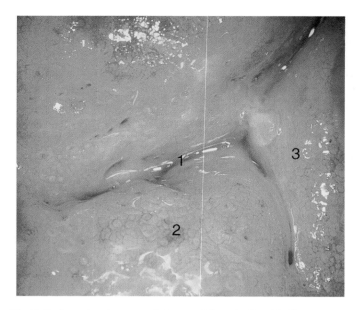

Fig. 7.66 An extensive area of abnormal (atypical) epithelium with extension high into the endocervix (1), onto the ectocervix at (2), and the vaginal fornix (3). Punch biopsies are performed at areas (2) and (3) to exclude the presence of invasion, after which these parts of the cervix were treated with vaporization. Because of the unsatisfactory nature of the central area (1) an excision procedure was performed.

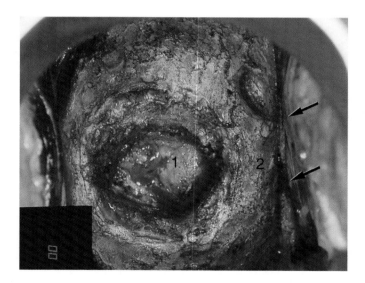

Fig. 7.67(a)

usually is, then a simple Ayre's or Aylesbury spatula smear is taken. If the squamocolumnar junction is within the endocervical canal, then a brush smear or endocervical curettage will give improved surveillance. However, Hughes *et al.* (1992) have suggested that the simple and well-tried Ayre's spatula can give just as good results as using the modern brush device. In a comparison study of 856 patients, 130 had histologically proven persistent CIN. Three consecutive cervical smears were taken using the Ayre's spatula, the Aylesbury spatula, and a brush device. Allocation of which spatula was to be used and the order of their usage at the first two post-treatment visits was randomized, and each patient was colposcoped immediately after the smear had been taken. There was no significant difference between the results obtained by use of the various devices, and Hughes *et al.* recommended that use of the Ayre's spatula is preferred for the follow-up of patients who have had local ablative or excisional treatment for CIN.

7.11 Hysterectomy in the treatment of CIN

Routine hysterectomy in the primary management of CIN is now rarely indicated. There are many thousands of cases reported in the literature, and the incidence of recurrence of clinical invasive cancer of the vaginal vault is surprisingly low. In most of these recurrences, there was a suspicion that there had been a failure at the initial examination to recognize the extension of the CIN onto the vagina, as shown in Figs 7.65 and 7.66.

The indications for hysterectomy have now been clearly defined and are as follows:

1 Preexisting benign gynecologic conditions, such as dysfunctional uterine bleeding, fibroids, endometriosis, uterovaginal prolapse, or the patient's request for sterilization. It should be remembered that histologic confirmation, in the form of a punch or cone biopsy, of a cervical lesion should be obtained prior to undertaking the procedure. If the whole transformation zone and abnormality are visible, punch biopsy may be used. However, if there is unsatisfactory colposcopy, with the lesion extending to within the cervical canal, and the possibility that an occult invasive carcinoma may be missed, then cone, biopsy must be performed. In these situations, the use of a frozen section has occasionally been advocated to exclude such occurrence (Hannigan et al., 1986).

2 Intraepithelial disease at the limits of the conization specimen, detected during histologic examination. This has been a standard indication in the past, but the authors can see only a limited place for its present-day employment. In young women with this condition it may not be necessary for hysterectomy to be carried out because, as mentioned previously, residual intraepithelial carcinoma in specimens after conization has been reported in 12–60% of cases, yet, paradoxically, these residual lesions do not seem to

progress to invasion except in a very few cases (Coppleson et al., 1992). Indeed, the number of cases of invasive carcinomas following treatment of carcinoma-in-situ (CIN 3) by performing hysterectomy is also incredibly low; Coppleson et al. (1992) reviewed a series of 22 studies and quoted a total of only 38 recurrent invasive carcinomas in 8910 patients who were subjected to a variety of hysterectomy procedures. However, it must be stressed that rigorous follow-up must be undertaken on any young women in whom residual CIN is suspected after local treatment (be it by local destruction or excision).

3 Persistent abnormal smears following conservative methods of management. This would seem to be an uncommon indication because any evidence of persistent disease, whether it be cytologically or colposcopically identified, would necessitate an excisional procedure (i.e. by cold knife, CO_2 laser, or loop diathermy).

4 Unusual technical reasons, such as a postmenopausal surprise positive smear in the presence of a small uterus, where a diagnostic cone biopsy may be difficult to perform and be less effective than vaginal hysterectomy.

5 A lesion may extend onto the vaginal vault and although a combined surgical and destructive technique may be used, as discussed in the previous section, in many cases hysterectomy may be an appropriate form of therapy. Use

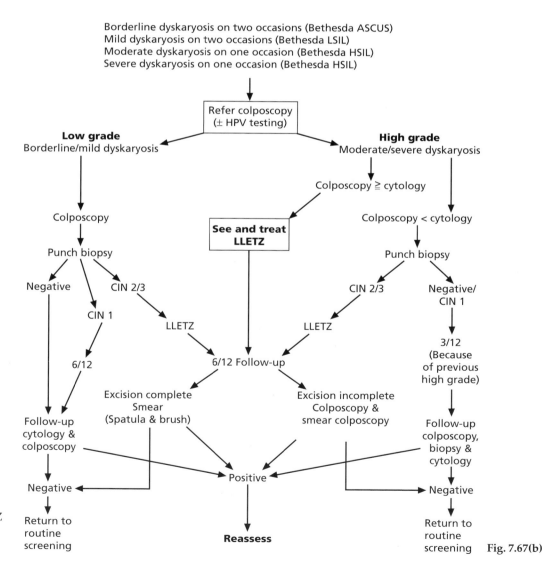

Fig. 7.67 (b) Algorithm for the management of patients with abnormal cervical cytology; LLETZ is used with a "see and treat" policy. From Murdoch et al. (1992b).

of the colposcope is essential to define the limits of the lesion and to establish the size of any vaginal cuff to be removed. An example of a lesion that could be treated by hysterectomy is shown in Fig. 7.66.

6 If the patient is fearful of more conservative methods, or where there are doubts about the follow-up for regular surveillance.

For the patient requiring hysterectomy, there is little doubt that the optimal therapy is to use either a vaginal hysterectomy or a minimal access technique, such as a laparoscopically assisted vaginal hysterectomy (LAVH). Such a technique allows accurate identification and delineation of the site of the cervical abnormal areas and reduces the risk of leaving a residue of precancer behind. This is of particular value for the patient who has a lesion which extends from the cervix onto the fornices of the vagina (2.4%) (Nwabinelli & Monaghan, 1991). The treatment of patients with persistant cytologic abnormalities using standard abdominal procedures is marred by a significant risk of leaving behind slivers of the cervix and vagina which harbor areas of CIN and may go on to develop invasive lesions at a later date. A significant advantage of the LAVH is the freedom given to the surgeon to remove the ovaries in those patients where it is appropriate to do so.

If hysterectomy is to be performed after conization, then it would seem that the procedure should be carried out immediately, or postponed for at least 6 weeks (Coppleson et al., 1992). In the follow-up of such patients, it is the authors' practice to visualize the vault with a colposcope at 4 and 12 months after hysterectomy, and then to undertake periodic vault cytology annually for 5 years and then every 2–3 years after that.

7.12 Summary: the optimal method of CIN treatment and of follow-up

On a number of occasions, reference has been made to the various success rates in the clearance of CIN using both local destructive methods and excisional techniques. There has lately been a dramatic increase in the use of the large loop diathermy for removal of CIN lesions (Wright et al., 1992a). The impetus in favor of this very simple device has meant that doubt has been cast on the efficacy of local destructive techniques, especially laser vaporization and cold coagulation. It is important to point out that although excisional techniques using the loop have indeed discovered early invasive lesions in excised specimens, it does not necessarily mean that the local destructive techniques are redundant (Benedet et al., 1992). It can be argued that many of the early microinvasive lesions now found by the use of excisional techniques would have been quite effectively destroyed by use of local destructive techniques. However, their presence is noted and has led to a number of authors suggesting that excision should be the primary technique used to deal with CIN (McIndoe et al., 1989; Buxton et al., 1991; Murdoch et al., 1991, 1992b). Another advantage of the loop excisional technique has been the introduction of a "see and treat" policy, where the patient is evaluated and treated in one visit. One of us (JM) has found it to be safe,

effective, efficient, and highly acceptable to both patients and colposcopists; it has been a major contributor to the efficiency with which colposcopy clinics are now run (Murdoch et al., 1992a). A protocol incorporating these various techniques is seen in Fig. 7.67b.

The criticism of the excisional techniques is that they impose an increased load on the pathologist because each specimen must be treated as though it were a formal conization. Another objection seems to be that large areas of the transformation zone can be easily removed with this simple device and, in inexperienced hands, excessive and unnecessary damage may be performed. The long-term study of Bigrigg et al. (1994) showed no increased effect on menstruation or fertility after LLETZ.

It would seem that the best results of therapy using either local destruction or excision depend on the correct selection of cases and on the expertise and experience of operators. It is only they who can make the decision as to which technique is suitable.

Follow-up of CIN management

Follow-up of the patient is traditionally by cytology and colposcopy and it would seem that recurrences occur primarily in the 1st and 2nd years, thus leading to the recommendation that the time of observation is primarily during these periods. It is recommended that the first two examinations occur at 4 to 6, and 12 months postoperatively; the first examination should involve both colposcopy and cytology. Colposcopy is important to assess the degree of constriction of the cervix, although a number of authors have suggested that cytology alone should be used and that this is effective in detecting any recurrence. In a colposcopic and cytologic follow-up of 1000 women treated with laser vaporization, Lopes et al. (1990) detected by colposcopy six out of 27 cases of residual disease, compared with an abnormal cytology in 26 of the 27 cases; 21 were detected as abnormal on the first visit after laser treatment. Recent work by Lavie et al. (personal communication) has questioned the need for routine colposcopic assessment in the review period following LLETZ. They found that colposcopy did not improve on cytology in detecting abnormalities in 711 patients. The only positive contribution was in patients with incompletely resected margins.

It is possible that the detection of high risk oncogenic HPV-DNA may be of use in the follow up of women over the age of 35 years, when a positive result most likely indicates the presence of persistance disease (ter-Harmsel et al., 1999).

7.13 Long-term complications of CIN treatment

Stenosis and constriction

Whenever surgical treatment is performed, the body heals the wound by repairing the tissue with collagen, and when this repair is excessive, then scarring occurs. On the cervix, the result of such scarring over a long period, that is, 6 to 12

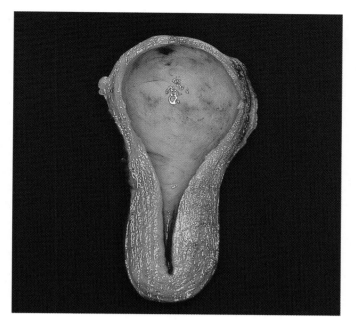

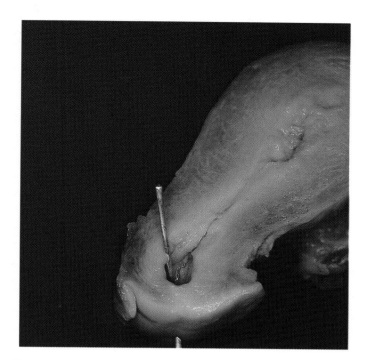

Fig. 7.69

Fig. 7.68 and 7.69 A hysterectomy specimen showing the presence of complete cervical stenosis following a cone biopsy 4 years earlier. In Fig. 7.68, a pyometra had developed in this postmenopausal woman. In Fig. 7.69, a probe has been forcibly passed through where the cervical canal previously existed.

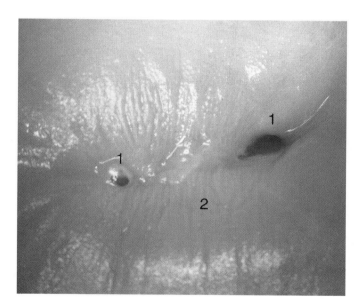

Fig. 7.70 Artificial twin ora (1) produced by the center of the cervix healing over following cryosurgical treatment. The typical radial ridging (2) seen after cryosurgery is present on the posterior lip of the cervix.

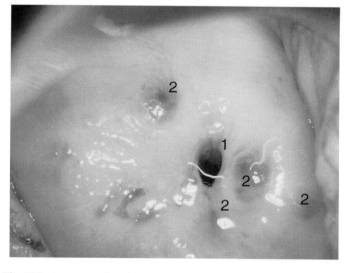

Fig. 7.71 A narrowed and scarred external os (1) surrounded by curious puncta that are the result of residual foci of glandular epithelium (2), following laser therapy. This is an example of cervical endometriosis.

months or more, is a narrowing of the cervical os; in its most extreme form this will completely seal the cervix (Figs 7.68 & 7.69). This problem tends to occur most frequently in postmenopausal and postpartum women, and may result in the development of a pyometra (Fig. 7.68). As a long-term complication in the younger woman, stenosis may lead to pelvic endometriosis following on a hematometra. This extreme enlargement may result in a diagnostic dilemma that can only be solved surgically, although with modern ultrasound techniques, the diagnosis can now be readily made without surgery.

Scarring and stenosis can occur following use of any of the described conservative techniques (Figs 7.70–7.74). Figure 7.70 shows artificial twin orifices that have developed after cryosurgery. Residual glandular epithelium can produce an unusual appearance, as shown in Fig. 7.71; dense white scarring is also seen in this case and this may confuse the clinician into believing that abnormal (atypical) epithelium exists.

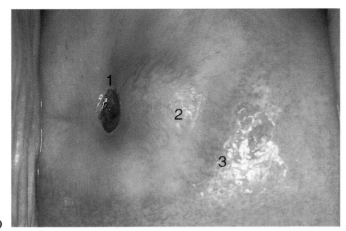

Fig. 7.72(a)

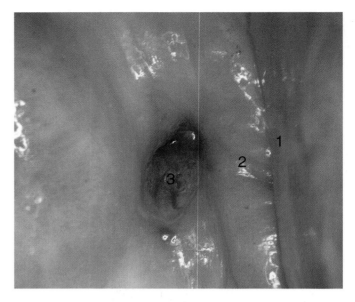

Fig. 7.74 The cervix shown in Fig. 7.73 is seen 6 months later. A large area of the left-hand side of the cervix is missing, with the cervix close to the left vaginal fornix (1). The residual ectocervix on the left is at (2). The cervical canal is at (3). Although excision of this large area (which was found to contain an early microinvasive lesion) lead to much deformity, the patient has had two normal vaginal deliveries since undergoing this procedure.

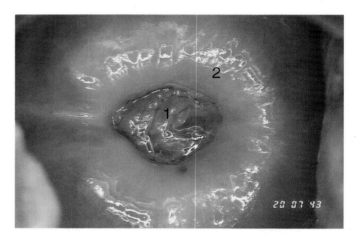

Fig. 7.72(b)

Fig. 7.72 (a) Severe constriction of the ectocervix existed until a cervical dilator, (b), was used to break down a small membrane covering the os (1). A large cone biopsy had previously been performed; the edge of the scarred treatment area is at (2), the remaining cervix at (3). (b) A cervical dilator (1), developed by Dr B. Mansell of London, and an endocervical brush (2); both should be used to dilate the cervical constriction.

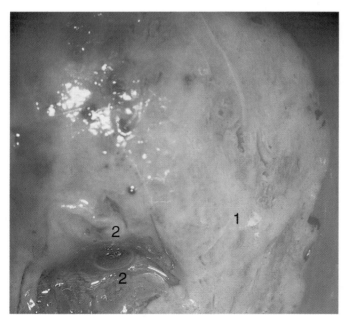

Fig. 7.75

Fig. 7.73 A large area of very abnormal (atypical) (Coppleson grade 3) epithelium exists on the ectocervix (1) and extends toward the left vaginal fornix; the upper limit can be clearly seen at (2). A large excisional procedure was employed, resulting in constriction and deformity of the cervix as shown in Fig. 7.74.

Large areas of the cervix on removal can lead to much subsequent deformity (Figs 7.73 & 7.74) with surprising preservation of function.

When stenosis has occurred (Figs 7.70–7.72a), the patient often presents with symptoms of painful and prolonged menstruation. Probably the most simple management method is to perform a dilatation of the cervix under general anesthesia. However, it may be possible to temporize by using a small dilator and injecting local anesthetic into the cervix; this technique was developed by Dr B. Mansell of London (Fig. 7.72b). Even use of a narrow endocervical brush may relieve the problem.

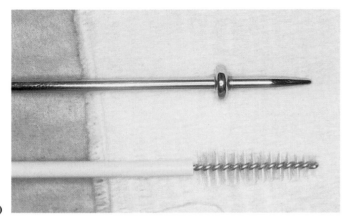

Surgical treatment and reconstruction following stenosis

Rarely, it may be necessary to reconstruct the cervix when it has been severely distorted by scarring or when symptoms are such that severe discomfort is regularly felt by the patient. Fig. 7.77 shows the operative appearance of a patient who required treatment for a high endocervical lesion. The results of this treatment were satisfactory with a deep central clearance for a microinvasive carcinoma. Unfortunately, some 6 months after treatment, the os had scarred to such an extent that the patient was experiencing severe discomfort during menstruation. The os was reduced to a mere pinhole (Fig. 7.78). A commonly used technique for management is cervical dilatation at regular intervals (Fig. 7.79).

In cases of complete stenosis (Fig. 7.80), the cervix can be infiltrated with local anesthetic and gently probed with a 21G needle (Fig. 7.81) in an attempt to aspirate retained menstrual blood thereby indicating the direction in which entry should be made into the site of the obstructed endocervix (Fig. 7.82). In Fig. 7.82, an incision has been made exposing the endocervical canal and a cervical dilator (Hegar 4) inserted into the endocervix. Countertraction is provided with a pair of tenaculum forceps.

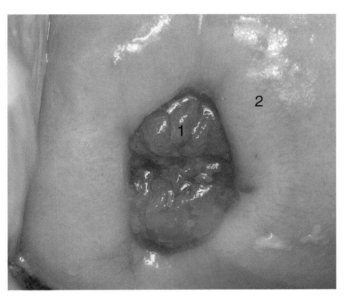

Fig. 7.76

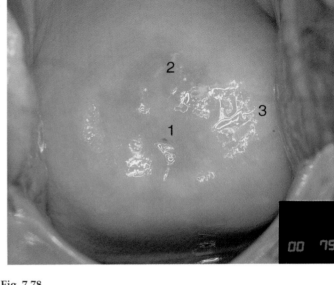

Fig. 7.78

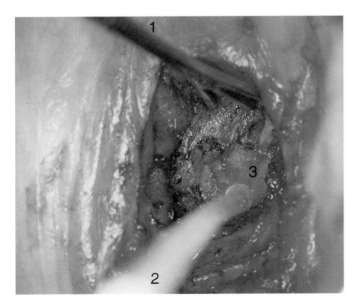

Fig. 7.77

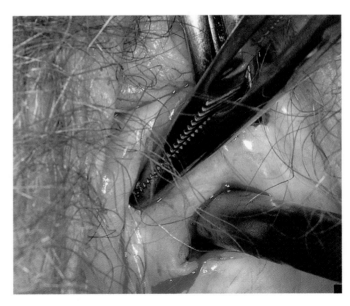

Fig. 7.79 The cervical canal is dilated.

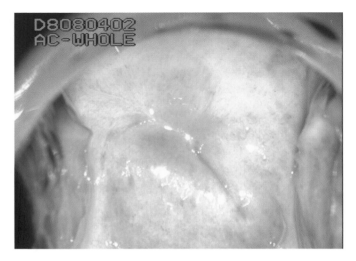

Fig. 7.80

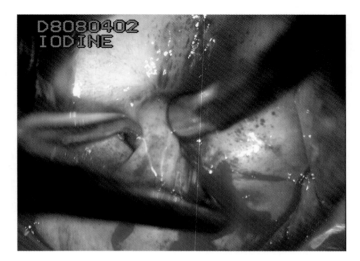

Fig. 7.82

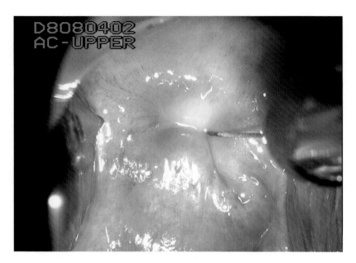

Fig. 7.81

Excessive eversion of the columnar epithelium (post-treatment)

During the early days of laser usage in the 1980s, a potent cause of recurrence was limited destruction of the CIN lesion. This resulted in recurrence of large areas of columnar epithelium on the ectocervix, which seemed to be prone to recurrent infection by the mutagenic agent that is responsible for CIN. This high rate of recurrence resulted in more radical destruction of the CIN and its surrounding tissue and this led to a dramatic improvement in results (Anderson, 1982; Townsend & Richart, 1983; Ali *et al.*, 1986). To avoid the development of such areas of columnar epithelium, it is suggested that the "top hat" configuration be adopted when removing the abnormal (atypical) epithelium within the transformation zone. An excellent example of this is seen in Fig. 7.67a. Comparison can be made with the cervices shown in Figs 7.75 and 7.76; both are within 6 months of treatment. Laser vaporization was used in the case seen in Fig. 7.75 and large loop diathermy was used in the case shown in Fig. 7.76. In both, the everted and exposed columnar epithelium is at (1) and the healed (treated) cervix at (2). It is suggested that women who

would seem to be at increased risk for the development of a new CIN lesion should be kept under close surveillance.

Subsequent pregnancy

There is always concern about subsequent fertility and pregnancy outcome following treatment for CIN. Bigrigg *et al.* (1991) found no effect on subsequent fertility or pregnancy outcome following loop diathermy treatment. However Blomfield *et al.* (1993), when examining pregnancy outcome following LLETZ (LEEP), found a higher incidence of low birthweight babies when compared with controls. More recently, other authors have shown that using the CO_2 laser, a cone biopsy greater than 10 mm in depth acts as an independent risk factor for the occurrence of preterm labor (Raio *et al.*, 1997).

Recurrence

Efficient follow-up surveillance

Although modern conservative therapies for the treatment of CIN are extremely successful, with clearance rates in the order of 95% or better, it is important to stress that the patient must take part in a regular surveillance program so that any residual or recurrent disease can be identified at an early stage and effectively dealt with. Six cases illustrating recurrent disease are presented in Figs 7.83–7.88.

The recommendations for surveillance protocols, some of which have been discussed above, are as follows:
1 Cytologic review should begin 4–6 months following treatment.
2 Colposcopy should be undertaken, at least at the first visit.
3 A smear should be taken with an appropriate sampling device.
4 Cytologic review should then be repeated 12 months post-treatment, and then at annual intervals for 5 years afterwards.
5 Thereafter, a return to triennial smear screening is sufficient.

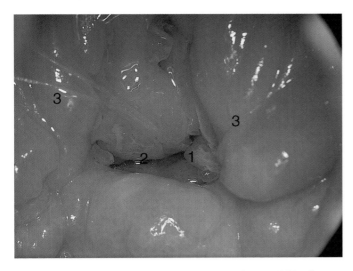

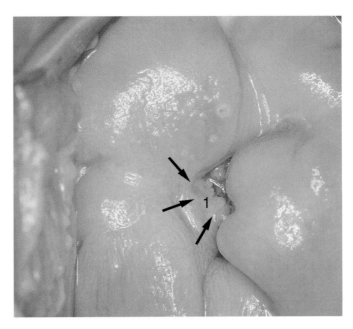

Fig. 7.83 An extremely scarred cervix, 5 years after a cold knife cone biopsy was used to treat cervical intraepithelial neoplasia (CIN) 3. An area of atypical epithelium within the endocervix is seen at (1) and there is a further small area within the lateral scar at (2). Two Sturmdorf sutures were used and the deformity caused by them can be seen at (3). An excisional procedure will be needed to diagnose and treat this lesion.

Fig. 7.84 Gross scarring of the endocervix following a cone biopsy some 4 years previously for cervical intraepithelial neoplasia (CIN) 3. Cytology, although negative for 3 years, suddenly became abnormal with the presence of a severe dyskaryotic smear. Abnormal (atypical) epithelium (1, and arrowed) can just be seen at the entrance to the endocervix. A further excisional procedure (laser cone biopsy) revealed the presence of CIN 3.

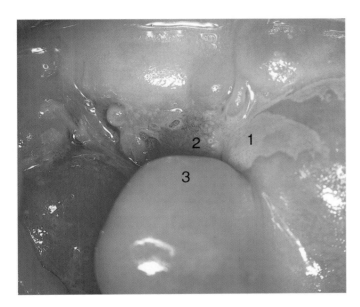

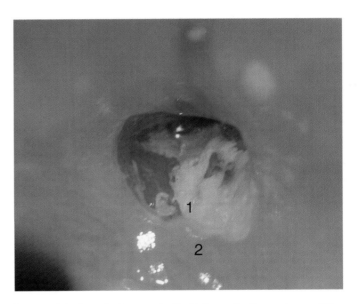

Fig. 7.85 An irregular scarred cervix following cone biopsy 4 years previously for cervical intraepithelial neoplasia (CIN) 3; a residual lesion (1) extends into the endocervical canal (2). Careful cytologic and colposcopic review with biopsy, and secondary excisional treatment is necessary. The distorted posterior cervical lip is present at (3).

Fig. 7.86 A lesion of colposcopically high-grade disease is seen (1) extending into the endocervical canal. The original cervical intraepithelial neoplasia (CIN) 3 lesion had been treated by laser vaporization some 3 years beforehand; the treated (healed) area is at (2).

In the UK, the National Health Cervical Screening Programme (NHSCSP) has reviewed the current state of evidence and have confirmed the review periods above (Duncan, 1997).

A continuing argument has centered around the need for colposcopy in the follow-up protocol. Murdoch *et al.* (1992b) have quantified the risks of recurrent cytologic abnormality after loop diathermy excision; the risk depended on where the residual disease was likely to occur, as judged by its position in the excision specimen. From this information, they were able to allocate follow-up by colposcopy and/or cytology. They recommended that patients with completely clear margins required only cytologic review, whereas those cases where the endocervical

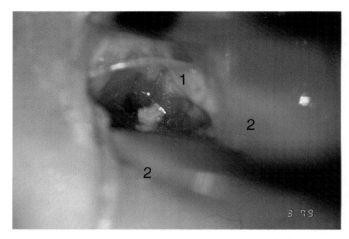

Fig. 7.87 A residual colposcopically major-grade lesion (1) is seen high within the endocervical canal; this occurred 2 years after laser vaporization. The treated (healed) cervix is at (2). A further excisional procedure will be needed for diagnosis and treatment.

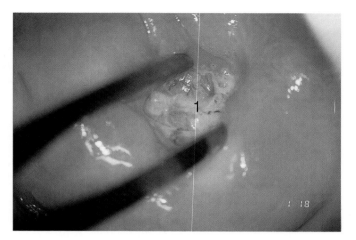

Fig. 7.88 A high-grade lesion (1) within the endocervix; the top of the lesion cannot be seen. It occurred 2 years after laser vaporization. Excision biopsy revealed the presence of cervical intraepithelial neoplasia (CIN) 3.

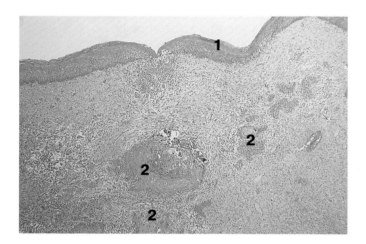

Fig. 7.89 A section through a loop diathermy cone, which was undertaken for a persistent cytologic abnormality 2 years after laser treatment. It shows an intact surface epithelium (1) overlying foci of microinvasive cancer (2), which must have developed after the laser treatment.

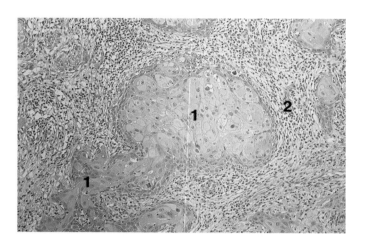

Fig. 7.90 High-power view of Fig. 7.89 showing the focus of microinvasive disease (1) and the intense stromal response at (2).

margin was not clear required brush cytology or endocervical curettage. Patients with incomplete ectocervical margins required colposcopy as well as standard cytology, and those without any clear margins required colposcopy and brush cytology with the addition of, endocervical curettage.

One of the most worrying risks following ablative conservative treatment is that of the development of an invasive cancer. Reports of such occurrences have been recorded following cryosurgery and laser treatment (Sevin *et al.*, 1979; Cullimore *et al.*, 1989; Pearson *et al.*, 1989; Soutter *et al.*, 1997). Figures 7.89 and 7.90 show the histologic findings following a loop diathermy excision. This procedure was performed because the patient had persistent cytologic abnormalities after receiving laser ablative therapy for CIN. The overlying epithelium is intact but in the deep tissues a small focus of microinvasive cancer is present (stage Ia1). The lesion was effectively removed by this procedure, so no further treatment was necessary.

Treatment of suspected recurrence

It is now accepted that when recurrence occurs, it should be treated by excision biopsy and not by repeat vaporization. Cullimore *et al.* (1989) found that within a group of females treated with laser vaporization, five cases of invasive carcinoma occurred within 12 months. During the short study period of 2 years, 1081 patients were treated with vaporization; in 40 cases (3.7%) a positive smear developed during the follow-up period. Eight patients had histologic evidence of CIN on colposcopic biopsy in the presence of a negative smear, three had colposcopic suspicion of invasive disease, and 29 had abnormal cytology on two occasions. The mean follow-up period was 13.5 months. Nearly three-quarters of the patients had a satisfactory colposcopy at follow-up. When cone biopsy was undertaken, two cases of unsuspected invasion and 29 of CIN were found. Nine cases were clear. The frequency of unsuspected invasive disease in patients treated by laser vaporization can be calculated from these figures to be 0.19%. In the study by Cullimore *et al.*, 19 of the 40 patients would not have been suitable to receive a second destructive treatment; this was due to the colposcopic findings in 16 cases and to the suspicion of invasive disease in three cases. Thus, excision becomes necessary. This study, like that by Benedet *et al.* (1985), points out the problems in colposcopic recognition of early invasive cancer. The signs of invasion can be subtle and easily missed, especially after prior treatment, when there may well be distortion of the cervix, or when early invasion exists within the endocervical canal.

7.13 Precancer in pregnancy

The occurrence of a cancer during pregnancy is relatively rare in developed countries, mainly because of the declining birth rate and the tendency to have families at an early age when cancer incidence is relatively low. Cancer of the cervix is the commonest pelvic cancer to occur during the reproductive years. However, the incidence remains low, being variably reported as occurring at a rate of one to 13 cases per 10 000 women. Figures from larger centers suggest an incidence of one case per 2000–2500 pregnancies, and an incidence of CIN 3 of one case per 750 pregnancies (Shepherd, 1990).

Management of invasive cervical cancer during pregnancy

In general, the cancer (Figs 7.91 & 7.92) should be managed as though the patient was not pregnant. Minor variations as to the timing of treatment may have to be made to give the possibility of producing a live child at the same time as effectively treating the cancer. In the first two trimesters, the general rule is that the cancer should be treated and the pregnancy sacrificed (Fig. 7.92). Difficulties arise when the pregnancy is some 22–26 weeks old, when there is a real possibility of survival if the fetus can be delivered alive (Singer, 1988; Nevin *et al.*, 1993). Fine judgments will be called for. The assistance of a highly skilled fetomaternal medical opinion is essential. Ultrasound will give a guide to fetal maturity and efforts should be made to improve fetal lung function before a decision to deliver is made. A delay of 1–2 weeks to improve fetal well-being will not make a significant difference to the prospects for maternal survival. Once the timing of delivery has been determined, a Cesarean Wertheim's radical hysterectomy is the treatment of choice. The ovaries can be preserved. A vaginal delivery should be avoided.

In later pregnancy, where concerns about potential fetal viability are less of a problem, the cancer should be treated in the most appropriate manner for the particular stage, once the fetus has been surgically delivered.

Management of the abnormal smear in pregnancy

For 10–15 pregnant women in every thousand, the news that their smear is abnormal will be a major concern. Fears for themselves, their unborn child, and other members of the family will be paramount. It is important that they are seen, counseled, and colposcoped as rapidly as possible.

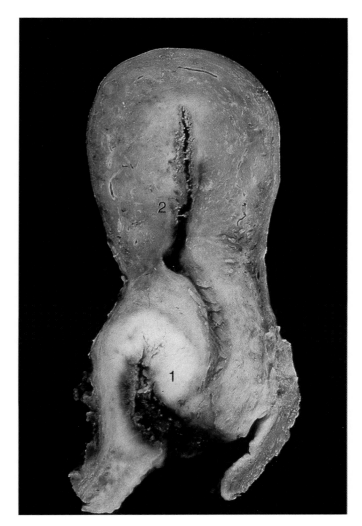

Fig. 7.91 A coronal section of a recently pregnant uterus; it shows a large stage Ib cancer of the anterior lip of the cervix (1). The decidua in the upper cavity can be seen at (2).

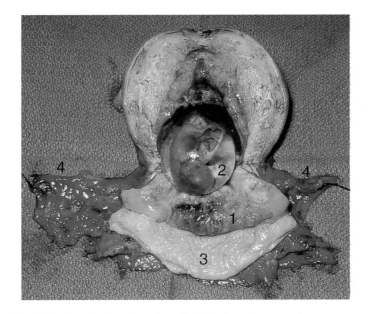

Fig. 7.92 A sagittal section of a radical hysterectomy specimen showing an exophytic stage Ib posterior lip cancer (1), with a small pregnancy sac (2). The large cuff of the vagina (3) and the paracolpos dissection (4) are also shown.

The main aim of this process is to be able to tell patients confidently that they do not have an invasive cancer and that management of the abnormal smear can be delayed until well after the delivery of the child.

Following the finding of an abnormal smear, colposcopy should be carried out at the earliest opportunity (Figs 7.93 & 7.94). In the first and second trimesters, there are usually no major technical difficulties in performing colposcopy, but later in pregnancy there may be some difficulties owing to the laxity of the vaginal wall; very late in pregnancy, when the fetal head has engaged, significant access problems may arise.

The most important factor for the clinician in performing colposcopy during pregnancy is to be gentle and sympathetic and to understand the many (often unspoken) concerns that the patient will have. An experienced colposcopist must view the cervix. Usually it is possible to eliminate the risk of an invasive cancer on colposcopic and cytologic grounds alone. These techniques will be described below. However, if there is the slightest suggestion of an invasive cancer, then an adequate biopsy (i.e. a wedge or cone biopsy) must be made. Sometimes it may be necessary to perform a simple punch biopsy.

The physiologic changes undergone by the cervix during pregnancy can sometimes aid in the detection of CIN lesions; the abnormal (atypical) epithelium appears white or has a mosaic or punctated appearance that, when viewed colposcopically, appears very prominent against the darkish blue background of the extremely vascular and engorged cervix. This can easily be seen in Fig. 7.93 where the abnormal (atypical) epithelium (1), present on the anterior lip, extends for a short distance into the endocervix (2). Eversion of the endocervical epithelium, which occurs from as early as the 10th week of pregnancy, allows the upper extent of the abnormal (atypical) epithelium to be more easily visualized, but occasionally this is not so; in Fig. 7.94, this epithelium (1) extends above the visual limits high into the endocervix (2).

However, in pregnancy, the progestogenic effect and subsequent decidualization of the cervix can result in problems with the interpretation of colposcopic findings (see Chapter 12, p. 313).

Colposcopic examination

Two important observations must be made during colposcopy: (i) the determination of the full extent of the abnormal (atypical) epithelium; and (ii) assessment of this epithelium as being consistent with precancer or early cancer. The full extent of the abnormal (atypical) epithelium within the transformation zone must be seen before a satisfactory colposcopic opinion can be given. This means that the upper extent of the lesion must be seen; if it cannot, then the presence of early invasion cannot be excluded. Whether the lesion is judged to be colposcopically inconsistent with a CIN stage will, to some extent, be determined by the experience of the examiner. Lesions that are not satisfactorily categorized must be submitted to biopsy.

Biopsy under colposcopic direction

If any doubt exists colposcopically regarding the presence of early invasive cancer, then a biopsy of the atypical epithelium must be taken for confirmation. This can be performed in one of three ways.

Punch biopsy

A punch biopsy, taken under colposcopic vision and without patient anesthesia, is used by many gynecologists to obtain histologic confirmation of CIN. Others dispense with this, so long as they are satisfied that they have excluded the possibility of early invasion. Again, the ability

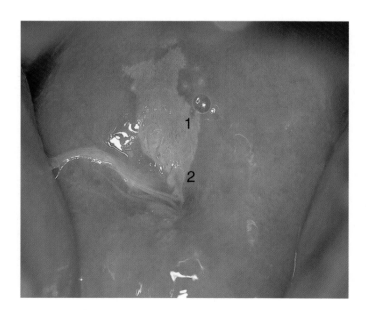

Fig. 7.93

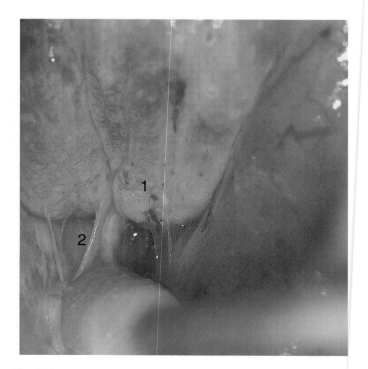

Fig. 7.94

to do this will depend on the observer. Although after punch biopsy the biopsy site seems exceedingly vascular, hemostasis can be obtained by simple pressure with a tampon after the application of silver nitrate or Monsel's ferric subsulfate solution for at least 3 minutes. These procedures are shown in Figs 7.95–7.97. In Fig. 7.95, two areas of abnormal (atypical) epithelium exist on the anterior (1) and posterior (2) cervix, and a small punch biopsy is being taken with Patterson's colon forceps (3). In Fig. 7.96, the two areas (1) and (1) that have been sampled have been treated with a 3-minute application of silver nitrate; this has left a characteristic darkened crater. In Fig. 7.97, a tampon is being placed directly onto the area to apply further pressure. Immediately after the biopsy has been taken, pressure can be applied with a simple swab stick placed directly in the crater, and this should be left there for at least 3 minutes.

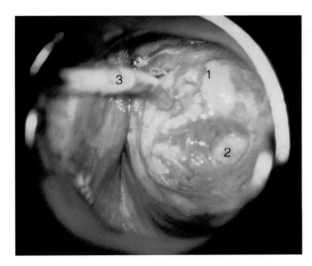

Fig. 7.95

Wedge biopsy

This biopsy is performed under colposcopic control and with the patient under anesthesia; it is usually taken in the form of a wedge. It not only accurately removes the suspicious tissue but also gives the pathologist an adequate amount of material with which to make a satisfactory diagnosis. The procedure can be seen in Figs 7.98–7.102 (see pp. 200–201).

Cone biopsy

The traditional method of obtaining a cervical biopsy when colposcopy is not available should be undertaken with care. There is a higher incidence of bleeding complications, both primary and secondary; perinatal mortality has also been attributed directly to conization during pregnancy (Mikuta *et al.*, 1968; Chao *et al.*, 1969; Boutselis, 1972; van Nagell, 1972; Jones *et al.*, 1979). Postpartum hysterectomies also show the high incidence of residual tumor that may exist in up to 50% of cases (Mikuta *et al.*, 1968), and a twofold increase in the residual tumor remaining after cone biopsy when intervention in the first and third trimesters is compared (Boutselis, 1972). Wedge biopsy would seem to offer a more accurate and relatively atraumatic alternative to cone biopsy, although with the advent of the CO_2 laser a more accurate, and also relatively atraumatic, modality is available if cone biopsy is deemed necessary.

Treatment

Without colposcopy, resorting to a "blind" cone biopsy becomes necessary with its attendant morbidity. If colposcopy suggests the presence of only precancer, then either a punch biopsy can be performed, as detailed above, or the patient can be observed conservatively. The expertise of the colposcopist is important. If biopsy has revealed the

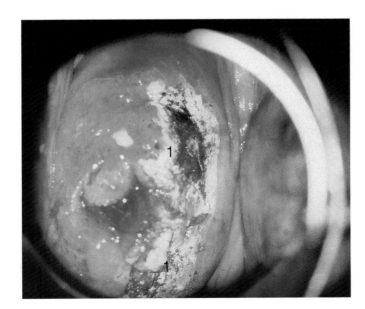

Fig. 7.96

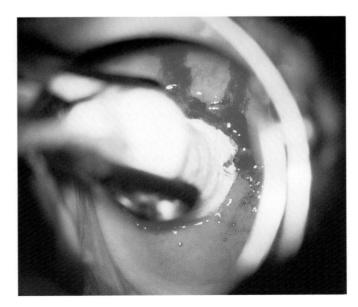

Fig. 7.97

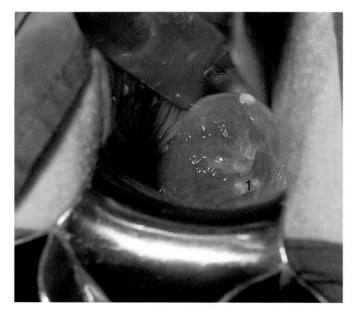

Fig. 7.98

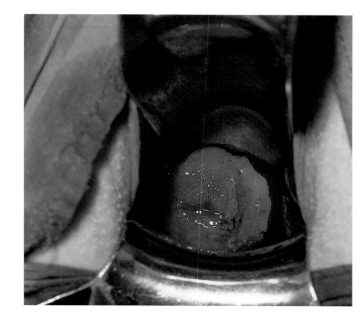

Fig. 7.99

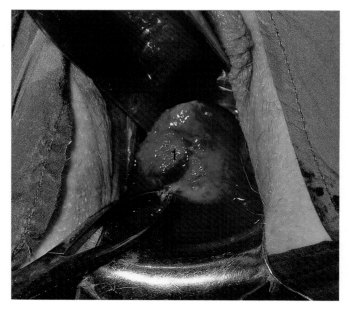

Fig. 7.100

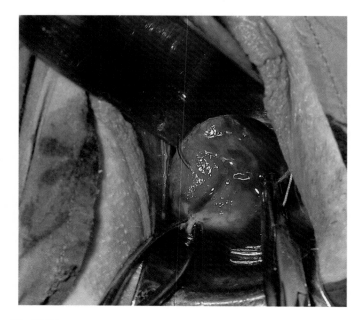

Fig. 7.101

Fig. 7.98–7.102 These figures show the removal of an atypical epithelium that was present in the cervix of a 32-year-old female, para 2, who presented with a severe dyskaryotic smear in early pregnancy. In Fig. 7.98, the colposcopy (undertaken using saline instead of acetic acid) shows abnormal (atypical) epithelium extending over the ectocervix and onto the posterior region of the endocervix (1). This latter area was regarded as suspicious of invasive cancer and warranted a wedge biopsy. In Fig. 7.99, Schiller's iodine solution has been applied and the atypical epithelium is seen at (1) with normal epithelium at (2). In Fig. 7.100, two elliptic incisions have been made to encompass the whole of the atypical area; the incision has been carried down 2 mm into the stroma to ensure adequate removal of the lesion. In Fig. 7.101, an interrupted suture using 3.0 material is used. If bleeding is excessive, then a hemostatic "figure-of-eight" suture can be inserted; Fig. 7.102 shows the suture being tied. In this instance, one other suture was needed for complete suture and hemostasis.

presence of CIN 3 or less and invasion has been excluded, then the patient can be allowed to deliver vaginally and can be reviewed at the 10th week postpartum.

If there is any colposcopic or cytologic suggestion of invasion, then cone biopsy or wedge biopsy must be performed with the patient under anesthesia. Histologic confirmation of CIN 3 or less would dictate a conservative form of management, but any suggestion of early invasion on the specimen presents the obstetrician with a difficult decision to make. If the invasive lesion penetrates less than 3 mm into the stroma and is less than 7 mm in linear length along the surface, has the most minimal involvement to the endothelial lined spaces, and if the margins of the cone are clear, then a conservative management program can be

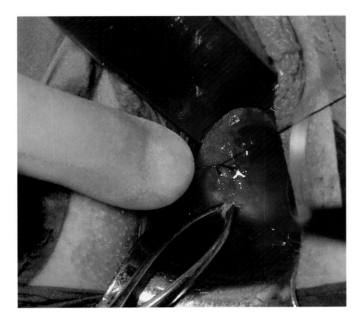

Fig. 7.102

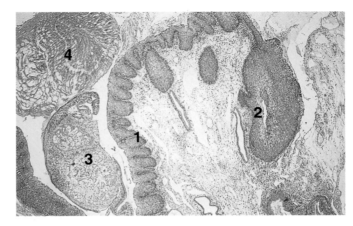

Fig. 7.103 (a) A wedge biopsy specimen taken during pregnancy. Cervical intraepithelial neoplasia (CIN) 3 is seen at (1) with extension into a glandular crypt at (2). The latter appearance is easily confused with that of early invasive disease, especially when a segment of CIN 3 has been isolated because of the plane of section of the specimen. This is what has happened in (3), but it is purely an extension of CIN 3 into the glandular crypt. However, no breach of the basement membrane, which would suggest early cancer, has occurred in any of this section. Microglandular hyperplasia is present at (4).

adopted. The patient would then be allowed to deliver vaginally and would be followed closely during the postpartum period with cytologic and colposcopic examinations. If, however, the lesion is more than 3 mm but less than 5 mm deep, above 7 mm in linear length, and infiltrates the endothelial lined spaces, then this lesion must be regarded as early invasion. Radical removal of the uterus and pregnancy needs to be undertaken. However, with the availability of expert neonatal resuscitation, Cesarean section can be performed followed by radical uterine extirpation. Fetal maturity assessment must be made by ultrasound. It is essential that each case must be considered individually and the expertise of pathologists, fetal medicine experts, radiologists and pediatricians is important in this respect. Sometimes it is necessary to sacrifice the fetus (Fig. 7.92).

A recent study (El-Bastawissi *et al.*, 1999) assessed the effect of carcinoma-in-situ for subsequent pregnancy outcome. A retrospective cohort study reviewed 1851 women diagnosed with CIS over an 8-year period between 1984 and 1992 and followed their subsequent delivery history, comparing them with a random sample of over 9000 women without CIS who gave birth during the same time. It was found that women with CIS who had had a cone biopsy had an increased risk of prematurity and a low birth weight infant compared with those women who had not had any treatment for CIS. Although there was an increased risk of Cesarean section within their cohort group, the authors were unable to determine whether the increased risk of operative delivery was caused by obstetrical complications or by the physicians' or women's choice. However, obstetrical complications could be a result of cervical dystocia secondary to endocervical tissue scarring.

Interpretation of a biopsy specimen during pregnancy

Typical epithelial changes during pregnancy include the condition of microglandular endocervical hyperplasia (MEH) (Singer, 1988). This is a combination of cellular changes in the endocervix and results from the progestogenic influence on the epithelium; it is seen predominantly in pregnancy but also occurs in females taking the oral contraceptive pill. It is produced by secondary gland formation with budding of the endocervical crypts. Between the glandular epithelial elements there may be cells that have the appearance of reserve cells that sometimes may be associated with the production of immature squamous metaplasia. Such an example is shown in Fig. 7.103a of a wedge biopsy taken during pregnancy.

7.15 Precancer in the HIV-positive patient

Infections with human immunodeficiency virus (HIV) have reached epidemic proportions around the world with an estimated 18 million HIV-infected adults by the turn of the century. Up to 40% of them will be women but in certain groups such as drug addicts, the percentage will be higher. Disturbingly, many adolescent girls will be amongst the sufferers.

It has now been recognized that invasive cervical cancer is an AIDS-defining condition in association with such conditions as opportunistic infections, central nervous system pathologies and tumors such as Kaposi's sarcoma, primitive CNS non-Hodgkin's lymphoma, and B-cell lymphomas with unfavorable histology.

There would seem to be three major areas in which HIV affects the cervix.
1 HIV-infected women have a high prevalence of abnormal Papanicolaou smears, cervical condyloma and CIN. The prevalence increases as the severity of the immunodeficiency increases (Branca *et al.*, 1995; Boccalon *et al.*, 1996; Bongain *et al.*, 1996; Fruchter, *et al.*, 1996; Olaitan *et al.*, 1997; Robinson *et al.*, 1997; Schulz *et al.*, 1996).
2 HIV-infected women have an unusually high prevalence

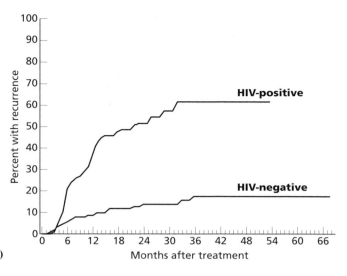

Fig. 7.103(b)

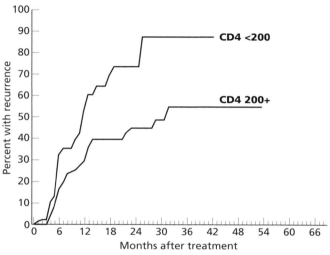

Fig. 7.103(c)

Fig. 7.103 (*Continued*) (b) Percentage of CIN recurrance in HIV positive/negative women while (c) shows CD4 counts in relation to recurrence.

of condyloma and intraepithelial neoplasia, involving not only the cervix but also the rest of the lower genital tract, namely, the vagina, vulva, perineum and anus (Korn *et al.*, 1996; Petry *et al.*, 1996).

3 HIV-infected women with CIN have unusually high rates of persistent and recurrent disease after treatment and high rates of progression if untreated (Fruchter *et al.*, 1996).

CIN/SIL (squamous intraepithelial lesions) in HIV-infected women

Numerous studies have clearly documented an association between HIV-infection and CIN/SIL. Many cytologic studies have reported abnormal PAP smears in a prevalence ranging between 52% to 63% amongst HIV-seropositive women (Wright, 1996). The prevalence of cytologic abnormalities in the HIV-seropositive group is up to 12.5 times that observed among the control HIV-seronegative women in these studies. Recently Wright *et al.* (1994) have used a combination of colposcopy and cytology to screen cohorts of HIV-infected and HIV-unaffected women for

cervical disease. They found that there were 13% of 389 HIV-seropositive women presenting with low-grade CIN compared with only 4% of 307 seronegative women. This was a highly significant difference, but more importantly high-grade CIN (CIN 2 to 3) was detected in 7% of HIV-seropositive women compared with 1% of HIV-seronegative women. Other authors have confirmed these findings (Fruchter *et al.*, 1996; Spinillo *et al.*, 1996). The predicted increase in invasive cancer amongst these women with cervical cancer precursors has not yet occurred in this HIV-infected population. There are reports that HIV-infective women have a more aggressive type of cervical cancer and also that the presence of HIV complicates progression to invasive cervical cancer in HIV-infected women (Klevens *et al.*, 1996).

Risk factors for the development of CIN in HIV-infected women

Wright *et al.* (1996), in his New York study mentioned above, found that biopsy-confirmed CIN in their women was significantly associated with HIV-seropositivity, CD4+ T-lymphocyte counts of less than 200 cells/μL, a history of treatment for CIN, a history of genital warts, detection of HPV-DNA, and an age greater than 34. They showed that in a multivariate analysis, four variables were found to be associated with CIN, and they were the cervicovaginal HPV infection, HIV-seropositivity, CD4+ T-lymphocyte counts of less than 200 cells/μL, and age >34. These findings suggest that HIV infection and HIV-associated immunosuppression are significant risk factors for the development of CIN.

HPV–HIV coinfection

Several studies have shown an increasing incidence of cytologic and/or histologic HPV-related lesions in the lower genital tract of HIV-infected women compared with HIV-negative women. This is not surprising in view of the analogous epidemiologic features of both diseases. However, it is unclear if the high incidence of HPV-related genital lesions in HIV-positive women is a consequence of the HPV infection. In HIV-infected women, the prevalence of HPV infection varies according to the presence of symptomatic HIV infection and a number of studies using various techniques to diagnose HPV infection have demonstrated that its prevalence was similar in HIV-negative women and in those with asymptomatic HIV infection (20 vs. 27%) while the prevalence in women with symptomatic HIV infection was 79%. Sun *et al.* (1995) detected HPV-DNA in 60% of the HIV-seropositive women enrolled in the New York study compared with 36% of the HIV-seronegative women. He suggested that latent HPV infections as well as clinically expressed HPV infections are significantly increased in HIV-seropositive women when compared with HIV-seronegative women.

It has been suggested that the molecular basis for the interaction between HIV and HPV resides in the HIV gene (*tat*) and the ability of this protein to induce the expression of E6 and E7 early transforming HPV genes through the LCR-regulating region stimulation. This finding would tend to suggest that this *tat* protein has an additive action in HPV-induced neoplastic progression (Vernon *et al.*, 1993; Boccalon *et al.*, 1996).

Screening for cervical disease in HIV-affected women

Because of the high prevalence of cervical cancer precursors and the proposed increased future risk of developing invasive cancer in HIV-infected women, it is obvious that they need to be screened for the presence of cervical disease (Wright, 1996). However, there is much controversy about how best to screen them, especially as some studies have reported a very high false-positive cytologic rate (Fink *et al.*, 1994; Robinson *et al.*, 1997). On the basis of this, it has been suggested that all HIV-infected women should undergo routine colposcopy. Olaitan *et al.* (1997) indicated that they had an increased prevalence of CIN by undertaking such screening (i.e. cytology and colposcopy) while Wright *et al.* (1995) does not believe that this form of screening is warranted. He states that colposcopic screening may actually result in the overdiagnosis and subsequent overtreatment of this population. The current recommendations from the Centers for Disease Control and Prevention (Atlanta, USA) are that HIV-infected women should be monitored for cervical disease using frequent PAP smears rather than colposcopy. Wright *et al.* (1996) have also shown that mild cytologic atypia are increased in HIV-infected women and they recommend that all HIV-infected women with mild cytologic atypia should be referred for colposcopy. They found a high prevalence of CIN amongst HIV-infected women with ASCUS PAP smears; with CIN detected by colposcopically directed biopsy in 38% of the HIV-infected women with mild cytologic atypia compared with 14% of HIV-uninfected women.

Treatment of CIN in HIV-infected women

It would seem as though colposcopically directed punch biopsies in HIV-positive women are poor predictors of the true nature of the CIN lesion (Del-Priore *et al.*, 1996). This is because of the associated intense inflammatory reaction within the cervical epithelium. Cone biopsy would certainly be a more accurate indicator of existing disease but only when indicated by appropriate cytology. Not surprisingly, there would also seem to be an increased risk of complications after standard treatment, be it laser vaporization or cone biopsy. In the study by Cuthill *et al.* (1995) there was an increase in excessive bleeding after therapy, as was there in the rate of cervicovaginal infections in the HIV-positive women.

The recurrence of CIN in women with HIV infections after treatment is, not surprisingly, increased. Fruchter *et al.* (1996) showed that amongst 127 HIV-infected CIN patients, 62% developed recurrent CIN by 36 months after treatment compared with 18% of the 193 HIV-negative CIN 1 patients. Recurrence rates reached 87% in 41 HIV-infected women

with CD4 counts <200 cells/mm³. Progression to higher grade neoplasia including one cervical cancer occurred by 36 months in 25% of HIV-infected women, but only 2% of HIV-negative women. After adjusting for age, CIN severity and treatment type, predictors of recurrence included HIV infection (rate ratio 4.4) (Fig. 7.103b,c) and in HIV-positive women, low CD4+ count (rate ratio 2.2). They also showed that in patients treated by excision, predictors of recurrence included HIV infection and residual CIN after treatment. With a second treatment, a second CIN recurrence developed in 14 of 33 HIV-infected and then in only one of 17 HIV-negative women. The presence of chronic condylomas was found in the long-term follow-up of 45% of treated HIV–CIN patients compared with only 5% of HIV-negative women.

Summary

It appears that there is a high prevalence of CIN in HIV infected women and that much of the CIN is high grade. Also there are high association rates between HPV and HIV in these women, suggesting that these women have the potential for the development of cervical cancer and should be monitored very quickly. The rapid progression rate from low-grade to high-grade CIN lesions must also be observed closely (Fink *et al.*, 1994; Olaitan *et al.*, 1997).

7.16 Management of early invasive squamous carcinoma of the cervix (FIGO stage I)

Early invasive squamous carcinoma of the cervix has been called by various names, including microinvasive carcinoma, occult carcinoma, preclinical carcinoma, and questionable or early stromal invasive carcinoma. With all these terms have come variations in the morphologic features, the most important of which is the depth of penetration of the early cancer into the underlying stroma. With so many variables it is not surprising that confusion has arisen in trying to obtain objective parameters by which to manage these lesions.

History of "microinvasion"

In 1985, FIGO (International Federation of Gynecology and Obstetrics) issued guidelines for the subdivision of early invasive squamous carcinoma, previously classified as stage Ia, into two types. These were stage Ia1, which was called early stromal invasion, and stage Ia2, called microinvasion. This meant the abandonment of terms such as occult cancer, which was merged with clinical stage I disease, and there was a reintroduction of the term preclinical invasive (colposcopically) overt/suspect cancer; some of these were indeed stage Ia or Ib. Further modifications of this subdivision were made in October 1988 (FIGO, 1988) when exact measurements were set for the stage Ia1 and Ia2 lesion (see Table 1.1b, p. 9). These dimensions included the depth of invasion and horizontal spread. In 1994, at the 14th Annual Meeting of FIGO, the definition of stage I cervical cancer was revised. This classification is shown in Table 7.1 (FIGO, 1995).

Part of the problem in the management of early invasive disease has been that many decisions on therapy are histologically based. This would be a satisfactory situation but for the fact that there is still inadequate evidence to indicate at what point (defined histologically) the lesion alters its biologic potential and enters the metastatic phase (Coppleson, 1992). This point may be able to be defined by examination of various morphologic parameters. However, the basic definition of early invasion can be difficult to make. Sedlis *et al.* (1979) for example, showed that 50% of cases of microinvasive cancer submitted to the Gynecologic Oncology Study Group in the USA did not conform to the original diagnosis of microinvasion and, indeed, 99 out of 132 cases showed no evidence of invasion whatsoever. Similar findings were evident in the study by the Royal College of Obstetricians and Gynaecologists in the UK (Morgan *et al.*, 1993).

It would therefore seem prudent to examine the various histologic parameters on which therapy decisions are presently made to see whether a consensus can be arrived at to enable a more scientific approach to be made concerning therapy management. These histologic parameters will now be considered individually.

Histologic parameters important for therapy decision-making

Depth of invasion

The literature abounds with publications attesting to the supposed depth of invasion that should be classified as microinvasion. These values vary from 1 to 9 mm and as Coppleson (1992) commented, "aside from the arbitrariness of setting such a parameter, abiding to it introduces new problems of subjectivity and thus imprecision." The problem of definition is further confused by two issues; namely, the plane of section of the specimen, and the finding of deeply involved clefts that do not appear to have any obvious connection with the surface in oblique sections. The intense inflammatory reaction that usually accompanies any membrane penetration further confuses the histologic picture, as does increasing squamous differentiation of the penetrating cells at the invasion site. Trying to determine the frequency of lymph node metastasis with such variable pathology has been difficult.

In many reports, the frequency of lymph node involvement varied from 0% to 7% in histologically defined microinvasion. Benson and Norris (1977), in a classic review of 41 cases covering 20 years, found only one in 98 cases and pointed out that the prevalence of nodal involvement could be increased by factors such as sampling error, especially when the biopsy was small, and by selecting the most advanced lesions for operative lymphadenectomy. A review of the literature shows that where there is penetration of 3 mm or less, lymph node metastases are very uncommon; indeed, Holzer (1982) quotes one in 338 cases; van Nagell *et al.* (1983) nil in 52; and Coppleson *et al.* (1992)

Table 7.1 Carcinoma of the cervix: FIGO staging (FIGO, 1995).

Stage 0	Primary tumor cannot be assessed. No evidence of primary tumor. Carcinoma-in-situ.
Stage I	Cervical carcinoma is strictly confined to the uterus (extension to corpus should be disregarded)
Stage Ia	Invasive cancer identified only microscopically. All gross lesions even with superficial invasion are stage IB cancers. Invasion is limited to measured stromal invasion with maximum depth of 5 mm and not wider than 7 mm. The depth of invasion should not be more than 5 mm taken from the base of the epithelium, either surface or glandular, from which it originates. Vascular space involvement, either venous or lymphatic, should not alter the staging
Stage Ia1	Measured invasion of stroma no greater than 3 mm in depth and no wider than 7 mm
Stage Ia2	Measured invasion of stroma greater than 3 mm and no greater than 5 mm and no wider than 7 mm
Stage Ib	Clinical lesions confined to the cervix or preclinical lesions greater than IA
Stage Ib1	Clinical lesions no greater than 4 cm in size
Stage Ib2	Clinical lesions greater than 4 cm in size

nil in 82. Coppleson *et al.* reviewed five major recent publications and totaled 404 women who were submitted to pelvic lymphadenectomy; only in two of them (0.5%) were there nodal metastases. When penetration extended to between 3 and 5 mm, the incidence, as quoted in Coppleson's review of the literature, was 12 (8%) out of 146 women. Hence the new FIGO staging (1995) takes close account of these data (see Table 7.1.)

Lymphovascular space involvement

It would seem that once tumor cells are present within the endothelial-lined spaces of the lymphatics and vascular system, the risk of lymph node metastasis should be increased. However, this, like the former parameter (i.e. depth of invasion), also presents a confusing picture in respect of reaching a therapy decision. In a careful study, Roche and Norris (1975) found that 57% of cases of microinvasion had lymphatic space involvement but none involved nodal metastasis. Simon *et al.* (1986) found in their review of the literature that 54 (14%) out of 373 females submitted to lymphadenectomy had LVS involvement, and only one of them (1.9%) had nodal metastasis. None of 213 women who received long-term follow-up had either local recurrence or death from the tumor. Creasman *et al.* (1985) reported that 39 out of 267 females had lymph node involvement, but only one had lymph node metastasis where the depth of invading tumor into the stroma was 3 mm or less. Where the penetration was 3–5 mm, nearly 50% had LVS involvement but only one had metastasis; the 56 women without lymph node involvement had a prevalence of positive nodes of 11% (six cases).

A number of studies (Table 7.4, p. 209) have demonstrated the correlation between the depth of penetration and LVS involvement, and in cases where the penetration is less than 1 mm this ranges from 0% to 10%; where the invasion is to between 3 and 5 mm, the rate varied from 6% to 43%. Coppleson (1992) has stated, that "the parameter of LVS permeation *per se* is irrelevant in forecasting or suspecting metastatic spread." Recent work has shown that using univariate analysis, stage, tumor size and LVS involvement were all significant prognostic factors for recurrence. However multivariate analysis has shown that only tumor size and LVS involvement are significant in the presence of complete surgical resection and negative lymph nodes (Comerci *et al.*, 1998).

Confluence

It has been suggested by various authors that invasion by "confluent masses of neoplastic cells" (Fidler & Boyes, 1959) was associated with an increase in recurrent invasive disease. There are also authors (Roche & Norris, 1975) who hold the opposite view, and it would seem as though a possible explanation for the high rate reported was the fact that most cases were of clinical, and not preclinical or early invasive disease (Coppleson, 1992).

Determining a correct management protocol

It must be obvious to any reader of the literature that, concerning the treatment of early invasive squamous cervical carcinoma, there is a paradox, in that the infrequent occurrence of lymph node metastasis, the recurrence of the lesions, and the subsequent death rate from cancer are difficult to balance against the morbidity and mortality from the radical surgical procedures that have been recommended for this condition. Coppleson (1992) has listed four reasons that are at the root cause of problems associated with determining a correct management protocol. These are:

1 A general "arbitrariness of definition in use, including the methods of arriving at them and the subjectivity involved in making these diagnoses."
2 A lack of, uniformity in reporting the results of recurrence and mortality rates.
3 The difficulty of assessing the correct incidence of lymph node involvement.
4 The morbidity and mortality of the actual surgical procedures.

As a result of examining each one of these factors, Coppleson has recommended a form of management protocol that emphasizes the combined use of the two major diagnostic modalities, namely colposcopy and pathology, thereby avoiding complete reliance on pathology. In the following section this protocol will be examined.

Recommended therapy

By using colposcopy and pathology it is possible to use objective parameters to determine the therapy. Adequate biopsy is essential in this assessment, and *a cone or large ex-cisional sample must be obtained*. Colposcopy is invaluable in directing this biopsy. Rarely, a vaginal hysterectomy may need to be substituted for a cone biopsy, especially if indications for this biopsy develop in the postmenopausal woman.

Conservative management can be confidently employed only after colposcopy has excluded the colposcopically overt (invasive) lesion, and after endocervical curettage has excluded the clinical cancer in the endocervical canal. Biopsy and curettage material should not be suspicious of carcinoma. The conservative treatment methods are either (i) cone biopsy by cold knife, LLETZ or laser or partial cervical amputation; or (ii) hysterectomy.

Cone biopsy

Cone biopsy or amputation of the cervix is especially suitable in young women who have early invasive lesions and where the pathology has shown the presence of stage Ia1 disease or invasion into the stroma of less than 3 mm with no LVS involvement and with the excision lines clear of disease. Burghardt (1992), while advocating conization as a standard treatment for stage Ia1 disease, is more discriminating in choosing conservative methods when dealing with stage Ia2. In some of his earlier work, Burghardt (1984) showed that by measuring the depth of invasion and the lateral extent along the surface of the lesion, it was possible to determine a semi-quantitative measure of tumor volume; he also showed that a specific tumor volume, that is, 350 mm³ was not associated with any risk of nodal involvement. These measurements have been accepted within the recent FIGO classification (Table 7.1) and it is now recommended that when using these two measurements, with limits of 5 mm for depth and 7 mm for horizontal spread, conservative management can be used to treat lesions falling within the definition of stage Ia2 disease. Lesions within these parameters are treated by either conization or cervical amputation, but any lesions that are more advanced than this should be treated by more radical measures. Mor Yosef (1990) has shown the efficacy of using LLETZ as a "cone biopsy" technique. Indeed the same department have gone on to show the value of the large loop cone biopsy coupled with laparoscopic lymphadenectomy in stage Ia2 microinvasive disease, thus allowing the preservation of the uterus.

Hysterectomy

Hysterectomy is usually performed when the criteria for conservative management no longer apply. For instance, in the case of extensive vascular involvement and penetration to 3–5 mm, there would be merit in recommending a conservative abdominal hysterectomy accompanied by pelvic lymphadenectomy without removal of the parametrial tissue or ureteric dissection. Certainly, adnexal conservation is paramount, especially in the premenopausal woman. Ideally, the hysterectomy should be undertaken by the vaginal route, except in those instances where lymphadenectomy is perceived to be necessary, that is, with extensive vascular involvement. Some authors insist that parametrial involvement can be disregarded (Holzer, 1982; Burghardt, 1992) in microinvasive carcinoma, and that the uncommon vaginal extension should be recognizable colposcopically. This would allow the safe employment of the vaginal route. There are others (Morrow, 1993) who advocate a modified abdominal hysterectomy, and the indications are listed below. In this procedure, the medial portion of the parametrium is taken, so as to include the paracervical nodes; also included is a small vaginal cuff and some resection of the uterosacral ligaments.

The Schauta operation, which is intermediate between the radical hysterectomy with pelvic lymphadenectomy and the conservative classic hysterectomy, has been recommended by some authors (Kovacic *et al.*, 1976; Burghardt & Holzer, 1977). Coppleson (1992) has summarized the dilemma that exists concerning the correct management of early invasive cancer. He insists that, "in the final analysis there is always a subjective element in the decision concerning management and it would seem that in difficult cases, nevertheless, the addition of colposcopy to traditional histologic assessment represents a small but positive advance, in that more women can be treated conservatively with assured safety than was previously possible."

Laparoscopic-assisted Schauta vaginal hysterectomy (LAVH) with the opportunity for lymph node sampling is now becoming recognized as a viable option for therapy in this condition.

For stage Ia1 (less than 3 mm of invasion) the risk of lymph node metastases are very close to zero. Thus for these patients it is usually found that if the diagnostic procedure, (cone biopsy etc) has completely resected the lesion then no further therapy is necessary. Ueki *et al.* (1994), using their own equivalent definition of stage Ia1 (microinvasive carcinoma, MIC) have confirmed that conservative therapy in the form of Nd-YAG laser conization is an appropriate and effective therapy. However where the patient has other gynecologic problems which suggest that a hysterectomy is appropriate then a vaginal or minimal access surgical procedure is optimal. Where excision of the stage Ia1 lesion is incomplete then further assessment is necessary. This may take the form of colposcopic assessment with loop diathermy biopsy or cone, so that the incomplete margins can be reviewed. Often the margins which were reported as involved have in fact been effectively dealt with by the initial procedure. However it is vital to eliminate the risk of a larger invasive cancer lying beyond the initial diagnostic biopsy, "the tip of the iceberg phenomenon" (Bolger *et al.*, 1996).

Where the lesion has extended between 3 and 5 mm the risk of lymph node metastases rises to low single figure percentages. If following the diagnostic cone biopsy the lesion has been reported as being completely excised, the LAVH with assessment of the pelvic lymph nodes will give considerable information and will effectively deal with this early invasive carcinoma of the cervix. In addition the procedure allows accurate delineation of any extension of the disease onto the outer cervix or vagina, thus decreasing the risk of persistent abnormal smears. The author's viewpoint has been partially confirmed in a retrospective review by Yaegashi *et al.* (1994) who stated that "conservative"

therapy in the form of conization and hysterectomy or extended hysterectomy can be used rather than radical hysterectomy in selected patients. Morrow (1993) has also advocated the use of modified radical hysterectomy to include a small section of parametrium.

Early invasive cancer spreads by lymphatic channel embolization rather than by permeation, thus leaving tissue between the primary tumor and the primary lymph nodes free. Conservation of this tissue does not jeopardize the patient's prognosis.

Therefore for the patient requiring hysterectomy with stage Ia1 cancer, an LAVH with or without ovarian removal depending on the wishes of the patient is the recommended course of action.

For stage Ia2, whether an LAVH should be carried out with or without removal of the ovaries and node sampling, or a comprehensive lymphadenectomy should be made remains unresolved. This dilemma was present long before the arrival of minimal access surgery.

Adenocarcinoma-in-situ and early invasive adenocarcinoma of the cervix

These conditions once thought to be relatively rare now present very frequently in large colposcopy clinics, particularly since the return of the widespread use of excisional methods of assessment and management (loop diathermy cone and excision biopsy).

Minimal access surgery is an ideal method to reduce the impact of surgery in these conditions in a very similar way to the applications for microinvasive squamous cancer.

The role of conservative therapy is well-recognized (Cullimore *et al.*, 1992); most patients with adenocarcinoma-in-situ will be effectively treated by the loop diathermy cone biopsy which has made the diagnosis. The only caveat to this recommendation has been the commonly held belief of the more disparate nature of adenocarcinoma-in-situ when compared with the more confluent nature of CIN. These reservations have been significantly overstated; the risk of there being a separate lesion after complete resection of the main focus is extremely small (Maini *et al.*, 1998). It is now generally recommended that adenocarcinoma-in-situ be managed as for CIN. Similarly an LAVH would be appropriate for the patient with additional reasons for performing a hysterectomy.

Early invasive adenocarcinoma of the cervix however presents difficult management problems. We do not have a clear definition of a "microinvasive" stage for this type of cancer (Östör *et al.*, 1997). Many clinicians are uncomfortable about the potentially disparate nature of the condition and its tendency to develop deep in the substance of the cervix resulting in large tumors before clinical diagnosis can be made. If a deep diagnostic cone is not performed then there is a significant danger of underdiagnosis of the true extent of the disease with a consequent undertreatment if a non-radical hysterectomy or LAVH is employed.

However, a number of authors have proposed that patients with microinvasive adenocarcinoma who meet criteria for FIGO stage Ia1, namely microscopically identifiable lesions up to 3 mm invasive depth, and up to

7 mm width, were candidates for non-radical surgery. Östör et al. (1997) found such disease confined to the cervix with no recurrences amongst 43 patients with up to 3 mm of invasion by cervical adenocarcinoma. Kaku et al. (1997) likewise reviewed 30 cases of microinvasive cervical adenocarcinoma who had hysterectomy (29) or cone (1), and among 21 with less than 3 mm invasion found no evidence of disease beyond the cervix and none developed recurrent disease. Schorge et al. (1999) reported 21 women with microinvasive carcinoma meeting the FIGO stage Ia1 classification. The mean age of the median range of follow-up was 76 months (30–172) and the median age of the patients 38 (24–75) years. Definitive treatment included radical hysterectomy, simple abdominal and vaginal hysterectomy or loop excision. Endocervical adenocarcinoma (FIGO stage Ia1) was present in 18, adenosquamous in two, and clear cell in one, and in none of them was there any evidence of parametrial invasion or lymph node metastasis. There was no disease recurrence. These authors insist that in those who meet the criteria for FIGO stage Ia1 cervical carcinoma with disease limited to the cervix, conservative surgery such as cone biopsy or simple hysterectomy might offer definitive treatment.

There has been some uncertainty about the true risk of metastases to the ovaries and thus the question of ovarian conservation has been vexed. Shingleton (1995), has shown a tiny risk of approximately 1–1.5% for both squamous and adenocarcinomas. Conversely the pressure to maintain ovarian function is reduced because concerns about the use of HRT following treatment of adenocarcinoma of the cervix are unfounded thus assisting the decision to remove ovaries as part of the definitive management.

Recent work by Maini et al. (1998) has focused on whether the status of the endocervical margins of LLETZ used in the treatment of CGIN can predict the status of the remaining cervix. The authors did demonstrate in a retro-spective study that LLETZ was an adequate primary management of CGIN and that the excision margin status did appear to be a prognostic factor for residual disease.

Stage Ib cancer of the cervix

Conservative surgery

In western society there has developed a pattern of life for young women where the development of a career has been given priority over childbearing. This has resulted in the frequently observed situation where a woman in the third or fourth decade of life has been found to have a cancer of the cervix. The traditional approach has been to perform a hysterectomy, usually radical. However there are now significant pressures to preserve fertility. Dargent et al. (1994) have developed a procedure which they have called a radical *trachelectomy* whereby the cervix is removed with the paracervical and upper vaginal support tissues up to the internal os. (Fig. 7.104a & b). This locally radical procedure combined with a pelvic lymphadenectomy has been demonstrated to be successful not only in treating the cancer but in preserving fertility in a selected group of patients. The procedure has now been performed on over 150 women worldwide with a significant number of successful pregnancies (Roy & Plante, 1998) and a reassuringly low recurrence rate. The assessment of the patient in the preoperative period is vital with the use of MRI increasingly important. Considerable experience of radical vaginal surgery and cervical cancer care is essential prior to embarking on such procedures. The long-term results are

Fig. 7.104 (a) A drawing showing the area that is removed (shaded) during a radical trachelectomy. In (b) this excised area can be seen with the cervical cancer (stage Ib1) at (1), ectocervix at (2) and vaginal valut at (3).

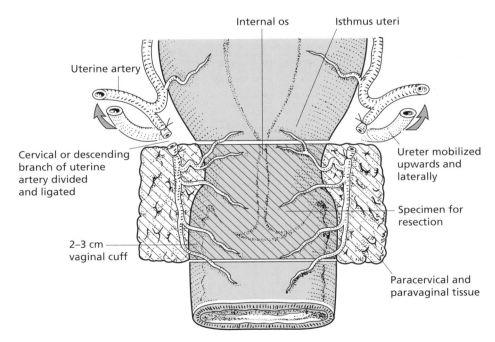

Fig. 7.104(a)

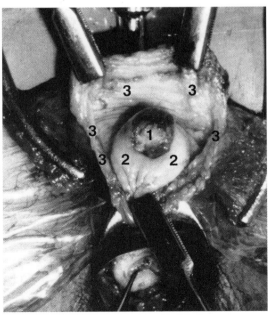

Fig. 7.104(b)

beginning to develop for this "niche market" in cancer surgery.

Radical surgery

For stage Ib disease because of the higher risk of local spread and lymph node metastases (15–25%), a more comprehensive local radical therapy is frequently necessary together with a full lymphadenectomy. Daniel Dargent has demonstrated the combination of a Schauta radical vaginal hysterectomy together with extraperitoneal dissection of the lymph nodes. More recently the radical Schauta hysterectomy with the addition of the laparoscopic transperitoneal resection of the pelvic and para-aortic lymph nodes has been demonstrated (Querleu, 1991; Childers et al., 1992; Nehzat et al., 1992; Kadar & Reich, 1993). These have shown the elegant use of monopolar diathermy for the removal of all pelvic and para-aortic lymph nodes. It is fascinating to see how reintroducing radical vaginal surgery such as the Schauta and adding modern minimal access surgery in the form of laparoscopic lymphadenectomy has countered many of the old arguments about the limited value of radical vaginal surgery in cancer care. Delgado (1994) has shown that using a combination of the Mitra approach to the pelvic lymph nodes carried deep into the pelvis so as to allow the lateral parts of the cardinal ligaments to be stapled, he can then simplify the performance of a Schauta procedure and significantly limit intraperitoneal contamination.

Sartori et al. (1995) have attempted to define more accurately the need for radical resection of the parametrial tissues by observing in a retrospective study the presence or absence of parametrial nodes and the survival performance of these patients. No significant survival difference was found in either those with involved parametrial nodes or those with negative nodes. The authors concluded that the extent of the radical hysterectomy should be based on a modern knowledge of the patterns of spread (sic). Kinney et al. (1995) from The Mayo Clinic reviewed a series of 387 patients over almost a 30-year period. Amongst this group, they identified a subset of 83 patients (21.4%) who had tumors invading deeper than 3 mm, but with a volume less than 4.19 cm^3, that is, a sphere of 2 cm in diameter and without evidence of angiolymphatic space involvement. None of these patients had parametrial node involvement. Five-year survival was 97.6%. The authors considered that this subset should be candidates for a modified radical procedure plus lymphadenectomy. The author would concur and extend the reduction in surgical impact by advocating performing the procedure using laparoscopic techniques. Koh and Greer (1995) in a well-argued editorial commenting on the Kinney paper (1995) drew attention to the difficulties of measurement, of the need for "generous" cone biopsies for accurate assessment and the current limitations of the use of MRI. The argument that the good results were possibly influenced by the radical hysterectomies which these patients underwent and that a reduction in radicality would be potentially dangerous is well-taken. There is continuing re-evaluation of the extent of radicality for all surgical procedures. The development of reduced-impact surgery to achieve the same cure rates with less morbidity is paramount.

Results of treatment

A number of studies have analyzed the recurrence rate according to the mode of treatment for stage Ia with divisions into stages Ia1 and Ia2 (Tables 7.2–7.4). Table 7.2 summarizes three major studies (Averette et al., 1976; Kolstad, 1989; Burghardt et al., 1991) which showed that the recurrence of invasive cancer in those cases that had originally been treated as stage Ia1 was extremely low; only one case occurred (i.e. in the series by Burghardt et al., 1991) some 12 years after a cone biopsy had been performed, and no evidence of LVS involvement was seen. In another review of the literature, Sevin et al. (1992) have analyzed the recurrence rate according to whether the stage was Ia1 or Ia2, and they showed a rate of 1.3% for the former and 4.2% for the latter. These accumulated figures (1799 women with stage Ia1 and 1176 with stage Ia2) encompassed all modes of therapy, from the most conservative to the most radical.

Cone biopsy for the treatment of stage Ia1 would seem reasonable in view of the low recurrence rate, but as for its use in the treatment of stage Ia2, some reservations must still exist as very few results concerning recurrence are yet

	Radical hysterectomy		Hysterectomy		Cone biopsy		Follow-up (years)
	n	Recur.	n	Recur.	n	Recur.	
Averette et al. (1976)*	162	0					1–15
Burghardt et al. (1991)	48	0	170	0	93	1†	5–30
Kolstad (1989)	98	0	57	0	3	0	3–17
Total	308	0	227	0	96	1	
Percentage		0		0		0.8	

Table 7.2 Invasive recurrence of stage Ia1 related to treatment for squamous cell carcinoma of the cervix.

These data are from patients with early stromal invasion (ESI) as defined by the 1985 FIGO classification.

*No lymph-vascular space (LVS) involvement.

†This recurrence was 12 years after a cone biopsy for stage Ib.

Table 7.3 Cone biopsy for stage Ia squamous carcinoma of the cervix.

| | Depth of invasion (mm) | n | Recurrence | | | Follow-up (years) |
			n	LVS involvement	Died of disease	
Coppleson (1992)	1–3	17	1	1	1	>5
Kolstad (1989)	1–5	15	1	0	–	3–17
Burghardt et al. (1991)	1–5	18	3	2	1	3–20
Morris (pers. comm.)	1–3	10	0	0	0	1.6 (med)
Andersen et al. (1993)	≤3	31	0	0	0	3.0
Total		91	5	3	2	–

Not all cases had negative cone margins.
At least four of the five recurrences had invasion ≤3 mm.
med; median.
From Morrow (1993).

Table 7.4 Squamous carcinoma of the cervix, stage Ia: depth of invasion and lymph-vascular space (LVS) involvement.

| Depth of invasion (mm) | n | LVS involvement (%) | |
		Mean	Range
≤1.0	197	8.6	0–10
1.1–3.0	263	21.3	3–25
3.1–5.0	121	22.3	6–39

From Sedlis et al. (1979), Hasumi et al. (1980), Creasman et al. (1985), Maiman et al. (1988), Burghardt (1992).

available. In Table 7.3, some 91 cases have been assembled and recurrence has occurred in five of them. Not all the 91 cases had negative cone margins and at least four of the five recurrences had invasion to a depth of 3 mm or less. This recurrence rate in the more advanced of these early invasive lesions is not surprising, in view of the known frequency of LVS involvement in relation to the depth of invasion, as is shown in Table 7.4. It can be seen that when the disease penetrates less than 1 mm, then LVS involvement is 8.6%, whereas when the invasion is between 3.1 and 5 mm, LVS involvement can be as high as 22.3%.

It appears that with increasing depth of invasion, there is a small but steady increase in death rates. This is summarized in Table 7.5.

Recommended treatment: summary

The treatment of stage Ia squamous carcinoma of the cervix must always be based on an adequate cone biopsy specimen:

Stage Ia1

• No lymphovascular space involvement, (LVSI): cone biopsy or simple vaginal or abdominal hysterectomy.
• With LVSI if cone margins are confidently clear no further action or simple vaginal or abdominal hysterectomy.

Table 7.5 Death rates related to depth of invasion.

	No. of cases	Died of cancer
Early stromal invasion (ESI)	1011	2 (0.2%)
1–3 mm invasion	572	7 (1.2%)
3–5 mm invasion	409	7 (1.7%)

After Burghardt et al. (1997).

Stage Ia2

• Where there is a need for preservation of fertility, a cone biopsy with adequate margins combined with a laparoscopic node dissection will be reassuring. If the margins are in doubt but all evidence including MRI assessment suggests a small tumor then a radical trachelectomy with laparoscopic pelvic lymph node dissection will be optimal therapy.
• For the patient where continuing fertility is unimportant, a laparoscopic Coelio Schauta procedure is optimal. Although a radical hysterectomy may still be performed it should be tailored "down" to reduce the impact of surgery.

7.17 References

Abdul-Karim, F., Fu, Y., Reagan, W. & Wentz, W. (1982) Morphometric study of intraepithelial neoplasia of the cervix. *Obstet Gynecol* **60**,210.

Ali, S.W., Evans, A.S. & Monaghan, J.M. (1986) Results of CO₂ laser cylinder vaporisation of CIN in 1234 patients. An analysis of failures. *Br J Obstet Gynaecol* **93**,75.

Anderson, M.C. (1992) Handling biopsy specimens. In: Anderson, M., Jordan, J., Morse, A. & Sharpe, F. (eds) *The Text and Atlas of Integrated Colposcopy*, p. 92. Chapman and Hall Medical, London.

Anderson, M.C. (1982) Treatment of cervical intraepithelial neoplasia with carbon dioxide laser: a report of 543 patients. *Obstet Gynecol* **59**,720.

Anderson, M. & Hartley, R. (1980) Cervical crypt involvement by intraepithelial neoplasia. *Obstet Gynecol* **55**,546.

Andersen, E.S., Husth, M., Joergensen, A. & Nielsen, K. (1993) Laser conization for microinvasive carcinoma of the cervix. Short-term results. *Int J Gynecol Cancer* **3**,183.

Anderson, S.E., Thorup, K. & Larsen, G. (1988) Results of cryosurgery for cervical intraepithelial neoplasia. *Gynecol Oncol* **30**,21.

Averette, H.E., Nelson, J.H. Jr., Ng, A.B. *et al.* (1976) Diagnosis and management of microinvasion (stage Ia) carcinoma of the uterine cervix. *Cancer* **38**,414.

Benedet, J.L., Anderson, G.H. & Boyes, D.A. (1985) Colposcopic accuracy in the diagnosis of microinvasive and occult invasive carcinoma of the cervix. *Obstet Gynecol* **65**,557.

Benedet, J.L., Miller, D.M. & Nickerson, K.C. (1992) Results of conservative management of cervical intraepithelial neoplasia. *Obstet Gynecol* **79**(1),105.

Benson, W.L. & Norris, H.J. (1977) A critical review of the frequency of lymph node metastasis and death from microinvasive carcinoma of the cervix. *Obstet Gynecol* **49**,632.

Bigrigg, A., Haffenden, D.K., Sheehan, A.L., Codling, B.W. & Read, M.D. (1994) Efficacy and safety of large-loop excision of the transformation zone. *Lancet* **343**,32.

Bigrigg, M.A., Codling, B.W., Pearson, P., Read, M.D. & Swingler, G.R. (1991) Pregnancy after cervical loop diathermy. *Lancet* **337**,119.

Blomfield, P.I., Buxton, J., Dunn, J. & Luesley, D.M. (1993) Pregnancy outcome after large loop excision of the cervical transformation zone. *Am J Obstet Gynecol* **169**,620.

Boccalon, M., Tyrelli, U. & Vacchere, E. (1996) Intra-epithelial and invasive cervical neoplasia during HIV infection. *Eur J Cancer* **32a**(13),2212.

Bolger, B., Lopes Ade, B. & Monaghan, J.M. (1996) The role of loop diathermy in the management of early invasive cancer of the cervix. *Int J Gynec Cancer*.

Bongain, A., Rampal, A. & Gilette, J.Y. (1996) Cervical intraepithelial neoplasia in women infected with human immunodeficiency virus. *Eur J Obstet Gynecol Reprod Biol* **65**(2),195.

Boonstra, H., Aalders, J., Koudstaal, J. & Janssens, J. (1990) Minimum extension and appropriate topographic position of tissue destruction for treatment of cervical intraepithelial neoplasia. *Obstet Gynecol* **75**,227.

Boutselis, J.G. (1972) Intraepithelial carcinoma of the cervix associated with pregnancy. *Obstet Gynecol* **40**,657.

Branca, M., Delfino, A., Rossi, E., Giacomini, G., Leoncini, L., Riti, M.G. *et al.* (1995) Cervical intraepithelial neoplasia and human papillomavirus related lesions of the genital tract in HIV positive and negative women. *Eur J Gynaecol Oncol* **16**,410.

Brown, J., Campion, M., Cuzick, J. & Singer, A. (1988) Psychosexual trauma of an abnormal smear. *Br J Obstet Gynaecol* **95**,175.

Burghardt, E. (1984) Microinvasive carcinoma in gynaecological pathology. *Clin Obstet Gynecol* **11**,239.

Burghardt, E. (1992) Pathology of early invasive squamous and glandular carcinoma of the cervix (FIGO stage 1A). In: Coppleson, M. (ed.) *Gynaecological Oncology*, Vol. 1, 2nd edn, p. 609. Churchill Livingstone, Edinburgh.

Burghardt, E., Cirardi, F., Lahousen, M., Pickel, H. & Tamussino, K. (1991) Microinvasive carcinoma of the uterine cervix (International Federation of Gynaecology and Obstetrics (stage Ia)). *Cancer* **67**,1037.

Burghardt, E. & Holzer, E. (1977) Diagnosis and treatment of microinvasive cancer of the cervix uteri. *Obstet Gynecol* **49**,641.

Burghardt, E., Östŏr, A. & Fox, H. (1997) The new FIGO definition of cervical cancer Stage 1A: a critique. *Gynecol Oncol* **65**,1.

Buxton, E.J., Luesley, D.M., Shafi, M.I. & Rollason, M. (1991) Colposcopically directed punch biopsy; a potentially misleading investigation. *Br J Obstet Gynaecol* **98**(12),1273.

Campion, M., McCance, D., Cuzick, J. & Singer, A. (1986) Progressive potential of mild cervical atypia; prospective geologic, colposcopic and virological study. *Lancet* **2**,237.

Cartier, R. (1984) Therapeutic choices in treatment. In: Cartier, R. (ed.) *Practical Colposcopy*, p. 162. Laboratoire Cartier, Paris.

Chanen, W. (1989) The efficacy of electrocoagulation diathermy performed under local anaesthesia for the eradication of precancerous lesions of the cervix. *Aust NZ J Obstet Gynaecol* **29**,189.

Chanen, W. & Hollyock, V. (1974) Colposcopy and the conservative management of cervical dysplasia and carcinoma in situ. *Obstet Gynecol* **43**,527.

Chanen, W. & Rome, R. (1983) Electrocoagulation diathermy for cervical dysplasia and carcinoma in situ; a fifteen-year survey. *Obstet Gynecol* **61**,673.

Chao, S., McCaffery, R.M., Todd, W.D. & More, J.G. (1969) Conisation in evaluation and management of cervical neoplasia. *Am J Obstet Gynecol* **103**,574.

Childers, J.M., Hatch, K. & Surwit, E.A. (1992) The role of laparoscopic lymphadenectomy in the management of cervical carcinoma. *Gynecol Oncol* **47**,38.

Comerci, G., Bolger, B., Flannelly, G. *et al.* (1998) Prognostic factors in surgically treated stage Ib–IIb carcinoma of the cervix with negative lymph nodes. *Int J Gynecol Cancer* **8**,23.

Coppleson, M. (1992) Early invasive squamous adenocarcinoma of the cervix (FIGO stage 1A); clinical features and management. In: Coppleson, M. (ed.) *Gynaecological Oncology*, Vol. 1, 2nd edn, p. 632. Churchill Livingstone, Edinburgh.

Coppleson, M., Atkinson, K.H. & Dalrymple, J.C. (1992) Cervical squamous and glandular intraepithelial neoplasia; clinical features and review of management. In: Coppleson, M. (ed.) *Gynaecological Oncology*, Vol. 1, 2nd edn, p. 594. Churchill Livingstone, Edinburgh.

Cox, J.T., Lorincz, A.T., Schiffman, M.H., Sherman, M.E., Cullen, A., Kurman, R.J. (1995) Human papillomavirus testing by hybrid capture appears to be useful in triaging women with a cytologic diagnosis of atypical squamous cells of undetermined significance. *Am J Obstet Gynecol* **172**,946.

Creasman, W.T., Hinshaw, W.N. & Clarke-Pearson, D.L. (1984) Cryosurgery in the management of cervical intraepithelial neoplasia. *Obstet Gynecol* **63**,145.

Creasman, W.T., Setter, B.F., Clarke-Pearson, D.L., Kaufmann, L. & Parker, R.T. (1985) Management of stage IA carcinoma of the cervix. *Am J Obstet Gynecol* **153**,164.

Cullimore, J., Luesley, D., Rollason, T., Byrne, P., Buckley, C., Anderson, M. *et al.* (1992) A prospective study of conization of the cervix in the management of cervical intraepithelial glandular neoplasia — a preliminary report. *Br J Obstet Gynaecol* **99**,314.

Cullimore, J.E., Woodman, C.B., Luesley, D. & Jordan, J. (1989) When laser vaporization for CIN fails, what next? *Lancet* **1**,561.

Cuthill, S., Maimon, M., Fruchter, R.G. & Cheng, C.C. (1995) Complications after treatment of CIN in women infected with HIV.

Cuzick, J., Terry, C., Ho, L., Hollingsworth, T. & Anderson, M. (1992) Human papillomavirus type 16 DNA in cervical smears as a predictor of high grade intraepithelial neoplasia. *Lancet* **339**,959.

Cuzick, J., Terry, G., Ho, L., Hollingworth, T. & Anderson, M. (1994) Type-specific human papillomavirus DNA in abnormal smears as a predictor of high-grade cervical intraepithelial neoplasia. *Br J Cancer* **69**,167.

Dargent, D., Roy, M., Keita, N., Mathevet, P. & Adeleine, P. (1993) The Schauta operation its place in the management of cervical cancer. (adstract). *Gynecol Oncol* **49**,109.

Dargent, D., Brun, J.L., Roy, M. & Remy, I. (1994) Pregnancies following radical trachelectomy for invasive cancer. *Gynecol Oncol* **52**,105.

de Cristofana, D., Fontana, P. & Pezzoli, C. (1988) Pathological study of the cervix after cold coagulation. *Am J Obstet Gynecol* **159**(5),1053.

Delgado, G. (1994) Radical vaginal hysterectomy with Mitra extra peritoneal lymph node dissection.

Delgado, G., Potku, R.K. & Dolan, J.R. (1995) Retroperitoneal radical hysterectomy *Gynecol Oncol* **56**,191.

Del-Priore, G., Gilmour, P.R. & Cheon, T.H. (1996) Colposcopic biopsies versus loop electrosurgical excision procedure, cone histology in human immunodeficiency virus-positive women. *J Reprod Med* **41**(9),653.

Duncan, I.D. (1997) (ed.) Guidelines for clinical practice and programme management, 2nd edn. *NHSCSP Publications No 8*, Sheffield.

El-Bastawissi, A., Becker, T. & Dalling, J. (1999) Effective cervical carcinoma in situ and its management on pregnancy outcome. *Obstet Gynecol* **93**,207.

Ferenczy, A., Franco, E. & Arseneau, J. (1996) Diagnostic performance of hybrid capture human papillomavirus deoxyribonucleic acid assay combined with liquid-based cytologic study. *Am J Obstet Gynecol* **175**,651.

Ferris, D.G., Wright, T.C., Litaker, M.C. *et al.* (1998) Triage of women with ASCUS and LSIL on pap smear reports; Management by repeat pap smear, HPV DNA testing, or colposcopy. *J Fam Pract* **46**(2),125.

Fidler, H.K. & Boyes, D.A. (1959) Patterns of early invasion from intraepithelial carcinoma of the cervix. *Cancer* **12**,673.

FIGO (1988) In: Pettersson, F. (ed.) *Annual Report on the Results of Treatment in Gynaecological Cancer.* Radium Hemmet, Stockholm.

FIGO (1995) Modifications in the staging for stage 1 vulvar and stage 1 cervical cancer. *Int J Gynecol Obstet* **50**,215.

Fink, M.J., Fruchter, R.G., Maimon, R., Sedlis, A. & Chen, P. (1994) The adequacy of cytology and colposcopy in diagnosing cervical neoplasia in HIV seropositive women. *Gynecol Oncol* **55**(1),133.

Flannelly, G., Langhan, H., Jandial, L., Mana, E., Campbell, M., Kitchener, H. (1997) A study of treatment failures following large loop excision of the transformation zone for the treatment of cervical intraepithelial neoplasia. *Br J Obstet Gynaecol* **104**,718.

Fruchter, R.G., Maimon, M., Sedlis, A. & Arrastia, D. (1996) Multiple recurrences of CIN in women with HIV. *Obstet Gynecol* **87**(3),338.

Giles, J.A., Hudson, E. & Walker, P. (1988) Colposcopic assessment of the accuracy of cervical cytological screening. *Br Med J* **296**,1099.

Giles, J.A., Walker, P.C. & Chalk, P.A. (1987) The treatment of CIN by radical electrocoagulation diathermy: five years' experience. *Br J Obstet Gynaecol* **94**,1089.

Goodman, J. & Sumner, D. (1991) Patient acceptability of laser and cold coagulation for premalignant cervical cancer. *Br J Obstet Gynaecol* **98**(11),1168.

Gordon, H.K. & Duncan, I.D. (1991) Effective destruction of cervical intraepithelial neoplasia (CIN III) at 100°C using the Semm cold coagulator: 14 years' experience. *Br J Obstet Gynaecol* **98**(1),14.

Hall, S., Lorincz, A., Shah, F. *et al.* (1996) Human papillomavirus DNA detection in cervical specimens by hybrid capture: correlation with cytologic and histologic diagnoses of squamous epithelial lesions of the cervix. *Gynecol Oncol* **62**,353.

Hannigan, E.V., Simpson, J.S., Cillard, E.A. & Dinh, T.V. (1986) Frozen section evaluation of cervical conization specimens. *J Reprod Med* **31**,11.

ter-Harmsel, B., Smedts, F., Kuijpers, J., van Muyden, R., Oosterhuis, W., Quint, W. (1999) Relationship between human papillomavirus type 16 in the cervix and intraepithelial neoplasia. *Obstet Gynecol* **93**,46.

Hasumi, K., Sakamoto, A. & Sugano, H. (1980) Microinvasive carcinoma of the uterine cervix. *Cancer* **45**,928.

Hatch, K.D., Schneider, A. & Abdel-Nour, M.W. (1995) An evaluation of human papillomavirus testing for intermediate- and high-risk types as triage before colposcopy. *Am J Obstet Gynaecol* **172**,1150.

Hatch, K.D., Hallum, A.V., III, Nour, M. (1996) New surgical approaches to treatment of cervical cancer. *J Natl Cancer Inst Monogr* **21**,71.

Holzer, E. (1982) Microinvasive carcinoma of the cervix — clinical aspects, treatment and follow-up. In: Burghardt, E. & Holzer, J. (eds) *Minimal Invasive Cancer (Microcarcinoma),* p. 78. W.B. Saunders, Philadelphia.

Holzer, E. & Pickel, J.H. (1975) Ausdehnung des atypischen pathologischen Plattenepithels an der Zervix. *Arch Geschwulstforsch* **44**,79.

Hughes, R.G., Haddad, N.G., Smart, G.E. *et al.* (1992) The cytological detection of persistent CIN after local ablative treatment: a comparison of sampling devices. *Br J Obstet Gynaecol* **99**(6),498.

Jarmnulowicz, M., Jenkins, D., Barton, S.E. & Singer, A. (1989) Cytological status and lesion size: a further dimension in cervical intraepithelial neoplasia. *Br J Obstet Gynaecol* **96**,1061.

Jones, J.M., Sweetman, P. & Hibbard, B.N. (1979) The outcome of pregnancy after cone biopsy of the cervix: a case control study. *Br J Obstet Gynaecol* **86**,813.

Jones, M.H., Jenkins, J. & Singer, A. (1992) Cytological surveillance for mild cervical dyskaryosis. *Lancet* **339**,1440.

Kadar, N. & Reich, H. (1993) Laparoscopically assisted radical Schauta hysterectomy and bilateral pelvic lymphadenectomy for the treatment of bulky Stage Ib carcinoma of the cervix. *Gynaecol Endoscopy* **2**,135.

Kaku, T., Kamura, T., Sakai, K. *et al.* (1997) Early adenocarcinoma of the uterine cervix. *Gynecol Oncol* **65**,281.

Kierkegaard, O., Byralsen, C., Hansen, K.C., Frandsen, K.H., Frydenberg, M. (1995) Association between colposcopic findings and histology in cervical lesions: the significance of the size of the lesion. *Gynecol Oncology* **57**(1),66.

Kinney, W.K., Hodge, D.O., Egorshin, E.V., Ballard, D.J., Podratz, K.C. (1995) Identification of a low-risk subset of patients with stage Ib invasive cancer of the cervix possibly suited to less radical surgical treatment. *Gynecol Oncol* **57**,3.

Klevens, R.M., Fleming, P.L., Mays, M.A., Frey, R. (1996) Characteristics of women with AIDS and invasive cervical cancer. *Obstet Gynecol* **88**(2),269.

Koh, W.J. & Greer, B.E. (1995) Making the surgery fit the disease — the search for the optimal extent of radical surgical treatment in early invasive cervical cancer. *Gynecol Oncol* **57**,1.

Kolstad, P. (1989) Follow-up study of 232 patients with stage 1a1 and 411 patients with stage 1a2 squamous cell carcinoma of the cervix (microinvasive carcinoma cervix). *Gynecol Oncol* **33**,265.

Kolstad, P. & Klem, V. (1976) Long-term follow-up of 1121 cases of carcinoma-in-situ. *Obstet Gynecol* **48**,125.

Korn, A.P., Abercrombie, P.D. & Costa, A. (1996) Vulvar intraepithelial neoplasia in women infected with HIV I. *Gynecol Oncol* **61**(3),384.

Kovacic, J., Novak, F., Stucin, M. & Cavic, M. (1976) The place of Schauta's radical vaginal hysterectomy in the therapy of cervical carcinoma. *Gynecol Oncol* **4**,33.

Lorincz, A. (1996) Hybrid capture method for detection of human papillomavirus DNA in clinical specimens. *Papillomavirus Rep* **7**,1.

Loobuyck, H.A. & Duncan, J. (1993) Destruction of CIN 1 and 2 with the SEMM cold coagulator: 13 years' experience. *Br J Obstet Gynaecol* **100**(5),465.

Lopes, A. de B., Mor-Yosef, S., Pearson, S., Ireland, D. & Monaghan, J. (1990) Is routine colposcopic assessment necessary following laser ablation of cervical intraepithelial neoplasia. *Br J Obstet Gynaecol* **97**,175.

Lopes, A. de B. *et al.* (1993) *Gynecologic Oncology* **49**,247.

Luesley, D.M., Cullimore, J., Redman, C.W. & Laughton, F.C. (1990) Loop diathermy excision of a cervical transformation zone in patients with abnormal cervical cytology. *Br Med J* **300**,1690.

Maiman, M.A., Fruchter, R.G., DiMaio, T.M. & Boyce, J.G. (1988) Superficially invasive squamous cell carcinoma of the cervix. *Obstet Gynecol* **72**,399.

Maini, M., Lavie, O., Comerci, G. *et al.* (1998) The management and follow up of patients with high grade cervical glandular intraepithelial neoplasia. *Int J Gynecol Cancer* **8**,287.

Manos, M.N., Kinney, W.K., Hurley, L.B. *et al.* (1999) Identifying women with cervical neoplasia-using human papillomavirus DNA testing for equivocal Papanicolaou results. *JAMA* **281**(17),1605.

Mansell, M.E., Ho, L., Terry, G., Singer, A. & Cuzick, J. (1994) Semiquantitative human papillomavirus DNA detection in the management of women with minor cytological abnormality. *Br J Obstet Gynaecol* **101**,807.

McIndoe, A., Robson, M., Tidy, J., Mason, P. & Anderson, M. (1989) Laser excision rather than vaporization: the treatment of choice for cervical intraepithelial neoplasia. *Obstet Gynecol* **74**,165.

Mikuta, J.J., Enterline, H.T. & Braun, T.E. (1968) Carcinoma-in-situ associated with pregnancy. *J Am Med Assoc* **204**,763.

Mitchell, H. & Medley, C. (1989) Evidence against diathermy as a beneficial treatment for human papillomavirus infection of the cervix. *Aust NZ J Obstet Gynaecol* **29**(4),439.

Monaghan, J.M., Kirkup, W., Davis, J.A. & Edington, P. (1982) Treatment of cervical intraepithelial neoplasia by colposcopically directed cryosurgery and subsequent pregnancy experience. *Br J Obstet Gynaecol* **89**,387.

Morgan, P.R., Anderson, M., Buckley, H. *et al.* (1993) Royal College of

Obstetrics and Gynaecology microinvasive carcinoma of the cervix study. *Br J Obstet Gynaecol* **100**,664.

Morrow, C.P. (1993) Tumours of the cervix. In: Morrow, C.P., Curtin, J.P. & Townsend, D. (eds) *Synopsis of Gynaecologic Oncology*, 4th edn, p. 127. Churchill Livingstone, Edinburgh.

Mor-Yosef, S., Lopes, A., Pearson, S., Monaghan, J.M. (1990) Loop diathermy cone biopsy. *Obstet Gynecol* **75**,884.

Murdoch, J.B., Crimshaw, R.N. & Monaghan, J.M. (1991) Loop diathermy excision of the abnormal cervical transformation zone. *Int J Gynecol Cancer* **1**,105.

Murdoch, J.B., Crimshaw, R.N., Morgan, P.R. & Monaghan, J.M. (1992a) The impact of loop diathermy on management of early invasive cervical cancer. *Int J Gynecol Cancer* **2**,129.

Murdoch, J.B., Morgan, P., Lopes, A. & Monaghan, J.M. (1992b) Histological incomplete excision of CIN after large loop excision of the transformation zone (LLETZ) merits careful follow-up, not retreatment. *Br J Obstet Gynaecol* **99**(12),990.

Nehzat, C., Nezhat, F. & Welander, C. (1992) Laparoscopic radical hysterectomy and pelvic and para-aortic lymphadenectomy in the treatment of carcinoma of the cervix. *Am J Obstet Gynecol* **166**,864.

Nevin, J., Soeters, K., DeHaeck, K., Bloch, B. & Van Wyk, L. (1993) Advanced cervical cancer associated with pregnancy. *Int Gynecol Cancer* **3**(1),57.

Nobbenhuis, M., Walboomers, J.M., Helmerhorst, T.J., Rozendaal, L. (1999) Relation of human papillomavirus status to cervical lesions and consequences for cervical-cancer screening: a prospective study. *Lancet* **354**,20.

Nwabinelli, J. & Monaghan, J.M. (1991) Vaginal epithelial abnormalities in patients with CIN: clinical and pathological features and management. *Br J Obstet Gynaecol* **98**,25.

Olaitan, A., Mocroft, A., Reid, W. & Johnson, M. (1997) Cervical abnormality and sexually transmitted disease screening in human immunodeficiency virus-positive women. *Obstet Gynecol* **89**(1),71.

Ostergard, D.R. (1980) Cryosurgical treatment of cervical intraepithelial neoplasia. *Obstet Gynecol* **56**,231.

Östör A (1993) Natural history of cervical intraepithelial neoplasia—a critical review. *Int J Gynecol Path* **12**,186.

Östör, A., Rome, R. & Quinn, M. (1997) Microinvasive adenocarcinoma of the cervix. A clinicopathologic study of 77 women. *Obstet Gynecol* **89**,88.

Paraskevaidis, E., Jandial, L., Mann, E.M., Fisher, P.M. & Kitchener, H.C. (1991) Patterns of treatment failure following laser for cervical intraepithelial neoplasia; implication for follow-up protocol. *Obstet Gynecol* **78**(1),80.

Partington, C., Turner, M., Soutter, P. & Griffiths, M. (1989) Laser vaporization versus laser excision conisation in the treatment of cervical intraepithelial neoplasia. *Obstet Gynecol* **73**,775.

Pearson, S.E., Whittaker, J., Ireland, D. & Monaghan, J.M. (1989) Invasive cancer of the cervix after laser treatment. *Br J Obstet Gynaecol* **96**,486.

Petry, K.U., Kochel, H. & Glaubitz, M. (1996) Human papillomavirus is associated with the frequent detection of warty and basaloid high-grade neoplasia of the vulva and cervical neoplasia among immunocompromised women. *Gynecol Oncol* **60**(1),30.

Prendiville, W., Cullimore, J. & Norman, S. (1989) Large loop excision of the transformation zone (LLETZ). A new method of management for women with cervical intraepithelial neoplasia. *Br J Obstet Gynaecol* **96**,1054.

Querleu, D. (1991) Hysterectomies enlargies de Schauta–Amreich et Schauta–Stoekel assistees par coelioscopie. *J Gynecol Obstet Biol Reprod* **20**,747.

Raio, L., Ghezzi, F., Di Naro, E., Gomez, R. & Luscher, K. (1997) Duration of pregnancy after CO_2 laser conization of the cervix: influence of cone height. *Obstet Gynecol* **90**(6),978.

Rasbridge, S., Jenkins, D. & Singer, A. (1990) A histological and immunohistological study of cervical intraepithelial neoplasia in relation to recurrence after local treatment. *Br J Obstet Gynaecol* **97**,245.

Richart, R.M. (1990) A modified terminology for cervical intraepithelial neoplasia. *Obstet Gynecol* **75**,131.

Robertson, W.H., Wood, M.B.E., Crozier, E.H. & Hutchison, J. (1988) Risk of cervical cancer associated with mild dyskaryosis. *Br Med J* **297**,18.

Robinson, W.R., Barnes, S.E., Adams, S. & Perrin, M.S. (1997) Histology and Cytological Discrepancies in HIV infected obstetric patients with normal pap smears. *Gynecol Oncol* **65**,430.

Roche, W.D. & Norris, H.J. (1975) Microinvasive carcinoma of the cervix. Significance of lymphatic invasion and confluent patterns of stromal growth. *Cancer* **36**,180.

Rome, R., Chanen, W. & Pagano, R. (1987) The natural history of human papillomavirus (HPV) atypia of the cervix. *Aust NZ J Obstet Gynaecol* **27**,287.

Roy, M. & Plante, M (1998) Pregnancies after radical trachelectomy for early stage cervical cancer. *Am J Obstet Gynecol* **179**(1),1491.

Sartori, E., Fallo, L., La Face, B., Bianchi, U.A. & Pecorelli, S. (1995) Extended radical hysterectomy in early stage carcinoma of the uterine cervix: tailoring the radicality. *Int J Gynecol Cancer* **5**,143.

Schiffman, M.H. (1993) Latest HPV findings: some clinical implications. *Contemp Obstet Gynecol* **38**(10),27.

Schorge J., Lee K.R., Flynn C.E., Goodman A. & Sheets E. (1999) Cervical 1A[1] cervical adenocarcinoma: definition and treatment. *Obstet Gynecol* **93**(2),219.

Schuessler, W.W., Vancaille, T.G., Reich, H. & Griffith, D.P. (1991) Transperitoneal endosurgical lymphadenectomy.

Schulz, T., Boschoff, C. & Weiss, R. (1996) HIV Infection and neoplasia. *Lancet* **343**(9027),587.

Sedlis, A., Sall, S., Tsukada, Y. *et al.* (1979) Microinvasive carcinoma of the uterine cervix; a clinical pathological study. *Am J Obstet Gynecol* **133**,64.

Seshadri, L. & Cope, J. (1985) The diagnosis, treatment and complications of CIN. *Aust NZ J Obstet Gynaecol* **25**,208.

Sevin, B., Ford, J.H., Girtanner, R.D. *et al.* (1979) Invasive cancer of the cervix after cryosurgery. Pitfalls of conservative management. *Obstet Gynecol* **53**,465.

Sevin, B., Naji, M., Averette, H.E. *et al.* (1992) Microinvasive carcinoma of the cervix. *Cancer* **70**,2121.

Shafi, M.I., Luesley, D.M., Jordan, J.A., Dunn, J.A., Rollason, T.P., Yates, M. (1997) Randomised trial of immediate versus deferred treatment stategies for the management of minor cervical cytological abnormalities. *Br J Obstet Gynaecol* **104**(5),590.

Shepherd, J. (1990) Cancer complicating pregnancy. In: Shepherd, J. & Monaghan, J. (eds) *Clinical Gynaecological Oncology*. Blackwell Scientific Publications, Oxford.

Shingleton, H.M. & Orr, J.W. (1995) Ovarian metastases. In: Singleton & Orr (eds) *Cancer of the Cervix*, p. 72. Lippincott.

Sigurdsson, K., Arnadottir, T., Snorradottir, M., Benediktsdottir, K. & Saemundsson, H. (1997) Human papilloma virus (HPV) in an Icelandic population: the role of HPV DNA testing based on hybrid capture and PCR assays among women with screen-detected abnormal PAP smears. *Int J Cancer* **72**,446.

Simon, N.L., Core, H., Shingleton, H.M. *et al.* (1986) Study of superficially invasive carcinoma of the cervix. *Obstet Gynecol* **68**,19.

Singer, A. (1988) Malignant and premalignant disease in the genital tract. In: Turnbull, A. & Chamberlain, B. (eds) *Obstetrics*, p. 657. Churchill Livingstone, Edinburgh.

Soutter, W.P., Fenton, D., Gudgeon, P. & Sharp, F. (1984) Quantitative microcolpohysterescopic assessment of the extent of endocervical involvement by cervical intraepithelial neoplasia. *Br J Obstet Gynaecol* **91**,712.

Soutter, W.P., Lopes, A. de B., Fletcher, A. *et al.* (1997) Invasive cervical cancer after conservative therapy for cervical intraepithelial neoplasia. *Lancet*.

Spinillo, A., Tente, P., Iasci, A. & D-Santolo, A. (1996) Cervical intraepithelial neoplasia in pregnant intravenous drug users infected with human immunodeficiency virus type 1. *Eur J Gynecol Reprod Biol* **68**,175.

Sun, X.W., Ellerbrock, T.V., Lungu, O., Chiasson, M.A., Bush, T.J., Wright, T.C. Jr. (1995) Human papillomavirus infection in human immunodeficiency virus-seropositive women. *Obstet Gynecol* **85**,680.

Syrjänen, K., Miantyjlarvi, R., Vlayrynen, M. *et al.* (1987) Human papillomavirus (HPV) infections involved in the neoplastic process of the uterine cervix as established by prospective follow-up of 513 women for two years. *Eur J Gynecol Oncol* **8**,5.

Sze, E., Rosenzweig, B., Birenbaum, D. *et al.* (1989) Excisional conisation of the cervix-uteri. *J Gynecol Surg* **5**,325.

Tabor, A. & Berget, A. (1990) Cold knife and laser conisation for cervical intraepithelial neoplasia. *Obstet Gynecol* **76**(4),622.

Terry, G., Ho, L., Jenkins, D. & Singer, A. (1992) Definition of human papillomavirus type 16 levels in low and high grade cervical lesions by simple polymerase chain reaction technique. *Arch Virol* **128**,123.

Tidbury, P., Singer, A. & Jenkins, D. (1992) CIN III: The role of lesion size in invasion. *Br J Obstet Gynaecol* **99**,583.

Townsend, D.E. & Richart, R.M. (1983) Cryotherapy and carbon dioxide laser management of cervical intraepithelial neoplasia; a controlled comparison. *Obstet Gynecol* **61**,75.

Turner, M.J., Rasmussen, M.J.J., Flannelly, C.M., Murphy, J.F. & Lenchan, F.M. (1992) Outpatients' loop diathermy conisation as an alternative to inpatient knife conisation of the cervix. *J Reprod Med* **37**,314.

Ueki, M. (1985) Examination of cervical vessels. In: Ueki, M. (ed.) *Cervical Adenocarcinoma — A Colposcopic Atlas*, p. 18. Ishiyaku Euro-America, St Louis.

Ueki, M., Okamoto, Y., Misaki, O., Seiki, Y. *et al.* (1994) Conservative therapy for microinvasive carcinoma of the uterine cervix. *Gynecol Oncol* **53**(1),109.

van Nagell, J.R., Greenwell, N., Powell, D.F. *et al.* (1983) Microinvasive carcinoma of the cervix. *Am J Obstet Gynecol* **145**,981.

van Nagell, J.R., Roddick, J.W., Cooper, R.M. & Triplett, H.B. (1972) Vaginal hysterectomy following conisation in the treatment of carcinoma-in-situ of the cervix. *Am J Obstet Gynecol* **113**,948.

Vergote, I.B., Makare, A.P. & Kjorstad, K.E. (1992) Laser excision of the transformation zone as treatment of cervical intraepithelial neoplasia with satisfactory colposcopy. *Gynecol Oncol* **44**(3),235.

Vernon, S.D., Hart, C.E., Reeves, W.C., Icenogle, J.P. (1993) The HIV-1 *tat* protein enhances E2-dependent human papillomavirus 16 transcription. *Virus Res* **27**,133.

Volante, R., Pasero, L. & Saraceno, L. (1992) Carbon dioxide laser surgery with colposcopy for cervico-vaginal intraepithelial neoplasia treatment: ten years' experience and failure analysis. *Eur J Gynecol Oncol* **13** (Suppl. 1),78.

Walton, L.A., Edelman, D.A., Fowler, W.C. & Photopulos, G.J. (1980) Cryosurgery for the treatment of cervical intraepithelial neoplasia during the reproductive years. *Obstet Gynecol* **55**,353.

Way, S., Hennigan, M. & Wright, V.C. (1968) Some experience of preinvasive and microinvasive cancer of the cervix. *J Obstet Gynaecol Br Commonwealth* **75**,593.

Woodman, C.B., Jordan, J.A., Mylotte, M.J., Gustafeson, R. & Wade-Evans, T. (1985) The management of cervical intraepithelial neoplasia by coagulation electrodiathermy. *Br J Obstet Gynaecol* **92**,751.

Wright, T. (1996) Papillomavirus infection and neoplasia in women infected with human immunodeficiency virus. In: Monsonego, J. (ed.) *Cervical Cancer*, p. 131. Greening Blackwells, Oxford.

Wright, T.C., Gagnon, S., Richart, R.M. & Ferenczy, A. (1992a) Treatment of cervical intraepithelial neoplasia using the loop electrosurgical excision procedure. *Obstet Gynecol* **79**(2),173.

Wright, T.C., Richart, R.M., Ferenczy, A. & Koulos, J. (1992b) Comparison of specimens removed by CO, laser conisation and the loop electrosurgical excision procedure. *Obstet Gynecol* **79**(1),1471.

Wright, T.C., Jr., Ellerbrock, T.V., Chiasson, M.A., Van-Devanter, N., Sun, X.W. (1994) Cervical intraepithelial neoplasia in women infected with human immunodeficiency virus: prevalance, risk factors, and validity of Papanicolaou smears. New York Cervical Disease Study. *Obstet Gynecol* **84**,591.

Wright, T.C., Sun, S.W., Koulos, J. (1995) Comparison of management algorithms for the evaluation of women with low-grade cytologic abnormalities. *Obstet Gynecol* **85**,202.

Wright, T., Moscalilli, R., Dol, P., Ellebrock, T. & Van der Vanter, N. (1996) Significance of mild cytological atypia in women infected with human immunodeficiency virus. *Obstet Gynecol* **87**(4),515.

Yaegashi, N., Sato, S., Inoue, Y., Noda, K. & Yajima, A. (1994) Conservative surgical treatment in cervical cancer with 3 mm to 5 mm stromal invasion in the absence of confluent invasion and lymphovascular space involvement. *Gynecol Oncol* **54**,333.

Zarcone, R., Cardone, G., Bullini, P., Raucci, F. & Minerva B. (1990) Incidence of HPV and CIN in HIV positive women. *Gynecology* **47**(11),477.

Chapter 8
Vaginal Intraepithelial Neoplasia

8.1 Introduction

Cancer of the vagina is a rare condition and represents approximately 1–3% of all gynecologic malignancies (DiSaia & Creasman, 1989a). The majority of these are squamous cell lesions, but some rarer conditions, such as clear cell adenocarcinoma and melanomas, occur from time to time. The majority of the invasive lesions are found when they produce clinical symptoms, and rarely occur subsequent to the management of true preinvasive conditions (Benedet *et al.*, 1983). The precancerous stage of the invasive squamous cell disease occurs in the form of an intraepithelial neoplastic condition termed vaginal intraepithelial neoplasia (VAIN) (DiSaia & Creasman, 1989b).

8.2 Natural history of VAIN

VAIN is uncommon, accounting for approximately 0.4% of lower genital tract intraepithelial disease (Cramer & Cutler, 1974) but, like vulvar intraepithelial neoplasia (VIN), has increased in recent years; it is now found in younger females and this rise seems to be associated with the increased prevalence of human papillomavirus (HPV) infections of the genital tract (Bornstein *et al.*, 1988; Townsend, 1991).

There appear to be four populations of women who are at increased risk of developing VAIN. The first, which forms the majority, is those women who have already undergone procedures to deal with a preexisting cervical precancer (cervical intraepithelial neoplasia; CIN) (Benedet & Sanders, 1984). Treatment may have been in the form of a local conservative procedure, using either the laser, loop diathermy, or cryotherapy. It is estimated that up to 1–3% of patients with cervical neoplasia have either coexisting VAIN or will develop it at a later date (Lee & Symmonds, 1976). The time at which this will occur may be as short as 2 years or may extend up to 17 years (Townsend, 1991). There also seems to be an increased risk of VAIN in those who have VIN (Benedet & Sanders, 1984; Bornstein *et al.*, 1988).

The second population constitutes those who have had radiation therapy for cervical cancer. This increased incidence of VAIN may take some 10 to 15 years to manifest itself after the initial radiation therapy (Rutledge, 1967); it has been suggested that the epithelium of the vagina may be sensitized by low-dose radiation for the subsequent development of neoplasia.

The third population are those who have had a hysterectomy as treatment for CIN, and in whom a vaginal abnormality is diagnosed during follow-up (Hoffman *et al.*, 1989, 1992; Sherman, 1990). This presentation was more common in the past, when relatively few patients had the advantage of a colposcopic assessment of their CIN before being treated by hysterectomy. In many cases, part of the preexisting cervical lesion extended into the vaginal fornix and was not included in the surgical resection. Recently, Nwabineli and Monaghan (1991) have shown that in some 2.5% of females cervical and vaginal forniceal intraepithelial lesions will coexist, and in some 67% of them a confluence between the two areas is present. It is in this area of abnormal (atypical) epithelium (with its extension of CIN) that the subsequent VAIN and invasive cancer would seem to develop (Woodman *et al.*, 1984; Romeo *et al.*, 1990).

The age range for those who may develop VAIN extends from 24 to 80 years (Hummer *et al.*, 1970). In the younger age group there has been a marked increase in association with other epithelial lesions of the genital tract, and this may be related to the increased presence of HPV (Bornstein *et al.*, 1988).

The fourth group consists of women who are immunosuppressed, either following renal or other transplants, or idiopathically, or in association with human immunodeficiency virus (HIV) infections.

The exact malignant potential of VAIN is still not known (Murad *et al.*, 1975). This contrasts with the situation for CIN, where approximately 30% of the major-grade lesions (CIN 3) will progress to malignancy over a 20-year period. It is assumed that VAIN progresses to invasive disease because of its similarity to intraepithelial disease of the cervix, but, unfortunately, it is difficult to determine either the number or the type of VAIN lesions that will indeed progress. Recently, Punnonen *et al.* (1989) have presented some evidence that both VAIN and invasive vaginal carcinoma have "molecular similarities." By using DNA flow cytometry and archival paraffin-embedded tissue of both VAIN and vaginal cancer, they were able to determine the overall frequency of DNA aneuploidy and also the existence of the S-phase fraction (SPF). They found that VAIN and cancer both had a high frequency of DNA-aneuploid stemlines and showed a high SPF. This would suggest that both were biologically extremely similar. Futher evidence comes from a case-control study of VAIN and vaginal cancer undertaken by Brinton *et al.* (1990). The study of 41 patients with VAIN or invasive cancer of the vagina was undertaken to identify potential risk factors. As with cervical cancer, poor education and low family income were risk factors for both types of vaginal lesion; in addition, a history of genital warts was strongly related [relative risk (RR) = 2.9]. Previous genital symptoms, such as vaginal discharge or irritation, increased the subsequent cancer risk (RR = 6.1). A previous abnormal pap smear likewise represented an increased risk for both (RR = 3.8), as did an early hysterectomy (RR = 6.7).

8.3 Etiology

It has been assumed for many years that both cervical and vaginal neoplasias share a common etiology, although the direct evidence has been difficult to document. However, indirect evidence comes from number of associations. The most notable is that vaginal and cervical neoplasias occur synchronously (Rose *et al.*, 1987); that cervical cancer survivors have an increased risk of developing vaginal neoplasia as a second primary tumor and vice versa (Kleinerman *et al.*, 1995); and that human papillomaviruses, which are now recognized as the viral agents involved in the pathogenesis of cervical neoplasias, are present in vaginal tumor tissue (Daling & Sherman, 1992). A multicenter case-controlled study of in-situ and invasive vaginal carcinomas by Brinton *et al.* (1990) found that certain parameters of sexual behavior were only modestly related to vaginal cancer risk and that even in women who had reported five or more sexual partners in a lifetime the risk of disease was only 1.4-fold increased. An early age of first intercourse was not found to be associated, and this was surprising given the consistency in the association of these factors with cervical cancer causation. However, in that study, women who reported a history of sexually transmitted diseases were found to be at excess risk of vaginal tumors and the effect was due mainly to the frequent reporting of genital warts. A more recent study by Hildesheim *et al.* (1997) clarified the place of sexually transmitted agents in the risk of vaginal neoplasia. They showed that in blood samples from patients with vaginal neoplasia, the presence of HPV 16 VLP antibodies invested the patient with a 3.5 increased risk of cervical neoplasia and those with high antibodies were at a 33-fold increased risk of disease. Likewise, lesser but increased risks were found with the presence of herpes simplex virus-II (HSV-II) and *chlamydia trachomatis* antibodies. They concluded that sexually transmitted agents played an important role in the etiology of vaginal neoplasia.

Bjorge *et al.* (1997) have also evaluated, by a prospective seroepidemiologic study, the role of HPV in non-cervical anogenital cancers in Finland and Norway. Analysing two large serum banks of 700 000 samples followed up for a mean of 8 years, they were able to show the odds ratio of developing non-cervical anogenital cancers by the presence of IgG antibodies to specific microorganisms was increased. Seropositivity for HPV 16 increased the risk of developing vulval and vaginal cancers by a factor of 4.5, and those seropositive for type 18 increased the risk of developing a preinvasive lesion of both vagina and vulva by a factor of 12. These data further support the role of HPV in the causation of vaginal neoplasia.

8.4 Clinical presentation

Vaginoscopy

Vaginoscopy is the magnified illumination of the vaginal mucosa using a colposcope. Before describing the vaginoscopic features of VAIN, it is important to stress the distribution of VAIN lesions within the vagina. The majority occur in the upper one-third, and the middle and lower thirds are involved by less than 10% of lesions. The majority are also multifocal (Hummer *et al.*, 1970). When found after a hysterectomy for CIN, they are usually associated with the folds at the vaginal vault in the 3- and 9-o'clock positions, the so-called dog ears.

Colposcopically, these lesions are usually acetowhite with sharp borders and a granular surface appearance. Occasionally, there is a fine punctation but mosaic or leukoplakic appearances are rarely found. Because of the loose nature of the vaginal mucosa, the contours of the actual lesions are irregular, making their diagnosis sometimes difficult. Vaginoscopy is carried out after the entire vaginal mucosa has been washed with a 5% acetic acid solution. Any excess fluid is wiped off, because the acetic acid causes a burning sensation in the vagina. The mucosal folds of the vagina do present difficulties and lesions may be obscured by prominent folds. When undertaking an examination, it is important to rotate the speculum with the blades fully opened through 360°, especially as it is withdrawn. It may be necessary for hooks to be used to expose those lesions that may be present within the vaginal vault area.

The application of Lugol's iodine solution is most important because VAIN lesions will usually stain light yellow and their sharp borders will be accentuated. Biopsies should be taken of any such lesion, although those present in the vault, especially when no cervix exists, cause problems because of the pain that is induced by sampling. The injection of local anesthetic before biopsy is important.

In postmenopausal patients, there is marked atrophy of the vaginal mucosa and interpretation may be difficult. Bleeding may occur as soon as the acetic acid is wiped onto the tissue, and an intense burning sensation may also be induced. The application of topical estrogen cream for up to 3 to 4 weeks before reexamination is recommended.

VAIN seen as an extension of the cervical atypical transformation zone

It is highly likely that most VAIN lesions in the upper vagina originate as an extension of a CIN lesion into the vaginal fornix. Minucci *et al.* (1995) have also shown that when VAIN existed, it was exactly the same pathologic type as a CIN lesion in 75% of cases. Nwabineli and Monaghan (1991) have shown that in some 2–2.5% of patients, abnormal (atypical) epithelium coexists in the cervix and upper vagina, and in 67% of these the lesions are confluent. This extension of the CIN lesion into the vaginal fornix will sometimes be difficult to diagnose, especially if there are redundant folds of vaginal skin covering the fornix. Figures 8.1–8.3 show examples of such lesions present in the vaginal fornix and associated with the cervical transformation zone. In Fig. 8.1, an area of acetowhite epithelium with a papillary surface is present at (1) high in the left vaginal fornix. It occurs in a 64-year-old woman in whom the cervical transformation zone is difficult to differentiate from the native cervical and vaginal epithelium. The canal is at (3) and the ectocervix at (2), and it has the same surface contour and configuration as the vaginal epithelium at (4). Initially, it would seem as though the abnormal (atypical) epithelium at (1) arose *de novo* in the vaginal fornix. However, displacement of the cervix to the patient's right side showed this area to be extensive and to occupy the lateral margins of the ectocervix, the vaginal vault, and a small part of the vaginal wall.

A similar case exists in Fig. 8.2, in which abnormal (atypical) epithelium (1) is likewise present in the left vaginal fornix. It originally was part of the atypical cervical trans-

formation zone, the lateral extension of which on the ectocervix can just be seen at (2). The endocervix is at (3) and vaginal epithelium at (4).

In Fig. 8.3, a very granular and acetowhite lesion (1) is present on the ectocervix and projects into the vaginal fornix. All the lesions demonstrated in Figs 8.1–8.3 have been proven by biopsy to be VAIN.

VAIN as seen in association with HPV lesions

VAIN is not uncommonly associated with subclinical papillomavirus infection (SPI) of the vagina. It may sometimes present diagnostic difficulties because of the exaggerated nature of the vaginal rugosity and of the papillary nature of the surface lesions. Examples are shown in Figs 8.4 and 8.5. In Fig. 8.4, an area of acetowhiteness with a papillary surface configuration is seen at (1); the ectocervix is at (2) and normal vaginal epithelium at (3). An obvious condylomatous lesion is seen at (4) and this may have the

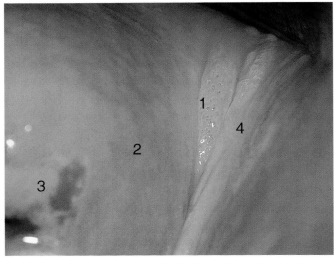

Fig. 8.1

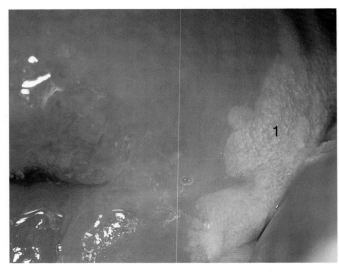

Fig. 8.3

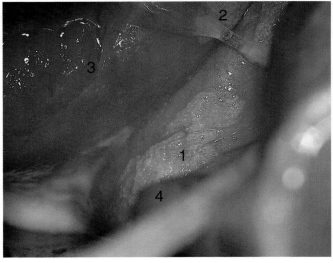

Fig. 8.2

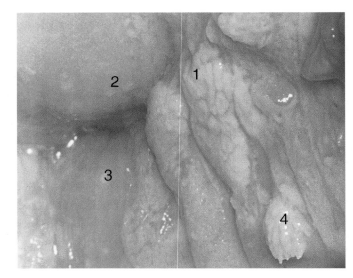

Fig. 8.4

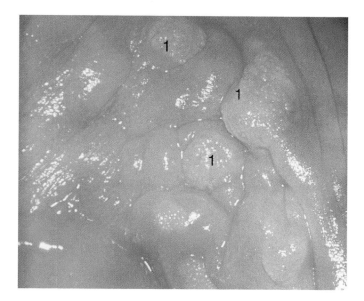

Fig. 8.5

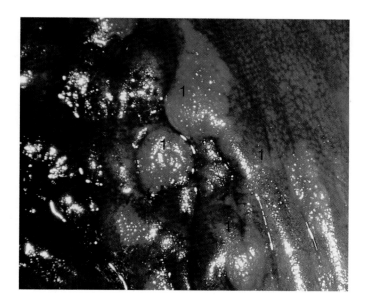

Fig. 8.6

same etiology as the lesion at (1), although punch biopsy of (1) shows it to be composed of a VIN 1/3 with evidence of HPV infection. Biopsy of (4) shows typical condylomatous features.

Figure 8.5 demonstrates the multifocal nature of VAIN. The three lesions labeled (1) also have a typical SPI configuration. Diagnosis without biopsy is impossible. Application of Lugol's iodine solution (Fig. 8.6) is of some help in differentiation. The partial uptake of the iodine stain by the lesion alerts the observer to the fact that this is of a lesser degree of epithelial atypia than major-grade lesions that possess a sharper border with more intense iodine-negative staining (see Fig. 8.8). Punch biopsy of the lesions stained with acetic acid in Fig. 8.5 and Lugol's iodine solution in Fig. 8.6 showed them to be of low-grade VAIN.

Vaginoscopy is essential to determine the distribution of VAIN within the vagina. The largest possible speculum should be used to perform the examination and should be repositioned frequently to allow inspection of all the mucosal surfaces. The examination of all four walls of the vagina, starting at the apex and working down to the introitus, should be carried out as separate and sequential steps. The speculum must be fully opened and rotated through a 360° circle, especially if the vaginal folds are prominent. The use of Q-tip swabs or hooks is also important in determining the position of the scattered multifocal loculi of VAIN.

Employment of such diagnostic aids can be seen in Fig. 8.7, where a Q-tip has been inserted between the lateral vaginal wall and the cervix. An acetowhite lesion with sharp borders and an obvious granular surface is seen on the side wall (1) with normal squamous vaginal epithelium at (2). The area of SPI is seen at (3). The Q-tip has been used to open up the area between the latter lesion and the abnormal (atypical) vaginal epithelium; if this had not been done,

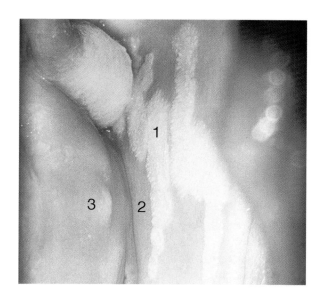

Fig. 8.7

the appearance would have suggested the extension of the cervical lesion onto the vaginal fornix. This would have prevented the full extent of the lesion becoming visible. The application of Lugol's iodine solution (Fig. 8.8) finally confirms the major-grade character of this lesion. The borders are sharp and no iodine has been taken up by the central area. A punch biopsy of this area can now be undertaken. However, it may be necessary to move the speculum down into the mid or lower vagina and retract the open blades, thereby allowing the mucosal folds, with the associated VAIN, to adopt a convex shape; in this situation, they are much easier to biopsy. When the VAIN lesion is "flattened," as in Fig. 8.7, it will be found that it is difficult to obtain a purchase upon the epithelium with the biopsy forceps, which will tend to slip off the surface. It is

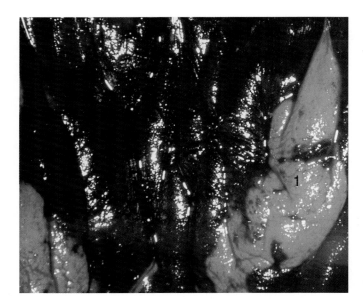

Fig. 8.8

therefore important to reposition the speculum, as described above.

8.5 VAIN following hysterectomy

VAIN following a hysterectomy for CIN is very uncommon; various authors quote between 1% and 3% as the prevalence of vaginal recurrence after hysterectomy when a similar lesion previously existed on the cervix. Some authors have quoted a higher frequency of this association; Ferguson and Maclure (1963) reported positive cytologic findings in 20% of patients previously treated for CIN. This large group, however, included invasive and in-situ cervical cancers that had been previously irradiated or removed by hysterectomy. Although the long-term recurrence rate for VAIN is uncertain, it is suggested by many authors that incomplete excision of the vaginal cuff at the time of hysterectomy for CIN may explain these early recurrences. The presence of such a lesion in the vaginal cuff area before 1 year after hysterectomy often represents a failure to diagnose and treat the vaginal component of cervical disease at the time of primary treatment; in many cases, histologic examination of the original uterine specimen reveals disease at the surgical margins (Mussey & Soule, 1959; Woodman et al., 1984).

Hoffmann et al. (1992) showed the propensity for the development of invasive vaginal cancer in women having had previous hysterectomy for cervical neoplasia. Thirty-one women had hysterectomy, of whom 25 had preexisting cervical neoplasia. Fourteen of them subsequently developed VAIN or vaginal HPV infection and all had upper vaginectomy. Surprisingly, nine were found to have invasive disease, four of a frankly invasive nature, and five with invasion to a depth of 2 mm. The authors concluded that upper vaginectomy was the treatment of choice for VAIN 3 diagnosed at the vaginal apex or in the region of the vaginal apex scar.

In a separate study Hoffman et al. (1989) have shown that the neoplastic process may be included within vaginal cuff inclusion cysts or sinuses. They showed that in 26 women who were treated for VAIN, 22 of whom had had a hysterectomy (15 for CIN 3 or cancer), five had a vaginal cuff inclusion cyst or sinus containing the neoplastic process; all of them eventually underwent upper vaginectomy as part of their treatment. Two of them were found to have an invasive squamous cell carcinoma of the vagina. It is stressed by the authors that any nodularity or distortion of the vaginal cuff is best treated by surgical excision, not only to treat the existing VAIN but also to discover any occult invasive cancer.

While most of these cases are diagnosed within a few years of surgery, a different pattern is seen in patients who have a history of previous radiotherapy. Palmer and Spratt (1956) reported an increased incidence of bowel, bladder, and vaginal cancer in patients who had received radiotherapy to the pelvis. They also found a higher rate of cancer in the group receiving lower doses of radiation. This raises the possibility that a sublethal dose of radiation, sufficient to cause cell damage but not cell death, may have been implicated in the etiology.

Preoperative colposcopy and staining of the upper vagina with Lugol's iodine solution should demonstrate the extension of any abnormal (atypical) cervical epithelium onto the vaginal fornix. This will allow a surgeon performing hysterectomy for CIN to determine accurately the amount of vaginal cuff to remove, whether the operation be by the abdominal or by the more preferable vaginal approach. Indeed, hysterectomy as a treatment for CIN is nowadays an uncommon event (see Chapter 7, p. 190).

Figure 8.9a shows a diagrammatic representation of the failure to evaluate preoperatively the extent of CIN. The vaginal angle clamp can be seen applied across an area of CIN that extends into the right vaginal fornix; obviously this extension had not been fully recognized preoperatively. The result is that residual disease is retained postoperatively in the angle of the vagina (Fig. 8.9b). It has been suggested that after these angle clamps are ligated, the vaginal vault should be left open, and mattress sutures should be avoided in the resuturing of the vault (Sharp & Saunders, 1990). Hemostasis is obtained by simply oversewing the vaginal edges. No prospective trial to evaluate the efficacy of this procedure has been undertaken.

Presentation after hysterectomy: value of cytology

A persistent abnormality in the vaginal smear will alert the gynecologist to the fact that residual disease exists. Vaginoscopy will therefore need to be undertaken. It must be remembered that postoperatively the vaginal vault usually contains recesses at the 3- and 9-o'clock positions; these may incorporate some abnormal (atypical) epithelium with residual disease. In the postmenopausal woman, it may be extremely difficult to visualize these recesses or "dog ears," and in such a case the procedure should be performed under a light anesthetic. Various ancillary aids,

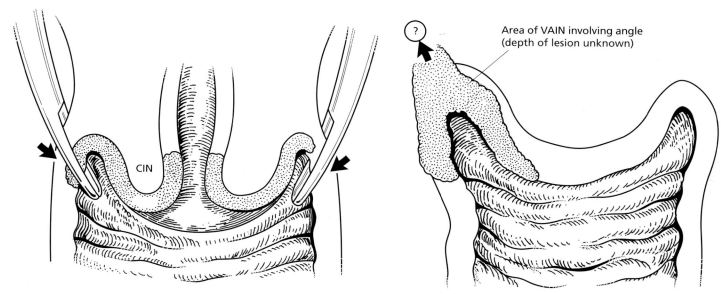

Fig. 8.9(a)

Fig. 8.9(b)

Area of VAIN involving angle (depth of lesion unknown)

such as a claw device or Desjardin's or Kogan's forceps, will need to be employed, as will the application of Lugol's iodine solution. It will also be important to take special note of those females who have an abnormal cytology following radiation for cervical carcinoma. According to DiSaia and Creasman (1989a), women treated in this way are at high risk of progression to invasive cancer of the vagina over a varying period of follow-up. The radiation changes induced within the vagina may be difficult to evaluate and multiple biopsies of any suspicious epithelium are mandatory.

In Figs 8.10–8.13a, the presence of VAIN is sought in a patient presenting with abnormal cytology 2 years after having a total abdominal hysterectomy for CIN 3. In Fig. 8.10, the vaginal vault recesses can be seen at (1) and (4) with the vaginal vault present in area (2). The recess on the patient's left is prominent, whereas that on the right is present initially as a longitudinal slit; this will need to be opened with Desjardin's forceps for a full examination. Normal squamous epithelium is present at that site but two small adjacent areas, marked (3) and (3), indicate the presence of focal acetowhite areas with sharp margins, suggesting the presence of major-grade disease. In Fig. 8.11, an examination of the left-hand recess has been undertaken. A small focal acetowhite lesion is visible at (1) with the vaginal vault at area (2). The further continuation of the recess is seen at (3). In Fig. 8.12, the right-hand recess has been opened and its upper extent can be seen at (1) with the vaginal vault epithelium at (2). Desjardin's forceps have been gently inserted into the recess, and in Fig. 8.13a these forceps have been opened wide and the base of the recess painted with Lugol's iodine solution. There is complete uptake of the iodine and therefore no abnormality exists at the apex of the recess. Obviously, excision biopsy of any abnormality found in this area is imperative.

A source of confusion in diagnosing possible VAIN arises with the presence of granulation tissue following hysterectomy. It can sometimes be difficult to differentiate, especially because of the abnormal vascularity existing in both

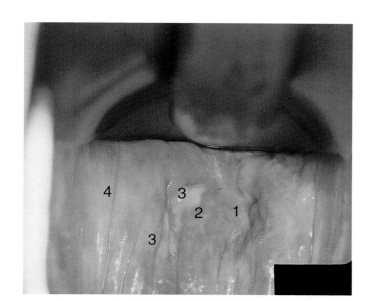

Fig. 8.10

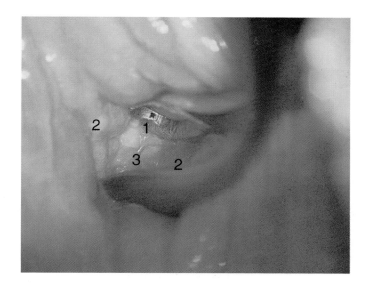

Fig. 8.11

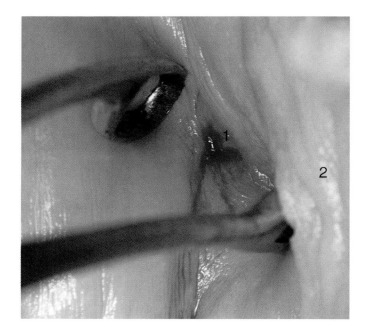

Fig. 8.12

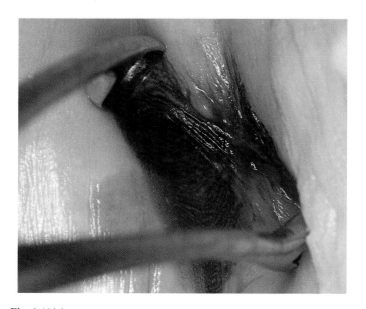

Fig. 8.13(a)

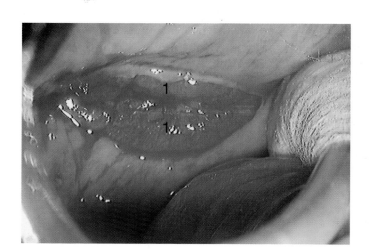

Fig. 8.13(b)

benign granulations and those associated with a poly-poidal type of VAIN. In Figs 8.13b and c, granulations developed in the vaginal vault (1) and angles (1) after abdominal hysterectomy in cases where persistent CIN made management difficult. Abnormal vessels (arrowed) can be seen in Fig. 8.13b and biopsy was essential in both cases to exclude the presence of neoplasia. However, in the case shown in Figs 8.13d and e, in a woman who had previously had four attempts at local destruction of a CIN 3 and who eventually had an abdominal hysterectomy, an area of

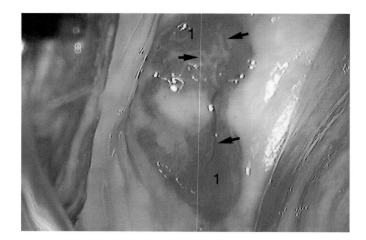

Fig. 8.13(c)

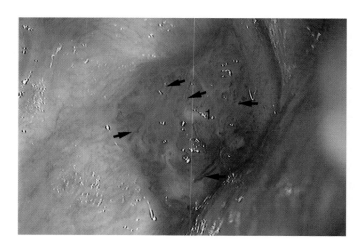

Fig. 8.13(d)

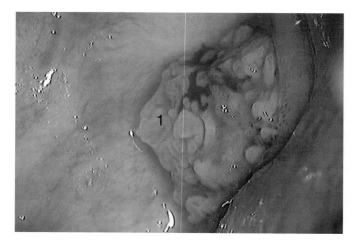

Fig. 8.13(e)

suspicious granulations (1) is seen in the left vaginal horn. In Fig. 8.13d, very abnormal vessels (arrowed) are seen and when acetic acid is applied, the vascularity is lost, but a dense acetowhiteness (1) develops in the tissue. Biopsy of these lesions showed the presence of VAIN with early invasion.

8.6 Biopsy of the VAIN lesion

Once the patient has been examined and the lesion defined, it is important to take a biopsy in order to produce tissue confirmation. From time to time in the patient who has had a previous hysterectomy and is postmenopausal, it will be difficult to gain access to the upper vagina. The use of acetic acid or iodine may produce further considerable discomfort to the patient because of the thinness and atrophic change in the vaginal skin. It is often worthwhile for the patient to use estrogen cream for 1 to 2 weeks before returning to the colposcopy clinic for a reexamination; by this time the vaginal skin will have markedly thickened. Sometimes, minor epithelial abnormalities will have disappeared and the major-grade VAIN lesions will be much easier to identify confidently and biopsy.

In the postmenopausal woman it may be extremely difficult to obtain an adequate cytologic sample of the vaginal vault epithelium because of marked atrophic changes; attempts to procure an adequate smear from this dry surface may induce bleeding, further obscuring and interfering with the cytologic specimen. In these cases, it is imperative to use estrogens in the form of cream instilled high into the vagina so that, after a few weeks, it will be possible and easier to obtain a satisfactory smear, and also to procure a punch biopsy.

The biopsy forceps used in the vagina are a matter of the clinician's personal preference. Mention has already been made of the need to readjust the vaginal speculum to make the mucosal surface and its accompanying abnormal (atypical) epithelium more accessible to the biopsy instrument. Such a situation can be seen in Fig. 8.14, where an Eppendorfer biopsy forceps is being used to remove an area of iodine-negative tissue (1) present high on the posterior vaginal wall (2). A full-thickness block of tissue can be satisfactorily removed and the pathologist is then able to identify any associated VAIN lesion. Bleeding of any significant degree is uncommon, and if it does occur then it can be easily stopped by the quick application of either silver nitrate or Monsell's solution (ferric subsulfate).

8.7 Pathology of VAIN: is it a precancerous lesion?

It is proposed that categories of histologic types of precancerous disease of the vagina be classified in a similar manner to those for CIN (Townsend, 1991). Mild dysplasia (VAIN 1) is characterized by the development of atypia in the lower third of the epithelial layer, whereas in moderate dysplasia (VAIN 2) the abnormality reaches into the upper third. In severe dysplasia and carcinoma-in-situ (CIS) (VAIN 3) there is full-thickness atypia that extends from the

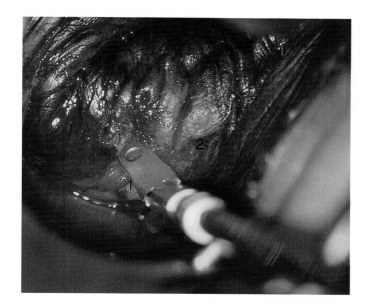

Fig. 8.14

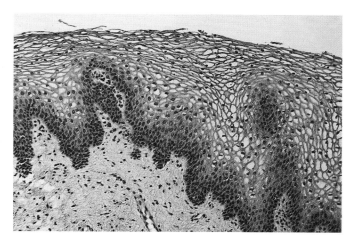

Fig. 8.15

basement membrane to the surface layer. The vaginal epithelium does not contain glandular skin appendages and therefore the diagnosis of these lesions presents very few problems to the pathologist.

It is important to recognize that the normal-appearing vaginal epithelium maturates and glycogenates as it differentiates (Fig. 8.15) and this is to be contrasted with the decrease in surface maturation that accompanies the increasing severity of the VAIN lesion. In Fig. 8.16, for example, a typical VAIN 3 lesion is seen with only a minimal amount of surface maturation and almost the entire thickness of the epithelium (1) is filled with atypical cells.

In Fig. 8.17, an area of frank invasive carcinoma of the vagina is seen in relation to a surface strip of a preexisting VAIN 3 (1). A pocket of invasion is seen deep within the stroma at (2).

The histologic diagnosis of VAIN 1 and VAIN 3 would seem to be straightforward, although there has been considerable discussion concerning the pathologic features and the malignant potential of VAIN 2. Its significance is therefore debatable. However, there seems to be no lack of evidence, both circumstantial and indirect, that VAIN 3 is

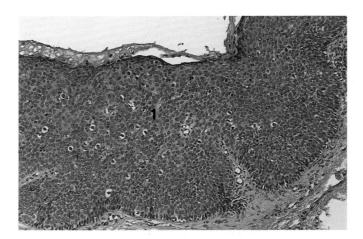

Fig. 8.16

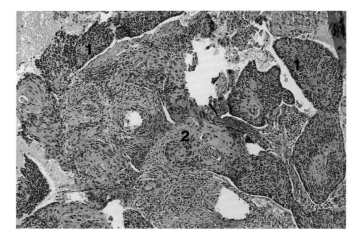

Fig. 8.17

indeed a precancerous condition (Gray & Christopherson, 1969; Murad *et al.*, 1975; Stuart *et al.*, 1981; Schmidt, 1987; Punnonen *et al.*, 1989; Brinton *et al.*, 1990). Such evidence includes the association with cervical and vulvar neoplasia, its occurrence after removal of a CIN lesion by hysterectomy, the similarities present in the pathology of VAIN and CIN which are identical except for the absence of glandular elements in VAIN lesion, and the association of HPV with VAIN (Bornstein *et al.*, 1988).

8.8 Vaginal precancer and cancer: part of the lower genital tract neoplastic syndrome

As has been discussed above, vaginal precancer and cancer is usually found in association with other malignancies in the anogenital tract. Vaginal carcinoma has been described in up to 8% of cases of vulvar carcinoma (Schmidt, 1987). However, these vaginal carcinomas are primary and satisfy the International Federation of Gynecology and Obstetrics (FIGO) criteria for the designation of the tumor as primarily vaginal. These criteria include the facts that the primary growth must be in the vagina, the cervix uteri is not involved, and there is no clinical evidence of metastatic disease. It has been proposed that the presence of these multiple precancers and cancers in the female anogenital tract should be classified as part of a lower genital tract

neoplastic syndrome (Schmidt *et al.*, 1982; Schmidt, 1987). The evidence suggests that there is a common neoplastic pathway involving these tissues and that this most likely involves the participation of HPV; these tumors all share a common origin in tissue developing from the urogenital sinus.

The occurrence of vaginal precancer in unusual hosts, such as those with immunosuppression (Simpkins & Hull, 1975), should also alert the clinician to the possibility of the coexistence of vaginal carcinoma.

Pathology

Primary vaginal malignancies may be of either a mixed epithelial, mesenchymal, or germ cell origin. The epithelial lesions are essentially those of the squamous cell type, but occasionally adenocarcinoma and melanomas may occur. Evidence suggests that squamous lesions arise from the VAIN lesions, which have been discussed above (Fig. 8.17). Their occurrence in women who have previously had hysterectomy is well documented. It would appear that vaginal malignancies arising from the primary VAIN appear at a later stage than those following CIN, i.e. posthysterectomy (Stuart *et al.*, 1981). This is usually because the latter group are submitted to intensive cytologic screening, whereas in the former group the occurrence *de novo* is essentially asymptomatic until symptoms of actual malignancy appear.

A case illustrating this is seen in Fig. 8.18a and b. The vaginal vault pictured is from a 46-year-old woman who had had an abdominal hysterectomy for CIN 3 some 3 years earlier. In Fig. 8.18a, colposcopy of the vaginal vault, in response to abnormal cytology, shows a dense area of acetowhite epithelium at (1), normal vaginal epithelium at (2), the vaginal fornices at (3), and the vaginal wall at (4). Some subepithelial hemorrhage and ulceration are already obvious in the vault and are associated with a punctate vascular pattern. Staining with Lugol's iodine solution, as seen in Fig. 8.18b, further suggests the presence of a major-grade lesion, in that the borders are sharp and iodine staining is not visible within the abnormal (atypical) area. Excision biopsy of this area revealed the presence of an early invasive carcinoma with infiltration to a depth of 4mm. In the case shown in Figs 8.18ci–iii, a similar early invasive lesion is seen in the vaginal vault some 4 years after a simple hysterectomy had been performed for microinvasive disease of the cervix. Dense acetowhite epithelium extends onto the anterior and posterior aspects of the upper third of the vagina (Fig. 8.18ci). Desjardin's forceps expose the apex of the vault (Fig. 8.18cii) within which can be seen epithelium containing abnormal vessels (Fig. 8.18ciii); biopsy of this epithelium revealed the presence of early invasive carcinoma.

The same situation can also be seen in the case shown in Fig. 8.18d; this woman had had microinvasive carcinoma of the cervix removed by cone biopsy some 3 years previously. Although the cervix (2) is free of disease, in the vaginal fornix at (1) there is an altered surface contour. There are small polypoid and papillary excrescences on the surface,

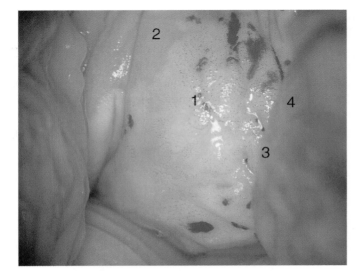

Fig. 8.18(a)

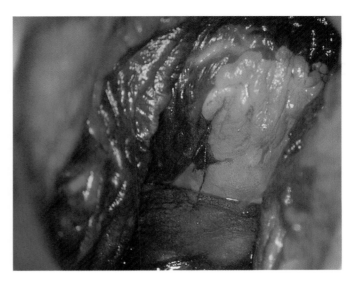

Fig. 8.18(b)

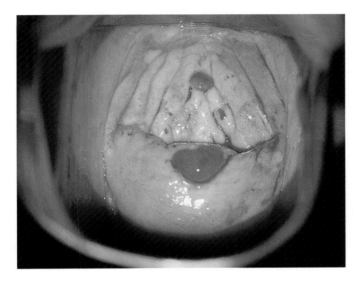

Fig. 8.18(ci)

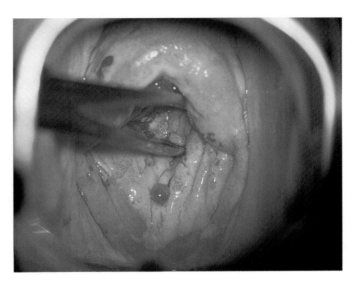

Fig. 8.18(cii)

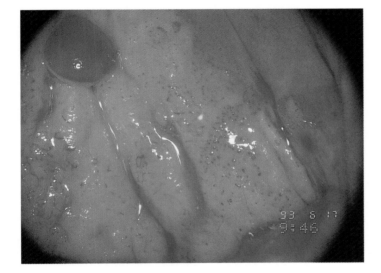

Fig. 8.18(ciii)

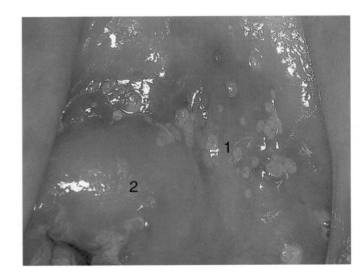

Fig. 8.18(d)

and excision biopsy confirmed the presence of early invasive carcinoma.

In Figs 8.19 and 8.20, vaginal carcinoma has appeared as ulcerative lesions in women who had had a hysterectomy for CIN 3 some 5 and 8 years beforehand. Neither patient had follow-up cytologic surveillance. In both, the ulcerative nature of the lesion (1) is made obvious by the characteristic raised border. Whelton and Kottmeier (1962) reported that more than half of the vaginal squamous carcinomas that they studied were ulcerated with raised borders and a penetrating lesion. In these lesions it is also helpful to apply Lugol's iodine stain to delineate the abnormal (atypical) epithelium; in Fig. 8.21 it is obvious that the stain has not been taken up by the central malignant area (1). In Figs 8.19–8.21 the vaginal fornix is at (2). An excision biopsy is necessary to confirm the diagnosis because, occasionally, especially in a premenopausal woman, a tampon-induced ulcer may be confused with an early ulcerative vaginal carcinoma.

Figure 8.22 shows a further vaginal carcinoma (1) in a deep recess of the vagina in a woman who had previously had a CIN lesion of the cervix removed by hysterectomy. This again shows the importance of examination of the vaginal vault recesses following hysterectomy.

In Whelton and Kottmeier's study, in 30% of vaginal cancers the lesions were mostly papillary and situated in the upper two-thirds of the posterior or lateral vagina. They emphasized that many of these lesions were small, soft, and easily missed by palpation. Hilgers (1978) also reported that lesions developed in the upper third of the vagina in about half the cases in his series; approximately 30% presented in the lower third and 20% in the middle third. The posterior vaginal wall is usually involved in 60% of cases, the anterior wall in 25%, and the lateral wall in about 15%.

Figure 8.23 is an operation specimen in which a radical hysterectomy and total vaginectomy had been performed on a female with neoplastic disease of the lower genital tract. A primary vaginal carcinoma is present at (1), but it is also obvious that there are further lesions of a lesser neoplastic nature present at (2) in the upper vagina. Some raised polypoid areas (3) exist within the vagina, and on biopsy showed not only HPV infection but also VAIN 3. CIN 3 was likewise present on the cervix (4). Vulvar in-situ

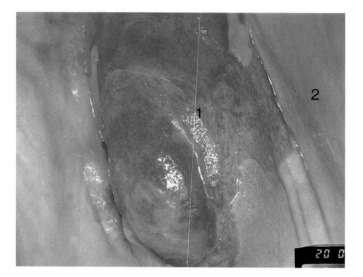

Fig. 8.20

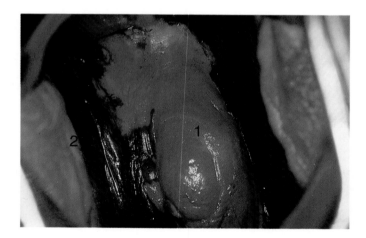

Fig. 8.21

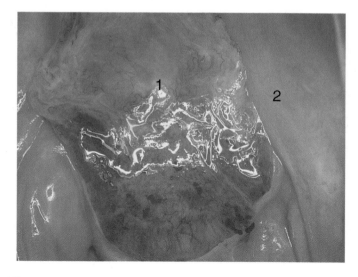

Fig. 8.19

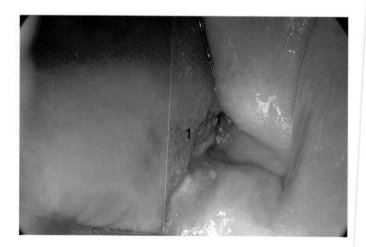

Fig. 8.22

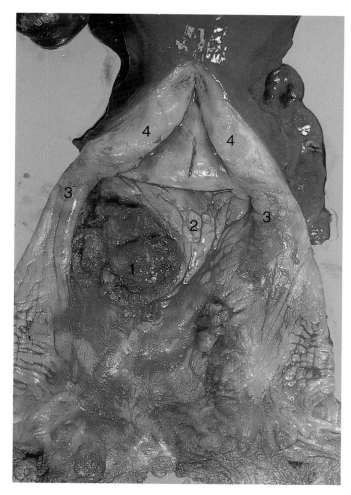

Fig. 8.23

carcinoma (VIN 3) was present at various sites; this woman has the condition that comes under the heading of the "lower genital tract neoplastic syndrome." Schmidt *et al.* (1982) reported on a large series; in which 27% of patients with primary malignant vulvar disease had one or more other primary tumors; 53.8% of these other malignant neoplasms arose within the reproductive system and 8.1% of these occurred as primary vaginal carcinomas.

Non-malignant lesions masquerading as vaginal neoplasia

There are a number of vaginal lesions that masquerade as neoplastic. It is only by using the colposcope and directed punch biopsy that their true nature can be determined and neoplasia excluded.

The lesions presenting this diagnostic dilemma are as follows.

1 The atrophic vaginal vault postradiotherapy.
2 Vaginal adenosis.
3 Extension of the cervical congenital transformation zone.
4 Ulceration caused by retained vaginal tampons.
5 Diethylstilbestrol (DES) changes in young women (see Chapter 11).

Appearances *postirradiation*, especially in the atrophic vagina, suggest the presence of vaginal carcinoma. Not

only can there be abnormal cytology as a result of the severe atrophic and postirradiation changes, but also colposcopically atypical and bizarre vessels are common. The thin white epithelium with its accompanying vasculature is extremely vulnerable to any trauma and this further complicates the diagnostic picture. Biopsy of any abnormal (atypical) epithelium or epithelium showing atypical vessels is mandatory to exclude the presence of invasive disease. Figure 8.24 shows the vaginal vault after irradiation for cervical carcinoma in a postmenopausal woman; the vessels show irregularity in caliber and branching and are not unlike those seen in invasive cancer. A punch biopsy of the area can be difficult to obtain and so it may be necessary to stabilize the tissue, using a claw device before a satisfactory biopsy can be taken.

Vaginal adenosis is defined as any condition in which columnar epithelium exists within the vagina. Colposcopic examination of most such areas shows them to be composed of either pure columnar or a mixed columnar and metaplastic epithelial tissue. Recently Dungar and Wilkinson (1995), studying the development of vaginal adenosis in women treated with topical 5-fluorouracil vaginal cream have found that columnar epithelium could develop on the vaginal surface where stratified squamous epithelium previously existed. Superficial vaginal glands (adenosis) were found to line the epithelium identical to the surface columnar epithelium of the cervix and they believe that these findings are consistent with evidence for a metaplastic process in which stratified squamous epithelium is replaced by columnar, representing columnar cell metaplasia or acquired vaginal adenosis. The areas that developed were unresolving, reddened areas in the upper third of the vagina and this was confusing for the clinician, who had initiated 5-fluorouracil vaginal therapy as a form of treatment for existing vaginal intraepithelial neoplasia.

Adenosis may be connected to the transformation zone or occur singly. In about 2–4% of females there is some extension of the typical transformation zone onto the vaginal vault (Kolstad, 1970; Nwabineli & Monaghan, 1991). However, metaplasia usually converts the glandular epithelium (present in these extensions into the vaginal fornix) to squamous epithelium, but in some cases where the vaginal vault is lax and the ability of the vaginal pH to penetrate these areas is limited, the result is that columnar epithelium may remain a purely mucus-producing area without undergoing metaplasia. Such an occurrence is shown in Fig. 8.25a, where the transformation zone is present at (1) and columnar and metaplastic squamous epithelium (2) extends to the lateral vaginal fornix at (3, and arrowed). A fold of the patulous vagina is at (4); this fold would normally cover the area at (2), thereby preventing the acid vaginal pH from initiating the conversion process. Without colposcopy and biopsy to confirm the benign nature of this tissue, this area appeared to be associated with a vaginal neoplasm.

The presence of isolated areas of vaginal adenosis within the vagina is uncommon, but when it occurs it may also be difficult to distinguish from primary vaginal carcinoma. Colposcopy with biopsy is indicated. A series of such lesions are illustrated in Fig. 8.25b–f.

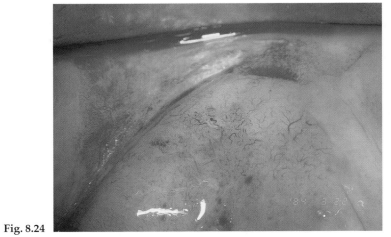

Fig. 8.24

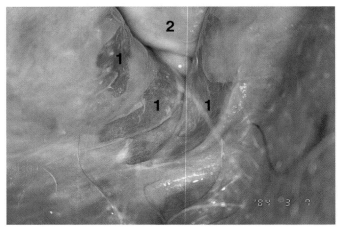

Fig. 8.25(ci)

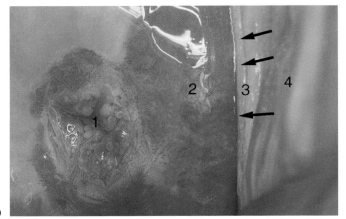

Fig. 8.25(a)

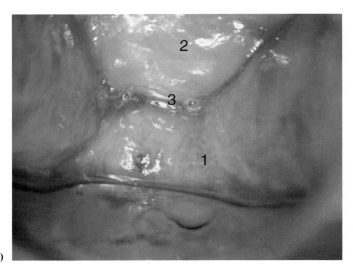

Fig. 8.25(b)

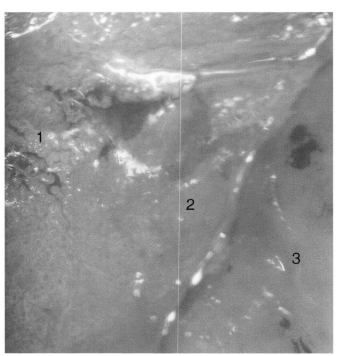

Fig. 8.25(d)

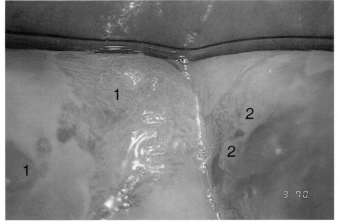

Fig. 8.25(ci)

Fig. 8.25(e)

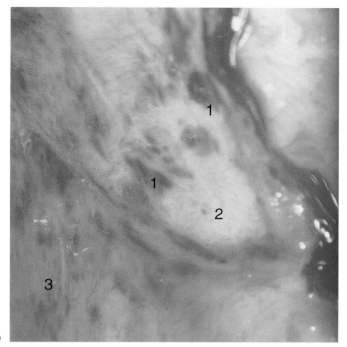

Fig. 8.25(f)

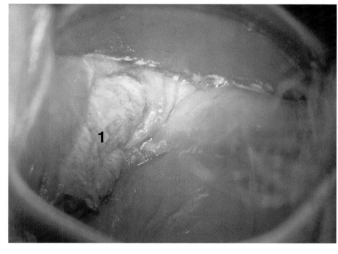

Fig. 8.25(g)

Fig. 8.25(h)

Fig. 8.25 (a) See text.

(b) Colposcopy of a 32-year-old woman, who presented with postcoital bleeding. An area of columnar epithelium exists at (1), at (2) is the anterior vaginal fornix and the cervix is at (3). This is an example of vaginal adenosis and only after colposcopy and biopsy was diagnosis possible.

(ci) A high-power view of area (1) in (b); this clearly shows villus-like structures extending across the posterior vaginal vault (1) and onto the lateral vaginal fornix at (2).

Biopsy confirms the benign nature of this tissue (cii) with columnar epithelium (1) on the vaginal surface where stratified epithelium would be expected. An extremely vascularized stroma exists at (2) with a small gland present in the stroma at (3).

(d) The vaginal introitus of a 30-year-old female who has vaginal adenosis (1) at the introitus. Such a situation is not uncommon and biopsy is indicated. Lichen planus and a neoplasm must be excluded, by such a biopsy. The anterior vaginal wall is at (2).

(e) Colposcopy of a 32-year-old woman, who presented with postcoital bleeding, showing a typical columnar epithelial area at (1) in the posterior vaginal vault. An area of metaplastic squamous epithelium is at (2) and the lateral side wall of the vagina at (3). Again, this area of vaginal adenosis could be confused with neoplasia. Its destruction, using the CO_2 laser, is shown in (f).

(f) The lesion of vaginal adenosis shown in (e), present within the posterior fornix, had been destroyed with the CO_2 laser 6 weeks earlier. The healing area is seen with new squamous epithelium at (1) and (2); the more mature of this new epithelium is at (2). The lateral vaginal wall is at (3). The CO_2 laser has effectively destroyed the diseased area in a safe manner. Glandular tissue may extend for 1–1.5 mm into the vaginal stroma. Visual identification of the glands during vaporization (seen as "bubbling" of the tissue) is necessary to ensure safe removal of the adenotic tissue. Follow-up at 4- to 6-week intervals after treatment is important so that adhesions may be broken down and constricture prevented.

Vaginal ulceration can obviously be caused by cancer (Figs 8.19, 8.20) but also by the retention of a tampon (Fig. 8.25g). Vaginal discharge with a pungent odor is not uncommon and after the tampon is removed, ulceration may be seen in Fig. 8.25h. It will take many weeks to heal, and more so in perimenopausal women. Biopsy is needed if any doubt exists as to the benign nature of this condition and reference has already been made to its differentiation from vaginal cancer in respect of Figs 8.19 and 8.20.

8.9 Treatment of VAIN

There are presently available a wide range of therapies to treat VAIN. Before any treatment is undertaken, the lesion will have been submitted to vaginoscopy and biopsy. The therapies available are as follows.

1 Local excision (biopsy).
2 Chemotherapy [intravaginal 5-fluorouracil (5FU)].
3 Physical destruction methods:
   (a) CO_2 laser.
   (b) cryosurgery.
   (c) electrocautery.

4 Radiation.

5 Major surgical procedures (partial vaginectomy, total vaginectomy with graft).

6 Conservative surgical removal.

It would seem prudent to treat only those lesions that have been diagnosed as VAIN 2 and/or 3. Lesser lesions, such as subclinical HPV and VAIN 1, are not considered to have a precancerous potential. An option would be to delay any active interference until after the initial biopsy results have been obtained, and to review at regular intervals.

Use of the CO_2 laser

For lesions that are localized and proven histologically to be VAIN 2 and/or 3, the CO_2 laser is a very efficient form of therapy (Townsend *et al.*, 1982; Stuart *et al.*, 1988; Volante *et al.*, 1992). Using low-power energy, i.e. about half that used on the cervix, the epithelium can be vaporized and removed to a depth of no more than 1 mm. The VAIN lesion is extremely shallow and does not penetrate any glandular structures, which are absent from the vagina. Prior to treatment, the lesion is injected with a local anesthetic mixture of 2% xylocaine; this acts as a protective buffer, preventing the laser beam from penetrating deeper than is necessary.

The CO_2 laser vaporization can be performed after this local anesthetic injection has been given or, if more extensive lesions are involved, a general anesthetic will be necessary. If this is the case, then saline can be used instead of local anesthetic to protect the underlying surface. Because of the irregular nature of the vaginal surface, the speculum has to be manipulated in both the horizontal and the vertical plane. Occasionally, the laser beam can be fired through the side openings of the speculum.

The outline of the lesion is marked by applying acetic acid followed by Lugol's iodine solution. The beam is passed quickly across the lesion and the depth of destruction can be measured visually. The correct depth has been reached when the straight fibers of the lamina propria of the vagina are visible (Fig. 8.27). In Fig. 8.26, a multifocal lesion, defined by Lugol's iodine solution, is present on the posterior vaginal wall (1); biopsy has revealed its nature as VAIN 2 and 3 with wart viral changes. This type of multifocal lesion is ideal for CO_2 laser vaporization, and in Fig. 8.27 such a procedure is being undertaken. The CO_2 laser has been used to evaporate the tissue to a depth of approximately 1 mm. The lesion has been outlined and vaporization has left carbon particles in the region of the vaporized epidermis (1). Gentle wiping has removed them at (2), allowing the underlying straight fibers of the lamina propria to be seen. The epithelial bridges of normal vaginal squamous tissue (3), which should be preserved, provide the vehicle from which epithelial regeneration will occur.

Two large studies have attested to the efficacy of using CO_2 laser vaporization for VAIN. Stuart *et al.* (1988) treated to a depth of some 2–3 mm in 27 women and noted a 78% success rate after one or two treatments. Volante *et al.* (1992)

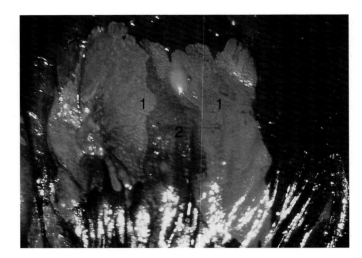

Fig. 8.26

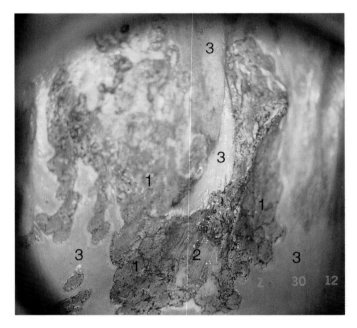

Fig. 8.27

described 334 patients treated with the CO_2 laser, none of whom subsequently developed invasive disease.

Partial vaginectomy

A partial vaginectomy is the universal recommendation (Ireland & Monaghan, 1988; Hoffman *et al.*, 1992) for treatment of VAIN lesions in the vault in cases where hysterectomy has been performed for cervical CIS. This operation can be performed either *per vaginam* or *per abdomen*, but does carry with it an appreciable morbidity. Extensive removal will also lead to shortening and narrowing of the vagina.

A number of studies have recently been published concerning the use of surgery in the form of upper vaginectomy for in-situ, occult or superficially invasive disease of the vagina (Ireland & Monaghan, 1988; Hoffman *et al.*, 1992). Hoffman and co-worker's study (Hoffman *et al.*, 1992) is described above and the recommendation of this group is that upper vaginectomy is necessary following the diagnosis of occult invasive carcinoma of the vagina, and for the treatment of VAIN 3 and superficially invasive carcinoma. In a previous study, Hoffman *et al.* (1989) describe the finding of the vaginal cuff inclusion cysts and recommend again that upper vaginectomy be used to remove such cysts and associated sinuses.

Local excision

Small areas of VAIN 3 are ideal for local excision using the CO_2 laser. This can be done either under local anesthesia, as described, or, where there are larger areas, under a general anesthetic. Sherman (1990) describes local treatment with the CO_2 laser for 143 patients who were diagnosed as having focal lesions containing VAIN. He describes a technique in which needles are inserted into the vaginal mucosa and fluid is subsequently introduced into the underlying submucosal areas, thereby allowing ballooning of the recesses and the scar tissue in that area. Furthermore, it positions the vaginal mucosa at right angles to the laser beam.

It has been the author's (AS) preference to use a local excision technique in cases where fully visualized residual VAIN 3 exists in the vaginal vault after an abdominal hysterectomy has been carried out for cervical CIN 3. An example of such a case is shown in Fig. 8.28. A postmenopausal woman presented, 5 years after an abdominal hysterectomy for cervical CIN 3, with a localized patch of VAIN 3 (1) that extended into the vaginal vault (2, and arrowed); the lateral margin of the area could not be outlined at the initial inspection. However, this margin can be seen if the claw device as seen in Fig. 8.30, is used to retract the area in a medial direction. Once this has been done, then the area can be locally resected using the CO_2 laser; this technique is described below.

The full extent of the lesion must be assessed beforehand. This involves a detailed viewing of the vaginal vault folds that exist in the 3- and 9-o'clock positions, seen at (2) and (2) in Fig. 8.29, which shows the situation in a patient who has had a hysterectomy. In this case, an area of a minor-grade nature exists at (1) but there has been no extension into the vault. The lateral vaginal walls are at (3). However, in another case (Fig. 8.30 and the high-power view of this lesion in Fig. 8.31) an area of VAIN 3 (1) is seen to extend into the vaginal vault. Using a three-pronged claw (2) to effect downward retraction in the line of the arrow, its right lateral margin can be easily seen in Figs 8.30 and 8.31; its extension into the left fornix is also made easier to view by using another claw device (3). This area is suitable for local excision.

Local excision of vaginal vault lesions

Local excision may be used to remove lesions in the vaginal vault, like those seen in Figs 8.28–8.31. In the sequence shown in Figs 8.32–8.34, an area of histologically confirmed VAIN 3 (1) within the vaginal vault of a 54-year-old woman, 4 years after abdominal hysterectomy for CIN 3,

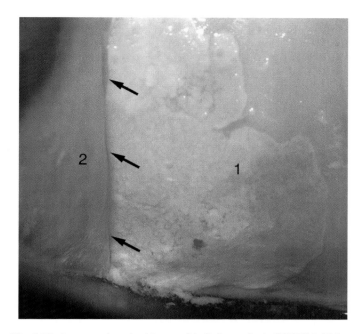

Fig. 8.28 An area of vaginal intraepithelial neoplasia (VAIN) 3 (1) in the vault of a patient who had had an abdominal hysterectomy for cervical carcinoma in situ (CIS) 5 years previously. The lateral margin (arrowed) was not visible initially, but downward retraction with a claw device exposed its full extent. The lateral vaginal wall in this postmenopausal woman is at (2).

has been outlined with Lugol's iodine solution (Fig. 8.32). Its extension into the lateral vaginal folds has been excluded.

Using the super pulse mode of the CO_2 laser (utilizing power densities of 750–1200 W/cm²), an incision is made around the abnormal area to a depth of about 2–3 mm. A three-pronged claw device (see Fig. 8.30) is then used to retract the outlined area in a medial (Fig. 8.33) and then lateral direction; the laser beam undercuts the area to be removed. Beforehand, saline is injected underneath the area to "cushion" the tissue and prevent the beam from deeper penetration. With strong retraction, it is possible to accomplish this "skinning" procedure with minimal blood loss. After removal of the diseased tissue, the area (1) is left open (Fig. 8.34) and the patient given antibiotics. Within 6 weeks the excised area has regained epithelium from the adjoining vaginal mucosa. Regular vaginal dilatation is encouraged to prevent any shortening or narrowing and ensure that the resultant vagina is pliable with minimal constriction. Regular observation at 6- to 8-week intervals for up to 6 months is recommended.

A full and detailed inspection must be made of the removed specimen; indeed, the examination should be regarded as though it was of a cervical cone biopsy specimen. This technique of local excision is essentially a large excision biopsy; the CO_2 laser allows very accurate removal of the abnormal tissue and its use should be considered as an alternative to more radical forms of therapy, such as partial vaginectomy and radiation (DiSaia & Creasman, 1989a; Hoffman *et al.*, 1989, 1992). Any finding of early invasive disease within the removed specimen will necessitate more radical forms of therapy. Obviously, the finding of

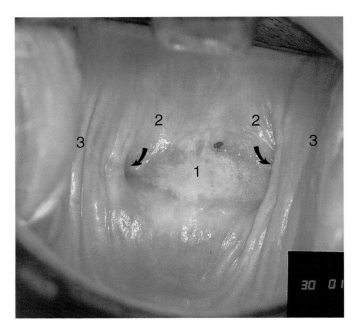

Fig. 8.29 A small area of minor-grade disease in the vaginal vault (1) with no extension into the vaginal horns (2, and arrowed). The vaginal wall is at (3). Because of the minor nature of this lesion (i.e. vulvar intraepithelial neoplasia (VIN) 1) no further treatment was undertaken, except regular surveillance using exfoliative cytology. The cytologic report indicated minor- (low-) grade disease but if any major-grade cytologic changes developed, then further examination and probable biopsy of this area would be required.

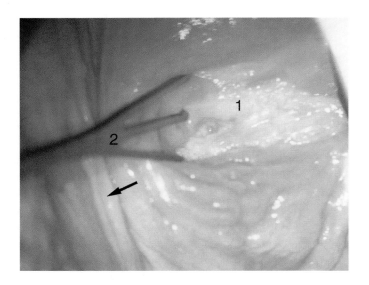

Fig. 8.30 Localized area of vaginal intraepithelial neoplasia (VAIN) 3 (1) in the vaginal vault of a female who had had a total abdominal hysterectomy for cervical intraepithelial neoplasia (CIN) 3. A three-pronged clawed device (2) is used to retract the right vaginal wall downward (arrow); this outlines the right lateral margin of the VAIN 3.

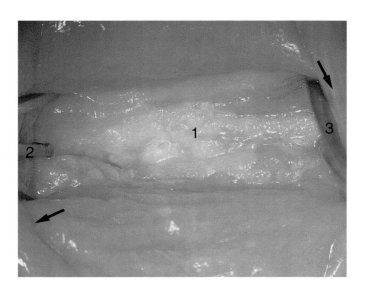

Fig. 8.31 A high-power view of Fig. 8.30, showing a patch of vaginal intraepithelial neoplasia (VAIN) 3 (1); two claw devices (2) and (3) are stretching the vault (in the direction indicated by the arrows). The full extent of the lesion in both vaginal folds is shown.

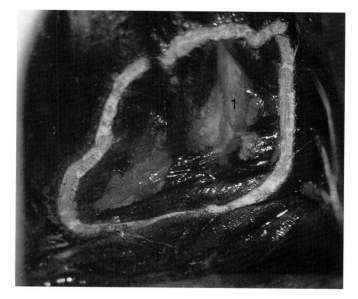

Fig. 8.32

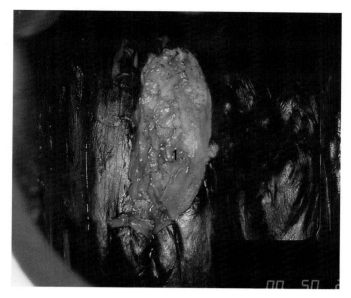

Fig. 8.34

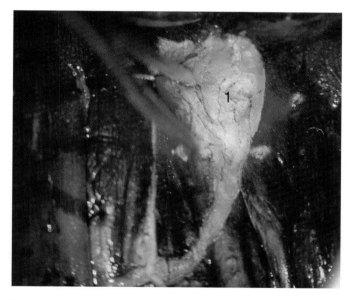

Fig. 8.33

incomplete removal would require frequent follow-up or, possibly, further more extensive removal.

This technique of partial laser vaginectomy has been successfully used by the author (AS) on 22 women over a 9-year period. In one case, early invasive cancer (less than 2 mm) was found but in all the others VAIN 3 was confirmed. To date, recurrence has occurred in four cases and all have been VAIN 3. Two inadvertent entries were made to the Pouch of Douglas, which healed spontaneously and no other complications were noted. Julian *et al.* (1992) have performed a similar procedure on 10 women, producing a low rate of complications with excellent healing. In their series, there were four women in whom invasive squamous cell carcinoma was diagnosed; in one, a recurrent squamous cell carcinoma of the cervix was found that was not diagnosed until the laser opened the upper vaginal vault and demonstrated the previously unseen cervix.

The alternative procedure to the one described above is

vaginectomy (Feroze, 1991). It is usually followed by vaginal restoration with a split-thickness skin graft, either immediately or after a few days. This is an extremely difficult operation to undertake; there is appreciable morbidity and a risk of the shortening and narrowing of the vagina.

8.10 References

Benedet, J.L. & Sanders, B.H. (1984) Carcinoma in situ of the vagina. *Am J Obstet Gynecol* **148**,695.

Benedet, J.L., Murphy, K.J., Fairey, R.N. & Boyes, D.A. (1983) Primary invasive carcinoma of the vagina. *Obstet Gynecol* **62**,715.

Bjorge, T., Dilner, J., Antilla, T., Ingerland, A. & Thoresen, S. (1997) Prospective sero-epidemiological study of role of human papillomavirus in non-cervical ano-genital cancer. *BMJ* **315**,646.

Bornstein, J., Kaufman, R.H., Adam, E. & Adler-Storthz, K. (1988) Multicentric intraepithelial neoplasia involving the vulva. Clinical features and association with human papillomavirus and herpes simplex virus. *Cancer* **62**(8),1601.

Brinton, L.A., Nasca, P.C., Mallin, K. & Richart, R.M. (1990) A case control study of in-situ and invasive carcinoma of the vagina. *Gynecol Oncol* **38**(1),49.

Cramer, D. & Cutler, S. (1974) Incidence and histopathology of malignancies of the female genital organs in the United States. *Am J Obstet Gynecol* **118**,443.

Daling, J.R. & Sherman, K.J. (1992) Relationship between human papillomavirus infection and tumours of anogenital sites other than cancer. In: Munoz, N., Bosch, F.X., Shah, K.V. & Meheus, A. (eds) *The Epidemiology of Cervical Cancer and Human Papillomavirus*, p. 223. International Agency for Research on Cancer, Lyon.

DiSaia, P. & Creasman, W.T. (1989a) Invasive cancer of the vagina and urethra. In: DiSaia, P. & Creasman, W. (eds) *Clinical Gynecologic Oncology*, p. 273. CV Mosby & Co., St Louis.

DiSaia, P. & Creasman, W.T. (1989b) Pre-invasive disease of the cervix, vagina and vulva. In: DiSaia, P. & Creasman, W. (eds) *Clinical Gynecologic Oncology*, p. 33. CV Mosby & Co., St Louis.

DiSaia, P.J., Morrow, C.P. & Townsend, D.E. (1975) *Synopsis of Gynaecologic Oncology*. Wiley, New York.

Dungar, C.F. & Wilkinson, E.J. (1995) Vaginal columnar cell metaplasia. An acquired adenosis associated with topical 5-fluorouracil therapy. *J Reprod Med* **40**(5),361.

Ferguson, J.H. & Maclure, J.G. (1963) Intraepithelial carcinoma dysplasia and exfoliation of cancer cell in the vaginal mucosa. *Am J Obstet Gynecol* **87**,326.

Feroze, R. (1991) Radical vaginal operations. In: Coppleson, M. (ed.) *Gynaecological Oncology*, 2nd edn, p. 1201. Churchill Livingstone, Edinburgh.

Gray, L.A. & Christopherson, W.M. (1969) In situ and early invasive carcinoma of the vagina. *Obstet Gynecol* **34**,226.

Hilgers, R.D. (1978) Squamous cell carcinoma of the vagina. *Surg Clin N Am* **58**(1),25.

Hildesheim, A., Han, C.L., Brinton, L., Schiller, J.T. *et al.* (1997) Sexually transmitted agents and risk of carcinoma of the vagina. *Int J Gynecol Cancer* **7**,251.

Hoffman, M.S., De Cesare, S.L., Roberts, W.S. *et al.* (1992) Upper vaginectomy for in-situ and occult superficially invasive carcinoma of the vagina. *Am J Obstet Gynecol* **166**(1),30.

Hoffman, M.S., Roberts, W.S., La Polla, J.P. & Kavanagh, D. (1989) Neoplasia in vaginal cuff epithelial inclusion cysts after hysterectomy. *J Reprod Med* **34**(6),412.

Hummer, W.K., Mussey, E., Decker, D.G. & Docherty, M.B. (1970) Carcinoma in situ of the vagina. *Am J Obstet Gynecol* **108**,1109.

Ireland, D. & Monaghan, J.M. (1988) The management of patients with abnormal vaginal cytology following hysterectomy. *Br J Obstet Gynaecol* **95**,973.

Julian, T.M., O'Connell, B.J. & Gosewehr, J. (1992) Indications, techniques and advantages of partial laser vaginectomy. *Obstet Gynecol* **80**(1),140.

Kleinerman, R.A., Boice, J.D., Storm, H.H. *et al.* (1995) Secondary primary cancer after treatment for cervical cancer—an International Cancer Registry Study. *Cancer* **76**,442.

Kolstad, P. (1970) Diagnosis and management of precancerous lesions of the cervix uteri. *Int J Obstet Gynecol* **8**,551.

Lee, R.A. & Symmonds, R.E. (1976) Recurrent carcinoma in situ of the vagina in patients previously treated for in-situ carcinoma of the cervix. *Obstet Gynecol* **48**,61.

Minucci, D., Cineal, A. & Oselladore, M. (1995) Epidemiological aspects of vaginal intra-epithelial neoplasia (VAIN). *Clin Exper Obstet Gynecol* **22**(1),36.

Murad, T.M., Durant, J.R. & Maddox, W.A. (1975) The pathologic behaviour of primary vaginal cancer and its relationship to cervical cancer. *Cancer* **35**,787.

Mussey, E. & Soule, E.H. (1959) Carcinoma in situ of the cervix. A clinical review of 842 cases. *Am J Obstet Gynecol* **77**,957.

Nwabineli, N.J. & Monaghan, J.M. (1991) Vaginal epithelial abnormality in patients with CIN: clinical and pathological features and management. *Br J Obstet Gynaecol* **98**(1),25.

Palmer, J.P. & Spratt, D.W. (1956) Pelvic carcinoma following irradiation for benign gynecological diseases. *Am J Obstet Gynecol* **72**,497.

Punnonen, R., Kallioniemi, O.P., Matill, J., Vayrynen, M. & Koivula, T. (1989) Primary invasive and in situ vaginal carcinoma. Flow-cytometric analysis of DNA aneuploidy and cell proliferation from archival paraffin-embedded tissue. *Eur J Obstet Gynecol Reprod Biol* **32**(3),247.

Romeo, R., Silento, N., Maffie, G. *et al.* (1990) Primary carcinoma of the vagina: case report. *Eur J Gynecol Oncol* **11**,481.

Rose, P.G., Heterick, E., Boutselis, J. & Sacks, L. (1987) Multiple primary gynaecological neoplasms. *Am J Obstet Gynecol* **157**,261.

Rutledge, F. (1967) Carcinoma of the vagina. *Am J Obstet Gynecol* **97**,635.

Schmidt, W.A. (1987) Pathology of the vagina. In: Fox, H. (ed.) *Obstetric and Gynaecologic Pathology* Vol. 3, p. 147. Churchill Livingstone, Edinburgh.

Schmidt, W.A., Mussman, M.G. & Edwards, C.L. (1982) Vulvar malignancy associated with multiple primary cancers. *Lab Investigation* **46**,73.

Sharp, F. & Saunders, N. (1990) The treatment of vaginal precancer. *Clin Prac Gynaecol* **2**(2),211.

Sherman, A.I. (1990) Laser therapy for vaginal intraepithelial neoplasia after hysterectomy. *J Reprod Med* **30**(10),941.

Simpkins, P.B. & Hull, M.G. (1975) Intraepithelial vaginal neoplasia following immunosuppressive therapy treated with topical 5-FU. *Obstet Gynecol* **46**,360.

Stuart, G.C., Allen, H.H. & Anderson, R.J. (1981) Squamous cell carcinoma of the vagina following hysterectomy. *Am J Obstet Gynecol* **139**,311.

Stuart, G.C., Flagler, E.A., Nation, J.G. & Duggan, M. (1988) Laser vaporisation of vaginal intraepithelial neoplasia. *Am J Obstet Gynecol* **158**(2),240.

Townsend, D.E. (1991) Intraepithelial neoplasia of the vagina. In: Coppleson, M. (ed.) *Gynaecological Oncology*, p. 493. Churchill Livingstone, Edinburgh.

Townsend, D.E., Levine, V., Crum, C.P. & Richart, R.M. (1982) Treatment of vaginal carcinoma in situ with the CO_2 laser. *Am J Obstet Gynecol* **43**,565.

Volante, E.R., Pisero, L. & Saraceno, L. (1992) Carbon dioxide laser surgery in colposcopy for cervico-vaginal intraepithelial neoplasia treatment. Ten-year experience and failure analysis. *Eur J Gynecol Oncol* **13**(1),78.

Whelton, J.J. & Kottmeier, H.L. (1962) Primary carcinomas of the vagina. *Acta Obstet Gynecol Scand* **41**,22.

Woodman, C.B.J., Jordan, J.A. & Wade-Evans, T. (1984) The management of vaginal intraepithelial neoplasia after hysterectomy. *Br J Obstet Gynaecol* **91**,707.

Chapter 9
Vulvar Intraepithelial Neoplasia

9.1 Introduction

The concept of intraepithelial neoplasia of the vulva has been with us since its description in the early part of this century. In recent years there has developed an increasing awareness of the characteristics of vulvar intraepithelial neoplasia (VIN) as more information on the epidemiology, pathology and clinical management has come to light. One of the most important developments of recent years has been the introduction of a revised classification of the condition, as a result of the 1987 recommendations of the committee on nomenclature of the International Society for the Study of Vulvar Diseases (ISSVD) (Table 9.1). This was confirmed by the committee on histological classification of vulvar tumors and dystrophies of the International Society of Gynaecological Pathologists (ISGYP). These august bodies recommend use of the term VIN to replace the very wide range of somewhat confusing terms that have been used in the past; these include Bowen's disease, leukoplakia, Bowenoid papulosis, squamous cell carcinoma-in-situ, and hyperplastic dystrophy (Ridley, 1989; Ridley et al., 1989a,b).

VIN is characterized in a similar way to its cervical counterpart, cervical intraepithelial neoplasia (CIN), in that it is made up of neoplastic cells that are confined by the boundaries of the epithelium. It is also recognized that VIN may, if untreated, progress to invasive cancer of the vulva, but, conversely, it has been known to regress spontaneously (discussed in detail below).

The broad similarity with CIN is maintained by division into three grades: VIN 1 is equivalent to mild dysplasia; VIN 2 to moderate dysplasia; and VIN 3 to severe dysplasia and carcinoma-in-situ (CIS). In recent years there has developed considerable interest in the role of the human papillomavirus (HPV) and its effects on and relationships to VIN. It would appear, however, that viral integration and the development of aneuploidy is essential for the progression of VIN toward an invasive carcinoma (Friedrich et al., 1980; Buscema et al., 1988; Kaufman et al., 1988; Pilotti et al., 1990; Rusk et al., 1991; Li Vigni et al., 1992). Similar attempts are being made in the field of VIN, as have been made in respect of CIN, to try to identify high- and low-grade lesions, that is, to identify those lesions with an increased or reduced risk of progression (Ferenczy, 1992).

The term VIN 3 or, as it was previously called "squamous cell carcinoma-in-situ" has been described by a variety of terms including Bowen's disease, erythroplasia of Queyrat,

carcinoma-in-situ simplex and squamous cell carcinoma-in-situ. It was believed that each one of these conditions had its own characteristic histopathology and that biologically they acted differently from one another (Abell & Gosling, 1961). However, it was Woodruff and Hildebrand in 1958 who insisted that there were no variations in histologic features between any of the types mentioned above, but that variations could occur in different areas of a single lesion. Thus, all the above terms are now grouped together as VIN 3, although recently, there has been a trend to call some pigmented lesions Bowenoid papulosis or Bowenoid dysplasia (Kaufman & Faro, 1994). It is suggested that Bowenoid papulosis or Bowenoid dysplasia are virally induced with no malignant potential and often spontaneously regress, although it is difficult morphologically to distinguish these essentially clinical descriptive types of in-situ epithelial change from VIN 3. Kaufman and Faro insist that they all must be "looked upon in the same light as VIN 3" (Kaufman & Faro, 1994).

9.2 Epidemiology and pathogenesis

Prevalence and incidence

It is difficult to be certain of the prevalence or incidence of VIN in a population because, to date, there have been no organized screening programs for the indentification of this condition. There is a general impression among all clinicians in the field that there has been an increase in both prevalence and incidence in recent years. As a result of a review of various cancer registries in the USA, Sturgeon et al. (1992) have recently found that the incidence rate of in-situ vulvar cancer nearly doubled between 1973 and 1976 and 1985 and 1987, whereas the rate of invasive squamous cell carcinoma remained stable. They felt that the possible reasons for this discordance could be related to the fact that women affected by the "sexual revolution" are not yet old enough to have invasive cancer, or that the early diagnosis and treatment of CIS has mitigated the anticipated increases in invasive vulvar carcinoma incidence. It could also be that in-situ and invasive carcinomas of the vulva have different causation, with the sexually transmitted HPV involved in the etiology of CIS and other factors involved with most invasive squamous cell carcinomas.

Other authors have also noted an increase in intraepithelial disease. Iverson and Tretli (1998), analyzing time trends in incidence of intraepithelial and invasive vulvar neopla-

Table 9.1 International Society for the Study of Vulvar Diseases (ISSVD) and International Society of Gynaecological Pathologists (ISGYP*) classification.

Non-neoplastic epithelial disorders of vulvar skin and mucosa
Lichen sclerosus (LS)
Squamous cell hyperplasia (formerly hyperplastic dystrophy)
Other dermatoses

Mixed epithelial disorders may occur. In such cases it is recommended that both conditions be reported. For example: LS with associated squamous cell hyperplasia (formerly classified as mixed dystrophy) should be reported as LS and squamous cell hyperplasia. Squamous cell hyperplasia with associated vulvar intraepithelial neoplasia (VIN) (formerly hyperplastic dystrophy with atypia) should be diagnosed as VIN.

Squamous cell hyperplasia is used for those instances in which the hyperplasia is not attributable to another cause. Specific lesions or dermatoses involving the vulva (e.g. psoriasis, lichen planus, lichen simplex chronicus, *Candida* infection, condyloma acuminata) may include squamous cell hyperplasia but should be diagnosed specifically and excluded from this category.

VIN
Squamous intraepithelial neoplasia
    VIN 1 (mild dysplasia)
    VIN 2 (moderate dysplasia)
    VIN 3 (severe dysplasia or carcinoma-in-situ)
    VIN 3 differentiated type, basaloid, Bowenoid (warty)

Nonsquamous intraepithelial neoplasia
    Paget's disease
    Melanoma level 1

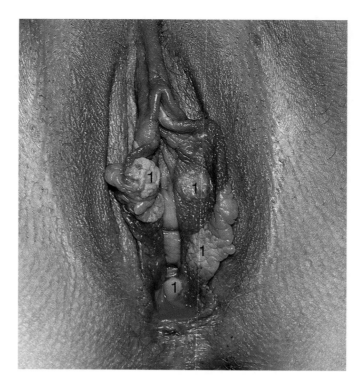

Fig. 9.1

sia and the transition of intraepithelial neoplasia to cancer in Norway, found that the incidence rate of intraepithelial neoplasia increased threefold from 1973–77 to 1988–92 and 3.4% changed into invasive disease. Multivariate analyses identified age as a significant variable and the age adjusted incidence rate for squamous cell cancer was constant for the whole period. The 5-year survival rates have not changed significantly over the period studied. They concluded that age was a strong prognostic factor showing an excess death rate by increasing age.

The stationary invasive cancer rate in respect of the rise in premalignant rate may be explained by the fact that transformation of HPV infection into malignant disease might take years if a long latency period is necessary. Other explanations offered might be that the two diseases have different etiologies as suggested by Sturgeon *et al.* (1992) or that HPV preinvasive lesions very seldom develop into invasive cancer, but remain as an in-situ lesion or, indeed, disappear. However, in the Iverson (1998) study, in-situ lesions were found to have a malignant potential because 3.4% progressed to cancer and this is exactly the same as previous reports by Iverson *et al.* (1981); these were in spite of surgical treatments. This is certainly evidence that in-situ lesions (VIN 3) can progress to invasive cancer.

Association between VIN and CIN

The association between VIN and CIN is close. Multicentric disease of the cervix and vulva, and occasionally of the vagina, is commonly found by clinicians. This pattern of multicentric disease is well demonstrated (Figs 9.1 & 9.2). In Fig. 9.1, a 48-year-old woman had not only VIN 3 (1) but also similar intraepithelial disease of both the cervix and the vagina. The 27-year-old female whose vulvar and perianal area is pictured in Fig. 9.2 had both intraepithelial and early invasive disease (microcarcinoma) affecting the cervix, vagina, and vulvar (1) and perianal (2) areas. She was not immunocompromised but was an extremely heavy smoker and had a long history (>10 years) of genital tract HPV infection. Indeed, condyloma acuminata can still be seen on the vulvar (3) and perianal (4) areas.

This increased risk of VIN in association with invasive and preinvasive conditions of the cervix is well documented (Buchler, 1975; Choo & Morley, 1980; Bornstein *et al.*, 1988; Fiorica *et al.*, 1988; Mitchell *et al.*, 1993). In the study by Bornstein *et al.* (1988), 16 out of 46 patients with VIN 3 were found to have an additional site of lower genital tract neoplasia, primarily in the cervix. They found that the frequency of multicentricity decreased significantly with age, and patients with multicentric disease (involving the vagina and/or cervix in addition to the vulva) had a significantly higher frequency of multifocal disease, involving more than one location on the vulva, and of recurrent disease than did patients without multicentric disease. The condition may be either synchronous or metachronous. It is therefore important that all patients with vulvar disease should be included in standard cervical screening programs. Conversely, patients who have had cervical lesions and exhibit vulvar symptomatology should

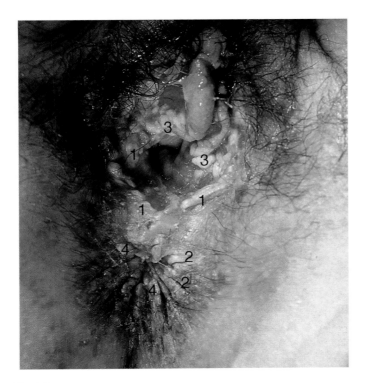

Fig. 9.2

be checked from time to time; vulvoscopy should be performed and any suspicious lesions biopsied. The age range of patients developing VIN is very wide; some patients are as young as 15 years of age and others as old as 90 years of age. In most series the mean patient age for developing VIN is the early thirties, although a wide mean age from 28 years through to 50 years has been reported (Friedrich *et al.*, 1980). There is about a 30-year difference in mean age between the precancerous (VIN) and cancerous forms of the disease.

Viral etiology

The strong association between HPV and cervical cancer, the multicentric nature of HPV-related diseases in the lower genital tract (Bornstein *et al.*, 1988), and the increased incidence of all anogenital tract cancers in immunosuppressed individuals (Sillman & Sedlis, 1991) strongly suggests that these tumors have a common etiologic factor in the presence of HPV. Since the early 1980s, it has been known that HPV is associated with anogenital neoplasma (Zachow *et al.*, 1981; Pilotti *et al.*, 1984), and the majority of studies carried out in the late 1980s, employing, as they did, DNA hybridization techniques to seek evidence of HPV, looked particularly for the presence of types 16 and 18 in clinical specimens or archival material (Gupta *et al.*, 1987; Daling & Sherman, 1992). Those studies in which tissues from patients with VIN 3 and invasive vulvar cancer were analyzed using in-situ hybridization techniques showed that 44% of VIN tissues were positive for HPV 16, whereas only 16% were positive for types 6 and 11. In the corresponding invasive cancers, HPV 16 was present in 45% and HPV 18 was present in only 11%. Using the Southern blot hybridization system, 70% of VIN 3 tissues were shown to

be positive for HPV 16, while only 18 and 67% of invasive cancers were positive for HPV 16 and 18, respectively (Daling & Sherman, 1992). There has been only one population-based study on the association of HPV with vulvar cancer, and in that study (Daling *et al.*, 1992) 72 out of 142 tumor tissues were shown to be positive for HPV, as detected by the polymerase chain reaction (PCR); the majority of these (76.4%) were positive for HPV 16.

Park *et al.* (1991) studied 30 cases of VIN 3 and looked for HPV types 6, 11, 16, and 18; they used in-situ hybridization of viral transcripts and also the new technique of PCR for the amplification of HPV and of the beta-globulin gene. They found evidence to suggest that there are at least two different types of VIN, with different clinical, pathologic, and viral profiles. These two types, which will be discussed below, are the Bowenoid and the basaloid; the former is seemingly associated both clinically and virologically with HPV. HPV16 DNA was the only type detected in 16 out of 30 (53%) cases of VIN 3 and in 15 out of 36 (40%) invasive cancers. This study by Park *et al.* (1991) suggests that there may be a subset of VIN 3 and invasive vulvar cancers that have a nonviral etiology. Similar findings have been suggested by Toki *et al.* (1991).

In the study by Park *et al.*, the HPV-positive women were younger than their HPV-negative counterparts (mean age of diagnosis, 49 versus 60 years) and their lesions more frequently demonstrated koilocytotic atypia (94 vs. 43%). Histologically, the Bowenoid lesions were more warty than the basaloid VIN lesions (65 vs. 30%). Pilotti *et al.* (1990) made similar findings, and Van Sickle *et al.* (1990) were able to show the progression of VIN 3 to carcinoma over a 9-year period in three women who possessed HPV 16 and 18 in their initial and later lesions. Husseinzadeh *et al.* (1989) found that VIN 3 in a multifocal form occurred in younger women, whereas the unifocal disease was found in older females. They concluded that VIN 3 was a disease that affects two patient populations: those with coexistent HPV, who were usually younger and had multifocal disease, and those with a variable history of HPV infection, who were older and more inclined to have unifocal disease. The possibility therefore exists that there may be separate genetic processes involved in the development of VIN 3 in younger women and the development of VIN 3 and cancer in older women.

It would seem as though the focality of the VIN 3 is dependent on viral infection with van Beurden *et al.* (1995) showing that there was a high prevalence of transcriptionally active HPV-DNA associated with multifocal and multicentric intraepithelial lesions. However, they did not find any correlation between different morphologic forms of VIN 3 and the presence of specific HPV-DNA. In their study, which involved 48 patients with a mean age of 37.7 years, 81% had multifocal VIN 3 and 66% multicentric. Forty-six per cent of biopsies were of the warty type, 17 of a basaloid type and 35% mixed with two differentiated types. When HPV analysis was performed, 92% were HPV-positive and 83% contained HPV-16 DNA. The HPV-DNA was more often present in the multifocal VIN 3 than in unifocal VIN 3 lesions and also more often in those that coexisted with other dysplastic multicentric lesions than in uni-centric VIN 3 lesions. They found that both types of VIN 3 often coexisted in the one lesion.

When, however, invasive lesions are considered, the presence of HPV-DNA is not always found. Toki *et al.* (1991) only found HPV-DNA in 21% of their well-differentiated keratinizing squamous carcinomas, but in 75% of those invasive lesions demonstrating basaloid morphology and in 100% with warty morphologic features. They concluded that vulval carcinoma can be found in two categories: a keratinizing squamous cell carcinoma, the classic morphologic type, which is rarely associated with HPV and predominates in older women, and a warty and basaloid cancer which is usually HPV-related, found in younger women and often associated with VIN 3.

Sexually transmitted diseases as etiologic factors

There does appear to be a strong relationship between certain sexually transmitted diseases (STDs) and VIN (Friedrich *et al.*, 1980; Beckmann *et al.*, 1988; Bornstein *et al.*, 1988; Sherman *et al.*, 1991). The most commonly associated STDs are condylomata acuminata, herpes simplex, gonorrhea, syphilis, trichomoniasis, and *Gardenerella vaginalis.* Indeed, Sherman *et al.* (1991), in a very detailed epidemiologic study involving 180 women with in-situ and 53 women with invasive vulvar cancer, found that females with vulvar cancer reported having had a greater number of sexual partners than did controls, and the risk of vulvar cancer was elevated among women who reported a prior history of condyloma (for in-situ cancer, the relative risk (RR) = 15.8; for invasive disease, RR = 17.3) or gonorrhea (for in-situ cancer, RR = 2.2; for invasive disease, RR = 5.0). Females who were seropositive for herpes simplex virus type 2 (HSV 2) were at greater risk for VIN 3 than were controls (RR = 2). Further a history of nonspecific vaginitis, trichomoniasis, syphilis, seropositivity, or cytomegalovirus was not related to case-control status. These results indicate that only a subset of STDs, particularly HPV, may play a role in the development of vulvar cancer. It may well be the case that the lesser grades of VIN are simply another clinical condition associated with sexual activity in younger patients.

In a study by Prabhat *et al.*, (1993) the cofactor role played by STDs in the etiology of cervical carcinoma was investigated by analyzing antibodies to HPV and other genital infectious agents. The results could probably be extrapolated to vulvar neoplasia. Serum from 219 women with cervical cancer and from 387 controls was analyzed for antibodies to infectious agents. HPV16-E7 and/or HPV18-E7 antibodies were significantly related to the risk of cervical cancer (RR 1.9) but antibodies to HSV 1 and HSV 2, *Chlamydia trachomonatis,* and to other multiple infectious agents were only associated with cervical cancer when seroprevalence rates in all cases and controls were compared. However, when HPV-seropositive cases and controls were compared, these associations were weaker and not significant. These findings suggest that past infection with sexually transmitted agents other than HPV may be

no more than surrogate markers of exposure to HPV, and of no separate etiologic significance.

The increased risk of development of VIN in immunosuppressed patients, such as those undergoing renal transplantation or those with lymphoproliferative disorders or systemic lupus erythematosus (SLE), is well documented (Wilkinson *et al.*, 1981; Sillman & Sedlis, 1991). Rare conditions, such as myelokathexis, have also been linked to an increased risk of VIN (J.M. Monaghan, pers. comm.).

Recent seroepidemiologic evidence relating to the role of human papillomavirus in non-cervical anogenital cancers has been forthcoming from a large study of some 700000 samples in a serum bank in Finland and Norway (Bjorge *et al.*, 1997). People who developed non-cervical anogenital cancers during the follow-up were identified by cancer registry linkage. Within this cohort, a nested case-control study was conducted based on the serologic diagnosis of infections with HPV 16, 18 and 33. There was a highly increased risk of developing both preinvasive vulvar and vaginal lesions amongst subjects who were seropositive for human papillomavirus type 16 (odds ratio ∞ (95% CI 3.8 to ∞)) and also among subjects seropositive for type 18 (odds ration 12 (95% CI 1.2 to 590)). They found that there was a high but non-significant increase in odds ratio for type 33 and *chlamydia trachomatis.*

Human immunodeficiency virus (HIV) and VIN 3

It was alluded to above that there was an increased risk of development of VIN in immunosuppressed patients. Since 1989, women with human immunodeficiency virus infection have been known to have a high incidence of cervical neoplasia, as described in Chapter 7. However, it is now becoming obvious that there is an increased risk of the development of intraepithelial vulval neoplasia in this group, especially those with a simultaneous HPV infection. Rose & Friare (1993) was the first to report a case of multiple primary gynecologic neoplasms in association with HIV, detailing the 5-year history of a young woman with simultaneous invasive cancer of breast, microinvasive carcinoma of cervix and intraepithelial neoplasia of vulva. Since that time, a number of studies have pointed up the increased risk of HIV in association with VIN 3. Korn *et al.* (1996) reviewed all cases of VIN 3 over a 4-year period at an inner city hospital and found that 8 of 28 women (29%) with VIN were infected with HIV. Chiasson *et al.* (1997) showed that the prevalence of vulvar vaginal condyloma was increased in women with HIV positivity and they found a small number of high grade VINs also in this group. Another by Petry *et al.* (1996), followed a total of 158 women who were either HIV-infected or under iatrogenic immunosuppression over a 4-year period to evaluate if certain vulval and/or cervical neoplasias had similar associated risk factors. They found two invasive vulval carcinomas and seven VIN 3 lesions and also an increased number of cervical precancers and cancers. Women who had more than five life-time partners were more likely to have HPV-DNA positive cervical swabs and vulval scrapes as well as cervical and/or vulval neoplasia. They showed that compared with

2.7% of the controls, 15.2% of patients with CIN had coexisting high-grade lesions of the vulva. With one exception, all patients with vulvar neoplasia either had symptomatic immunodeficiency or had received immunosuppressive drugs for more than 10 years. They concluded from this study that cervical and Bowenoid/basaloid vulval neoplasias seem to have a similar HPV-related origin and this may be indicative of some malfunction of the cellular immune response which appeared to be a cofactor in the genesis of HPV-associated neoplasia in both cervix and vulva.

The extent of the prevalence of VIN in the HIV population is still difficult to determine but a retrospective study of 38 HIV-infective women who were screened with colposcopy showed that 14% of them had VIN on biopsy and an additional 50% had abnormal PAP smears with 24% having biopsy evidence of CIN. This study, by Abercrombie and Korn (1995), showed the relatively high prevalence of VIN in HIV women.

Smoking risk

As with CIN, smokers appear to be at higher risk for the development of VIN and invasive cancer of the vulva. This may be mediated through the tendency to find a reduced immunosurveillance mechanism in patients who are habitual smokers (Wilkinson et al., 1988; Brinton et al., 1990; Sherman et al., 1991).

9.3 Natural history of VIN: the rationale for treatment?

The relationship between VIN and invasive vulvar cancer is far from clear and this makes difficult any consideration of the natural history and subsequent recommendations for the management of VIN. The problem with many of the studies of VIN that purport to show progression to malignancy is that the follow-up is of patients that have already been treated, and as such one would not expect to find progression. However, in the study by Jones and McLean (1986) there was progression in four out of five untreated patients who had high-grade VIN and were followed over a period of 7–8 years (Fig. 9.3a–d). There is considerable discussion as to whether the conditions of VIN 1 and 2 are true precancerous conditions, and whether there is a sequential progression from VIN 1 to 2 to 3. The considerable spatial disparity between the peak incidence of VIN 3 (35 years) and the peak incidence of invasive carcinoma of the vulva (68 years) leads to the conclusion that these two conditions may not be directly related in all circumstances. It is also noted that VIN 3 is commonly multifocal, whereas cancerous conditions of the vulva in the older patient are most frequently unifocal. When cancer occurs in younger women, it tends to be multifocal, suggesting development from VIN 3 and an association with HPV (Husseinzadeh et al., 1989; Pilotti et al., 1990; Van Sickle et al., 1990; Park et al., 1991; Rusk et al., 1991).

It is clear that the behavior of VIN 3 does not seem to be comparable with that of CIN 3; progression to malignancy is considered to be low at between 2% and 4% (Gardner et al., 1953; Woodruff et al., 1973; Friedrich et al., 1980; Benedet & Murphy, 1982; Jones & McLean, 1986). In a study by Buscema et al. (1980a), of 102 females who had VIN 3 and who were followed for up to 15 years, four patients went on to develop invasive disease after treatment for VIN, two of them after local excision and two after simple vulvectomy. Of these patients, two were under 40 years of age; both were immunosuppressed and one was receiving long-term steroid therapy for sarcoidosis. In the study by Jones and McLean (1986) (Fig. 9.3a–d), four of five patients with VIN 3, and who were observed without treatment, progressed to invasive disease over a period of 7–8 years. Bernstein et al. (1983) reported a different experience, where eight of 13 women with CIS, and who were observed without treatment, had persistent disease but no evidence of progression; the remaining five had complete spontaneous regression of their lesions.

This spontaneous regression of VIN 3 has also been documented by others; the rate is quoted as between 10% and 38% in patients under 35 years and who have multifocal or pigmented lesions (Friedrich, 1972; Skinner et al., 1973; Friedrich et al., 1980). In the study by Friedrich et al. (1980), 80% of patients in whom regression occurred were pregnant at the time of diagnosis; this contrasts with the subsequent study by Bernstein et al. (1983), in which no patients were pregnant when diagnosed. The fact that at the time of diagnosis these lesions were definitely intraepithelial neoplasia is confirmed by the finding that the lesions were initially aneuploid but, on regression, reverted to normal ploidy (Friedrich et al., 1980). It has been shown by Bergeron et al. (1987) that aneuploid VIN 3 lesions have an increased risk of progression to cancer and a reduced chance of spontaneous regression.

Increasing evidence suggests that the vulvar equivalent of CIN, when associated with HPV, seems to have the same characteristics. Nuclear aneuploidy and abnormal mitotic figures—features typical of neoplastic cells—are common to both VIN and CIN. HPV 16 is also found in both conditions and when present it is often episomal (extrachromosomal) in VIN; when VIN is associated with early invasion, there is integration into the cellular genome in both intraepithelial and the coexistent invasive cancer foci (Fu et al., 1981; Crum et al., 1982; Bergeron et al., 1987). It would also seem that the type of HPV is important in terms of progression, i.e. the possession of HPV16-positive aneuploid lesions of the vulva places the individual at increased risk for progression (Van Sickle et al., 1990) compared with those who have HPV 6/11 and nuclear polyploidy; in the latter, persistence or possibly regression, rather than malignant transformation, would be the rule. The clinical implications of an HPV 6/11 infection of the vulva seem to be an associated increased susceptibility to the acquisition of the HPV 16 oncogenic virus (Li Vigni et al., 1992). The finding of mixed lesions, incorporating both type 6/11 and type 16, would tend to support this contention (Bergeron et al., 1987; Gupta et al., 1987; Pilotti et al., 1990; Park et al., 1991; Li Vigni et al., 1992).

The difficulty of extrapolating this natural history to

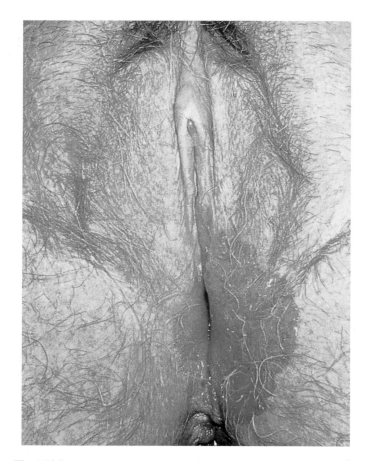

Fig. 9.3(a)

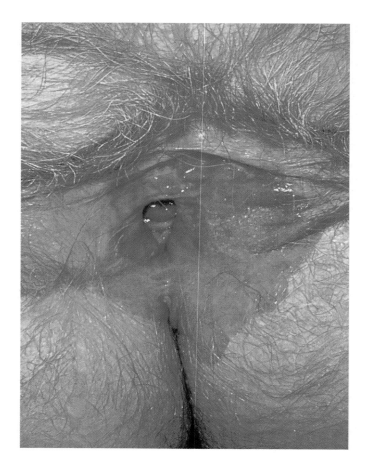

Fig. 9.3(b)

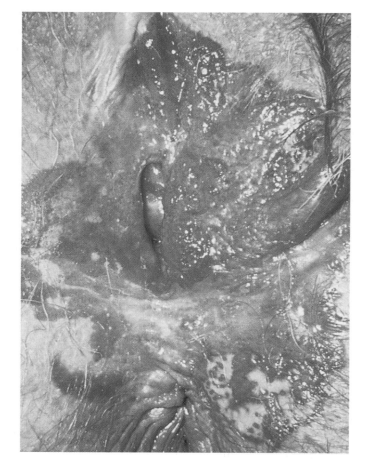

Fig. 9.3(c)

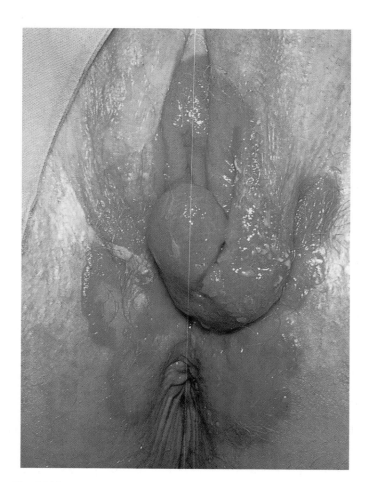

Fig. 9.3(d)

management protocols is made all the more problematic by the finding of occult invasive disease in biopsies that are obtained at the time of surgical treatment in cases in which the initial diagnosis had shown only VIN 3. Indeed, early stromal invasion of the vulva may be more common than is imagined. Pickel (1989), in an analysis of 151 vulvectomy specimens and 154 biopsies from the vulva, found that 17% of cases showed early stromal invasion. His cases included those with "dysplasias", "carcinoma-in-situ," or "invasive squamous carcinoma." Stromal invasion was distributed through all these cases and the invasion was also found in the margins. Table 9.2 shows the incidence of occult invasion found at the time of excisional treatment; there is a range of 6–9.5%. In the majority of cases, the invasive lesion was of an "early" squamous cell carcinoma with a depth of invasion less than 5 mm. In the study by Friedrich et al. (1980) three such cases were noted, but none subsequently recurred after local excision. It would therefore seem prudent, in view of the limited risk of progression, for treatment protocols to favor conservative methods, but emphasis should be placed on excisional techniques that allow histologic material to be obtained, so as to avoid missing the presence of occult invasive disease.

An example of this is seen in the study of van Beurden et al. (1998b), who showed that 9% of 47 patients with VIN 3 had a superficially invasive vulval carcinoma invading to less than 1 mm. Modesitt et al. (1998) likewise showed that in their group of 73 women aged 20–86 years (median age 43) with biopsy proven VIN 3, 17 of them (22%) had an occult invasive lesion on examination of a widely excised specimen of the VIN 3. A 15-year retrospective study has been reported by Herod et al. (1996a). They observed 133 women with a primary diagnosis of VIN, in whom evidence of papillomavirus existed in 78%. Nineteen (14%) of their patients were followed by observation, but 81% had surgery. They found that progression to invasive disease occurred in nine patients (7%) in the surgical group and four deaths occurred in this group with three from gynecologic malignancies of the lower genital tract.

Hording et al. (1995) likewise followed 73 women who had been treated for VIN for 5 years, during which time 26 (36%) developed one or more vulvar recurrences. Microinvasive carcinoma developed in 12 patients (16%), of whom three later developed frankly invasive cancer. HPV-16 DNA was found in 90% of the VINs. It would therefore appear that the evidence of these two studies, namely, Herod et al. (1996) and Hording et al. (1995) suggests that the risk of invasion may be higher than had previously been anticipated.

Within the natural history of VIN discussion, it is important to note that there would seem to be one morphologic variant of VIN which, in the opinion of Kaufman (1995) has proven to be an extremely aggressive lesion with occasionally a short progression time to development of invasive carcinoma. He refers to the well-differentiated variety of VIN which is not frequently seen. The morphologic features of this lesion are quite distinct and different from the two varieties already mentioned, namely basaloid and the warty VIN 3 which is described on p. 240. The squamous epithelial cells in these lesions tend to be mature and deep within the epithelial folds, with abnormal cell keratinization being noted (Fig. 9.5c). Because of the well-differentiated appearance, their significance is often overlooked.

9.4 Pathology

As has already been mentioned, the VIN terminology is partly based on that of CIN and on the desire to abolish imprecise terms such as "mild dysplasia" and "carcinoma-in-situ." The most important reason for the introduction of the VIN concept was the demonstration by Fu et al. (1981), as a result of using Feulgen micro-spectrophotometry, that in many cases of low-grade atypia (i.e. mild and moderate atypia) the abnormal cells were aneuploid, having a chromosome content that was not an exact multiple of 23. Also, there was no correlation between these degrees of minor-grade abnormality within the squamous epithelium and their neoplastic potential (Ferenczy, 1992), Friedrich et al. (1980) had previously shown, and this was confirmed by Fu et al. (1981), that the majority of vulvar CIS was indeed aneuploid, but there was no evidence that the aneuploid atypia of the minor-grade lesions and CIS differed biologically, except in their degree of maturation and differentiation.

Histologically, VINs contain an exaggeration of the epithelial proliferations (acanthosis) that lead to minute excrescences appearing on the surface of the epithelium. These are represented clinically by the papillary or granu-

Table 9.2 Incidence of occult invasion.

Reference	No. of cases of VIN 3	Occult invasion found at time of treatment (%)	Definition of "microinvasion" utilized
Collins et al. (1970)	41	4 (9.5)	Not defined
Woodruff et al. (1973)	44	3 (6.7)	Not defined
Friedrich et al. (1980)	50	3 (6.0)	<1 mm
Rettenmaier et al. (1987)	42	3 (7.1)	<1.5 mm
van Beurden et al. (1998b)	47	4 (9)	<1 mm
Modesitt et al. (1998)	73	17 (22)	0.2–10.0 mm (Median 1.0 mm Mean 1.7 mm)

Fig. 9.3 (*Opposite*) The series of four photographs, courtesy of Dr Ron Jones of Auckland, New Zealand, showing the development of invasive cancer over a 4-year period from an obvious vulvar intraepithelial neoplasia (VIN) 3 lesion.

(a) Vulva (April 1972) shows a red lesion on the labia minora and posterior labia majora.

(b) By December 1973, the lesion has enlarged and biopsy shows the presence of VIN 3.

(c) By January 1975, biopsy reveals the presence of VIN 3 and possibly early invasive disease.

(d) By September 1976, obvious cancer has developed and the full progression from an intraepithelial lesion to a malignant lesion can be seen.

lar surface of the VIN lesions. Also exaggerating the clinical appearance is the hyper- and parakeratosis that is normally associated with these lesions and which accounts for the increased white color tone. The cell nuclei are hyperchromatic and demonstrate a loss of organization, maturation, and cohesion. Mitotic figures are generally numerous and abnormal forms are often present. Less commonly, the neoplastic cells may be uniform, but usually they are multinucleate, pleomorphic, and contain agglutinated nuclear DNA—the so-called corps ronds. In many of them there is also evidence of HPV infection with koilocytosis; the cells demonstrate cytoplasmic cavitation and nuclear atypia, as well as cytoplasmic keratinization, the so-called dyskeratosis. It is well known that a pleomorphic nuclear morphology correlates with hypertetraploid aneuploid modal values (Wilkinson *et al.*, 1981).

Abnormalities of maturation and disturbances of the normal cellular stratification are characteristics of atypia within vulvar squamous epithelium. Two basic morphologic types of VIN are seen. One involves the proliferation of basal- or parabasal-type cells that extend into the upper layers of the epidermis; the so-called *basaloid VIN*. The other type, characterized by premature cellular maturation, often occurring in association with epithelial multinucleation, corps ronds, and koilocytosis, is a hallmark of papillomavirus infection. This second type is called *Bowenoid VIN*. In both types, all the characteristics of abnormal and bizarre mitotic figures can be found, as can cellular and nuclear pleomorphism, irregular clumping of nuclear keratin, and either parakeratosis or hyperkeratosis. Not surprisingly, the Bowenoid VIN is common in women with current or previous wart viral infections of the vulva. It is not unusual for both patterns of VIN to coexist. Reference has already been made to the study by Park *et al.* (1991) of the differences between these two types of VIN in respect of the clinical presentation, the presence of koilocytotic atypia, and the finding of HPV 16. This has led to the conclusion that there are at least two different types of VIN and that these have differing clinical, pathologic, and viral profiles.

Although the histologic definition of VIN has become considerably clearer in recent years, there is still a major difficulty in diagnosing the lesser grades of abnormality i.e. VIN 1/2. This is because many of these lesions are associated with koilocytosis, corps ronds, hyperkeratotic cells and other cellular characteristics which may be confused with higher grade lesions.

Figures 9.4 and 9.5a and b, typical examples of the histology of VIN, show VIN with the characteristic loss of architecture, superficial hyperkeratosis of varying degree, marked nuclear and cytoplasmic pleomorphism, altered maturation, hyperchromic nuclei and abnormal mitotic figures, and corps ronds. Very hypertrophic and somewhat acanthotic rete ridges are commonly found (Figs 9.4 & 9.5a), although it is not uncommon to observe a uniform band of pleomorphic cells extending from the surface epithelium to the base of the rete ridges. Varying degrees of differentiation will occur with widely varying levels of keratosis in the superficial layers.

It is also important to realize that there may be associated

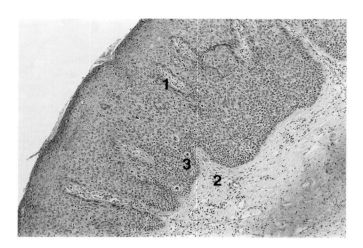

Fig. 9.4 An example of a basaloid-type vulvar intraepithelial neoplasia (VIN) 3 characterized by pleomorphic cells (1), which extend from the deep epithelial layers to the surface, with a minor covering of hyperkeratotic cells. There is some subdermal hyalinization (2) with abnormal mitoses noted at (3) in the lower levels of the epithelium.

changes within the skin surrounding both VIN 3 and obvious carcinoma. Barbero *et al.* (1990) examined 60 cases of VIN 3 and found that in 24 (40%) there were pathologic alterations in the adjacent epithelium; 23 of these contained hyperplasias and one lichen sclerosus. Another study by Borgeno *et al.* (1988) showed that adjacent to vulvar carcinomas there were "dystrophic changes" in 60% and VIN 3 in 20% of cases.

Reference has already been made to the third type of intraepithelial neoplasia, namely the well-differentiated variety. Abell and Gosling (1961) described it in terms of carcinoma-in-situ simplex, but it was later referred to as a well-differentiated variety of intraepithelial neoplasia. Seen in Fig. 9.5c, the epithelial cells are mature and deep within the epithelial folds and abnormal cell keratinization is noted. In Fig. 9.5d this keratinization has formed a pearl-like structure (arrowed). It is usually an aggressive lesion with a rapid progression to invasive cancer.

Differential diagnosis of VIN

Many conditions may mimic the preneoplastic or neoplastic vulvar lesions. The flat or papular condylomata, which have been described previously, and the squamous cell hyperplasia (formerly hyperplastic dystrophy) both present problems of differentiation from VIN. Table 9.3 shows the distinctive biomorphologic features of these three conditions. Other conditions that may cause confusion are those related to podophyllin-treated condylomata, VIN that extends into the pilosebaceous units, tangentially sectioned VIN, seborrheic keratosis, and basal cell carcinoma. The podophyllin-treated condylomata may show cytonuclear degeneration and an increased number of mitoses, but all these mitoses are normal and most are in the metaphase stage. If there is doubt as to the significance of these changes, it is suggested that a repeat biopsy be deferred for some 7 to 10 days after therapy.

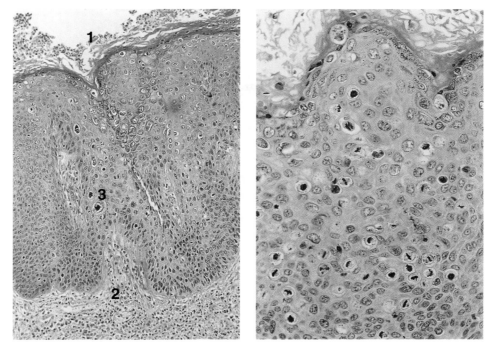

Fig. 9.5(a)   Fig. 9.5(b)

Fig. 9.5 (a) An example of a Bowenoid-type vulvar intraepithelial neoplasia (VIN) 3 with the cellular atypia characterized by the presence of koilocytes, corps ronds, and frequent mitoses. The differences from the lesion shown in Fig. 9.4 are that the superficial layers have a much better developed layer of keratinization (1) and the subdermal layers (2) possess marked lymphocyte infiltration. There are corps ronds present at (3). (b) A high-power view of (a) showing the surface with hyperkeratosis and within the epithelium there are corps ronds with many abnormal mitoses and multiple hyperkeratotic and dyskeratotic cells.

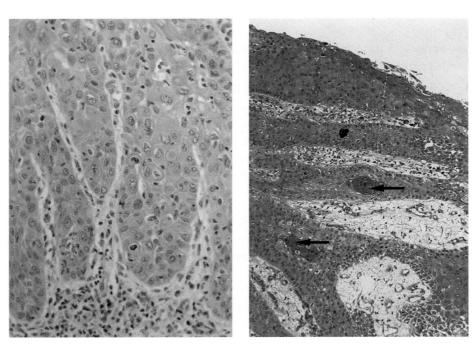

Fig. 9.5(c)   Fig. 9.5(d)

Seborrheic keratosis and the basal cell carcinoma of the superficially invasive type both originate from basal cells in otherwise normal epithelium. The cells are uniform with peripheral palisading in the basal cell carcinoma, whereas the seborrheic keratosis contains numerous keratin cysts that are absent from the VIN. Finally, VIN may present with elongated rete ridges that have squamous pearl formations at their tips; these may produce difficulties in determining whether the lesion is entirely intraepithelial, because oblique and transverse sectioning may give the impression that invasion has already begun. Careful orientation of the biopsy specimen is essential, and if in doubt a larger and further sample should be removed for assessment.

9.5 Clinical presentation

Considerable variation in the clinical presentation of VIN occurs with patterns of varying color, surface configuration, and topography. These various patterns will be considered individually here.

There seem to be two distinct clinical forms of VIN (Husseinzadeh *et al.*, 1989; Pilotti *et al.*, 1990; Park *et al.*, 1991; Ferenczy, 1992). The first, occurring in younger women, is multifocal and multicentric, whereas the second type, which occurs in older patients, is commonly unicentric. The premenopausal form appears to be more frequent than its postmenopausal variant.

Feature	VIN	Condyloma	EH
Cellular disorganization and loss of cohesion	Yes	No	No
Cellular pleomorphism	Yes	No	No
Surface koilocytosis	Yes/no	Yes†	No
Dyskeratosis	Often	Often	Rare
Mitosis in upper two-thirds of epithelium	Yes	No	No
AMFs	Yes	No	No
Pilosebaceous unit involvement	Yes	No	No
Nuclear DNA	Aneuploid	Polyploid	Diploid–polyploid
HPV DNA	Yes (type 16)	Yes (type 6/11)	Absent

Table 9.3 Distinctive biomorphologic features of vulvar intraepithelial neoplasia (VIN), condyloma*, and epithelial hyperplasia (EH).

*Condyloma: histology of both subclinical and clinical lesions.
†One-third to two-thirds of upper epithelium.
AMFs, abnormal mitotic figures; HPV, human papillomavirus.
Reproduced with permission from Ferenczy (1992).

Vulvoscopy: magnified illumination of the vulva with a colposcope

One important difference between VIN and CIN is that VIN is commonly symptomatic, producing pruritus to a varying degree. This will be seen in some 60–70% of patients. The remainder are asymptomatic and lesions are discovered during routine examinations. The use of the colposcope to perform vulvoscopy has been shown to be an essential adjunct to inspection techniques. The application of 5% acetic acid will greatly facilitate identification of areas of VIN. The acetic acid should be applied for a considerably longer period than when it is used on the cervix. Some patients may find it painful when a 5% solution is used, and so a 2% solution or gentle daubing of the vulva with a small cotton-tipped applicator or Q-tip may be necessary. The epithelium takes it up rather more slowly but a marked reaction is easily obtained. Similar characteristics of punctation, mosaic development, and acetowhiteness are noted on the vulva as on the cervix. It is, however, important that the vulva is carefully inspected before acetic acid is applied in order to outline preexisting areas of white skin that are usually due to hyperkeratosis. Following acetic acid application, a systematic examination must be made of the vaginal introitus, labia minora and majora, and perineum. Finally, inspection of the clitoris, terminal urethra, and perianal area and anal canals is undertaken.

The effect of application of acetic acid can be readily seen in Figs 9.6 and 9.7. Figure 9.6 shows the clinical appearance of the vulva; some regions (1) demonstrate circumscribed elevated areas that exhibit a fine punctate pattern produced by enlarged superficial vessels. Area (2) shows hyperkeratosis and a white appearance that is characteristic of superficial hyperkeratosis. In Fig. 9.7, acetic acid has been applied and areas (1) now show a hard white pattern with a fine stippled appearance; this confirms the punctation

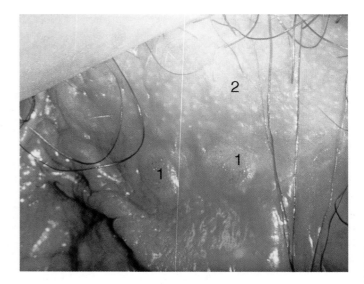

Fig. 9.6

noted in Fig. 9.6. Area (2) remains essentially the same with its typical hyperkeratotic pattern. The areas marked (1) show histologic evidence of VIN 3.

Vulvoscopy is a recent addition to the techniques used to examine the vulva. No attempt has been made to classify vulvoscopic findings and so that authors have used the only classification that is suggested at this time, namely that of Coppleson and Pixley (1992). It is as follows.
1 Color: (i) normal; (ii) white; (iii) acetowhite; (iv) red; (v) brown; (vi) other pigmentation.
2 Blood vessels: (i) absent; (ii) punctation; (iii) mosaic; (iv) atypical.
3 Surface configuration: (i) flat; (ii) raised; (iii) micropapillary; (iv) microcondylomatous; (v) villiform; (vi) papular; (vii) hyperkeratotic (leukoplakia).

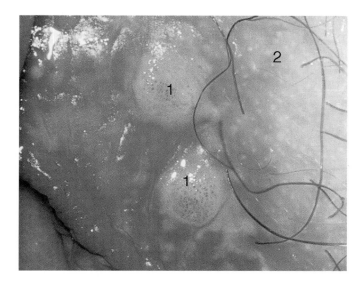

Fig. 9.7

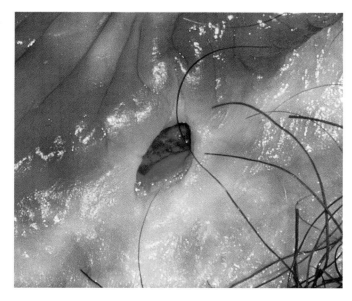

Fig. 9.8

4 Topography: (i) unifocal; (ii) multifocal; (iii) multisited, e.g. perianal, urethral, vaginal, or cervical.

Vulvoscopy, although important in women with suspected VIN has recently been used in a study to observe the vulva of healthy women without vulval complaints to determine the accuracy of acetic acid staining as a sign of precancer (van Beurden *et al.*, 1997). Photographs were taken before and after acetic acid and results showed that after the application of 5% acetic acid, there was an acetowhite staining of the vestibule in all women. However there were no hyperkeratotic areas found and mucosal and skin surfaces were smooth. Twelve women (30%) had acetowhite lesions outside the vestibule and six women (15%) were positive for HPV-DNA. However, the presence of HPV-DNA did not correlate with vestibular erythema or vestibular papillomatosis, which in themselves were present in 13 women (33%) and are normal constituents of the vaginal introitus. There was only a weak association between HPV-DNA and acetowhite lesions outside the vulva. The conclusion from this study was that acetowhite staining of the smooth vulvar skin is common in healthy women without vulvar complaints and therefore cannot be used as a definitive test for diagnosis of VIN.

Notwithstanding the findings in this study, it is accepted that hyperkeratotic lesions are the most likely to be associated with VIN or more extensive disease.

It is hoped that in the future the major international bodies interested in cervical pathology and vulvar diseases will agree upon a common terminology that can be used for the magnified and illuminated inspections of cervix, vagina, and vulva.

Collins toluidine blue test

Use of the Collins toluidine blue test has been advocated by many clinicians in an attempt to demonstrate abnormal maturation. This is usually in relation to parakeratosis, which is defined as retention of nuclear chromatin material in the usually acellular keratin layer of the epithelium. These changes can be identified by using the toluidine blue

test, in which a 1% aqueous solution of dye is applied to the external genital area (Collins *et al.*, 1966). Toluidine blue is a nuclear stain and will become fixed to the superficial nuclei in ulcers, fissures, and parakeratosis. After being left to dry for 2–3 minutes, the area is discolored with a solution of 1% acetic acid. Areas of parakeratosis and suspicious foci of increased nuclear atypia will retain the dye and acquire a deep blue tinge. The normal tissue accepts little or none of the dye. The problem is that hyperkeratotic lesions, although often neoplastic, stain poorly, whereas benign excoriations usually stain in brilliant colors; this gives rise to a high false-positive and also false-negative rate. Figure 9.8 shows such an event with an ulcerated area in the center of the figure having taken up the dye, giving rise to a false-positive picture.

Figure 9.9 shows some of the problems that may be encountered with the application of toluidine blue. In this patient, multiple condyloma acuminata and some areas of VIN were present around the vaginal introitus and fourchette. A 1% aqueous solution of toluidine blue was applied to the vulva with a large cotton swab. Even though the vulva was rinsed with a 1% aqueous solution of acetic acid and the dye wiped off, the resulting denseness of the stain can still be seen and there is no decoloration. This test has given a false-positive result because conditions that involve a rapid turnover of cells (and associated parakeratosis), like the condyloma acuminata in this case, stain positive with this nuclear dye.

The presence or absence of cancer can be confirmed only by biopsy, and so a colposcopic examination must be made before the toluidine blue test is performed. With the exception of some basal-cell cancers, most early squamous neoplasias do exhibit a surface layer of either hyperkeratosis or parakeratosis. Any ulcerated areas associated with these will stain a deep royal blue, but often the depth of the blue color is not dramatic; this is still an indication of parakeratosis and such an area should be biopsied. The vagina and the vestibular portion of the vulva are lined by squamous epithelium of a nonkeratinizing type, wherein the uppermost layer consists of nucleated squamous cells. These

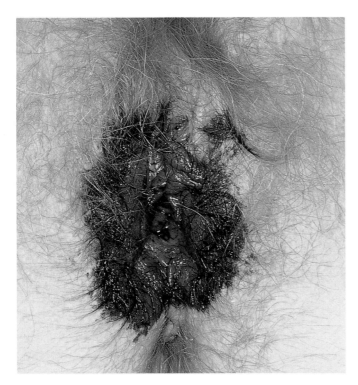

Fig. 9.9

structures should then be expected to stain lightly in the normal situation.

Although the toluidine blue test has been used for many years, its role, the authors feel, is limited. It has been stated by Friedrich (1983a) that "all cancer is not parakeratotic, all keratosis is not cancer." He, like other authors, insists that any area that looks suspicious, whether it be white, gray, red, dark, raised, or flat, should be biopsied. However, Friedrich felt that toluidine blue should be used to identify foci of parakeratosis that may occur outside the larger areas of abnormality that would obviously be biopsied. Certainly, vulvoscopy with acetic acid staining is a more accurate diagnostic technique than use of toluidine blue. Unequivocal evidence for the existence of VIN or invasion comes only from histology, obtained by either biopsy or surgical excision.

9.6 Biopsy of the vulva

A biopsy can be carried out with local anesthesia. Once the anesthetic has been administered, a sample of tissue is taken in all cases where a suspicion of clinical cancer exists or where the preclinical lesions of VIN have been diagnosed by vulvoscopy. The features suggestive of invasive cancer and which warrant biopsy are as follows.
1 Rapidly enlarging lesions.
2 Areas of ulceration or bleeding.
3 Exuberant tissue with abnormal vascularity.
In all these cases, a sample is taken with the intention of obtaining tissue to a depth of at least 5 mm.

The tissue to be sampled can be infiltrated beforehand with local anesthetic in the from of 1% xylocaine or lidocaine; this is injected into the subepithelial or subepidermal papillary dermis. The recent development of a new lidocaine–prilocaine cream, which is applied to the skin 10–15 minutes before the biopsy is taken, has made the final injection of local anesthetic very acceptable and painless. This EMLA (eutectic mixtures of local anesthetic) cream is applied to the area from which the biopsy will be taken, and sometimes this is all that is needed. However, the insertion of local anesthetic will elevate the skin so that the actual biopsy is made easier. Such biopsies are being taken in Figs 9.10–9.12.

In Fig. 9.10a, a simple outpatient technique, utilizing local anesthetic infiltration, is being used to obtain a biopsy of a lesion (1). In these circumstances, a fine dental needle (2) is inserted beneath the lesion to be biopsied and 1–2 ml local anesthetic are injected, thereby elevating the area. EMLA cream is applied prior to this injection. Utilizing either a punch biopsy, a knife, or a proprietary punch, such as a Keyes punch, a small biopsy can be obtained. Figure 9.10b shows a suspicious hyperkeratotic area (1) that can be biopsied rapidly and relatively painlessly using a sharp biopsy forceps, as shown in Fig. 9.11. A Kevorkian or Eppendorfer biopsy forceps (2) (in Fig. 9.11) will produce a satisfactory sample with an adequate depth of 2–5 mm; this will allow the pathologist to give an accurate comment on the nature of the lesion.

The 0.5- to 1-cm defect that is produced can be either left granulating or closed with a single stitch of 3.0 suture material. Healing is usually completed in about 2 weeks. After the specimen has been removed, some authors suggest that it be placed "end on;" the dermis side with serum-wet surface is placed on lens paper or Teflon and the surface epithelium lies face up (Ferenczy, 1992). To increase the adherence of specimens, Ferenczy applies a fine layer of lubricant (KY jelly) to the paper towel or Teflon. The adhered specimen and paper towel or Teflon are then placed in either 10% buffered formalin solution or Bouin's solution fixative. It is most important that the specimen is properly oriented so that tangential sectioning does not lead to difficulty with histologic diagnosis.

The Keyes instrument can also be used to obtain punch biopsies after EMLA cream has been applied and local anesthesia given. The Keyes punch (Figs 9.12 & 9.13) works very much like a cork borer and removes a circumscribed plug of skin, the diameter of which depends on the size of the instrument. In Figs 9.12 and 9.13 a variety of instruments are displayed but the usual one chosen is that which gives a 4- to 5-cm core of skin [(1) in Fig. 9.12]; the depth of tissue removed depends on the pressure employed and the sharpness of the instrument.

In Fig. 9.12, a circular biopsy incision is being carried out. The clinician maintains the pressure and rotation until the subcutaneous tissue is reached. The depth of the biopsy also depends on the epidermal thickness and the factors mentioned above. When the dermis is entered there is a sensation of decreased resistance, and if the biopsy penetrates too deep, then there will be excessive bleeding. If a

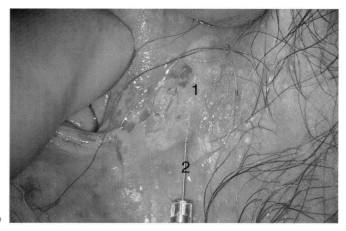

Fig. 9.10(a)

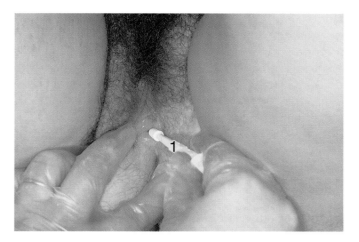

Fig. 9.12

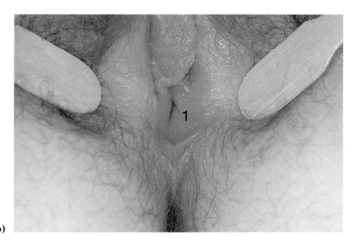

Fig. 9.10(b)

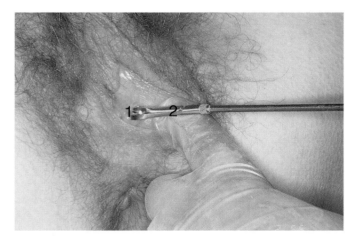

Fig. 9.11

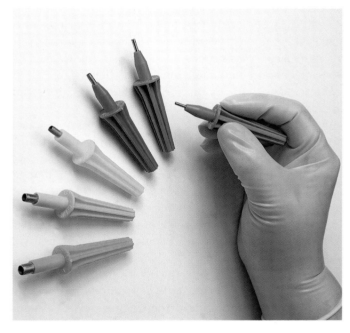

Fig. 9.13

9.7 Clinical appearances of VIN

The clinical appearance and situation on the vulva of VIN lesions is highly variable (Kaufman, 1991). Approximately 70% of them are multifocal. Their color ranges from white through to black, with shades of red and pink in between. It is estimated that approximately one-third of patients with this disease have hyperpigmented lesions with sharp borders. Lesions may also be dry or moist, and not infrequently they resemble condyloma acuminata with which they are often associated. They are characteristically papular, being raised above the surrounding skin, and over half exhibit superficial parakeratosis, giving rise to the

shallow biopsy is taken, then a fragmented and rather inadequate specimen is obtained.

After its removal, the specimen is grasped with some fine-toothed forceps and the dermal tissue is cut, with either a small scalpel or scissors. This leaves a circular or elliptic defect and occasionally some bleeding, which may be stopped using Monsell's (ferric subsulfate) solution or insertion of a single 3.0 suture.

changes that may be seen when the toluidine blue test, described above, is used. Contiguous structures may be superficially involved and of these, the perineal skin, perianal area, and indeed the anal canal are involved in between 14% and 35% of cases; particularly those in which the posterior part of the vulva is most severely affected (Schlaerth *et al.*, 1984).

When examining VIN lesions, the following characteristics must be observed.
1 Topography (i.e. uni- or multifocal).
2 Surface configuration (i.e. flat, raised, or micropapillary).
3 Color tone (i.e. white, red, or dark).
4 Degree of acetowhite change.
5 Blood vessels (i.e. absent, punctate, or mosaic).

The colposcopic features of the epithelium are affected by the thickness of vulvar skin, which in turn affects the opacity of the epithelium. This thickness varies from lesion to lesion and from area to area; for example, the skin of the labia majora hair-bearing keratinized area is thicker than that of the nonhair-bearing labia minora. If a VIN lesion is present, then obviously the thickness and opacity will be increased, and such variations will be accentuated by any associated parakeratosis, acanthosis, or thickening. Associated wart viral infections with their characteristic papillomatosis will, in turn, also affect the colposcopic appearance.

As has been mentioned above, the color tone of lesions is variable and many lesions will be colposcopically indistinct until acetic acid is applied; this produces obvious acetowhitening and defines the lesion (Figs 9.6 & 9.7). Changes in the angioarchitecture are not as well defined as those seen in comparable lesions on the cervix; however, punctation and mosaic patterns can occur. Punctation can be seen on the inner labia minora in some patients presenting with chronic vulvar irritation.

Although vulvoscopy aids the determination of the exact location of precancerous lesions, it is impossible without biopsy to predict accurately the degree of VIN change within the epithelium. A change of skin thickness and coloration are the most accurate colposcopic characteristics associated with VIN changes and these occurred in some 84% of 50 women studies in the author's unit (A. Singer & A. Mitchell, unpublished observations). The presence of acetowhite change in the absence of associated skin thickening and changing color tone is recognized to have very little discriminatory value in respect of VIN diagnosis (van Beurden *et al.*, 1997) and may, in many cases, be associated with subclinical papillomavirus infections (SPI) or occur as a result of coital trauma or scratching (Coppleson & Pixley, 1992).

In the following sections, the different colored VIN lesions, i.e. white, red, and dark, will be considered individually.

White lesions

White lesions on the vulva are not necessarily precancerous. However, the following three factors operate in producing this white appearance.

1 Surface keratin.
2 Any degree of depigmentation.
3 The relative avascularity of the tissue.

When surface keratin becomes moist, it will become opaque and appear either white or gray. The thicker the keratin layer, the more pronounced is this effect. This is one reason why vulvoscopy is not particularly accurate when used to examine vulvar lesions, compared with those found on the vagina and cervix. Depigmentation occurs when the basal-layer melanocytes are lost or destroyed, or when they are unable to manufacture melanin pigment (vitiligo). Relative avascularity of the tissue occurs when superficial vessels become constricted and when the distance between them and the surface is increased; this occurs in the sclerotic processes of lichen sclerosus (LS).

A biopsy must be taken to differentiate the precancerous VIN lesions from other white lesions that occur on the vulva. In the past these white lesions, including VIN, have traditionally been classified in three major groups, dependant on their histologic morphology. These three lesion groups are:
1 VIN.
2 Non-neoplastic epithelial disorders.
3 HPV infections.

The non-neoplastic epithelial disorders comprise those lesions described as LS, squamous cell hyperplasia (formerly hyperplastic dystrophy), and other dermatoses such as intertrigo. Figures 9.14 to 9.20 show examples of white lesions with associated precancerous change. In Fig. 9.14, a combination of condyloma acuminata (1) and thickened white epithelium (2) exist over a large part of the vulva, including labia minora and majora, clitoris, and periurethral areas. A biopsy (Fig. 9.15) of the area at (2) shows it to be of a VIN 3 type with a typical uniform neoplastic cell population of the epithelium with hyperkeratosis, and acanthotic rete pegs with numerous mitoses. Figure 9.16

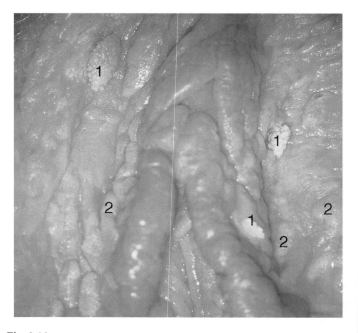

Fig. 9.14

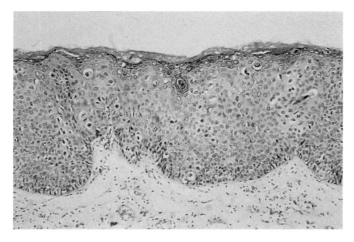

Fig. 9.15

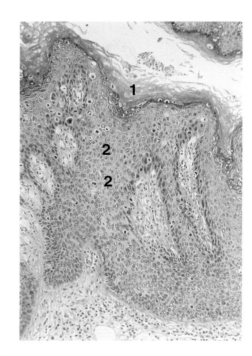

Fig. 9.17

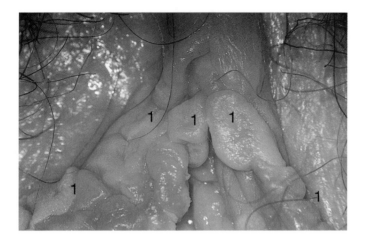

Fig. 9.16

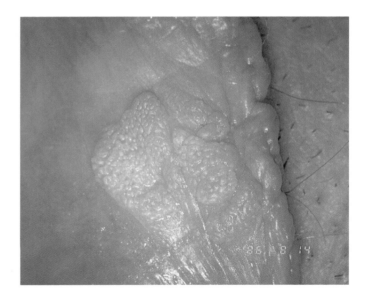

Fig. 9.18

shows the multifocal nature of a VIN 3 lesion, again with a thickened and granular surface. The associated pathology (Fig. 9.17) shows the very hyperkeratotic layer (1), overlying a neoplastic growth that shows disturbed maturation with pleomorphic and hyperchromatic nuclei, abnormal mitotic figures, and obvious crops ronds (2). The undulating surface of the biopsy corresponds with the clinical picture and could lead to these lesions being confused with those of condyloma acuminata. The value of a biopsy in making a correct diagnosis of these lesions is obvious.

In Figs 9.14 and 9.16, involvement of the clitoris and its hoods can be seen. It is only with the magnified and illuminated vision of vulvoscopy that this involvement can be accurately assessed.

Figures 9.18 to 9.20 show further examples of granular white lesions that give the impression of a condylomatous nature, whereas they are in fact associated with VIN 3. Figure 9.18 shows the outer labia minora of a female whose supposed condylomatous lesion had been treated with podophyllin for a number of years. It was only when a biopsy was taken that the true VIN 3 nature of the lesion was determined. Podophyllin-related changes can produce cytonuclear degeneration and an increased number of mitoses; however, Ferenczy (1992) states that mitotic figures produced in this manner are not abnormal and most of them are in metaphase. Ferenczy believes that this phe-

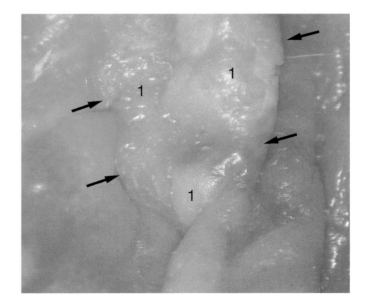

Fig. 9.19

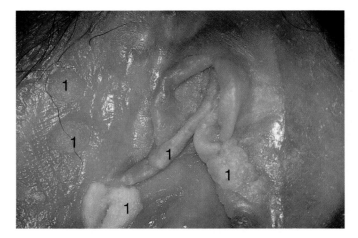

Fig. 9.20

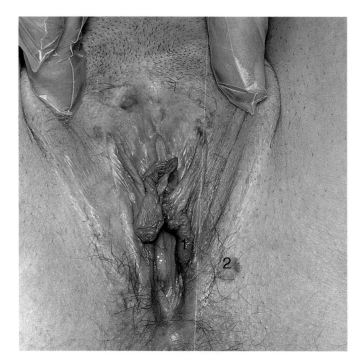

Fig. 9.21

nomenon is due to the action of podophyllotoxin, which prevents sliding of the microtubules of the mitotic spindle. If there is any doubt about the nature of these podophyllin-related lesions, then biopsy should be repeated 7 to 10 days after therapy, by which time the podophyllin effect may have subsided (Ferenczy, 1992).

In Figs 9.19 and 9.20 obvious condylomatous lesions (1) (arrowed in Fig. 9.19) are seen, and biopsy revealed the presence of VIN 3. In Fig. 9.20, the clitoris and its hoods are again involved (as in Figs 9.14 & 9.16).

Red lesions

The normal redness of the skin is due to reflected light coming from the superficial vasculature through the overlying epidermis. Any increase in this capillary bed will result in an erythematous appearance to the tissue; this appearance will likewise be modified by the thickness of the underlying epithelium, as discussed in Chapter 3. Vasodilation of the underlying vessels may be part of a local immune or inflammatory response to such conditions as candidal infections, allergic responses, seborrheic, dermatitis, folliculitis, and vestibular adenitis (Friedrich, 1983a).

Precancerous red lesions have an increased vascularity and have to be differentiated from other lesions, such as those associated with psoriasis, Paget's disease, and acute reactive vulvitis. The redness of these lesions is accentuated because of a decreased number of cell layers existing between the surface, and the increased vascularity within the dermal papillae (Friedrich, 1983b). As Friedrich points out, in these red lesions there is an evident characteristic histologic pattern with an upward proliferation of the papillae and only a few cells existing between the granular zone and the stratum corneum that intervenes between the surface and the dilated and twisted capillary loops in the papillary apex. This pattern is not only characteristic of the erythroblastic variety of VIN 3 but is also present in psoriasis, where it accounts for the characteristic Auspitz's sign

(the induction of fine capillary bleeding points on the surface of the lesion after it has been scraped with a blunt instrument).

Figures 9.21 and 9.22 are low- and high-power views of a midvulvar red lesion (1) that is raised and resembles red velvet. There are elevated white patches [(2) in Fig. 9.22a] and, more peripherally, pigmented areas in the upper labia majora and on the lower left part of the vulva [(2) in Fig. 9.21]. These variations in clinical pattern were all biopsied to produce a comprehensive record of the status of this patient's vulva. The red lesion was confirmed as VIN (Fig. 9.22b), as were the white and pigmented lesions. Where the lesions are so widespread and extensive, as in this case, some form of excisional technique should be used to ensure that an early invasive cancer is not missed. In the pathology of the VIN lesion shown in Fig. 9.22b there is a thin layer of surface parakeratosis, hence the red clinical appearance of this type of intraepithelial neoplasia. The neoplastic cells contain pleomorphic nuclei and there are several abnormal mitotic figures.

Many of these red lesions are symptomatic and induce pruritus, pain, and occasional bleeding that results from the fragility of the superficial capillaries. A diffuse erythematous change of the vulva is usually associated with a benign process, but a localized red lesion, like that seen in Figs 9.21 and 9.22, is suspicious for neoplasia. It must also be differentiated from lesions that result from contact dermatitis as a result of the sensitization of the vulva and perineal skin to a specific agent. It may be necessary to resort to use of the patch test to exclude a varied number of chemical and mineral substances that may be involved in this sensitization. Other causes, such as psoriasis, seborrheic dermatitis,

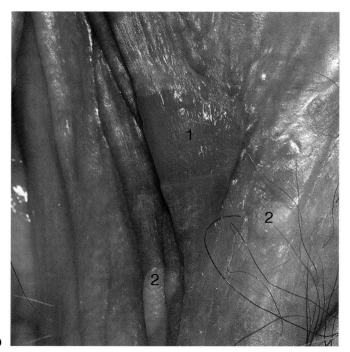

Fig. 9.22(a)

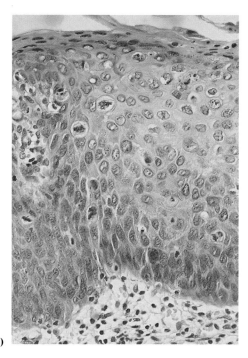

Fig. 9.22(b)

and cutaneous candidiasis, of red vulvar lesions must be excluded.

Dark lesions

In many VIN 3 lesions, intraepithelial melanin, intradermal melanin, or both are present with the result that the lesion may be dark brown or black (Fig. 9.23). They have been variously described as a multiple, discoid, flat or gray-brown lesion (Kimura *et al.*, 1978; Kimura, 1980), hyperpigmented raised lesions (Friedrich *et al.*, 1980; Estrada & Kaufman, 1993), reddish-brown verrucous-type lesions (Wade *et al.*, 1979), or papillary lesions (Hilliard *et al.*, 1979). Melanin synthesis in many of these lesions is often increased in the

epidermal melanocytes and the excess melanin is then extruded into the underlying papillary dermis, from where it is taken up (phagocytosed) by melanophages. This mechanism is called "melanin incontinence" and results in the pigmented appearance of many VIN lesions.

A number of dark lesions of a papillary or spiky condylomatous type have been described as multicentric pigmented Bowen's disease (Kimura *et al.*, 1978) or as Bowenoid papulosis (Wade *et al.*, 1979) (Fig. 9.24a–d). These lesions, with their discrete papular form, preserve the histologic features of Bowen's disease of the cutaneous epithelium. In that condition, multinucleation, dyskeratosis, individual cell keratinization, abnormal mitosis and corps ronds predominate (Fig. 9.25). Koilocytotic atypia exists, but in contrast to that seen in condylomata the koilocytes are confined to the most superficial layers of the epithelium, are few in number, and their delicate perinuclear halos are replaced by compact concentric clear spaces around the obviously abnormal nuclei (Crum *et al.*, 1982). These lesions, however, appear primarily in young individuals and were believed to be clinically innocuous; they were reported to regress spontaneously after sampling (Bhawan, 1980). However, some authors have described more advanced nuclear changes than those reported in the original descriptions; they quote the presence of enlarged nuclei, multinucleation, and aneuploidy within these lesions (Ulbright *et al.*, 1982). It is therefore possible that the lesions are more significant than was previously reckoned, and their common clinical appearance, in conjunction with typical VIN lesions, suggests that Bowenoid papulosis cannot be excluded from the spectrum of precancerous vulvar lesions (Wilkinson, 1987). They have also been associated with a simultaneously occurring cervical intraepithelial lesion (Stafford *et al.*, 1990).

The term Bowenoid papulosis has been used by a number of clinicians to describe a predominantly multifocal pigmented lesion which runs a benign course, with a proportion undergoing spontaneous remission (60%), and is found predominantly in young sexually active women. Clinically, as can be seen in Fig. 9.24(b) there are scattered or variously colored lesions covering the perineum, appearing adherent to the skin, with many having a "warty" surface. Sometime they can be smooth and shiny, as seen in 9.24a. In 9.24(c), localized areas are seen on both sides of the labia minora in a 19-year-old woman. There is an uncommon form of a very florid Bowenoid papulosis, as seen in 9.24(d), in which the whole of the vulva is covered with warty hyperkeratotic lesions varying in color, some areas being white, some red and others dark brown. These lesions are called confluent Bowenoid papulosis and would seem to occur in immunocompromised patients. They should be investigated intensely as they commonly occur in association with early microinvasive disease.

The term Bowen's disease has been used in the past to describe solitary plaques, usually in older women. The lesions, although essentially pigmented, may occasionally be white, red and spontaneous remission does not occur. This type of solitary lesion may progress to invasive disease. Such an area is seen in 9.23a and b.

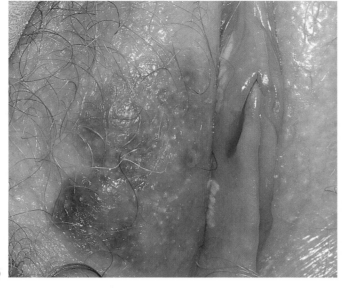

Figs 9.23(a)

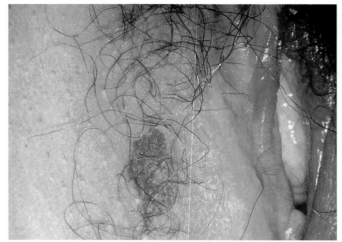

Fig. 9.23(b)

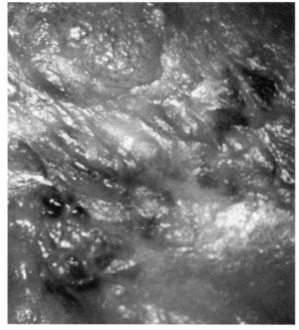

Fig. 9.24(a)

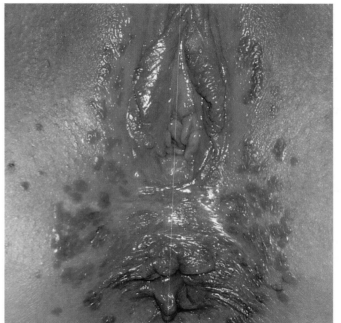

Fig. 9.24(b)

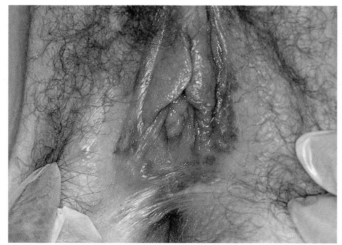

Fig. 9.24(c)

Fig. 9.24(d)

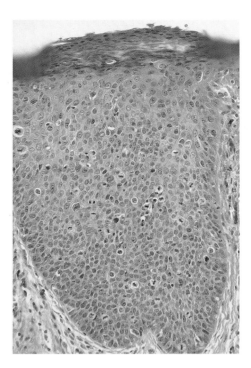

Fig. 9.25

Although rare, melanomas of the vulva account for 10% of all vulvar cancers. The vulva constitutes only 1% of the total skin surface, yet approximately 5% of all melanomas in the female arise in this region. Melanomas may present as a superficial spreading lesion (Fig. 9.26a) that occupies an extensive area. They can arise anywhere on the vulva but are most likely to occur in non hair-bearing areas, especially around the labia minora and clitoris (Fig. 9.26b). They may also develop in the area of the urethral miatus and/or vagina and this, in the past, has led to a small number being misclassified. Approximately 10% of them are nonpigmented. An uncommon presentation is as a nodular lesion

---

Figs 9.23–9.25 In Fig. 9.23a and b (*opposite*) an extensive but localized melanotic area exists on the labia majora; excision biopsy showed it to be VIN 3.

Figure 9.24a (*opposite*) shows the dark changes which are characteristic of vulvar intraepithelial neoplasia (VIN) 3 but may, from time to time, be confused with melanotic changes. Such an appearance has also been referred to as Bowenoid papulosis. A wide local excision is necessary, and careful analysis by the pathologist is indicated to differentiate VIN 3 from a more sinister melanotic lesion.

The histology of a lesion similar to that shown in Fig. 9.24a is presented in Fig. 9.25 (*above*) and shows it to be VIN 3 of a type that is also described by some authors as characteristic of Bowenoid papulosis. The pathology of this lesion (Fig. 9.25) is highlighted by a uniform configuration of neoplastic cells throughout the acanthotic epithelium with many mitotic figures at all levels of the neoplastic epithelium. In addition to the surface parakeratosis, there are multiple melanophages in the adjacent stroma (right and left) and these are responsible for the pigmented clinical appearance of this type of VIN (also referred to as Bowenoid papulosis).

that is raised with an irregular surface, and this carries an ominous prognosis (Fig. 9.27a). The prognosis is directly related to the depth or level of cutaneous invasion (Fig. 9.27b), rather than to the size of the lesion.

Experience in the surgical management of cutaneous melanoma has relied on the level of invasion according to the schema of Clark *et al.* (1969) and the measurement of tumor thickness proposed by Breslow (1970). Breslow measured the tumor thickness from the granular layer to the deepest point of invasion and both his and Clark's measurements seem to be the most reliable predictors of local recurrence and regional lymph node spread. Chung *et al.* (1975) reviewed melanomas of the vulva utilizing the microstaging techniques of Clark and Breslow and found that they were unsuitable for microstaging melanoma of the vulva, and in turn have produced a more rationalized classification. However, it is imperative that all vulval melanomas be classified by one or all of the three techniques listed above.

Diagnosis depends on the realization that any pigmented lesion of the vulva could be malignant. As most vulval nevi are junctional, it is recommended that prophylactic removal be employed (Curtain & Morrow, 1992). However, the features of impending malignancy in a pigmented lesion are those of recent and rapid growth, change in color, bleeding or pruritis. Biopsy of any such lesion should be excisional, with a margin of normal skin, but if the lesion is extensive, then a wedge biopsy should be preferred. There is no place for any locally destructive measures in respect of these lesions.

9.8 VIN affecting the pilosebaceous unit

The vulva is composed of both hair-bearing and nonhair-bearing skin. This is important to remember when considering the extent of involvement of the pilosebaceous units that are associated with these types of skin, for it is within these units that extensions of VIN may be found.

The mons pubis, the lateral and exposed aspects of the labia majora and perianal skin, are covered with hair-bearing skin. The hair follicles, the hair and sebaceous glands, and the apocrine glands form a distinct functional unit throughout these areas of the perianal skin. Also, eccrine sweat glands are found in the labia majora.

Nonhair-bearing areas are usually those related to the inner aspects of the labia majora as well as to the whole of the labia minora, the frenulum, and the prepuce of the clitoris. Within these areas there are sebaceous glands that open directly onto skin. However, they are rarely involved with apocrine or eccrine glands.

VIN in pilosebaceous units has been extensively studied. When it extends into the underlying dermal hair follicles and/or sebaceous glands, it is in all respects similar to the CIN that obtrudes into endocervical glands. In the vulva, the lesion may be in direct histologic continuity with the underlying pilosebaceous system. It has been shown (discussed later), by Baggish *et al.* (1989), Schatz *et al.* (1989), and Benedet *et al.* (1991), that when VIN 3 is present within the pilosebaceous unit it extends to a depth of not more than about 2 mm in both hairy and nonhairy skin.

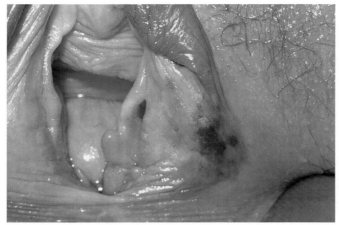
Fig. 9.26(a)

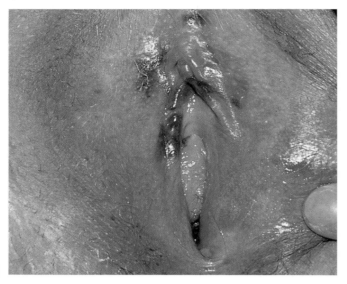
Fig. 9.26(b)

Fig. 9.26 (a) A melanoma-in-situ with the dense black epithelium clearly demarkated. This condition must be excised with a wide margin and a careful assessment of its deeper margins must be made. (b) An early invasive melanoma diagnosed after an extensive biopsy of the pigmented areas.

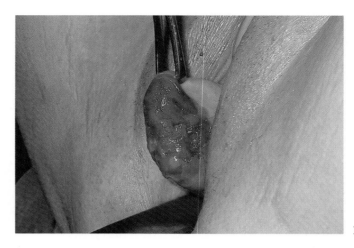
Fig. 9.27(a)

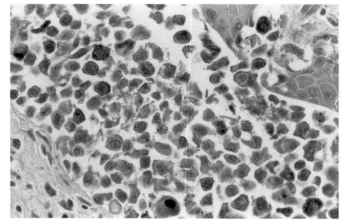
Fig. 9.27(b)

Fig. 9.27 (a) A melanoma presenting as a small nodular lesion with an irregular surface and contour at the base of the left labia minora.
(b) The pathology shows cutaneous invasion to level 3 (Clark's Classification) which has been determined by measurement from the granular layer of the vulval skin or the outermost epithelial layer of the squamous mucosa, to the depth of invasion. Level 3 corresponds to approximately 1–2 mm involvement of the dermis.

In Fig. 9.28, a raised pearly white papular lesion extends from the lower border of the labia minora (1) into the inner aspect of the labia majora (2). After the hair has been removed by shaving, the entrance to the hair follicles (arrowed) can be clearly seen within this VIN lesion, which extended in the unit to a depth of about 1.5 mm. Figure 9.29 shows an intraepithelial neoplastic lesion extending into a pilosebaceous unit (arrowed). Figure 9.30 shows the problems that may arise in the diagnosis of VIN in skin appendages. In this figure there are minimal epithelial abnormalities (1) within this squamous cell hyperplastic surface lesion, which has extended deep into the appendages (2) (3) and could be interpreted as VIN.

9.9 Early invasive carcinoma of the vulva

There is no agreement about use of the term microinvasive or early invasive carcinoma of the vulva in respect of the characteristics of the epithelial lesion and of the depth of

penetration into the underlying dermis (Wilkinson, 1990, 1992). The term microinvasive carcinoma was originally proposed by Kneale *et al.* (1981): "a squamous cell carcinoma 2 cm or less in diameter with no more than 5 mm of stromal invasion where the depth of invasion is the maximum measured in any one high-power field. The presence of confluence, vascular channel permeation or cellular neoplasia does not exclude the case from this category." The maximum depth of microinvasion as 5 mm was based on the study by Wharton *et al.* (1974); 25 patients with vulvar carcinoma that had invaded to 5 mm or less had no nodal disease or recurrence, and all survived. Twenty others, whose neoplasm invaded beyond that depth, had a 25% risk of nodal lymph spread and a 15% mortality rate. However, the 5-mm line suggested by Wharton *et al.* has been challenged by others, and Wilkinson *et al.* (1982) showed that 12% of patients with tumor invasion to a depth of 5 mm or less had inguinal node metastasis. Ridley *et al.* (1988a) suggest that the only truly valid concept of vulvar microinvasive carcinoma "is one which, though seen histologically to have broken out from the confines of the epithe-

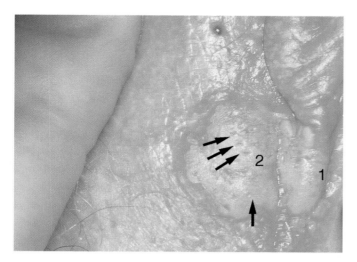

Fig. 9.28

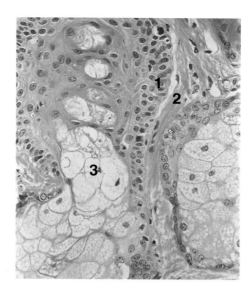

Fig. 9.30

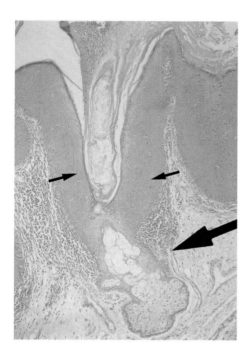

Fig. 9.29

lium, is only invading the stroma to such an extent that it carries no risk of lymph node metastasis. Therefore a definition of 5 mm as a maximum depth of invasion is insufficiently stringent and is associated with an unacceptably high nodal involvement rate." It would seem from many other reports that only those tumors that invade to a depth of 1 mm or less are associated with a virtual absence of lymph node involvement. In those carcinomas invading up to 1.5 mm, there seems to be a very low risk (Wilkinson *et al.*, 1982; Hacker *et al.*, 1983). As will be described later, the ISSVD has proposed a substage of the FIGO (International Federation of Gynecology and Obstetrics) stage I, which identifies those tumors that invade to a depth of 1 mm or less. This substage, proposed as stage Ia, identifies as a solitary squamous carcinoma of 2 cm or less in diameter and

with a depth of invasion of 1 mm or less. The depth of invasion is defined as the measurement of the tumor from the epithelial stromal junction of the adjacent most superficial dermal papillae to the deepest point of invasion. Tumors with and without vascular space involvement are included in this definition (Kneale, 1983).

It has been reported that there has been an increase in the percentage of such early invasive lesions (Elliott, 1992). This most likely reflects the increase in the reported incidence of the precursive lesions of VIN 3 as well as an increasing awareness by pathologists and gynecologists of the existence of these early lesions.

It has latterly been reported that there is a significant but still small early invasive carcinoma found in areas where there is extensive VIN 3. This has been previously detailed (p. 239) (Hording *et al.*, 1995; Modesitt *et al.*, 1998; van Beurden *et al.*, 1998b).

Clinical features

The clinical features are the same as those described for VIN 3, except that some of these early invasive lesions may be more raised, roughened, and pigmented. Lesions are multifocal in up to 30% of cases and as many as five separate macroscopic, and even microscopic, lesions have been reported in one vulva (Magrina *et al.*, 1979; Kneale *et al.*, 1981). It is not unusual to find other conditions, such as lichen sclerosus and squamous cell hyperplasia, occurring in conjunction with early invasion (Borgeno *et al.*, 1988; Barbero *et al.*, 1990; Elliott, 1992). In Elliott's (1992) series, 62% of cases possessed these associated conditions and a further 24% contained VIN 3 with or without HPV changes.

The lesions shown in Figs 9.31 and 9.32 are associated with early invasive disease. In each, there has been long-standing and chronic irritation with marked hypertrophy of all the vulvar structures. Figure 9.31 shows a large lesion that affects the labia (1) and extends into the perianal region; this is causing marked hypertrophy in both sites. In Fig. 9.32, the extent of the lesion onto the labia majora and further laterally is arrowed; it likewise projects into the perianal area. Careful assessment of the remainder of the genital tract and anus is mandatory in such cases. Extensive excision biopsies were carried out on these two patients and showed VIN 3 with invasion to less than 1 mm existing in multiple sites across the vulva.

Risk of nodal spread: depth and volume measurements

It would seem from many studies that tumor volume, rather than the depth of tumor invasion, relates more accurately to the risk of nodal metastasis (Burghardt, 1984). Very little is known about the volume of early invasive disease of the vulva in terms of the correlation between depth of invasion and tumor mass. It would appear that the tumor volume remains below 1000 mm^3 when the depth of invasion is less than 1.5 mm, but extension beyond that depth is associated with a wide range of tumor volumes that do not correlate with the depth of invasion (Wilkinson et al., 1982; Burghardt, 1984). In the large-area lesions as seen in Figs 9.33–9.35b, various areas of microinvasion may be present when eventual excision is undertaken.

It is extremely difficult to measure the exact tumor volume of many lesions and it has been suggested that the maximum diameter of an early invasive carcinoma would be a better indicator of nodal spread. DiSaia et al. (1979) suggested that 1 cm should be the limit for a "microinvasive carcinoma" but Magrina et al. (1979) noted that 10% of patients with tumors measuring 1 cm or less in diameter developed nodal metastasis. Kneale et al. (1981) found a 4% incidence of lymph node involvement and a 16% incidence of local recurrence in association with neoplasms of 1 cm or less in diameter. Others consider that depth of invasion is a better indicator of lymph node involvement than is the

diameter, and that tumor volume is irrelevant (Hoffman et al., 1983).

Assessment of the pathologic specimen

In an examination of the excised specimen, not only must the depth of invasion be measured but also such features as vascular space involvement, confluence, degree of tumor differentiation, and, if possible, tumor volume, must be estimated so that an accurate prognosis can be given. It would seem that invasion of vascular-type spaces significantly increases the risk of nodal metastasis in early invasive lesions; Kolstad et al. (1982) showed that 40% of patients in whom vascular space involvement was present had nodal metastasis, whereas only 3% without such involvement had nodal spread. Wilkinson et al. (1982), however, did not show any clear-cut relationship between nodal metastasis and vascular space involvement in such early lesions. The relationship between tumor differentiation and risk of metastasis is also controversial; Kolstad et al. (1982) and Woodruff (1982) showed that there was no association between these two parameters.

The ISSVD (Kneale, 1983) recommended that the term micro-invasive carcinoma of the vulva be discontinued, and that a new classification of stage Ia be used to describe "those solitary lesions confined to a maximum of 2 cm in diameter and 1 mm depth of invasion." This definition would replace the previous terminology.

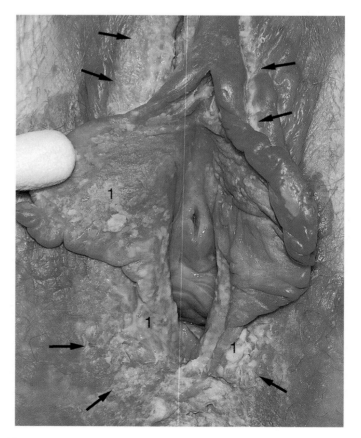

Fig. 9.32

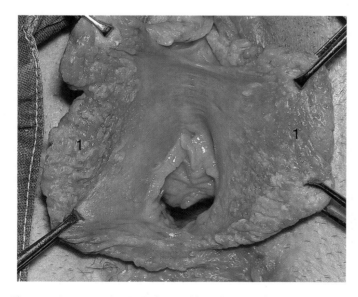

Fig. 9.31 An extensive VIN 3 lesion (1) with areas of early invasion (<1 mm) involving the labia and extending to the perianal area.

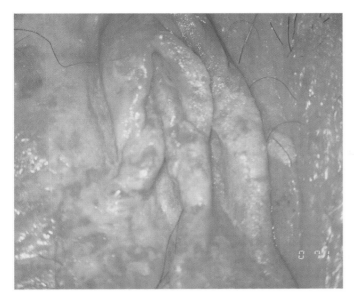

Fig. 9.33 An extensive area of hyperkeratotic white tissue involving the periclitoral area, labia majora, and labia minora. A large excision procedure was carried out and a small focus of early invasive carcinoma (<1 mm) was found in the periclitoral area.

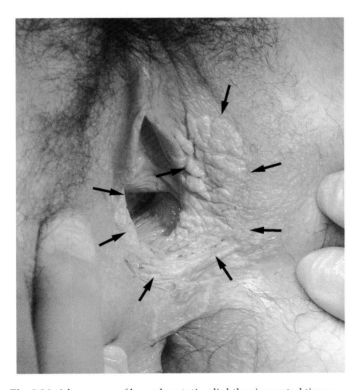

Fig. 9.34 A large area of hyperkeratotic, slightly pigmented tissue (arrowed) extends across the labia minora and majora on both sides. A small area of invasion (<1 mm) was found after an extensive local excision procedure was carried out.

The subject of early invasive carcinoma of the vulva is still controversial and future studies are required to define accurately the risk from these very early lesions.

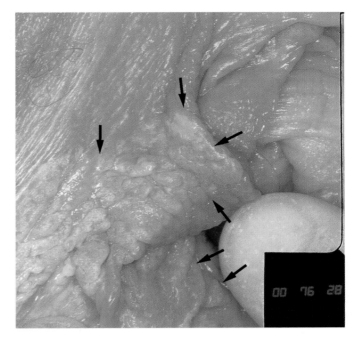

Fig. 9.35(a)

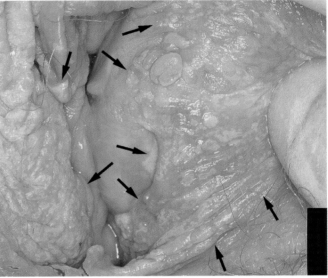

Fig. 9.35(b)

Fig. 9.35 An extensive hyperkeratotic white area (arrowed) existed on (a) the outer and (b) the inner aspects of the labia minora, with extension onto the labia majora (arrowed). Three small foci of very early invasive malignancy (<1 mm) were found after a wide local excision was performed.

Diagnosis

Diagnosis cannot be made clinically but can only be suspected from the features, described above and observed during the vulvoscopic examination (Figs 9.31–9.35b); histologic confirmation follows biopsy. An excision biopsy must be performed and should include a margin of 1 to 2 cm of normal, or apparently normal, vulvar skin. Such wide local excision biopsies present few problems with isolated solitary and well-defined lesions but with extensive lesions there is a need for multiple biopsies. It may also be that an elective simple vulvectomy or a skinning maneuver (described below) would be an effective and satisfactory alternative.

In Fig. 9.36, a very dense, keratinized area can be seen around the clitoris (1) and upper labia minora (2). A biopsy taken from area (2) showed the presence of VIN 3 (Fig. 9.37). However, close examination of the area to the left of the clitoris showed a small area with a faintly abnormal and vascular pattern (3). Lateral to this a further area of more obvious abnormal vascularity existed (Fig. 9.38).

The vascular pattern is difficult to visualize in the presence of such dense keratotic areas, but a thin smear of lubricant applied to this area will aid individualization of the vasculature. Vessels may be seen in the usual punctation or mosaic patterns that characterize CIN, vaginal intraepithelial neoplasia (VAIN), or early invasive disease. It is uncommon to see them in vulvar lesions because of the presence of thickened epithelium. However, in very early invasive lesions, not only punctation or mosaic patterns but also corkscrew vessels may exist and run parallel to the overlying epithelial surface; some irregular dilatation of these vessels may indicate the presence of early invasive cancer.

In Fig. 9.38 such vessels can be seen in two papular areas. Excision biopsy of the area marked (1) in Fig. 9.38 and its surrounds, showed the existence of very early invasive cancer penetrating to a depth of 0.8 mm. Figure 9.39a–c are of similar cases and show very early and superficial invasion. In cases 9.39a and b, invasion is less than 1 mm while in 9.39c the depth of penetration is 1.5 mm.

Recurrence of early invasive vulvar carcinoma

One of the characteristics of early invasive vulvar cancer is the frequency with which recurrent disease occurs. This can be either within a year or two of the initial procedure or at times ranging up to 15 years later. It has been suggested by some authors that the word recurrence should only be used for lesions that recur within 2 years of primary treatment, and that reoccurrence should be used to refer to the "postoperative appearance of a second vulvar carcinoma-in-situ

or invasive carcinoma so remote in time or location from the original process as to be considered unrelated" (Wharton *et al.*, 1974). Other authors (Elliott, 1992) suggest that the terms "second" or "new" cancer should be used for those tumors that recur 3 years or later after primary treatment.

The rate of recurrence is approximately 16%, as adjudged from eight series quoted by Elliott (1992). The range was

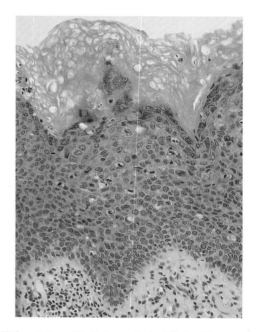

Fig. 9.37 Vulvar intraepithelial neoplasia (VIN) with extensive surface hyperkeratosis, hence the white clinical appearance of the lesion. Note the numerous mitotic figures, which have a transepithelial distribution, and nuclear pleomorphism.

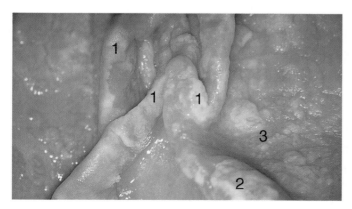

Fig. 9.36

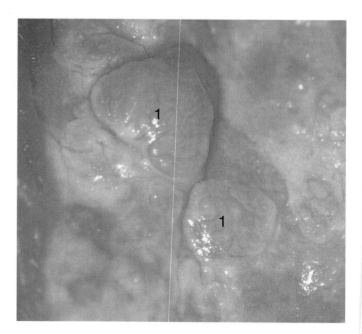

Fig. 9.38

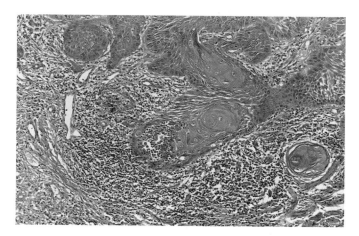

Fig. 9.39(a)

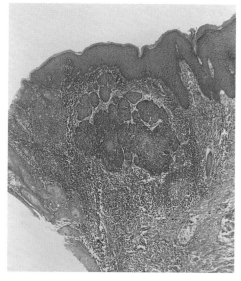

Fig. 9.39(b)

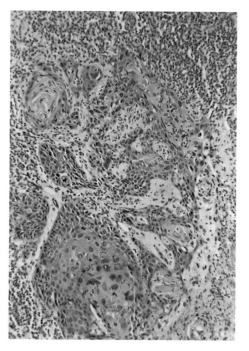

Fig. 9.39(c)

from 0% to 26.5%, involved 437 cases, and included both recurrence and reoccurrence of tumors. In another series of four cases, also described by Elliott (1992), the time of recurrence during follow-up ranged from 1 to 15 years. He suggests that one of the reasons for the increasing frequency of these late-developing cancers is "the continuing and meticulous follow-up that allows accrual of more long-term data than in earlier studies." It would appear from analysis of many studies that neither the size of the original lesion, anaplasia, lymphatic vascular permeation, or microscopic confluence, nor the extent of the primary surgery for the initial early invasive lesion correlates in any way with the early or late development of vulvar precancer or early invasion. However, the site of the tumor may correlate with development. In Elliott's series of 132 patients treated in Australia, 19 had tumors in the clitoral and urethral area and seven (37%) of these showed recurrence; in comparison, there were 28 (26% of 113) cases of recurrence for tumors sited elsewhere in the vulva.

Other factors that may indicate a propensity for recurrence include lymph node metastasis, found at the time of the original operation, and depth of stromal invasion. For instance, in 330 cases from four series (Elliot, 1992), there were 20 recurrences where the stromal involvement was less than 2 mm, and 39 where the invasion was from 2 to 5 mm. Elliott (1992) further suggests that the presence of HPV in association with VIN 3 is a very strong indicator for the later development of recurrent disease. Elliott also points out that those cases "associated with HPV" would seem to have a good chance of long-term survival. However, further studies are needed to confirm these preliminary findings.

Herod *et al.* (1996a) studied the long-term outcome of patients presenting with VIN with superficially invasive disease. Twenty-six women in the study were identified during a 15-year period. Treatment was primarily by local excision with a mean follow-up of $5\frac{1}{2}$ years. Disease persisted after primary treatment in five women (19%) with the histology of the recurrence being either VIN or early invasive disease. Symptomatic recurrences occurred in 38% and all occurred within 3 years. Overall, 12 of the group (46%) relapsed either histologically or symptomatically with a mean time of only 18 months. Fourteen patients or 54% were managed satisfactorily by their initial treatment.

In this series, one patient died of recurrent cervical cancer but more importantly, three progressed to frankly invasive disease; two (aged 33 and 39) of cancer of the vulva and one (aged 34) with carcinoma of the perianal margins. They concluded from this study that patients with superficially invasive cancer of the vulva could be safely treated by local excision without recourse to lymphadenectomy, but they added that relapse after primary treatment was common and there appeared to be a small but significant risk of progression to frankly invasive carcinoma.

9.10 Lichen sclerosus (LS)

It is not uncommon for the area adjacent to a cancerous or precancerous vulvar lesion to show evidence of a long-standing epithelial disorder. Many such women will present with symptoms in the surrounding areas and it is not unusual to discover a history of ineffective treatment applied to this skin, and also occasional biopsy and excision. The commonest coexistent skin lesions are LS and squamous cell hyperplasia. Both are classified as nonneoplastic epithelial disorders of the vulvar skin and mucosa. There may also be a mixture of these lesions and occasionally VIN 3. The finding of these areas in relation to neoplastic disease gave rise to the assumption that they may be precancerous. However, there is no evidence that LS is indeed a precancerous condition, although in a careful study by Wallace (1971) the incidence of neoplasia in the vulvas of patients with LS was in excess of that which would have been expected from the normal population. In another recent review of 132 cases of early invasive cancer of the vulva (Elliott, 1992), chronic vulvar dystrophy (as Elliott describes these surrounding lesions) was found in 82 (62%) cases. Close examination revealed that 15 (18%) were pure LS. In 30 (36%) cases squamous cell hyperplasia was present, and a mixture of these two lesions was found in the remaining 37 (46%) cases. The age range in Elliott's series was 31 to 88 years and the mean was 66.9 years. McAdam and Kissner (1958) found in 46 (11%) out of 400 cases of cancer either pure LS or a lesion classed as "leukoplakia" and which they considered could be LS. Other chronic dermatoses with sclerosus were found in this study; some may have been LS, and so could have pushed the percentage higher. Buscema *et al.* (1980a) found that approximately one-half of squamous cell carcinomas in their study had an associated area defined as "dystrophy," and it is possible that some of these were LS. Zaino *et al.* (1982) found 32 of 60 cases of squamous cell carcinoma to have "atypical hyperplastic dystrophy;" 15 possessed pure LS, while 14 others had hyperplastic dystrophy, nine mixed dystrophy, and nine CIS. Hewitt (1984) found LS in 96% of 104 cases of squamous cell carcinoma, and Dottenwille (1982) found 100% of 40 cases of squamous cell carcinoma to have an associated LS. The existence of LS has been noted in a vulva where VIN 3 was also present (Buckley *et al.*, 1984), and Ridley (1988a) describes two cases of LS in which vulvar condyloma existed and eventually progressed to VIN 3; in both women, extensive areas of LS existed.

Clinical presentation

LS may occur in extragenital sites, such as the truncal skin, but in about 60% of cases of women with vulvar lesions, the condition is confined only to the vulvar and perianal area. It is asymptomatic from an early stage, when there will be minimal clinical findings, but as it develops flat, ivory and slightly erythematous polygonal papules develop; these eventually become confluent and form larger plaques that coexist with associated atrophy. The result is that the skin develops a fine cigarette-paper-type wrinkling in which hemorrhage may develop, and with the associated scratch-ing and trauma due to the intense pruritis, there may develop hemorrhagic bullae, purpura or petechiae. Occasionally, there is hyperkeratosis, and eventually marked epidermal atrophy and local erosion may arise.

Histopathology

In Fig. 9.40 the classic histologic features of LS are seen; these include a broad zone of hyalinization and edema in the papillary and reticular dermis. In the absence of rete ridges the epidermis (1) is flattened and there may sometimes be hyperkeratosis. The dermis (2), besides being edematous and hyalinized, usually contains at its lower border some inflammatory cells (3). Atrophy may also extend to the dermis and subcutaneous tissues.

Management

In the management of patients with LS, it is important to inspect and sample by biopsy, twice-yearly, all non-healing ulcers and/or newly developed white hyperkeratotic lesions; this will allow carcinoma to be detected at an early and treatable stage. It must be emphasized that it can be extremely difficult to recognize the development of cancer in patients with LS owing to the associated ulceration and fissuring.

In the following figures, the development of malignancy is added to the background of existing LS changes. Figure 9.41a shows a vulva with a focus of invasive cancer (1) in a patient with extensive LS (2). There is obvious marked clitoral fold fusion as well as labial atrophy. It must be stressed that despite the coexistence of these two lesions, they are not thought to be related etiologically. In Fig. 9.41b and c, a malignant lesion presents as a red nodular regular area on the surface of the right labia minora. There is associated LS in the labial and clitoral areas, and in Fig. 9.41c the lesion has been elevated to show its internal attachment, which is just lateral to the urethra.

Pruritus accompanies almost all cases of LS from the outset; it induces vigorous scratching with subsequent ulceration and the formation of ecchymoses. This sometimes causes difficulty in diagnosis and such an example is

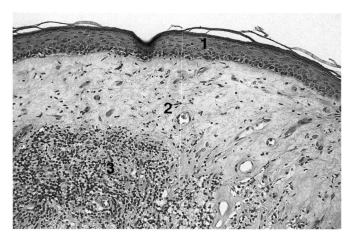

Fig. 9.40

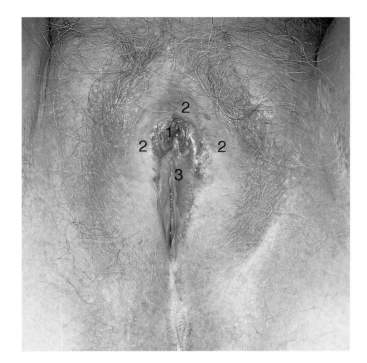

Fig. 9.41(a)

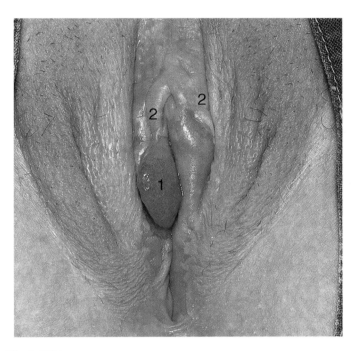

Fig. 9.41(b)

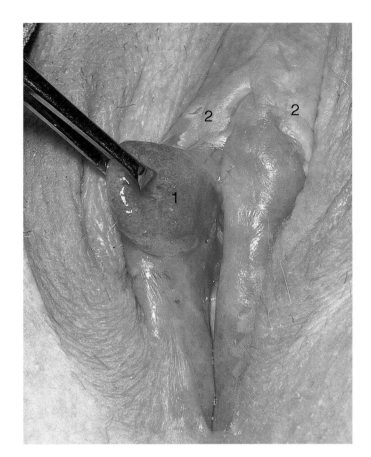

Fig. 9.41(c)

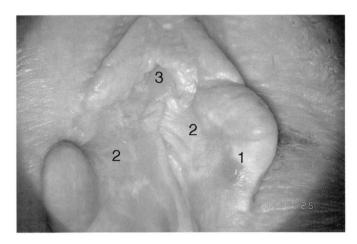

Fig. 9.42

seen in Fig. 9.42. This 68-year-old woman was treated with local applications of steroids and testosterones for a number of years for extremely symptomatic and progressive LS. A small ulcerated area at (1) was observed without being biopsied for over 1 year; this area was considered to have been induced by scratching. Eventually, biopsy revealed the presence of early invasive cancer. Other signs of LS are present; there is fusion of the inner labial folds over the urethra (2) and virtual obliteration of the clitoris at (3). In Fig. 9.43, the gross appearance of LS can be seen in this simple vulvectomy specimen which, at first appearance, would seem to be that of a vulva with early invasive

cancer. However, this patient suffered for many years with progressive LS and simple vulvectomy was carried out for symptomatic relief. The gross changes mimic invasive cancer but there was none in the specimen; it was the continual trauma induced by scratching that produced these changes.

In the following three cases (for which figures were kindly provided by Professor Raymond Kaufman) a superimposed malignancy is present against a background of LS. In Fig. 9.44, a raised, reddish lesion (1) is situated in the right labia minora region in a postmenopausal woman in whom LS is obvious. Very thin and atrophic tissue covers the inner labia minora (2) and the clitoris has been completely covered by the conglutination of its hoods (3).

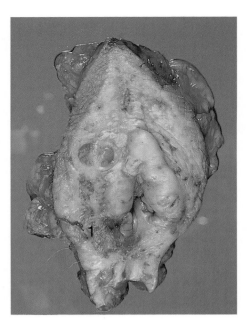

Fig. 9.43

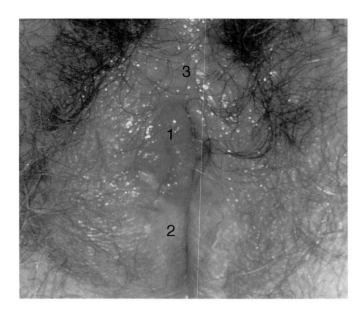

Fig. 9.44

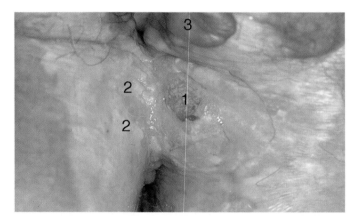

Fig. 9.45

Biopsy of area (1) revealed it to be a squamous cell carcinoma. In Fig. 9.45, a shallow ulcerative lesion (1) lies within an area of very atrophic perineal skin; obvious hyperkeratotic areas (2) are associated with the smooth surface of the labia minora (3). The lesion at (1) is a squamous cell carcinoma that developed 15 years after an area of VIN 3 had been excised. Viral typing showed this invasive lesion to contain HPV-DNA types 16 and 18.

In Fig. 9.46, an obvious ulcerative and histologically confirmed malignant lesion (1) involves the labia minora and majora on the left, and the labia minora and clitoral areas on the right in a postmenopausal woman whose vulva shows typical features of LS. There is very white, atrophic epithelium at (2) and the clitoral area has been completely obliterated by fusion of the overlying structures (3).

Figure 9.47 shows a biopsy taken from the edge of the ulcerative area (1) in Fig. 9.46; there is an obvious pattern of invasive squamous cell carcinoma. Viral typing of this malignancy showed it to contain HPV-DNA types 16 and 18.

9.11 Paget's disease (non-squamous intraepithelial neoplasia)

In 1874, Sir James Paget published the first description of this disease; his original cases were of disease involving the nipple and areola, and were associated with breast cancer. Later cases, associated with disease of the vulva, were also reported and in 1955 Woodruff collected the world literature, which amounted to only 23 cases. Paget's disease is considerable more common, involving multiple organ sites. Helwig and Graham (1963) described 98 cases of vulvar Paget's disease, of which 25 were associated with or preceded frank malignancy. The most common association is with a vulvar adnexal carcinoma or other local tumors, for example in Bartholin's gland; of the more distant neoplasms breast cancer is the most common, followed by

cancer of the vulva, cervix, and vagina (Lee *et al.*, 1977). In the 20–30% of women in whom there is an associated invasive neoplasm of the vulva or adjacent organs, the cells are believed to have migrated or metastasized from the tumor into the surrounding epidermis (Woodruff, 1977). The vast majority of Paget's disease lesions of the vulva appear to be of the autochthonous type; however, some develop from sweat ducts or embryonal remnants. These intraepithelial lesions may remain confined to the epidermis, or may invade the dermis to become invasive cancer.

In the largest retrospective series of Paget's disease patients, Fanning *et al.* (1999) examined 100 women, median age 70, who had been treated at eight institutions. Twenty of the women had a total of 26 non-vulvar malignancies. There had been symptoms of severe pruritus for 2 years prior to removal of the perineal lesion which was extensive in 16 of them. In this group a recurrence developed at the median time of 3 years in 34 of them. In 31 of these women with intraepithelial disease (Paget's), one had an invasive Paget's disease of the vulva, and two had

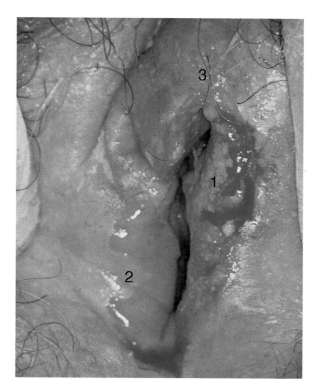

Fig. 9.46

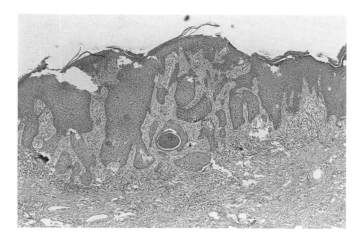

Fig. 9.47

extravulvar adenocarcinoma. There was a 12% prevalence of Paget's disease and a 4% prevalence of associated vulvar adenocarcinoma, with one patient dying of associated vulvar adenocarcinoma.

Clinical presentation

The characteristic clinical appearance (Fig. 9.48a, bi, bii, biii) is of a classic "weeping Paget's disease" involving a moist vulva in which there are patches of hyperkeratotic tissue (1) interspersed with rivulets of raw, reddened tissue (2). There is intense soreness and irritation. For disease occurring in hair-bearing areas of the vulva, the lesion is usually treated as though it were a local infection and this leads to a consequent delay in diagnosis. In Fig. 9.48bii & iii, the variable nature of Paget's disease is seen. The perianal

lesions exhibit an erythematous eczematoid surface with scales and crust.

Histopathology

The histopathology is absolutely characteristic; a good example can be seen in Fig. 9.48c where the superficial layer of hyperkeratotic epithelium is covered by a layer of round Paget cells (1) that run in a line or nest close to the basal layer. There is occasional heaping, but the cells are often laid out in single file along this layer. The cells may also be found within the hair follicles and the apocrine and eccrine ducts. As the epithelium matures, the cells are found at progressively higher levels, and when they reach the surface they are shed alongside the keratinized squamous. The Paget's cells stain positively with mucicarmine, aldehyde, fuchsin, and periodic acid Schiff (PAS) reagent; the latter reaction remains positive after diastase digestion. Specific immunopathologic staining using immunoperoxidase has shown cytoplasmic positivity for carcinoembryonic antigen (CEA), epithelial membrane antigen (EMA), certain low molecular weight keratins (LMK), gross cystic disease fluid protein (GCDFP), and casein (Nadji *et al.*, 1982; Moll & Moll, 1985; Ganjei *et al.*, 1990). Ganjei *et al.* (1990) have recently reported on 19 patients in whom biopsy proved the presence of Paget's disease of the vulva. They attempted to determine whether immunocytochemistry was helpful in assessing the surgical margins of the excised tissue and found that none of the histologically proven negative margins reacted to CEA, EMA, or LMK. However, CEA appears to be a valuable marker for extramammary Paget's disease; EMA and LMK are also expressed by the majority of such cases. None of the markers tested, however, was of added value in identifying Paget cells in surgical margins if those margins appeared normal on routine hematoxylin–eosin staining.

Management

Prior to treatment, a careful assessment of other sites for cancer must be made, but the management of the local disease consists essentially of performing a wide excision. If there is evidence for the presence of invasive cancer, radical procedures with femoral/inguinal lymphadenectomy may be necessary. The disease is frequently multifocal and a careful assessment must be made of the vulva, lower vagina, and perineum.

9.12 Vulvar lesions masquerading as cancer or precancer

A number of vulvar lesions mimic the appearances of cancer or precancer. They are mainly of an infective nature, being predominantly related to wart viral infections, and have been frequently reported as accompaniments to vulvar cancer. Other specific and associated infective conditions include granulomatous venereal disease and syphilis. Elliott (1992) has pointed out that these infections have a distinct geographic, ethnic, and socioeconomic bias

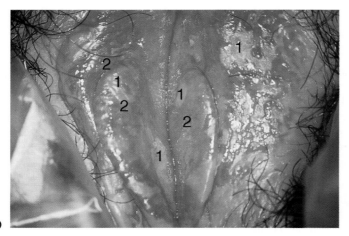

Fig. 9.48(a)

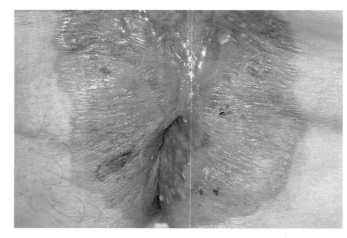

Fig. 9.48(b)

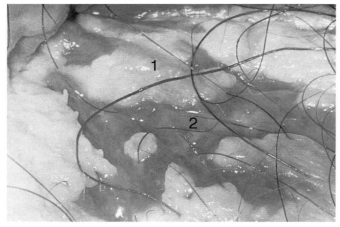

Fig. 9.48(bi)

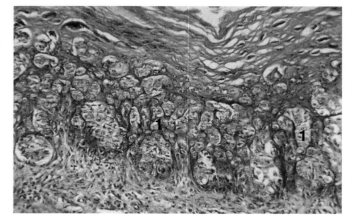

Fig. 9.48(c)

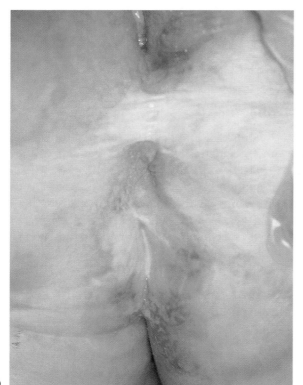

Fig. 9.48(bii)

in their association with vulvar cancer (Salzstein *et al.*, 1956; Hay & Cole, 1969; Sherman *et al.*, 1991).

Syphilis

The incubation period for this infectious disease, caused by *Treponema pallidum*, is between 10 and 90 days; it is commonly about 2 weeks and the untreated primary stage may last from 3 to 8 weeks. The first lesion to appear is a macule that soon becomes papular with ulceration to form a primary chancre. The indurated painless ulcer with a dull red base [as seen at (1) in Fig. 9.49] forms the classic presentation of a chancre; regional lymph nodes become enlarged within a week of the appearance of the oval lesion. These nodes are usually painless, firm, and smooth. However, the symptoms and signs of early syphilis are variable and there may be more than one chancre present (Fig. 9.49). Variations usually occur as a result of superimposed secondary infection. The labia majora seems to be a very common site for the primary chancre; in Fournier's original (1906) series some 46% occurred in this site, 22% occurred on the labia minora, and only 5% on the cervix.

It is obvious that the chancre may be mistaken for not only a squamous cell carcinoma but also conditions such as genital herpes, pyogenic lesions, infected injuries, chancroid, lymphogranuloma venereum, and Donovanosis. Drug-induced eruptions and Behçet's disease (Fig. 9.50a & b) must also be considered.

The laboratory tests for the diagnosis of early syphilis depend on dark-ground examination for *T. pallidum* and on

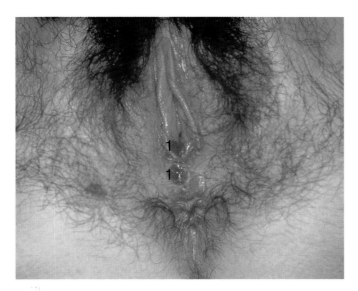

Fig. 9.49

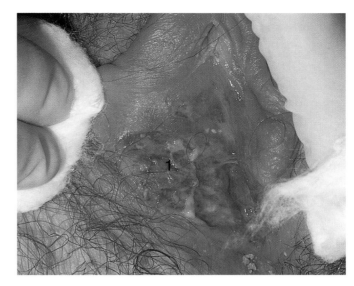

Fig. 9.50(a)

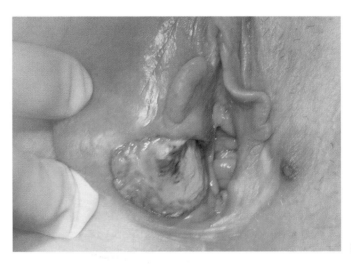

Fig. 9.50(b)

serologic tests. When there are ulcers or papular lesions of the skin or mucous membranes, dark-ground microscopy is a highly accurate and specific technique. To undertake such a test, the area must first be cleaned with normal saline. If the lesion is dry, it is scarified at the edges to cause bleeding and after the blood has clotted, a drop of serum is examined. If the lesion is moist enough, serum can be obtained by applying pressure. Magnification at 400 or 900× with dark-ground illumination will allow the treponemes to be detected. If, on examination of a suspicious lesion no organisms are seen, microscopy should be repeated daily for 2 to 3 days. Serologic tests for syphilis, such as VDRL (venereal disease research laboratory) or RPR (rapid plasma reagin), must also be performed, and they give positive results in up to 70% of patients with primary syphilis. They are also positive in high titers in secondary syphilis, after which the titer slowly falls, but becomes positive again in late syphilis. The specific treponemal test, such as FTA-ABS (fluorescent treponemal antibody absorption), is reactive in up to 90% of patients with primary syphilis; TPHA (treponemal haemagglutination) is also reactive in up to 87% of cases. Both tests are positive in virtually all cases of secondary syphilis, and remain positive indefinitely in more than 95% of untreated patients (Wende, 1971; King *et al.*, 1980).

Behçet's disease

The occurrence of genital ulceration, which may be confused with vulvar cancer or precancer, is also associated with oral and ocular inflammation. It was first described by the Turkish dermatologist Behçet in 1937 and was associated with conditions such as arthritis, thrombophlebitis, acneform skin eruptions, neurologic abnormalities, and ulcerative colitis.

A virus is considered to be involved in its causation, although it has been suggested that it may be an immunopathologic response to an HSV type 1 infection (Eglin *et al.*, 1982) as circulating immune complexes have been found in the blood.

The genital lesions are usually very striking and highly destructive, resulting in fenestration and scarring with progressive loss of the vulvar tissue. Even when small, the lesions are notable for their depth, and many are relatively tender. These vulvar lesions are usually painless, and the ulcers may be of varying sizes and persist for weeks or months. Scarring is usual but not inevitable. The labia minora is a common site of involvement and a typical lesion encompassing all the features just described is shown at (1) in Fig. 9.50a & b. Viral bacterial cultures will test negative, as will the dark-ground examination; the serologic tests for syphilis (mentioned above) will be nonreactive. Biopsy will show a nonspecific chronic inflammatory process with associated vasculitis. Oral lesions occur on the lips, tongue, buccal mucosa, and palate, and appear like common aphthous ulcers.

It is most important to exclude invasive squamous cancer by employing the tests described above to exclude syphilis. Recurrent herpes and recurrent untreated syphilis have to be considered, as does pemphigus, which may cause lesions of both the genitalia and the mouth. Pemphigus can be excluded by using specific immunofluorescent stains on fresh tissue samples.

Condylomata acuminata

The association between HPV infection and cervical, vaginal, and vulvar neoplasia has already been described. The presence of lesions caused by this virus on the vulva can produce difficulty in diagnosis, not only of the precancerous lesion, namely VIN 3, but also of invasive cancer. In a recent study by Daling and Sherman (1992), 72 out of 142 vulvar tumor tissues were positive for HPV as detected by PCR; a majority of these (76.4%) were positive for HPV 16. Indeed, many other studies (as quoted by Daling and Sherman, 1992) have analyzed tissues of patients with in-situ and invasive vulvar cancer for evidence of HPV; in-situ hybridization techniques have been used and have shown prevalence rates of 16, 44, and 11% of VIN 3 tissues that are positive for HPV types 6/11, 16, and 18 respectively. The corresponding prevalence rates for the same HPV types in invasive cancers were respectively 29, 44, and 11% positive. Using the more sensitive Southern blot hybridization technique, 70% of VIN 3 tissues were positive for HPV 16, whereas 18 and 67% of invasive cancer tissues were positive for HPV types 16 and 18 respectively. However, there have recently been reports (Li Vigni *et al.*, 1992) that almost 60% of invasive lesions and 47% of preinvasive lesions lack HPV 16 or 18, as judged by the extremely sensitive nonspecific PCR technique; this has given rise to suggestions that there is a subset of VIN 3, and invasive cancers, that has a non-viral etiology (Husseinzadeh *et al.*, 1989; Pilotti *et al.*, 1990; Rusk *et al.*, 1991; Toki *et al.*, 1991; Park *et al.*, 1991; Li Vigni *et al.*, 1992). It was noted that in many of these studies there were differences in the pathologic characteristics of tumors with and without HPV. It was also reported that females with tumors lacking HPV 16 and 18 were 10 to 20 years older than those women who had detectable HPV-DNA in their tumors.

Clinical features

Condylomata acuminata form multiple papillary or verrucous lesions, or may present as sessile rough-surfaced plaques on the skin or mucous membranes of the vulva, perineum, and perianal region. They occur frequently along the edges of the labia minora and may extend into the interlabial sulcus or around the introitus. Their color varies enormously, from flesh-colored to pigmented lesions that appear either gray-brown or almost black.

In Fig. 9.51, multiple flat and spiky condylomata, mostly pigmented, can be seen extending across the whole vulva and including the perianal area. They also extend into the interlabial sulcus. Close examination will reveal variations in the surface configuration but it is virtually impossible to determine whether these are indeed pigmented condylomata acuminata, a pigmented form of VIN 3, or the pigmented lesions described as Bowenoid papulosis (see p. 249). It is obvious that colposcopy and biopsy must be performed on all pigmented lesions to exclude the multifocal hyperpigmented variety of VIN 3 and, in some cases, early invasive malignancy. Figure 9.52a shows a typical exuberant condyloma acuminata that, on biopsy (Fig. 9.52b),

shows typical HPV changes with koilocytosis, elongation of the rete pegs, marked acanthosis, and increased mitotic activity. However, the mitotic figures are not abnormal, and the typical pleomorphic hyperchromatic nuclei with associated corps ronds, which are so characteristic of VIN 3, are missing in this lesion. It is usual in many condylomata for papillomatosis to occur, but the flat nature of this particular lesion is obvious. This contrasts with the spiky papillomatous type of condyloma seen in Fig. 9.53a and its associated pathology in Fig. 9.53b.

In Fig. 9.54a the difficulty of diagnosis of VIN 3 in the presence of condyloma acuminata is obvious. Although some classic condylomata acuminata are present on the outer labial areas (1), the central introital and fourchette region contains dense white lesions that are indistinguishable from the VIN 3 lesions (2) described previously. It is only with biopsy that differentiation can be made, and in this particular case multiple areas of VIN 3 were found in association with condyloma acuminata. Occasionally, one may also find other infective lesions that may be difficult to distinguish from warts; these include molluscum contagiosum, the papules and condylomata of secondary syphilis, and the vulvar lesions of Donovanosis. Differentiation from syphilis has already been described. Molluscum contagiosum has a slightly different appearance to the condylomatous lesion, and forms a firm pearly hemispheric papule that is usually 2–5mm in diameter and has a dimpled center, from which cheesy material may be squeezed. There may be multiple lesions that infect not only the vulva but also the lower abdomen, pubis, and adjacent skin. Solitary molluscum contagiosum may resemble a basal-cell carcinoma of the vulva. Diagnosis is made on clinical examination, but if the clinician is unsure, biopsy will reveal acanthotic prickle-cell epithelium, in which surface cytoplasmic virus particles produce the typical molluscum contagiosum body that occupies the central core of the lesion. Ridley (1988a) describes a diagnostic test in which the core

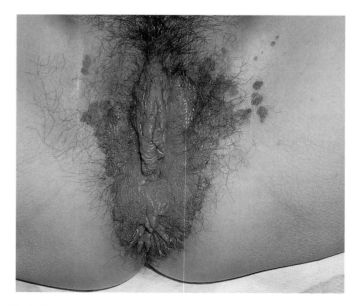

Fig. 9.51

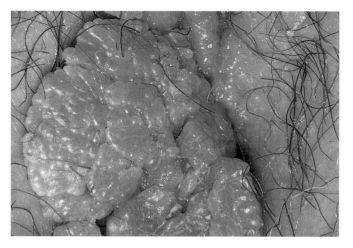
Fig. 9.52(a)

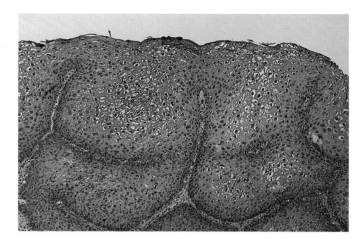
Fig. 9.52(b)

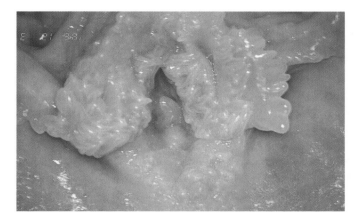
Fig. 9.53(a)

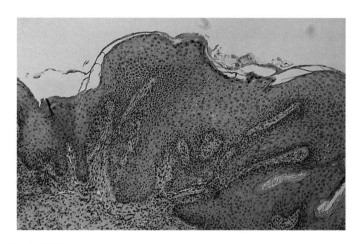
Fig. 9.53(b)

of the lesion is curetted out and mixed with a drop of 10% potassium hydroxide (KOH) on a slide; at a magnification of 400×, molluscum bodies appear as irregular masses that are about 35 μm in diameter.

The distinction of wart viral lesions from VIN and invasive cancer is of such importance that biopsy of all vulvar lesions whose nature and characteristics are uncertain, must be advocated. Also, it must be stressed that any condyloma acuminata that does not respond to treatment must be sampled. Any papular lesions should be viewed with suspicion and biopsy undertaken before treatment is commenced.

A biopsy of classic condylomata acuminata (Fig. 9.52b & 9.53b) will reveal papillomatosis with acanthosis, elongation of the rete pegs, koilocytosis and, as in this case, dense dermal inflammatory infiltrate. Parakeratosis will be present, especially on the surface of the epithelium, and less frequently there will be hyperkeratosis. The nuclear abnormalities are not evident in these cases; the nuclei show no hyperchromasia and have a uniform

structure. Mitotic activity is increased but the mitotic figures are not of the abnormal type such as is found in VIN 3.

Granuloma inguinale

This condition, which occurs in people who live in tropic and subtropic countries, may be presented by patients with a vulvar lesion that appears very similar to a malignancy. It is caused by the organism *Calymmatobacterium granulomatis*, a Gram-negative encapsulated rod of uncertain bacteriologic status; diagnosis is made by taking tissue smears in which the organism can be demonstrated within the cytoplasm of large mononuclear cells and occasionally in polymorphonuclear leukocytes. The condition that it causes is also known as Donovanosis.

The lesion occurs after an incubation period of 7 to 30 days and presents as a papular or nodular lesion on either the labia minora, fourchette or mons. The overlying skin that is associated with the papular or nodular lesions breaks down, giving rise to a soft, granulating ulcer that progressively spreads and may eventually involve large areas of both the perineum and anus (9.54b). There is associated lymphedema. The granulations may extend into the lower genital tract as far as the cervix, and there may be granulomatous lesions in the skin overlying the lymph nodes.

The diagnosis is made by demonstrating the presence of the infecting agent in tissue smears; Ridley (1988c) believes that the best specimens are obtained from "biopsy or curettings of the ulcer base that are then stained with Leishman's or Giemsa stains." A histologic examination is also important to exclude malignancy. As has already been mentioned, these lesions may resemble those of the condylomata of secondary syphilis and this condition must be excluded by serologic testing.

Lichen planus

Another condition which must be excluded as neoplastic is that of lichen planus which results in simultaneous orogenital ulceration affecting women between 30 and 60 years of age. In 25%, the lesion is limited to the mucus membranes and characteristically involves the vagina and vestibule, causing a desquamative vaginitis. This leads to acute inflammation of the vagina which appears denuded of epithelium. Biopsy of this tissue shows basal cell liquefaction at the dermoepidermal junction with a heavy band-like subepidermal lymphocytic infiltration. A more intense erosive type of lichen sclerosis has been described associated with gingival lichen planus and is called the syndrome of Hewitt and Pelisse (Hewitt *et al.*, 1985). In this stage, vacuolation of all the basal cells and incipient blister formation are characteristic of this tissue superimposed on the classical histology of lichen planus.

Adhesions begin to form in the upper part of the vagina and a gray pseudo-membrane may be noted, also on the surface. As the disease progresses, the vagina may become totally obliterated. The vestibular mucosa is frequently eroded, as seen in Fig. 9.54c, with resultant complaints of soreness and dyspareunia and obviously contact bleeding.

The oral manifestations show the reticulated gray, lacy pattern of what the author called *hyperkeratotic Wickham's striae of the buccal mucosa*. The gingival tissues also become swollen with interdental accentuations or appear acutely eroded with red scalloped borders to the gingival margins of the teeth as seen in Fig. 9.54d.

The vulvovaginal lesions usually predate the erosive or ulcerative mouth lesions by months or even years and about one-third of those with vulvovaginal disease do not experience the oral lesions. Lesions which involve the vulva are usually found on the inner aspects of the labia minora where the gray-white lacy strands of Wickham's hyperkeratosis may also be seen and resemble the ones described above for the buccal mucosa.

Biopsy is important, not only to differentiate these appearances from neoplasia but also from squamous cell hyperplasia or hyperkeratotic lichen sclerosis. Although a distinction is made between lichen planus and erosive

lichen planus, it is now clear that the desquamative vaginitis is, in fact, one form of erosive lichen planus (Kaufman & Faro, 1994).

Subclinical epithelial changes

There are a number of subclinical epithelial changes that can only be seen effectively with the magnification afforded by vulvoscopy and that may cause confusion with the diagnosis of VIN. Biopsy is necessary to determine the exact nature of the epithelium. These epithelial changes are of three types:
1 Acetowhitening of the epithelium.
2 Filamentous lesions.
3 Acetowhite microcondylomata.

Acetowhite epithelium

With the application of acetic acid, the vulvar skin may appear white (so-called acetowhite); this change is frequently found around the vaginal introitus and on the perineum. As has been shown above, major-grade VIN produces a very intense white coloration with the application of 5% acetic acid to the skin. These acetowhite changes, especially in the presence of skin thickening and changes in color tone, are significant and may indicate VIN, but there are a number of other acetowhite changes without these features that are of very little significance. A number of studies (Coppleson & Pixley, 1992) have shown that only some of them are associated with wart viral infections. Many are caused by constant scratching and rubbing, which produces a lichenification of the skin with corresponding excoriation. Such an example of a rather non-specific acetowhite change is shown in Fig. 9.55; this change takes on a characteristic horseshoe-shaped appearance around the inner aspect of the labia minora and posterior aspect of the vaginal introitus and adjoining perineum (arrowed). Frequently, these changes may extend into the vagina to blend indistinctly with normal vaginal epithelium or may extend over the length of the vagina. At other times, this acetowhite skin can be seen anterior to the urethra, on the clitoris or even on the mons. It is, as men-

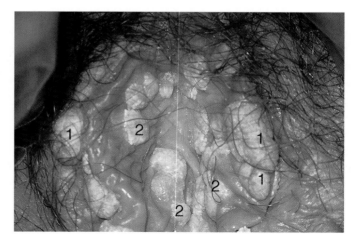

Fig. 9.54(a)

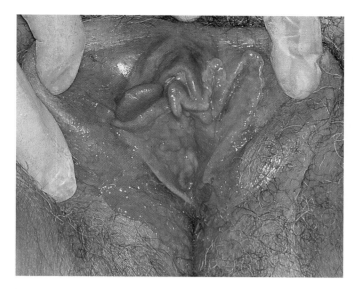

Fig. 9.54(b)

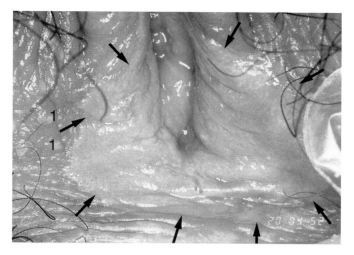

Fig. 9.55

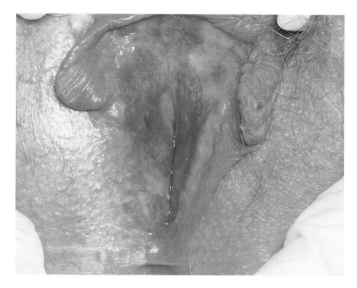

Fig. 9.54(c)

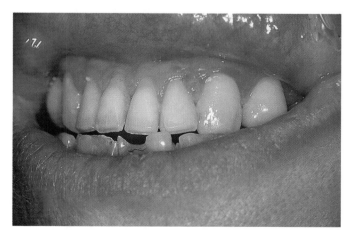

Fig. 9.54(d)

tioned above, a variant of changes in the normal epithelium but in some cases it may be associated with wart virus infection.

Filamentous lesions

A filamentous lesion may be found around the introital area and be confused with condyloma or occasionally VIN. Such lesions may be multipapillary or villiform and can be found in virginal females; they are called vestibular papillae or micropapilloma labialis (Fig. 9.56a). In sexually active females, they may be extensive and completely encircle the introitus (Fig. 9.56b & c) (Friedrich, 1983a; Woodruff & Friedrich, 1985). Some authors believe them to be associated with HPV (Campion, 1987) but others have failed to confirm this observation (Bergeron *et al.*, 1990). The histology of these micropapilloma labialis lesions is typical with a central capillary core surmounted by a thickened layer of squamous cells that give rise to the intense acetowhitening found when acetic acid is applied to these lesions. In Fig. 9.56d, the central capillary is marked (1) and the apical tip of squamous cells is at (2).

Acetowhite microcondylomata

These lesions are another form of SPI of the anogenital region. After the application of acetic acid, discrete acetowhite spots [(1) in Figs 9.55 & 9.57a] or acetowhite microcondylomata [(2) in Figs 9.57a & b] develop. Biopsy shows them to have the stigmata of HPV (Figs 9.58a & b). They range from a few in number to large numbers that may be so extensive as to cover the whole of the introital and perianal area, sometimes extending to the clitoris, labia majora, and adjacent skin. Occasionally, they are seen in the gluteal cleft. On close examination, it is seen that the discrete acetowhite spots may be associated with hair follicles, and intense pruritus develops. It is suggested that they and the microcondylomata may represent a latent state, or even a carrier phase of viral infection, in that they are frequently found when similar HPV changes exist in the vagina and cervix (Planner & Hobbs, 1987; Zhang *et al.*, 1988). They have been reported as occurring in conjunction with VIN in some 10% of cases (Planner & Hobbs, 1987, 1988).

These three epithelial types are classified as subclinical lesions, because they can be assessed only after acetic acid has been applied and vulvoscopy undertaken. They may be asymptomatic but in many women their presence is associated with itching and burning (Reid *et al.*, 1988). Many patients are diagnosed as having had recurrent genital moniliasis infection and there are usually other symptoms, such as dyspareunia. A naked-eye view of the area shows it to be completely normal and usually vaginal smears and cultures fail to demonstrate any fungal infection. It is estimated that about half these lesions will regress, and a conservative approach is recommended (Coppleson & Pixley, 1992). However, the severely symptomatic patient will need treatment, especially if the papillomavirus infections develop into frank condylomata. At times, adequate biopsies may need to be taken to exclude the presence of VIN.

9.13 Skin and accessory appendages that are important for the management of VIN

The vulvar skin is of a stratified squamous type that is highly specialized and composed of an epidermis, a papillary dermis, and reticular dermis with overlying subcutaneous fat. It possesses a number of appendages, including superficial sweat glands, pilosebaceous ducts that lead to hair follicles deep in the reticular dermis and fat layers, sebaceous glands, and other specialized structures such as Bartholin's gland and duct. Figure 9.59a and b shows these structures and their corresponding depth from the surface; in Fig. 9.59b (from Baggish, 1989) their involvement by VIN has been measured.

An appreciation of the extension of VIN into any of these skin appendages is important because a failure to destroy VIN in any of these structures would run the theoretic risk of recurrence. Mene and Buckley (1985) described the extension of VIN into skin appendages. Its involvement of hair follicles was to a mean depth of 1.2 mm with a range

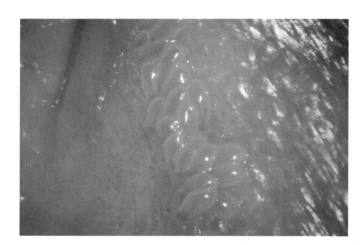

Fig. 9.56(a)

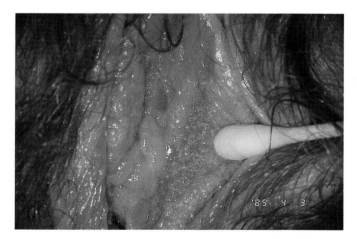

Fig. 9.56(b)

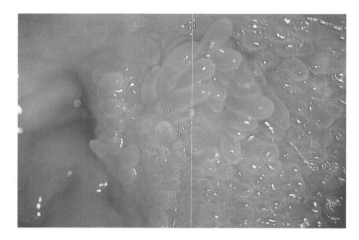

Fig. 9.56(c)

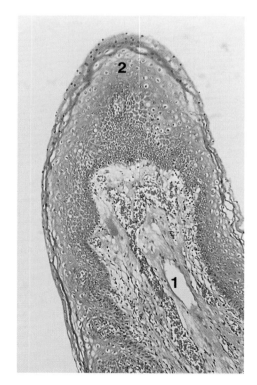

Fig. 9.56(d)

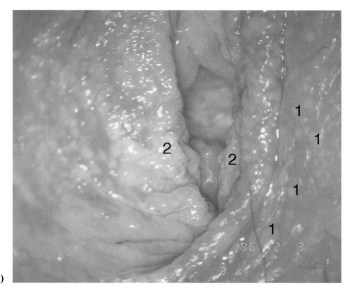

Fig. 9.57(a)

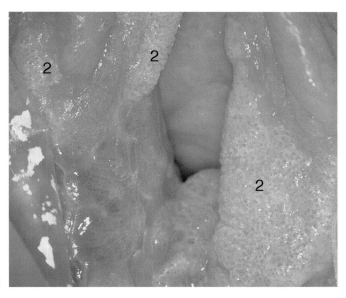

Fig. 9.57(b)

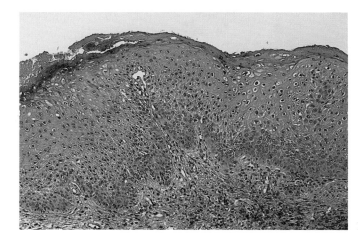

Fig. 9.58(a)

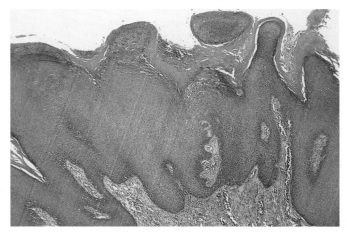

Fig. 9.58(b)

Figs 9.57 and 9.58 In Fig. 9.57, (a) shows discrete acetowhite spots at (1) with areas of dense acetowhite microcondylomata (2); the latter are also present in Fig. 9.57(b) where their surface contour is accentuated. Figures 9.58(a) and (b) are biopsies taken from the microcondylomatous areas in Figs 9.57(a) and (b) respectively; (a) shows human papillomavirus (HPV) chages, while (b) shows similar features but with associated hyperkeratosis and surface projections corresponding to the surface contour.

of 4.6 mm, and this involvement was related to the severity of the disease; VIN 3 extended to a maximum depth of 2.5 mm. When VIN 3 was present with microinvasion it extended to 3 mm, and when it was present with foci of invasive cancer that penetrated to less than 3 mm, it extended to 4.6 mm within the hair follicles.

Baggish *et al.* (1989) and Shatz *et al.* (1989) have published detailed measurements of the extent of superficial and deep-skin appendages involved with VIN. They showed that when these appendages contain VIN they do not penetrate as deeply as had previously been imagined; therefore, use of laser vaporization and other skinning techniques

were indeed safe and, more importantly, nonmutilating. Figure 9.59b (from Baggish, 1989) shows the mean depth of uninvolved superficial appendages to be 1.63 mm. Baggish measured the epidermis and found it to be only 0.31 mm deep. Further measurements showed the mean depth of deep appendages to be 3.6 mm; the deepest hair follicles measured 5 mm and were situated in the subcutaneous fat. Eighteen out of 50 patients with VIN 3 showed involvement of the skin appendages to a mean depth of 1.53 ± 0.77 mm, suggesting that laser vaporization (with the anticipated additional thermal necrosis) to a depth of 2.5 mm will eliminate appendages involving VIN 3 in 95% of instances. The most common sites of skin-appendage involvement were the labia majora or minora and interlabial folds.

Shatz *et al.* (1989) produced similar data to that of Baggish; with a calibrated microscope they measured the thickness of VIN and the depth to which it extended into the underlying pilosebaceous units of the vulvar skin. In 329 histologic sections from 62 cases, the mean thickness of VIN was 0.38 mm; 99.5% of all VIN measured less than 0.77 and 0.69 mm in the hairy and nonhairy skin, respectively. Sebaceous gland and hair follicle involvement by VIN was 21% and 32%, respectively. The mean depth of sebaceous gland involvement was 0.77 mm in hairy skin and 0.50 mm in nonhairy skin; 99.5% of all VIN extended less than 2.03 and 1.07 mm in the hairy and nonhairy skin, respectively.

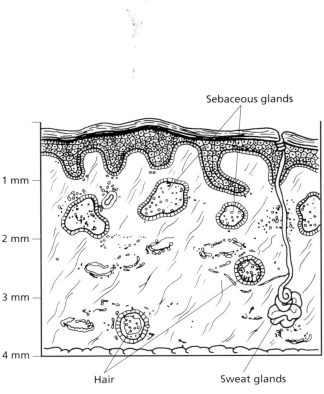

Fig. 9.59(a)

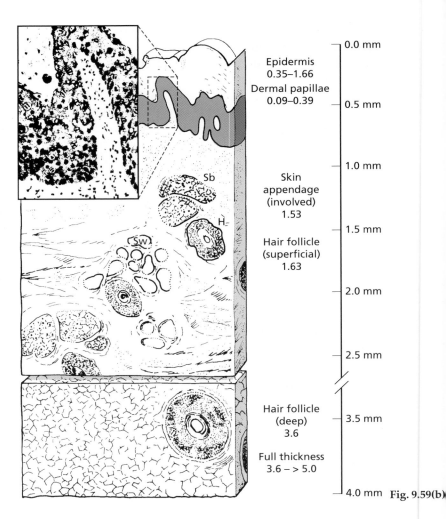

Epidermis
0.35–1.66

Dermal papillae
0.09–0.39

Skin
appendage
(involved)
1.53

Hair follicle
(superficial)
1.63

Hair follicle
(deep)
3.6

Full thickness
3.6 – > 5.0

0.0 mm

0.5 mm

1.0 mm

1.5 mm

2.0 mm

2.5 mm

3.5 mm

4.0 mm Fig. 9.59(b)

The mean depth of hair follicle involvement was 1.04 mm; 99.5% of all hair follicles showed less than 2.55 mm involvement. These findings, combined with those by Baggish, suggest that the removal of VIN to a depth of 1 and 2 mm in the nonhairy and hairy skin, respectively, would be appropriate for successful treatment.

In a recent study, Benedet *et al.* (1991) measured the thickness of the "dysplastic epithelium" and the depth of involved and uninvolved skin appendages with the ultimate aim of providing a morphometric basis on which to base laser therapy for VIN. They found that the mean thickness (±SD) of the epithelium for all grades of VIN was 0.5 ± 0.23 mm with a range of between 0.10 and 1.90 mm; there was only a small variation in thickness of the involved epithelium in relation to the location of the lesion. They commented that from a therapy point of view the difference in thickness between the various grades of VIN was not of practical clinical significance. The measurements suggested that laser vaporization to a depth of only 1 mm, including the zone of thermal necrosis, should be sufficient to destroy epidermal lesions with skin-appendage involvement. They stated that if the initial biopsy revealed involvement of adjacent hair follicles or sebaceous glands, then deeper tissue destruction would be necessary to achieve theoretically a greater than 90% elimination of the disease.

9.14 Management of VIN

The optimum management of VIN has yet to be determined because the natural history of the disease is still uncertain. Various treatment options, ranging from the conservative to the radical, will be discussed here. It must be remembered that many patients will be young and the emotional trauma of any procedure is considerable (Theusen *et al.*, 1992). The distribution of the disease itself also induces an element of variability. Its presence in either hair- or nonhair-bearing areas has an influence on the type of procedure performed. This being so, it is important to understand the anatomy and distribution of the structures discussed in Section 9.13.

Rationale for treatment

Determining the management of patients with VIN 3 is often difficult and a challenge to the gynecologist. Most patients who eventually are diagnosed with VIN 3 seek medical help because of longstanding symptoms such as itching and burning pain. Herod *et al.* (1996b) recently showed that nearly 70% of these patients presenting with VIN 3 had severe pruritus vulvae and although extensive surgery such as vulvectomy is less popular nowadays, its counterpart in the form of extensive vulval tissue removal is still being used for symptomatic areas. As has been alluded to above, even with extensive surgical procedures, recurrences of VIN are common. Reference has also been made above to recurrence rates that can be as high as 60%, especially if the margins of the excised area are involved with disease; and likewise, with multifocal disease, up to 40% recurrence rates have been reported in some series (Andreasson & Bock, 1985). To add to the difficulties of extensive surgical procedures, there is the risk of the development of psychosexual disease. It would seem as though the rationale for treatment is twofold:

1 To relieve the symptoms of disease.
2 To avoid recurrences and the risk of invasive cancer.

Over the last 30 years, there has been a gradual trend towards conservative therapy and it is agreed that when treatment is carried out, it should be directed towards preservation of a normal anatomy and function of the vulva. Kaufman (1995) makes a plea for the individualization of treatment on the basis of location and extent of lesion, insisting that when lesions involve the perineum or perirectal area, that it is critical that the anal canal be examined, as up to 20% of women with VIN have an accompanying disease in the anal canal.

Treatment options and procedures

A number of treatment options will be discussed and the results of each technique presented. The options that will be considered are as follows.

1 Conservative management.
2 Wide local excision using a knife or laser.
3 Skinning vulvectomy and skin grafting.
4 Simple vulvectomy.
5 Wide local excision with vaginal advancement.
6 Laser treatment.
7 Medical therapy (5-fluorouracil; 5-FU).

Before any treatment option is embarked upon, preoperative vulvoscopy and biopsy are essential to aid the decision as to which method will be employed to treat the VIN. Vulvoscopy is used to:

1 Define the extent of disease.
2 Direct biopsies to the area of most clinically severe abnormality.
3 Exclude overt invasive cancer.
4 Direct, if necessary, laser treatment through visualization of anatomic landmarks, thereby allowing the depth of vaporization to be determined.

Conservative management

The initial question to ask is, "is treatment necessary?" A study of the natural history of VIN shows that there is a low risk of progression and, indeed, there are case reports of spontaneous regression of VIN in young women. The majority of gynecologists currently treat VIN by conservative methods such as wide local excision and laser vaporization; the recurrence rate does not differ significantly with any one particular method.

It must be remembered that young women subjected to these forms of treatment run the risk of psychosexual sequelae. There is much evidence to suggest that in the management of both cervical and vulvar precancer, there is a significant increase in psychologic stress, postoperative social adjustment, and sexual dysfunction (Anderson & Hacker, 1983; Campion et al., 1988; McDonald et al., 1989; Jones, 1990; Theusen et al., 1992). When an expectant policy is undertaken, the patient must be willing to attend for long-term follow-up, and this will involve frequent biopsies and vulvoscopy to exclude malignancy. The patient has to be aware of the commitment that is necessary for this conservative observation of the lesion.

Vulvoscopy and mapping of lesions is performed at each visit, and any new lesions or existing lesions that alter in appearance must be biopsied. The significance of VIN and its relationship to vulvar malignancy is not so well defined that treatment for VIN can be advised in every case. Perhaps treatment should be confined to cases considered to be at high risk of malignant transformation: these include the elderly, the immunosuppressed patient, and lesions that are obviously aneuploid. Treatment in younger women may be confined to those in whom the disease is symptomatic, where biopsy suggests any change toward more advanced pathology, or in those lesions where it is felt that the overlying keratin layer is so thick that it is difficult to assess the underlying pathology. Obviously, in these cases frequent biopsy will aid in making the correct decision.

Wide local excision (using either knife or laser)

Wide local surgical excision is used to treat unifocal or multicentric lesions in nonhairy or hairy areas. Primary closure is usually obtained. However, in treating lesions in the perianal region, where there is less laxity than in the surrounding tissue, the wound may either be left to heal by secondary intention, or grafted, as will be discussed later; wide excision with vaginal advancement may also be considered. With use of wide local excision, the reported recurrence rate is 12–30% (Woodruff et al., 1973; Friedrich et al., 1980; Andreasson & Bock, 1985; Bornstein & Kaufman, 1988; Simonsen, 1989); recurrent disease is usually associated with involvement of the excision margins, and a margin of excision between 0.8 and 1.0 cm has been suggested. Even with the former margin, Friedrich et al. (1980) reported an 18% recurrence rate. The results from studies involving wide excision are given in Table 9.4.

When surgical excision is performed, the removed specimen should, in ideal circumstances, be sent to the laboratory to obtain frozen sections from the margin because despite the removal of up to a centimeter of normally appearing surrounding skin and mucosa, the margins may still be involved with intraepithelial neoplasia. The recurrence rate, as mentioned above, may be as high as 60%. Andreasson and Bock (1985), who followed 49 women treated with local excision found that in 23 in whom the margins were free of disease, only 1 (4.3%) developed a recurrence, whereas 11 of 19 (60%) with involved margins developed recurrence. Multifocal disease is well-known for being associated with recurrence and of their 22 patients, nine (40%) had recurrence compared with four (16.7%) of 24 with unifocal disease. The relatively high recurrence rate

Table 9.4 Results of studies using wide local excision.

Reference	No. of cases treated	No. of recurrences	Failure rate (%)
Woodruff *et al.* (1973)	15	2	13.3
Forney *et al.* (1977)	11	0	0.0
Friedrich *et al.* (1980)	17	3	17.6
Buscema *et al.* (1980a)	63	23	32.0
Caglar *et al.* (1982)	23	2	8.6
Bernstein *et al.* (1983)	16	2	12.4
Andreasson and Bock (1985)	43	13	30.0
Simonsen (1989)	23	0	0.0

Reproduced with permission from Singer and Mitchell (1990).

in individuals with multifocal disease is as a result of the fact that these patients, some 55%, had involved resection margins compared with only 29% of the patients with unifocal disease.

The impact of margin status on disease recurrence and incidence of occult cancer in women with VIN 3 has been highlighted by a study from Modesitt *et al.* (1998). They examined 73 women who were diagnosed preoperatively with VIN 3 by vulval biopsy and were treated with surgical resection with at least 1–2 cm of surgical margin. The mean age of these women was 45 years; 37% of them had had prior genital warts. What was worrying was that an underlying squamous vulval cancer with a median depth of invasion of 1 mm and a mean of 1.7 mm was found in 22% of patients when final analysis of the initial surgical specimen was undertaken. In respect of follow-up, 59 women were seen at least 7 months after surgery and of these, 66% (39/59) had positive surgical margins of whom 46% (18/39) had developed recurrent disease. There were 31% (18/59) who had negative margins and of those only 17% (3/18) had recurrent disease. This was a statistically significant difference. There were 3% who had unknown margins (2/59) and it was noted that multifocal disease and a history of genital warts also corresponded with a risk of VIN 3 recurrence.

Kaufman (1995) insists that it is important that a frozen section be taken from the margins of excised tissue and if they are positive, further tissue should be resected until no evidence of disease is noted along the edges of the removed specimen. He believes that even when large areas of skin or mucosa were removed from the vulva, it is almost always possible to achieve a primary closure following undermining of the edges of the defect or with the development of skin and subcutaneous flap.

Wide local excision using a laser is very popular because it employs the unique properties of this modality, namely, removal of precision-measured portions of tissue involved with VIN, and minimal trauma (Simonsen, 1989). Baggish (1989) has popularized the so-called skinning technique, which is also used for the treatment of VAIN and is described on p. 281. The technique involves the initial delineation of the affected area of VIN 3 as shown in Fig. 9.60a (see arrows) and b. The incision is then deepened to about 2.5 mm to allow the epidermis and dermis to be

undercut (Fig. 9.60c & d). When the laser is used with the rapid super pulse or chopped wave mode (Reid, 1992) a minimum of thermal injury is inflicted on the tissue. In Fig. 9.60d, there is a narrow, sharply defined rim of coagulation that is due to the radiant energy overload; the crater shows no carbonization, except where a small capillary has been coagulated. The undercutting process shown in Fig. 9.60c has resulted in the small area of VIN being removed, and the edges of the wound can be approximated with fine, absorbable sutures (Fig. 9.60e)

In the Fig. 9.61a–d such a technique of skinning the vulval surface as a wide local excision can be seen. In Fig. 9.61a an extensive area of hyperkeratotic skin extends across the outer surface of the right labia minora (1) on to the skin of the labia majora at (2). An ulcerated area is seen at (3) at the base of the labia minora. In Fig. 9.61b, using a rapid super-pulse mode on the CO_2 laser, a skinning technique is being employed which sweeps the skin with the diseased portion laterally in the direction of the arrows, removing the diseased area with a wide normal margin as marked (dashed line). Minimal damage to the tissues has been inflicted by the laser as seen by the sharpness of the incision line. In Fig. 9.61c the diseased area has been removed and primary closure can now begin. In Fig. 9.61d primary closure of the right labial wound has been undertaken and is arrowed. On the left side a hyperkeratotic area similar to that on the right was present on both the inner and outer aspects of the labia minora. A skinning technique removed all the disease and the end result is seen. Postoperatively there will be some swelling which may last for up to 4–6 weeks. The excised area showed the presence of VIN 3, but in the area marked (3) in Fig. 9.61a there was a very small focus of early microinvasive carcinoma.

Skinning vulvectomy with skin grafting

A skinning vulvectomy with split-thickness skin grafting and clitoral preservation was first described in 1968 by Rutledge and Sinclair. The reported recurrence rate after this procedure has been carried out is between 12% and 30%; failure is primarily due to the existence of positive excision margins (DiSaia & Rich, 1981; Bernstein *et al.*, 1983; Caglar *et al.*, 1986; Rettenmaier *et al.*, 1987). Cases of recurrent disease occurring within the grafted skin have now been reported (Cox *et al.*, 1986). The donor graft is taken up by the recipient site in over 85% of patients, and the majority seem able to resume coitus within 8 weeks. In DiSaia and Rich's (1981) study of 39 women, none reported dyspareunia after a period of 6 months. Dudzinsky and Rader (1990) have reported use of the mons pubis as an excellent graft donor site.

The technique has been recommended primarily for use in young women with multicentric disease that extends into the hair-bearing areas of the vulva, and in whom laser treatment would not be applicable because the necessary depth of treatment would not produce a good cosmetic result. Such a lesion can be seen in Fig. 9.62, in which an extensive area of VIN 3, previously confirmed by biopsy, is outlined by arrows. This technique is useful in cases where there is a wide area of unifocal disease and where excision

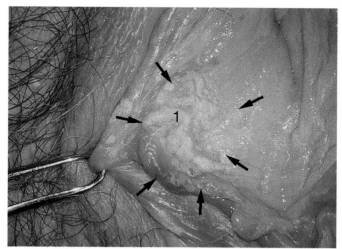

Fig. 9.60(a)

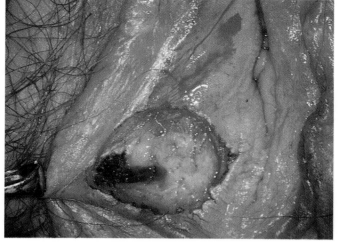

Fig. 9.60(d)

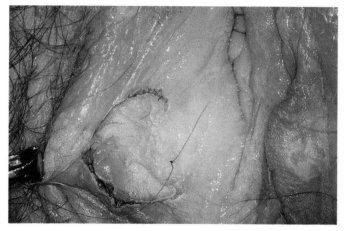

Fig. 9.60(b)

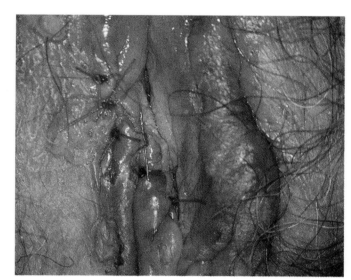

Fig. 9.60(e)

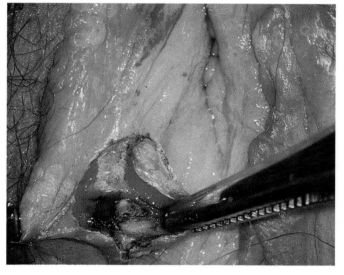

Fig. 9.60(c)

with primary closure would be technically difficult. The procedure does involve more prolonged hospitalization because a second scar usually results from removal of the graft from either the medial aspect of the thigh or the anterior abdominal wall. This scarring can, in itself, produce problems in young women but it does give a better functional and cosmetic vulvar result. Results of the studies employing this technique are given in Table 9.5.

A series has been published by Thomas *et al.* (1996), in which he and his group have shown that vulvoperineal reconstruction is possible after excision of large areas of multifocal intraepithelial disease in the anogenital area. They have followed, over a 7-year period, 12 women who were submitted to a radical surgical approach for extensive disease, one of whom is featured in Figs 9.62a and b and 9.63a–d. A multispeciality team was involved with gynecologists, general and plastic surgeons working together with an initial colostomy being performed followed by definitive vulvoperineal resection and simultaneous vulval reconstruction, using meshed split skin grafts or a combination of skin grafts and local flaps, as seen in the series of photographs Figs 9.62a and b and 9.63a–d. Seventeen vulvoperineal reconstructions were done for 12 patients, three of whom had incomplete histopathologic clearance at the initial operation. Apart from these three patients, one had recurrence of symptoms alone, without any evidence of multifocal intraepithelial disease, which was probably due to HPV infection. One patient developed a malignant squamous invasion 4 years later which was cured with surgical excision and reconstruction. The colostomy closure was done after achieving local control of the disease. This group believe that this staged approach achieves the objectives of eliminating disease, alleviating symptoms, preserving function and attempting to reconstruct normal

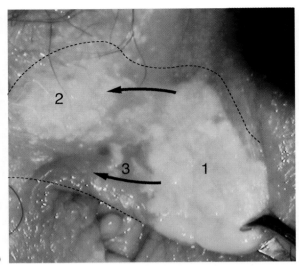

Fig. 9.61(a)

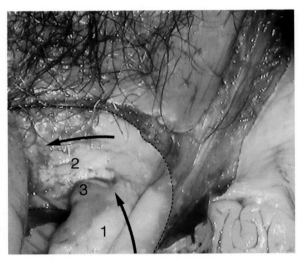

Fig. 9.61(b)

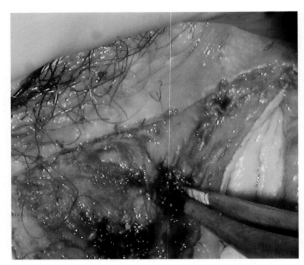

Fig. 9.61(c)

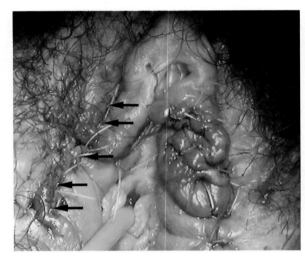

Fig. 9.61(d)

anatomy (as seen at 10 weeks post operatively in Fig. 9.63dii), without compromising the principles of surgical oncology. They insist that it results in a high patient satisfaction.

However, an alternative view will be presented later, arguing that a lesser procedure such as advocated by van Beurden *et al.* (1998b) and which involves vulvoscopy combined with a mapping procedure specifically to detect superficially invasive cervical cancer in patients with multifocal VIN 3 who are not symptomatic and who do not have preliminary evidence of superficial invasion, is a much better, more patient-satisfying procedure.

The authors feel that although there may be a place for this technique, an alternate method involving local excision by laser may offer a higher success rate and lower morbidity. This technique is described below and uses wide local excision with vaginal advancement.

Simple vulvectomy

A simple vulvectomy is a mutilating procedure for a young woman to undergo and it does not significantly reduce the recurrence rate. It is associated with a high incidence of postoperative psychosexual problems and is generally no longer popular. Many women will say that they would

Table 9.5 Results of studies using skinning vulvectomy with grafting.

Reference	No. of cases treated	No. of recurrences	Failure rate (%)
Forney *et al.* (1977)	8	1	12.5
DiSaia and Rich (1981)	39	15	39.0
Bernstein *et al.* (1983)	8	1	12.5
Wolcott & Gallup (1984)	13	7	53.8
Caglar *et al.* (1986)	24	2	8.3
Rettenmaier *et al.* (1987)	48	13	27.0

Reproduced with permission from Singer and Mitchell (1990).

"rather have a deformed vulva than no vulva at all" (Theusen *et al.*, 1992). More conservative measures are performed in young women with VIN, but there may be a place for this procedure in older patients who have extensive and symptomatic VIN 3. In these cases, it will be used to relieve symptoms and exclude occult invasion.

Wide local excision with vaginal advancement

In many instances, the excisional techniques described above are associated with significant morbidity in respect of postoperative healing, pain, hospitalization, and the

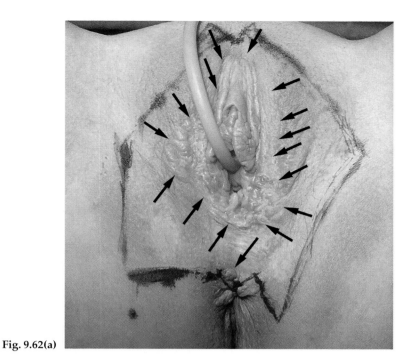

Fig. 9.62(a)

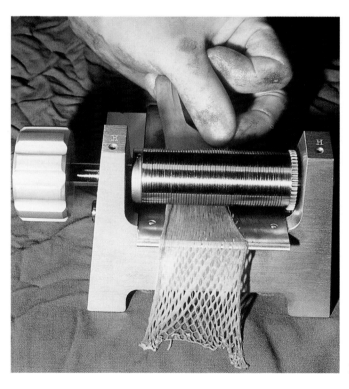

Fig. 9.62(b)

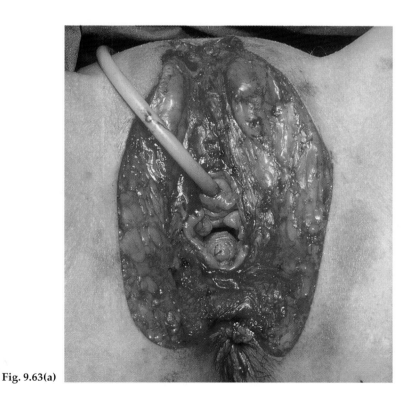

Fig. 9.63(a)

Fig. 9.63(b)

eventual cosmetic result. The use of a technique in which the lesion is locally and widely excised with the advancement of the vaginal mucosa to cover the defect, presents many advantages. Based on the original vaginal advancement technique described by Woodruff and Parmley (1983), it involves a two-part procedure in which the area of VIN 3 is first outlined, using vulvoscopy, and excised, and then the vagina is undercut and advanced.

The technique is especially suitable for lesions that involve the vaginal introitus, fourchette, or labia minora (Figs 9.34, 9.35a & b, 9.64 & 9.65) and in those cases where the perineum is involved to within 1.5 cm of the anal margin. In the two cases shown, there was severe pruritis and the patient was young. Close examination of Fig. 9.64 will show that the lesion extends to the hymenal margin at

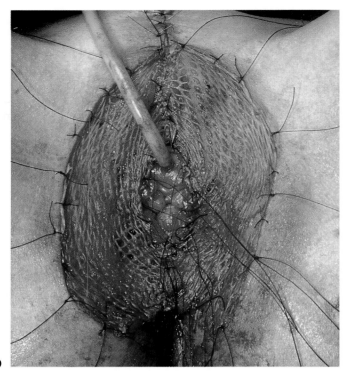

Fig. 9.63(c)

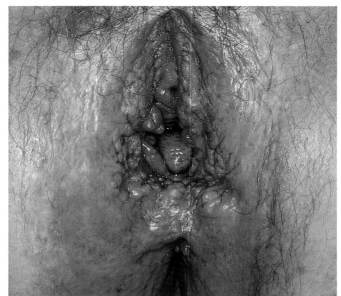

Fig. 9.63(d)

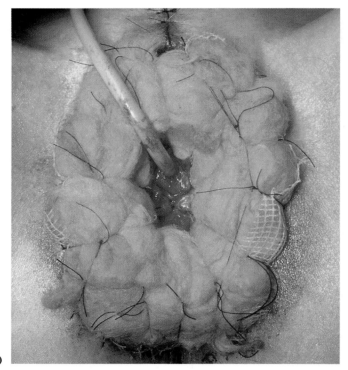

Fig. 9.63(di)

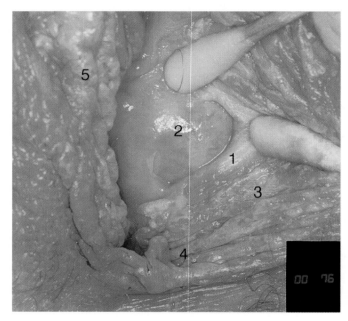

Fig. 9.64

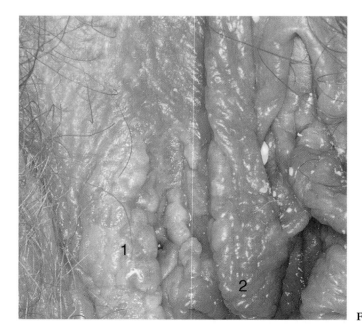

Fig. 9.65

(1), at which point it abuts an enlarged Bartholin's cyst (2). The hyperkeratotic area (3), a punch biopsy of which revealed VIN 3, extends posteriorly across the vestibule and fourchette (4) and involves the labia minora (5). Three areas of early invasion (<1 mm) were found after the wide excisional specimen was reviewed. In Fig. 9.65 VIN 3 is present in a hyperkeratotic area (1) on the labia majora; the lesion also extends to the labia minora (2), posterior vestibule, and fourchette.

Technique

The two parts of the technique are: (i) excision; and (ii) vaginal undercut and advancement.

In part one of the procedure excision is undertaken using the precision afforded by the CO_2 laser in the super pulse mode; it is also possible to use a scalpel if a laser is not available. There should be a margin of at least 1 cm around the lesion and the incision is deepened to at least 10–20 mm. Figure 9.66 shows a large area being removed in a young immunocompromised patient who had extensive VIN 3 of the fourchette and posterior vulva. The super pulse mode of the laser is used at a 40-W setting. The power density developed is in the region of $1500\,W/cm^2$. The lower parts of the labia minora, which were extensively involved with the lesion, have also been removed.

Part two of the technique involves undercutting and advancing the vagina. The vagina is cut between 1 and 3 cm above the hymenal ring and is then advanced to cover the area. Both superficial and deep sutures are inserted with approximation of the edges, as shown in Fig. 9.67. In this immunosuppressed woman, where a high chance of wound breakdown existed, non-absorbable black silk sutures were used. In the usual clinical condition, very fine 4-0 polyglycolic sutures are employed.

Figures 9.68 and 9.69 show the pre- and postoperative results in a 23-year-old female who had extensive VIN 3. In Fig. 9.68, VIN 3 can be seen on the upper part of the labia minora (1), labia majora (2), and part of the perineum (3); its outline is demarkated by the arrows. This patient also had extensive condylomata acuminata, and some lesions surrounding the perianal area are clearly visible (4). There was no precancerous disease in any of these latter lesions. The patient was suffering severe pain, which made inter-course impossible, and no form of medical treatment was effective.

Figure 9.69 shows the excellent cosmetic outcome of this procedure. An outer line of very fine sutures (1) delineates the excised area. The vagina (2) has been brought down to a point about halfway between the posterior fourchette and the anal margin. The anal condylomata have been destroyed with laser vaporization. Postoperatively, the woman was discharged from hospital within 24 hours and was encouraged to use sea-salt baths and dry the skin immediately after washing. Recuperation takes about 10 days and patients are advised to avoid long periods of standing during this time. Intercourse is discouraged for at least 6 weeks.

In Fig. 9.70, a very extensive lesion is seen to involve the labia minora and majora, and to extend onto the perineum.

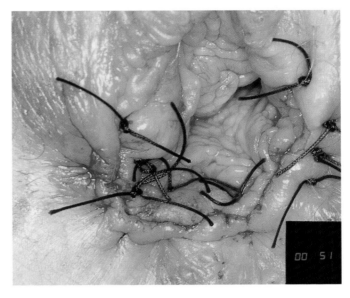

Fig. 9.67

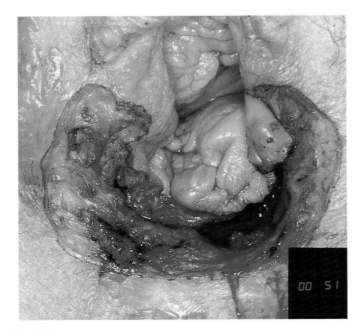

Fig. 9.66

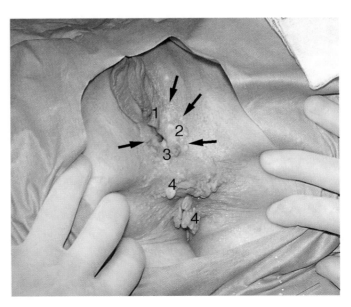

Fig. 9.68

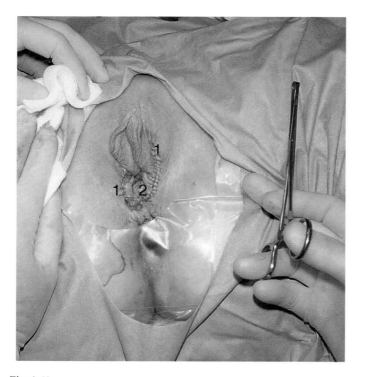

Fig. 9.69

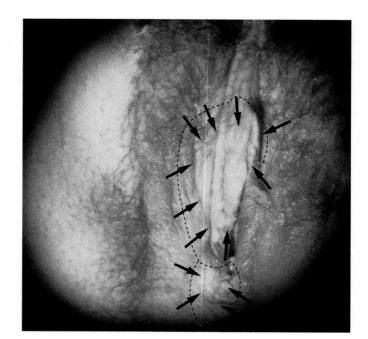

Fig. 9.70

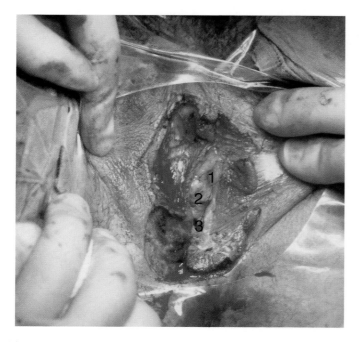

Fig. 9.71

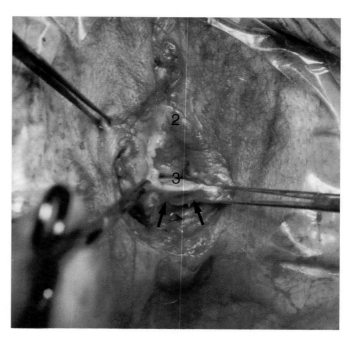

Fig. 9.72

Its outline is arrowed and the line of excision is indicated by the broken line. Multiple punch biopsy showed it to be a VIN 3. In Fig. 9.71, an extensive removal has already been performed; this has involved both the right and left labia majora and a small part of the minora, and has extended downward into the perineum. The clitoris has been preserved at (1) with the urethra at (2) and the vagina at (3). Most of the left-side labia minora and majora have been

preserved and only the disease with a 1-cm surrounding margin has been removed. In Fig. 9.72, partial resuture of the periclitoral and labia majora defect has been performed, especially on the patient's right side; the urethra can be seen at (2) and the undercut vagina at (3). Its under-surface is arrowed and in Fig. 9.73 it has been brought down and laid over the excised area. Figure 9.74 shows the final result. The vagina (3) is attached to the apex of the sutured perineal

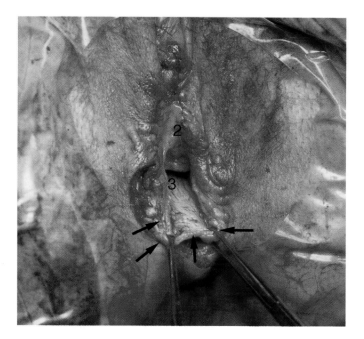

Fig. 9.73

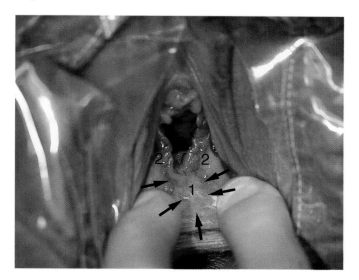

Fig. 9.75

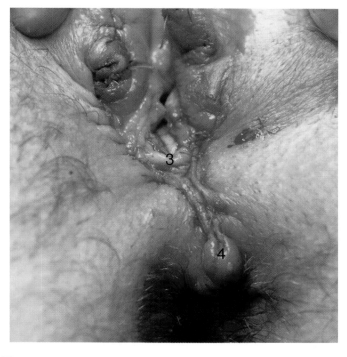

Fig. 9.74

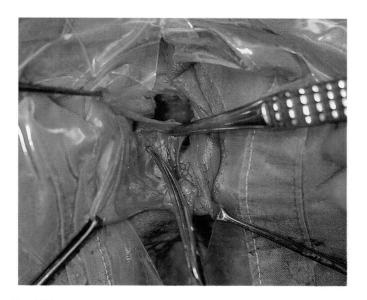

Fig. 9.76

wound, which has been united in a vertical fashion. Its lower end abuts the anal verge (4).

In Figs 9.75–9.82 the technique can be seen in detail. A description of the various stages follows.

Figure 9.75 shows the preoperative condition, with an extremely symptomatic VIN 3 lesion (confirmed by biopsy) existing in the posterior fourchette (1); the arrows indicate its extent. This 35-year-old woman also had extensive vestibulitis, and the erythema around the vestibular glands can be seen at (2) and (2); it is more obvious on the right

than on the left. The patient experienced extreme pain when the area was gently touched with a cotton-tip bud. Discomfort from this condition had not been lessened by any medication, and indeed had commenced at around the time when multiple local antimycotic agents were given for an associated vulvovaginal moniliasis. The vestibular glands were removed at the same time as was the VIN 3 lesion. This procedure is very similar to the vestibulectomy that was originally described by Woodruff and Parmley (1983).

Figure 9.76 shows the first part of an elliptic incision being made on the patient's right side. It is developed into the subcutaneous tissues, sweeping them in a medial

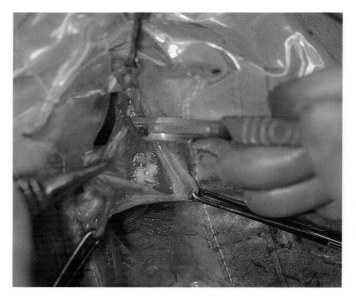

Fig. 9.77

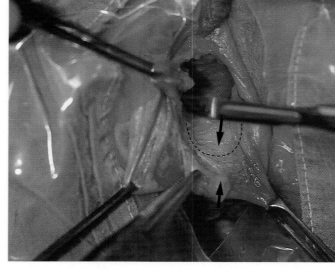

Fig. 9.79

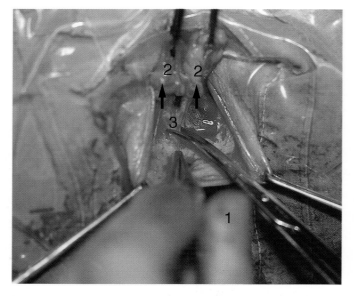

Fig. 9.78

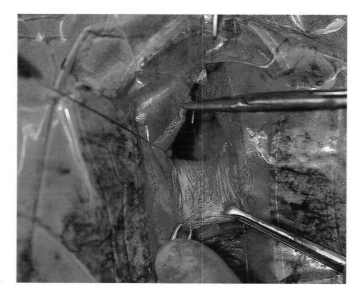

Fig. 9.80

direction. This procedure undercuts both the vestibular gland and the Bartholin's duct and gland that lie adjacent to the former structure.

Figure 9.77 shows the same type of incision being made on the patient's left side; gentle undercutting of the duct and glandular systems is carried out.

In Fig. 9.78, undercutting of the vagina has commenced. The operator's index finger (1) is inserted into the rectum while an assistant holds up the vagina (2). Small cuts are made in the tissue between the rectum and vagina (3), sweeping the tissue upward in the direction of the arrows.

In Fig. 9.79, an inner incision is made approximately 1.5 to 2cm above the hymenal ring (along the line, as indicated). In this case it will sweep from the patient's

right to left side. It is sometimes helpful to split the undermined vaginal skin in the midline (arrowed) as this will make the excision easier. The excised tissue is then removed.

In Fig. 9.80, the undermined vagina has been brought down to cover the defect in the vestibule and posterior fourchette. As can be seen, there is no excessive tension on this flap and it is certainly adequate to cover the excised area.

In Fig. 9.81, a suture has been inserted between the vaginal flap and the vaginal and vulvar skin; 4-0 polyglycolic acid sutures are employed. The initial resuture starts at the apex of the wound in the region of the excised vestibular glands, just lateral to the posterior part of the labia minora. It was continued to the 4- and 8-o'clock

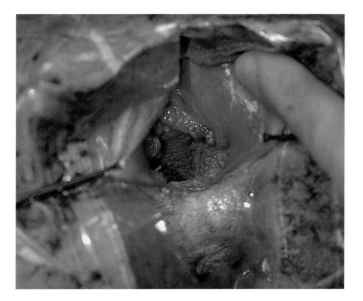

Fig. 9.81

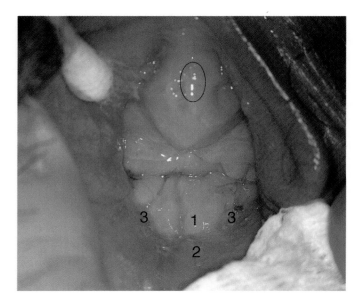

Fig. 9.82

positions. At that stage some deep sutures can be inserted in the midline to obliterate the space between the vagina and rectum. Meticulous hemostasis must be performed, and after these deep sutures have been placed, the final suture of the vaginal flap to the vulvar tissues in the posterior fourchette between the 4- and 8-o'clock positions can be undertaken. The initial resuture involves a continuous 4-0 polyglycolic acid suture but the last stages of the incision in the fourchette can be closed with interrupted sutures.

Figure 9.82 shows the healing area some 2 months after the operation; the vaginal mucosa (1) is attached to the posterior fourchette (2). The lateral suture lines (3) and (3) can just be seen. The patient was completely cured of the symptoms. Although the Bartholin's apparatus had been removed, little superficial dyspareunia is encountered. With sexual excitement the vagina becomes moist, and in its "everted" position there does not seem to be any interference with intercourse.

Results

One of us (AS) has performed 50 of these procedures over a 9-year period on women suffering from proven VIN 3. Pathology of the excised lesions revealed that microinvasion existed in two cases; penetration of the invasive cells was to a depth of 0.4–0.6 mm. To date, there have been eight small areas of recurrence; all have occurred at the junction of vaginal mucosa with vulvar skin, and all have been removed by local excision.

CO_2 laser vaporization

CO_2 laser vaporization treatment of VIN is associated with a recurrence rate of 5–40%. Recurrence is purely as a result of ineffective treatment in either depth or lateral extent. It is possible that HPV, a known etiologic agent for VIN 3, exists

Table 9.6 Results of studies using laser vaporization.

Reference	No. of case treated	No. of recurrences (%)
Baggish and Dorsey (1981)	35	3 (8)
Townsend et al. (1982)	33	2 (7)
Ferenczy (1983)	11	3 (27)
Bernstein et al. (1983)	18	1 (6)
Leuchter et al. (1984)	42	7 (17)
Baggish (1985)	228	82 (34) [1977–1981] 20 (9) [1983–1985]
Wright & Davies (1987)	29	12 (40) (hair-bearing area) 7 (25) (nonhair-bearing area)

Reproduced with permission from Singer and Mitchell (1990).

in normal tissue adjacent to the lesion and as such may reinfect the healing tissue. Ferenczy et al. (1985) have shown that involvement of the lateral margins of condylomatous lesions with HPV, as assessed by HPV-DNA hybridization studies, was associated with an increased risk of recurrence of condylomata. They showed that when a 15-mm margin of normal-appearing skin adjacent to the lesion was vaporized, recurrence rates were comparatively lower than when a 5-mm or less margin was taken.

A number of studies showing the success of laser treatment have appeared in the literature (Table 9.6), but many lack long-term follow-up. In early studies, laser vaporization was felt to be inadequate and was not recommended for VIN 3 when it involved the hairy skin of the vulva. The recommendations were made on inappropriately measured or unmeasured pilosebaceous-unit involvement. As has been explained above, as a result of the work of Baggish et al. (1989) and Shatz et al. (1989), excellent therapeutic and cosmetic results may be obtained with laser vaporization of the hairy and non-hairy skin to depths of 2 and 1 mm, respectively. Postlaser recurrence rates may be significantly reduced by the extended laser vaporization procedures (laser epidermectomy) that are now recommended (Reid, 1992).

Technique

The technique of laser ablation involves the use of a microscopically controlled method for depth control so that the VIN within the surface epithelium and pilosebaceous ducts can be eradicated. The involvement is generally limited to the superficial portions of the pilosebaceous ducts, making laser ablation to the midreticular level of the skin an ideal treatment in most instances. Reid (1992) believes that the "intended depth of destruction should be individualized by examining representative histological sections. "However, in the rare event of deep pilor extension, a surgical procedure, rather than a superficial vaporization, would be indicated. The preliminary biopsy of the tissue may give some indication of this rare occurrence.

Reid (1985) has described the existence of three surgical planes within the vulva that need to be identified for efficient laser vaporization of this tissue. Each one has specific morphologic characteristics.

Destruction of the *first plane* removes only the surface epithelium to the level of the basement membrane. The laser beam is placed within the prickle cell layer and destruction is achieved by rapid oscillations of the micromanipulator such that the helium–neon spot describes a roughly parallel series of lines. Each passage of the laser beam will reveal bubbles of silver opalescence beneath the charred surface squames, and this is associated with a distinctive crackling sound as the prickle layer is destroyed. Penetration of the basement membrane is, according to Reid (1992), accompanied by loss of these two characteristic signs. When the laser has destroyed the prickle cell layer, the basal cells can then be wiped from the basement membrane (see Fig. 9.59a), producing a plane of cleavage. Moist gauze is used to wipe away these cells and immediately the smooth intact surface of the papillary dermis is exposed, as shown in Figs 9.83 and 9.84. The dermal papillae give a shiny surface and diffused pink color to the tissues. This is readily visible in these two photographs in the areas marked (1); the edge of the lasered area is arrowed. Healing will be completed within 5 to 14 days, depending on the energy delivered, and in Fig. 9.85 such an event is seen occurring 7 days after laser ablation at a power density of 1000 W/cm². In this figure, islands of squamous epithelium (1) have already appeared within the treated area (2). There is minimal, if any, edema at the edges (arrowed) or in the surrounding tissues (3). The vaginal introitus is at (4). Complete healing was evident in this case on the 16th postoperative day.

The *second surgical plane* involves removal of both the epidermis and the loose network of fine collagen and elastin fibers that comprise the papillary dermis. Rapid oscillations, where the beam is moved so quickly that the laser scorches (rather than craters) the exposed chorion, will very

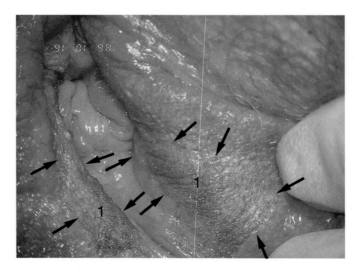

Fig. 9.83

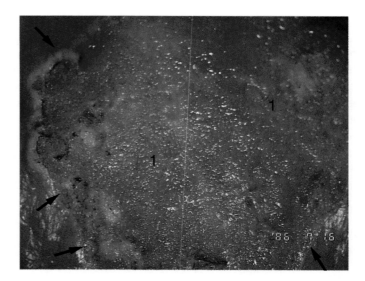

Fig. 9.84

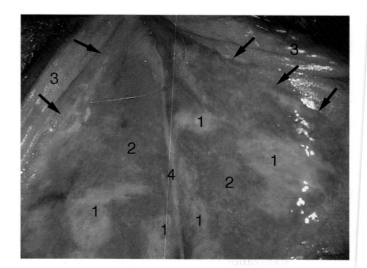

Fig. 9.85

quickly show the finely roughened, contoured, and yellowish cover, which is somewhat reminiscent of a chamois cloth, that is the second surgical layer. This clinical appearance indicates that the zone of coagulation necrosis will lie within the papillary dermis and there will be only minimal thermal injury to the underlying reticular dermis. In cases of extensive condylomata, destruction to this level is sufficient. In Fig. 9.86, three surgical planes are shown. The first plane, with a few dermal papillae and their shiny surface, can be seen at (1). The second surgical plane exists in the areas designated (2), while entry into the third plane, to be described below, is at (3). A sharp demarkation line at the edge of the lesion is arrowed. In Fig. 9.87, the second surgical plane can be clearly seen (1); the dermal papillae have been wiped away and the dense collagen of the midreticular dermis, accounting for the stark white color of the third surgical plane, is visible at (2).

The *third surgical plane* involves the destruction of the epidermis, the upper portions of the pilosebaceous duct, and a part of the reticular dermis. Reid has described the correct depth control at this level by recognition of three characteristic landmarks. First, there are the mid-reticular layers with their coarse collagen bundles that can be seen through the operating microscope as gray-white fibers "resembling water-logged cotton threads" [(1) in Fig. 9.88]. Second, after wiping the area with iced saline, the bright alabaster-white cover of other basal collagen plates becomes recognizable, and this also reveals the network of prominent arterioles and venules that run horizontal to the epithelial surface (Reid, 1992).

The technique of micromanipulator control in ablating this third layer involves using much slower and more deliberate movement of the micromanipulator. Reid believes that "the speed of a cut is coordinated to the visual recognition of a fibrous grain within the crater base and that this will not be exposed if the beam is moved too rapidly." Moving the beam slowly will uncover skin appendages within the deep reticular dermis, and once these have been uncovered, hair follicles and sweat glands will become readily visible as tiny refractile granules that resemble grains of sand. Regeneration will occur from the keratinocytes within the skin appendages and the third surgical plane represents the deepest level from which optimum healing will occur. Laser vaporization of the third surgical plane would certainly be sufficient to obliterate VIN.

Postoperative care

After treatment, the area should be infiltrated with bupivicaine. To prevent superinfection, the patient is asked to bathe in a sitz or sea-salt bath at least three times a day. Some authors apply silver sulfadiazine cream or nitrofurazone soluble dressings to prevent conglutination of the denuded surfaces, as are obvious in Fig. 9.85. Where extensive areas have been laser treated, use of a suprapubic

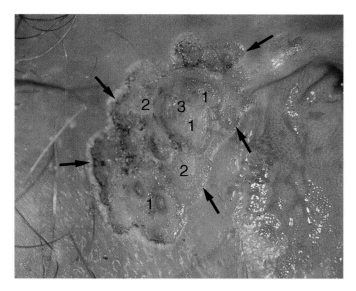

Fig. 9.86

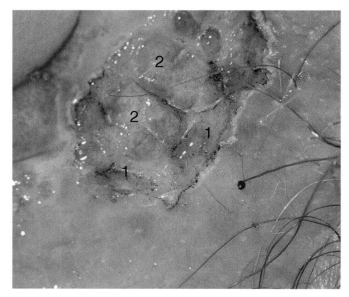

Fig. 9.87

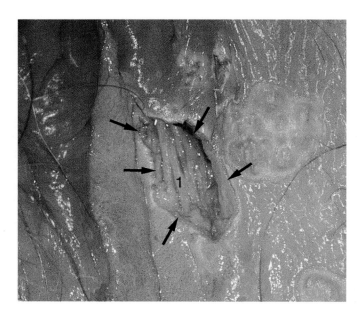

Fig. 9.88

catheter is recommended. A prophylactic antibiotic is usually employed in such circumstances. Patients without a suprapubic catheter are advised to apply a local anesthetic gel (i.e. 2% lignocaine) to the urethra and surrounding areas 5 minutes prior to micturition in order to reduce discomfort. Washing the vulva with tepid sea-salt water or taking sitz baths, and the application of antibacterial cream are the most important methods for reducing postoperative infection and for promoting satisfactory and rapid healing. Some patients find it beneficial to use a spray bottle filled with sea-salt water to rinse the vulva during and after micturition. This method is popular with patients because they can carry the spray bottle with them for use in public conveniences or at work. In the longer term postoperatively, sexual relations are usually difficult for up to 3 months. It should be explained to patients, preferably with their partners present, that there may be some psychosexual difficulties when intercourse is recommended. Patients are seen at 2-week intervals until the 6th postoperative week; this enables the physician to assess healing, prevent or release adhesion formation, and treat, by the application of 85% trichloracetic acid, any recurrent warts that may occur within this period. Patients are then seen at 4 months, at 1-year, and thereafter at 1-year intervals.

Medical therapy

Medical treatment of VIN includes the use of chemotherapy in the forms of 5-FU, dinitrochlorobenzene (DNCB) cream, and interferon. Photodynamic therapy, involving photochemical destruction of cells sensitized with a light-activator compound, such as hematoporphyrin, is undergoing trials at this time.

Initially encouraging reports for 5-FU treatment have been displaced by later evidence suggesting that it is of very little use in VIN treatment (Sillman et al., 1981, 1985; Krebs, 1987). Of women undergoing 5-FU treatment for vulvar lesions, 75% stop treatment after 10 days as a result of discomfort and ulceration; other studies have also reported a failure rate of up to 90% in those with VIN. Krebs (1986) administered it after treatment at 2-week intervals for 6 months. Among treated women, only 13% developed recurrent disease compared with 38% in the untreated group.

Which approach for treating VIN 3?

It would seem that the radicality of some procedures may not be successful in clearing the disease, no matter how expert the surgical technique. If the surgical margins are positive, as has been mentioned above, irrespective of the type of procedure performed, there will be a high rate of recurrence. Bearing this in mind, it is clear that there has to be another approach that takes into account the problem of positive margins with extensive disease. Van Beurden (1998b) and his group have suggested a number of alternatives which should be considered.

They have managed patients with VIN 3 by adapting the extent of the surgery to the individual patient and her

symptoms. Hence, their patients were characterized according to the focality of VIN 3, the existence of symptoms and the presence of superficially invasive cancer. They found that in unifocal VIN 3, they chose wide local excision irrespective of symptoms, since unifocality is a substantial risk factor for progression to invasive cancer, as shown by de Belilovsky & Lessana-Leibowitch (1993). Van Beurden and his group believe that extensive surgery in his patients is usually not mutilating because the amount of involved vulval skin is significantly smaller in unifocal VIN 3 than in multifocal VIN 3, extensive removal of multifocal VIN 3 was only chosen by them in those patients who suffered from symptoms covering all involved skin or in whom superficially invasive cancer was proven.

In all other patients with multifocal VIN 3, but without superficially invasive disease, they only removed involved vulval skin that was causing symptoms and by doing so they relieved symptoms and also avoided in many cases the psychological and sexual side-effects resulting from extensive surgery. The symptoms, especially of pain, could be localized easily by most of the patients.

The important factor was that this policy resulted in a subgroup of patients with VIN 3 for which an expectant management was adopted, as these patients neither had symptoms nor had a superficially invasive cancer. This individualized approach has much merit, with vulvoscopically directed biopsies from all lesions that were mapped playing a central role in the detection of invasive disease. By a mapping and biopsy process, they found superficially invasive cancer in 9% of patients while, on the other hand, in 26% of lesions they detected minor degrees of VIN, and in 10% did not find any lesion whatsoever. They believe that mapping and biopsy is a safe instrument for identifying superficially invasive disease. They only had one superficially invasive vulval cancer detected in one of their extensively operated patients during follow-up. Their results are very noteworthy. They emphasize symptoms and showed that only patients with unifocal VIN 3 were helped by extensive removal of the affected skin, whilst symptoms in all the other extensively operated-upon patients, had recurrence of symptoms. In contrast to these findings, almost 75% of patients who underwent their restricted form of surgery benefited from their therapy even after long-term follow-up. In these cases, as much vulval skin as possible was saved in contrast to the extensively operated-upon patients.

Van Beurden and his group insist that their protocols are an appropriate form of management for VIN 3. Vulvoscopy combined with mapping was a safe method by which to detect superficially invasive cervical cancer in patients with multifocal VIN 3. In these patients, who often had severe and long-lasting symptoms, restricted surgery was successful in relieving symptoms and also avoiding, in many cases, the psychosexual side effects resulting from extensive surgery.

This management protocol has raised comment and it has been suggested by others (Jones, 1998) that this essentially conservative technique could have potentially adverse effects. They argue that the time period for examination of progression of VIN 3 to possibly cancer is too small, (i.e. 11 and 5 months in the cases managed expectantly), and also that there could be a different natural history for both symptomatic and asymptomatic lesions. Jones also warns that there could be increasing incidence of VIN 3-related cancer in younger women, and he does not believe that "up to 12 months" follow-up is adequate for such women under observation as van Beurden *et al.* (1998b) suggest.

9.15 Treatment of early invasive vulvar carcinoma

The definition, clinical features, and prognosis, especially in respect of recurrence and reoccurrence, of vulvar microinvasive carcinoma have already been discussed. The management of these lesions has undergone dramatic changes over the last few years, with the emphasis now being placed on conservative management (Hacker, 1992; Kelley *et al.*, 1992). It would seem adequate to remove at least 1 cm of normal skin around any lesion where biopsy has suggested the presence of early invasion. The incision is carried to the deep fascia and this would appear to be adequate treatment with virtually no risk of lymph node metastasis associated with such lesions. In Fig. 9.89 such a procedure has been undertaken. A small area of early invasion has been diagnosed by an excision biopsy; the tumor penetrates to less than 1 mm. A wide excision of a surrounding area of VIN 3, in which the early invasion was diagnosed, has been undertaken down to the deep fascia, and includes at least a 1-cm margin of normal skin around the area. A frozen section was taken to confirm clear margins. The lateral margin is the labiocrural fold and the medial margin is just within the introitus.

The incisions are elliptic to allow satisfactory closure. In this instance a laser has been used, but a scalpel or the cutting mode of an electrosurgical unit can also be employed; the coagulation mode is used for the remainder of the procedure so as to reduce blood loss. Where a more

posterior perineal lesion exists, it may be necessary to identify the anal sphincter; the distal rectum and the rectovaginal space will then need to be dissected. In such a case an assistant maintains upward traction on the perineal specimen by using two pairs of Allis forceps; meanwhile, very sharp scissors are used to resect it from the rectovaginal space. It is usually possible to close the defect in two layers. If the perineal defect is too large for primary closure, then bilateral rhomboid flaps or local skin flaps (Hoffman *et al.*, 1990) may be used to advance the tissue forward to cover the defect.

Where the lesion exists on the labia, then the incision is again carried down to the deep fascia. The inferior fascia of the urogenital diaphragm is composed of two fascial layers. It is connected with the fascia lata of the thigh and also with the fascia overlying the pubic symphysis. Once the plane on the fascia has been reached, a finger or artery forceps can be passed along the deep fascia to define the deep margins of resection. This, in turn, allows the tissue to be elevated and resected. The medial and lateral margins can be dissected by gripping the edges with forceps, thereby maintaining traction. As with the perineum, the defect is closed in two layers.

Is lymphadenectomy necessary?

It would seem that gland resection can be omitted in patients with early invasion where the involvement is to a depth of 1 mm or less. All other patients, however, should ideally have a unilateral groin dissection, if the tumor is laterally located, or a bilateral dissection, if it is centrally located. This is also the recommended management for stage I vulvar carcinoma (i.e. those lesions that are less than 2 cm in diameter). If dissection of the groin is undertaken, then this is usually through an incision between 10 and 12 cm long; it starts at the anterior border of the anterior superior iliac spine and extends to a point 4 cm below the pubic tubercle. It is important always to use bony landmarks.

Results

Results of this conservative treatment of early invasion, and indeed of early stage I carcinoma of the vulva, are excellent. Krupp (1992) describes 100% survival after 5 years in 34 cases of early stage I carcinoma of the vulva, including a number of microinvasions, treated in this conservative manner. The individualization of management (Iversen *et al.*, 1981; Hacker *et al.*, 1984) for these very early invasive lesions would spare many women the significant morbidity associated with more radical surgical therapy used to treat such early disease.

9.16 References

Abell, M.R. & Gosling, J.R. (1961) Intraepithelial and infiltrative carcinoma of the vulva: Bowen's type. *Cancer* **14**,318.

Abercrombie, P.D. & Korn, A.P. (1995) Multifocal lower genital tract neoplasia in women with HIV disease. *Nurse-Pract* **20**(5),68.

Anderson, B.L. & Hacker, N.F. (1983) Psychosexual adjustment after vulvar surgery. *Obstet Gynecol* **62**,457.

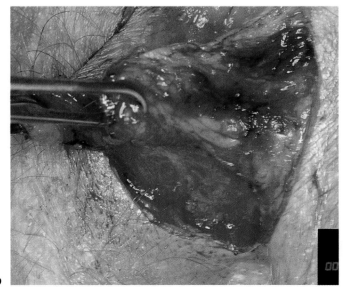

Fig. 9.89

Andreasson, B. & Bock, J.E. (1985) Intraepithelial neoplasia in the vulvar region. *Gynecol Oncol* **21**,300.

Baggish, M.S. (1985) Improved laser techniques for the elimination of genital and extragenital warts. *Am J Obstet Gynecol* **153**,545.

Baggish, M. (1989) Using the CO_2 laser in genital surgery. *Contemp Obstet Gynecol* **34**,125.

Baggish, M.S. & Dorsey, J.H. (1981) CO_2 laser for the treatment of vulvar carcinoma in situ. *Obstet Gynecol* **57**,371.

Baggish, M., Sze, E., Adelson, M., Cohn, G. & Oates, R. (1989) Quantitative evaluation of the skin and accessory appendages in vulvar carcinoma in situ. *Obstet Gynecol* **74**,169.

Barbero, M., Micheletti, L., Preti, M. *et al*. (1990) Vulvar intraepithelial neoplasia. A clinico-pathologic study of 60 cases. *J Reprod Med* **35**(11),1023.

Beckmann, A.M., Kiviat, N.B., Daling, J.R., Sherman, K.J. & McDougall, J.K. (1988) Human papillomavirus type 16 in multifocal neoplasia of the female genital tract. *Int J Gynecol Pathol* **7**,39.

Benedet, J.L. & Murphy, K.G. (1982) Squamous carcinoma in situ of the vulva. *Gynecol Oncol* **14**,213.

Benedet, J.L., Wilson, P.S. & Matisic, J. (1991) Epidermal thickness and skin appendage involvement in vulvar intraepithelial neoplasia. *J Reprod Med* **36**(8),608.

Bergeron, C., Ferenczy, A., Richart, R. & Guralnick, M. (1990) Micropapillomatosis labialis appears unrelated to human papillomavirus. *Obstet Gynecol* **76**(2),281.

Bergeron, C., Naghashfar, Z., Canaan, C. *et al*. (1987) Human papillomavirus type 16 in intraepithelial neoplasia (Bowenoid papulosis) and coexistent invasive carcinoma of the vulva. *Int J Gynecol Pathol* **6**,1.

Bernstein, S.G., Kovacs, B.R., Townsend, D.E. & Morrow, C.P. (1983) Vulvar carcinoma-in-situ. *Obstet Gynecol* **61**,304.

Bhawan, J. (1980) Multicentric pigmented Bowen's disease. A clinically benign squamous cell carcinoma in situ. *Gynecol Oncol* **10**,201.

Bjorge, T., Dillner, J., Antrilla, T. *et al*. (1997) Prospective seroepidemiological study of role of human papillomavirus in non-cervical anogenital cancers. *Br Med J* **315**,646.

Borgeno, B., Micheletti, L. & Barbero, M. (1988) Epithelial alterations adjacent to 111 vulvar carcinomas. *J Reprod Med* **33**(6),500.

Bornstein, J. & Kaufman, R.H. (1988) Combination of surgical excision and carbon dioxide laser vaporisation for multifocal vulvar intraepithelial neoplasia. *Am J Obstet Gynecol* **158**,459.

Bornstein, J., Kaufman, R.H. & Adam, E. (1988) Multicentric intraepithelial neoplasia involving the vulva. Clinical features and association with human papillomavirus and herpes simplex virus. *Cancer* **62**(8),1601.

Breslow, A. (1970) Thickness, cross-sectional areas and depth of invasion in the prognosis of cutaneous melanoma. *Ann Surg* **172**,902.

Brinton, L.A., Nasca, P.C., Mallin, K. *et al*. (1990) Case control study of cancer of the vulva. *Obstet Gynecol* **75**,859.

Buchler, D.A. (1975) Multiple primaries and gynecologic malignancies. *Am J Obstet Gynecol* **123**,376.

Buckley, C.H., Buttle, E.B. & Fox, H. (1984) Vulvar intraepithelial neoplasia and microinvasive carcinoma of the vulva. *J Clin Pathol* **37**,1201.

Burghardt, E. (1984) Microinvasive carcinoma in gynaecological pathology. *Clin Obstet Gynecol* **11**,239.

Buscema, J., Naghashfar, Z., Sawada, E. *et al*. (1988) The predominance of human papillomavirus type 16 in vulval neoplasia. *Obstet Gynecol* **71**,601.

Buscema, J., Stern, J. & Woodruff, J.D. (1980a) The significance of the histological alterations adjacent to invasive vulvar carcinoma. *Am J Obstet Gynecol* **137**,902.

Buscema, J., Woodruff, J.D., Parmley, T.H. & Genadry, R. (1980b) Carcinoma in situ of the vulva. *Obstet Gynecol* **55**,225.

Caglar, H., Delgado, G. & Hreshchyshyn, M.M. (1986) Partial and total skinning vulvectomy in treatment of carcinoma in situ of the vulva. *Obstet Gynecol* **68**,504.

Caglar, H., Tamer, S. & Hreshchyshyn, M.M. (1982) Vulvar intraepithelial neoplasia. *Obstet Gynecol* **60**,346.

Campion, M. (1987) Clinical manifestations of HPV infection. *Obstet Gynecol Clin N Am* **14**,368.

Campion, M.J., Brown, J.R., McCance, D.J. & Singer, A. (1988) Psychosexual trauma of an abnormal cervical smear. *Br J Obstet Gynaecol* **95**,175.

Chiasson, M., Ellebrock, T., Bush, T., Sun, X.W. & Wright T.C. (1997) Increased prevalence of vulvo-vaginal condyloma and vulvar intraepithelial neoplasia in women infected with the human immunodeficiency virus. *Obstet Gynecol* **89**(5),690.

Choo, Y.C. & Morley, G.W. (1980) Multiple primary neoplasms of the anogenital region. *Obstet Gynecol* **56**,365.

Clark, W.H., From, L., Bernardino, E.A. & Mihm, M.C. (1969) The histogenesis and biological behaviour of primary human malignant melanomas of the skin. *Cancer Res* **29**,705.

Chung, A.F., Woodruff, J.M. & Lewis, J.L. (1975) Malignant melanoma of the vulva. *Obstet Gynecol* **45**,638.

Collins, C.G., Hansen, L.H. & Theriot, E. (1966) A clinical stain for use in selecting biopsy sites in patients with vulvar disease. *Obstet Gynecol* **28**,158.

Collins, C.G., Roman-Lopez, J.J. & Lee, F.Y. (1970) Intraepithelial carcinoma of the vulva. *Am J Obstet Gynecol* **108**,1187.

Coppleson, M. & Pixley, E.C. (1992) Colposcopy of vulva and vagina. In: Coppleson, M. (ed.) *Gynecological Oncology*, Vol. 1, 2nd edn, p. 325. Churchill Livingstone, Edinburgh.

Cox, S.M., Kaufman, R.H. & Kaplan, A. (1986) Recurrent carcinoma in situ of the vulva in a skin graft. *Am J Obstet Gynecol* **155**,177.

Crum, C.P., Igawa, K., Fu, Y.S. *et al*. (1982) Intraepithelial squamous lesions of the vulva: biologic and histological criteria for the distinction of condyloma from vulvar intraepithelial neoplasia. *Am J Obstet Gynecol* **144**,77.

Curtain, J.P. & Morrow, C.P. (1992) Melanoma of female genital tract. In: Coppleson, M. (ed.) *Gynecological Oncology*, Vol. 2, 2nd edn, p. 1061. Churchill Livingstone, Edinburgh.

Daling, J.R. & Sherman, K.J. (1992) Relationship between human papillomavirus infection and tumours of anogenital sites other than the cervix. In: Muñoz, N., Bosch, F.X., Shah, K.V. & Meheus, A. (eds) *The Epidemiology of Cervical Cancer and Human Papillomavirus*, p. 223. International Agency for Research on Cancer (IARC), Lyon.

Daling, J.R., Sherman, K.J., Hislop, T.G., Maden, C. & Weiss, N.S. (1992) Cigarette smoking and risk of anogenital cancer. *Am J Epidemiol* **135**,180.

de Belilovsky & Lessana-Leibowitch, M. (1993) Maladie de Bowen et papulosis bowenoide: Donnees cliniques virologiques et evolutives comparatives. *Contracep Fertil Sex* **21**,231.

DiSaia, P.J. & Rich, W.M. (1981) Surgical approach to multifocal carcinoma in situ of the vulva. *Am J Obstet Gynecol* **140**,136.

DiSaia, P.J., Creasman, W.T. & Rich, W.M. (1979) An alternate approach to early cancer of the vulva. *Am J Obstet Gynecol* **133**,825.

Dottenwille, M.N. (1982) Cancer invasif de la vulve et lichen scléreux vulvaire. In: Hewitt, J. (1984) Conditions étiologiques du carcinome invasif d'emblée de la vulve. Possibilité d'un traitement proplylactique? *J Gynécol Obstet Biol Repro* **13**,297.

Dudzinsky, M.R. & Rader, J.S. (1990) The mons pubis, an excellent graft donor site in gynaecological surgery. *Am J Obstet Gynecol* **162**(3),722.

Eglin, R.P., Lehner, T. & Subak-Sharpe, J.H. (1982) Detection of RNA complementary to herpes simplex virus in mononuclear cells from patients with Behçet's syndrome and recurrent oral ulcers. *Lancet* **2**,1356.

Elliott, P.M. (1992) Early invasive carcinoma of the vulva; definition, clinical features and management. In: Coppleson, M. (ed.) *Gynaecological Oncology*, Vol. 1, 2nd edn, p. 465. Churchill Livingstone, Edinburgh.

Estrada, R. & Kaufman, R. (1993) Benign vulvar melanosis. *J Reprod Med* **38**(1),5.

Fanning, J., Lambert, L., Hale, M., Morris, P., Schuerch, C. (1999) Paget's disease of the vulva—prevalence of associated vulvar adenocarcinoma, invasive Paget's disease and recurrence after surgical excision. *Am J Obstet Gynecol* **180**(1,1),24.

Ferenczy, A. (1983) Using the laser to treat vulvar condylomata acuminata and intraepidermal neoplasia. *Can Med Assoc J* **128**,135.

Ferenczy, A. (1992) Intraepithelial neoplasia of the vulva. In: Coppleson, M. (ed.) *Gynaecological Oncology*, Vol. 1, 2nd edn, p. 450. Churchill Livingstone, Edinburgh.

Ferenczy, A., Mitao, M., Nagai, N., Silverstein, S.J. & Crum, C.P. (1985) Latent papillomavirus and recurring genital warts. *N Engl J Med* **313**,784.

Fiorica, J.V., Cavanagh, D., Marsden, D. *et al.* (1988) Carcinoma in situ of the vulva; 24 years' experience in south west Florida. *S Med J* **81**(5),589.

Forney, J.P., Morrow, C.P., Townsend, D.E., DiSaia, P.J. (1977) Management of carcinoma in situ of the vulva. *Am J Obstet Gynecol* **127**,801.

Fournier, J. (1906) Quoted by: Stokes, J.H. (1944) *Modern Clinical Syphiology*. W.B. Saunders, Philadelphia.

Friedrich, E.G. (1972) Reversible vulval atypia: a case report. *Obstet Gynecol* **39**,173.

Friedrich, E.G. (1983a) Diagnosis and therapy. In: Friedrich, E. (ed.) *Vulvar Diseases*, 2nd edn, p. 41. W.B. Saunders, Philadelphia.

Friedrich, E.G. (1983b) Red lesions. In: Friedrich, E. (ed.) *Vulvar Diseases*, 2nd edn, p. 109. W.B. Saunders, Philadelphia.

Friedrich, E.G. (1983c) The vulvar vestibule. *J Reprod Med* **23**,773.

Friedrich, E.G., Wilkinson, E.J. & Fu, Y.S. (1980) Carcinoma in situ of the vulva: a continuing challenge. *Am J Obstet Gynecol* **136**,830.

Fu, Y.S., Reagan, J.W., Townsend, D.E. *et al.* (1981) Nuclear DNA study of vulvar intraepithelial and invasive squamous neoplasms. *Obstet Gynecol* **57**,643.

Ganjei, P., Gueraldo, K.A., Lampe, B. & Nadji, M. (1990) Vulvar Paget's disease. Is immunocytochemistry helpful in assessing the surgical margins? *J Reprod Med* **35**(11),1002.

Gardner, S.H., Stout, F.E., Arbogast, J.L. & Huber, C.P. (1953) Intraepithelial carcinoma of the vulva. *Am J Obstet Gynecol* **65**,539.

Gupta, J., Pilotti, S., Shah, K.V., Di Paolo, G. & Rilke, F. (1987) Human papillomavirus associated early vulval neoplasia investigated by in situ hybridization. *Am J Surg Pathol* **11**,430.

Hacker, N.F. (1992) Conservative surgery for stage 1 carcinoma of the vulva. In: Coppleson, M. (ed.) *Gynaecological Oncology*, Vol. 2, 2nd edn, p. 1185. Churchill Livingstone, Edinburgh.

Hacker, N.F., Berek, J.S., Legasse, L.D. & Nieberg, K. (1984) Individualisation of treatment for stage 1 squamous cell vulvar carcinoma. *Obstet Gynecol* **63**,155.

Hacker, N.F., Nieberg, R.K., Berek, J.S. *et al.* (1983) Superficially invasive vulval cancer with nodal metastasis. *Gynecol Oncol* **15**,65.

Hay, D.M. & Cole, F.M. (1969) Primary invasive carcinoma of the vulva in Jamaica. *J Obstet Gynaecol Br Commonw* **76**,821.

Helwig, E.B. & Graham, J.H. (1963) Anogenital (extramammary) Paget's disease. *Cancer* **16**,387.

Herod, J.J., Shafi, M.I., Rollason, T.P. *et al.* (1996a) Vulvar intraepithelial neoplasia with superficially invasive carcinoma of the vulva. *Br J Obstet Gynaecol* **103**(5),21.

Herod, J.J., Shafi, M.I., Rollason, T.P. *et al.* (1996b) Vulvar intraepithelial neoplasia: long term follow up of treated and untreated women. *Br J Obstet Gynaecol* **103**(5),446.

Hewitt, J. (1984) Conditions étiologiques du carcinome invasif d'emblée de la vulve. Possibilité d'un traitement prophylactique? *J Gynecol Obstet Biol Reprod* **13**,297.

Hewitt, J., Polisse, M., Lessen-Leibowitch, M. *et al.* (1985) Le syndrome vulvo-vagino au gingival. *Rev Stomatol Chir Maxillofac* **86**,57.

Hilliard, G.D., Massey, F.M. & O'Toole, R.V. (1979) Vulvar neoplasia in the young. *Am J Obstet Gynecol* **135**,185.

Hoffman, J.S., Kumar, N.B. & Morley, G.W. (1983) Microinvasive squamous carcinoma of the vulva: search for definition. *Obstet Gynecol* **61**,615.

Hoffman, M.S., La Polla, J.P., Roberts, J.S. & Kaufner, D. (1990) Use of local flaps for primary anal reconstruction following perianal resection for neoplasia. *Gynecol Oncol* **36**(3),348.

Hording, U., Junge, J., Poulsen, H. & Lundval, F. (1995) Vulvar intraepithelial neoplasia—III: a viral disease of undetermined progressive potential. *Gynaecol Oncol* **56**(2),276.

Husseinzadeh, N., Newman, N.J. & Wesseler, T.A. (1989) Vulvar intraepithelial neoplasia: a clinico-pathological study of carcinoma-in-situ of the vulva. *Gynecol Oncol* **33**(2),157.

Iverson, T. & Tretli, S. (1998) Intraepithelial and invasive squamous cell neoplasia of the vulva: trends in incidence, recurrence, and survival rate in Norway. *Obstet Gynecol* **91**(6),969.

Iversen, T., Abeler, V. & Aalders, J. (1981) Individualised treatment for stage 1 carcinoma of the vulva. *Obstet Gynecol* **57**,85.

Jones, M. (1990) Genital precancers and emotional trauma. In: Singer, A. (ed.) Premalignant Lesions of the Lower Genital Tract. *Clin Prac Gynaecol* **2**(2),285.

Jones R.W. (1988) Management of VIN3. *Int J Gynecol Cancer* **8**,509.

Jones R.W. & McLean, M.R. (1986) Carcinoma in situ of the vulva; a review of 31 treated and 5 untreated cases. *Obstet Gynecol* **68**,499.

Kaufman, R.H. (ed.) (1991) Vulvovaginal disease. In: *Clinical Obstetrics and Gynecology*, Vol. 34, No. 3, p. 581. J.B. Lippincott, Philadelphia.

Kaufman, R.H. (1995) Intraepithelial neoplasia of the vulva. *Gynecol Oncol* **56**,80.

Kaufman, R. & Faro, S. (1994) Intraepithelial neoplasia of the vulva and vagina. In: *Benign Diseases of the Vagina and Vulva*, 4th edn, p. 140. Mosby, St Louis.

Kaufman, R.H., Bornstein, J., Adam, E. *et al.* (1988) Human papillomavirus and herpes simplex virus in vulval squamous cell carcinoma in situ. *Am J Obstet Gynecol* **158**(4),862.

Kelley, J.L., Burke, T.W., Tornos, C. *et al.* (1992) Minimally invasive vulvar carcinoma: an indication for conservative surgical therapy. *Gynecol Oncol* **44**,240.

Kimura, S. (1980) Condylomata acuminata with pigmented papular lesions. *Dermatologica* **160**,390.

Kimura, S., Hirai, A., Harada, R. & Nagashima, M. (1978) So-called multicentric pigmented Bowen's disease. *Dermatologica* **157**,229.

King, A., Nicole, C.S. & Rodin, P. (1980) *Venereal Diseases*, 4th edn. Baillière Tindal, London.

Kneale, B.L. (1983) Microinvasive cancer of the vulva; report of the International Society for the Study of Vulvar Disease Task Force. In: Proceedings of the Seventh World Congress of the ISSVD. *J Reprod Med* **29**,454.

Kneale, B.L.G., Elliott, P.M. & MacDonaid, I.A. (1981) Microinvasive carcinoma of the vulva: clinical features and management. In: Coppleson, M. (ed.) *Gynaecological Oncology*, Vol. 1, p. 320. Churchill Livingstone, Edinburgh.

Kolstad, P., Iverson, T., Abeler, V. (1982) Microinvasive carcinoma of the vulva—definition and treatment problems. *Clin Oncol* **8**,355.

Korn, A.P., Abercrombie, P.D. & Foster, A. (1996) Vulvar intraepithelial neoplasia in women infected with human immunodeficiency virus-1. *Gynecol Oncol* **61**(3),384.

Krebs, H.B. (1986) Prophylactic topical 5-fluorouracil following treatment of human papillomavirus-associated lesions of the vulva and vagina. *Obstet Gynecol* **68**,837.

Krebs, H.B. (1987) Treatment of vaginal condylomata acuminata by weekly topical application of 5-fluorouracil. *Obstet Gynecol* **70**,68.

Krupp, P.J. (1992) Invasive tumours of the vulva: clinical features, staging and management. In: Coppleson, M. (ed.) *Gynaecological Oncology*, Vol. 1, 2nd edn, p. 487. Churchill Livingstone, Edinburgh.

Lee, S.C., Roth, L.M. & Ehrlich, C. (1977) Extramammary Paget's disease of the vulva. *Cancer* **39**,614.

Leuchter, R.S., Townsend, D.E., Hacker, N.F. *et al.* (1984) Treatment of vulvar carcinoma in situ with the CO_2 laser. *Gynecol Oncol* **19**,314.

Li Vigni, R., Turano, A., Colombi, M. *et al.* (1992) Histological human papillomavirus-induced lesions: tryptization by molecular hybridization techniques. *Eur J Gynecol Oncol* **13**(3),236.

McAdam, A.J. & Kissner, R.W. (1958) Relationship of chronic vulvar disease, leukoplakia and carcinoma-in-situ to carcinoma of the vulva. *Cancer* **11**,740.

McDonald, T.W., Neutens, J.J., Fisher, C.M. & Jessee, D. (1989) Impact of CIN diagnosis and treatment on self-esteem and body image. *Gynecol Oncol* **34**,345.

Magrina, J.F., Webb, M.J., Gaffey, T.A. & Symonds, R.E. (1979) Stage I carcinoma of the vulva. *Am J Obstet Gynecol* **134**,453.

Mene, A. & Buckley C.H. (1985) Involvement of the vulval skin appendages by intraepithelial neoplasia. *Br J Obstet Gynaecol* **92**,634.

Mitchell, M.F., Prasad, C.J., Silva, E.G. *et al.* (1993) Second genital primary squamous neoplasms in vulvar carcinoma—viral and histopathologic correlates. *Obstet Gynecol* **81**(1),13.

Modesitt, S.C., Waters, A.B., Walton, L., Fowler, W.C. & Van Le, L. (1998) Vulvar intraepithelial neoplasia III: occult cancer and the impact of margin status on recurrence. *Obstet Gynecol* **92**(6),962.

Moll, I. & Moll, R. (1985) Cells of extramammary Paget's disease express cytokeratins different from those of epidermal cells. *J Invest Dermatol* **84**,3.

Nadji, M., Morales, A.R., Girtanner, R.E., Ziegels-Weissmann, J. & Penneys, N.S. (1982) Paget's disease of the skin. A unifying concept of histogenesis. *Cancer* **50**,2203.

Park, J.S., Jones, R.W., McLean, M.R. *et al.* (1991) Possible aetiological heterogeneity of vulvar intraepithelial neoplasia. A correlation of pathologic characteristics with human papillomavirus detection by in-situ hybridization and polymerase chain reaction. *Cancer* **67**(6),1599.

Petry, K., Kochel, H., Bode, U. & Kuhnle, H. (1996) Human papillomavirus is associated with the frequent detection of warty and basaloid high-grade neoplasia of the vulva and cervical neoplasia among immunocompromised women. *Gynecol Oncol* **60**,30.

Pickel, H. (1989) Early stromal invasion of the vulva. *Eur J Cynecol Oncol* **10**(2),97.

Pilotti, S., Delle-Torre, G., Rilke, F., Di Paolo, G. & Shah, K.V. (1984) Immunohistochemical and ultrastructural evidence of papillomavirus infection associated with in situ and microinvasive squamous cell carcinoma of the vulva. *Am J Surg Pathol* **8**,751.

Pilotti, S., Rotola, A., Di-Amato, L. *et al.* (1990) Vulvar carcinomas; search for sequences homologous to human papillomavirus and herpes simplex virus DNA. *Mod Pathol* **3**(4),442.

Planner, R.S. & Hobbs, J.B. (1987) Human papillomavirus infection and associated intraepithelial neoplasia of the cervix, vagina and vulva. *Obstet Gynecol* **27**,132.

Planner, R.S. & Hobbs, J.B. (1988) Intraepithelial and invasive neoplasia of the vulva in association with human papillomavirus infection. *J Reprod Med* **33**,503.

Prabhat, K.S., Beral, V., Peto, J. *et al.* (1993) Antibodies to human papillomavirus and to other genital infectious agents and invasive cervical cancer risk. *Lancet* **341**,1116.

Reid, M., Greenberg, M.D., Daoud, Y., Hussain, M. & Wilkinson, E. (1988) Colposcopic findings in women with vulvar pain syndromes: a preliminary report. *J Reprod Med* **33**,523.

Reid, R. (1985) Superficial laser vulvectomy III, a new surgical technique for appendage-conserving ablation of refractory condyloma and vulvar intraepithelial neoplasia. *Am J Obstet Gynecol* **152**(5),504.

Reid, R. (1992) Laser surgery in the lower genital tract. In: Coppleson, M. (ed.) *Gynaecological Oncology*, Vol. 2, 2nd edn, p. 1094. Churchill Livingstone, Edinburgh.

Rettenmaier, M.A., Berman, M.L. & DiSaia, P.J. (1987) Skinning vulvectomy for the treatment of multifocal vulvar intraepithelial neoplasia. *Obstet Gynecol* **69**,247.

Ridley, C.M. (1988a) General dermatological conditions and dermatoses of the vulva. In: Ridley, C.M. (ed.) *The Vulva*, p. 173. Churchill Livingstone, Edinburgh.

Ridley, C.M. (1988b) Dermatological conditions in the vulva. In: Ridley, C.M. (ed.) *The Vulva*, p. 185. Churchill Livingstone, Edinburgh.

Ridley, C.M. (1988c) Infective conditions. In: Ridley, C.M. (ed.) *The Vulva*, p. 97. Churchill Livingstone, Edinburgh.

Ridley, C.M. (1989) ISSVD new nomenclature for vulvar disease. *Am J Obstet Gynecol* **160**,769.

Ridley, C.M., Frankman, Q., Jones, I.S.C. & Wilkinson, E.J. (1989a) New nomenclature for vulvar disease. International Society for the Study of Vulvar Disease. *Hum Pathol* **20**,495.

Ridley, C.M., Frankman, O., Jones, I.S.C., Pincus, S.H. & Wilkinson, E.J. (1989b) New nomenclature for vulvar disease. Report of the Committee on Terminology, International Society for the Study of Vulvar Disease. *Int J Gynecol Pathol* **8**,83.

Rose, P.G. & Friare, A.E. (1993) Multiple primary gynaecological neoplasms in a young HIV positive patient. *J Surg Oncol* **53**(4), 269.

Rusk, D., Sutton, G.P., Look, K.Y. & Roman, A. (1991) Analysis of invasive cell carcinoma of the vulva and vulvar intraepithelial neoplasia for the presence of human papillomavirus DNA. *Obstet Gynecol* **77**(6),918.

Rutledge, F. & Sinclair, M. (1968) Treatment of intraepithelial carcinoma of the vulva by skin excision and graft. *Am J Obstet Gynecol* **102**,806.

Salzstein, S.L., Woodruff, J.D. & Novak, E.R. (1956) Post-granulomatous carcinoma of the vulva. *Obstet Gynecol* **7**,80.

Schlaerth, J.B., Morrow, C.P., Nalick, R.H. & Gaddis, O. (1984) Anal involvement by carcinoma in situ of the perineum in women. *Obstet Gynecol* **64**,406.

Shatz, P., Bergeron, C., Wilkinson, E. & Ferenczy, A. (1989) Vulvar intraepithelial neoplasia and skin appendage involvement. *Obstet Gynecol* **74**,769.

Sherman, K.J., Dalien, J.R., Chu, J. *et al.* (1991) Genital warts, other sexually transmitted diseases and vulval cancer. *Epidemiology* **2**(4),257.

Sillman, F.H. & Sedlis, A. (1991) Anogenital papillomavirus infection and neoplasia in immunodeficient women; an update. *Dermatol Clin* **9**,353.

Sillman, F.H., Boyce, J.G., Macaset, M.A. & Nicastri, A.D. (1981) 5-Fluorouracil/chemosurgery for intraepithelial neoplasia of the lower genital tract. *Obstet Gynecol* **58**,356.

Sillman, F.H., Sedlis, A. & Boyce, J.C. (1985) 5-FU/chemosurgery for difficult lower genital intraepithelial neoplasia. *Contemp Obstet Gynecol* **30**,79.

Simonsen, E.F. (1989) The CO_2 laser used for carcinoma-in-situ/Bowen's disease (VIN) and lichen sclerosus in the vulvar region. *Acta Obstet Gynecol Scand* **68**(6),551.

Singer, A. & Mitchell, H. (1990) Treatment of vulvar premalignancy. *Clin Prac Gynaecol* **2**(2),231.

Skinner, M.S., Sternberg, W.H., Ichinose, H. & Collins, J. (1973) Spontaneous regression of Bowenoid atypia of the vulva. *Obstet Gynecol* **42**,40.

Stafford, E.M., Greenberg, H. & Miles, P.A. (1990) Cervical intraepithelial neoplasia III in an adolescent with Bowenoid papulosis. *J Adol Health Care* **11**(6),523.

Sturgeon, S.R., Brinton, C.A., Devesa, S.S. & Kurman, R.J. (1992) In situ and invasive vulvar cancer trends (1973–1987). *Am J Obstet Gynecol* **166**(5),1482.

Theusen, B., Andreasson, B. & Bock, J.E. (1992) Sexual function and somatophysic reactions after local excision of vulvar intraepithelial neoplasia. *Acta Obstet Gynecol Scand* **71**(2),126.

Thomas, S.S., Chenoy, R., Fielding, J.W. *et al.* (1996) Vulvo-perineal reconstruction after excision of ano-genital multi-focal intraepithelial neoplasia. *Br J Plast Surg* **49**(8),539.

Toki, T., Kurman, R.J., Park, J.S. *et al.* (1991) Probable non-papillomavirus aetiology of squamous cell carcinoma of the vulva in older women; a clinico-pathological study using in-situ hybridization and polymerase chain reaction. *Int J Gynecol Pathol* **10**,107.

Townsend, D.E., Levine, R.U., Richart, R.M., Crum, C. & Petrilli, E.S. (1982) Management of vulvar intraepithelial neoplasia by carbon dioxide laser. *Obstet Gynecol* **60**,49.

Ulbright, T.M., Stehman, F.B., Roth, L.M. *et al.* (1982) Bowenoid dysplasia of the vulva. *Cancer* **50**,2910.

van Beurden, M., ten Cate, F.J. & ter Schegget, J. (1995) Multifocal vulvar intraepithelial neoplasia grade III and multicentric lower genital tract neoplasia is associated with transcriptionally active human papillomavirus. *Cancer* **75**(12),2879.

van Beurden, M., van de Vanger, N., de Craen, A.J. *et al.* (1997) Normal findings in vulvar examination and vulvoscopy. *Br J Obstet Gynaecol* **104**(3),320.

van Beurden, M., de Vange, N., ten Cate, F. & Lammes, F. (1998a) Multifocal vulvalar intraepithelial neoplasia grade III and multicentric lower genital tract neoplasia is associated with transcriptionally active human papillomavirus. *Cancer* **75**,2879.

van Beurden, M., van de Vanger, N., Ten Kate, F.J.W. *et al.* (1998b) Restricted surgical management of vulvar intraepithelial neoplasia 3: focus on invasion and on relief of symptoms. *Int J Gynecol Cancer* **8**,73.

Van Sickle, M., Kaufman, R.H., Adam, E. & Adler-Storchz, K. (1990) Detection of human papillomavirus DNA before and after development of invasive vulvar cancer. *Obstet Gynecol* **76**(3),540.

Wade, T.R., Kopf, A.W. & Ackerman, A.B. (1979) Bowenoid papulosis of the genitalia. *Arch Dermatol* **115**,306.

Wallace, H.J. (1971) Lichen sclerosus et atrophicus. *Trans St John's Hosp Dermatol Soc* **57**,9.

Wende, D. (1971) The VDRL slide test in 322 cases of dark field positive primary syphilis. *S Med J* **64**,50.

Wharton, J.T., Gallager, S. & Rutledge, F.N. (1974) Microinvasive carcinoma of the vulva. *Am J Obstet Gynecol* **118**,159.

Wilkinson, E.J. (1987) Vulvar intraepithelial neoplasias. In: Wilkinson, E.J. (ed.) *Pathology of the Vulva and Vagina*, p. 85. Churchill Livingstone, Edinburgh.

Wilkinson, E.J. (1990) The 1989 Presidential Address, International Society for the Study of Vulvar Disease. *J Reprod Med* **35**,981.

Wilkinson, E.J. (1992) Normal histology and nomenclature of the vulva, and malignant neoplasms, including VIN. *Dermatol Clin* **10**,283.

Wilkinson, E.J., Cook, J.C., Friedrich, E.G. & Massey, J.K. (1988)

Vulvar intraepithelial neoplasia, association with cigarette smoking. *Colpos Gynecol Laser Surg* **4**,143.

Wilkinson, E.J., Friedrich, E.G. & Fu, Y.S. (1981) Multicentric nature of vulvar carcinoma in situ. *Obstet Gynecol* **58**,69.

Wilkinson, E., Rico, M. & Pearson, K. (1982) Microinvasive carcinoma of vulva. *Int J Gynecol Pathol* **1**,29.

Wolcott, H.D. & Gallup, D.G. (1984) Wide local excision in the treatment of vulvar carcinoma in situ: a reappraisal. *Am J Obstet Gynecol* **150**,695.

Woodruff, J.D. (1955) Paget's disease of the vulva. *Obstet Gynecol* **5**,175.

Woodruff, J.D. (1977) Paget's disease. *Obstet Gynecol* **49**,511.

Woodruff, J.D. (1982) Early invasive cancer of the vulva. *Clin Oncol* **1**,349.

Woodruff, J.D. & Friedrich, E.G. (1985) The vestibule. *Clin Obstet Gynecol* **12**,134.

Woodruff, J.D. & Hildebrand, T.E.E. (1958) Carcinoma in situ of the vulva. *Obstet Gynecol* **12**,414.

Woodruff, J.D. & Parmley, T.H. (1983) Infection of the minor vestibular gland. *Obstet Gynecol* **62**,609.

Woodruff, J.D., Julian, C.D., Puray, T., Mermut, S. & Katayama, P. (1973) The contemporary challenge of carcinoma in situ of the vulva. *Am J Obstet Gynecol* **115**,677.

Wright, V.C. & Davies, E. (1987) Laser surgery for vulvar intraepithelial neoplasia: principles and results. *Am J Obstet Gynecol* **156**,374.

Zachow, K.R., Astrow, R.S., Bender, M. & Watts, S. (1981) Detection of human papillomavirus DNA in anogenital neoplasias. *Nature* **300**,771.

Zaino, R.J., Husseinzade, N., Nahhas, W. & Mortel, R. (1982) Epithelial alterations in proximity to invasive squamous carcinoma of the vulva. *Int J Gynecol Pathol* **1**,173.

Zhang, W.H., Coppleson, M., Rose, B.R. *et al.* (1988) Papillomavirus and cervical cancer: a clinical and laboratory study. *J Med Virol* **26**,163.

Chapter 10
Perianal and Anal Intraepithelial Neoplasia

10.1 Epidemiology

The natural history of perianal and anal in-situ intraepithelial neoplasia is uncertain in comparison with cervical intraepithelial neoplasia (CIN), where the progression to invasive cancer occurs in about 36% of cases over a 20-year period (McIndoe et al., 1984). Anal carcinoma is much less common than its cervical counterpart so the progression rate would certainly be lower for grade 3 intraepithelial neoplasia of the anus than of the cervix. However, there would seem to be evidence that the rate of anal carcinoma is indeed increasing, especially in the USA (Wechsner et al., 1988), and it may only be a matter of time before the same occurs in Europe. The only way of possibly reducing this potential risk with its corresponding morbidity and mortality would be to introduce a program of diagnosis and eradication of the intraepithelial disease. There is circumstantial evidence that the anal intraepithelial neoplasias and anal carcinoma are part of one spectrum (Scholefield et al., 1989, 1992), and this chapter will be concerned with presenting the clinical features and characteristics of these lesions and recommending appropriate management.

10.2 Etiology

There has been evidence for a number of years that human papillomavirus type 16 (HPV 16) has an important role in the etiology of most lower genital tract precancers and cancers, including those related to the perianal and anal areas (Palmer et al., 1989). It is suggested that the transmission of the HPV infection throughout the genital tract is by direct spread from adjacent areas and in this situation it would be from the vulva to the perianal and anal areas (Goorney et al., 1987; Sonnix et al., 1991). The presence of HPV 16 DNA in perianal and anal preneoplastic lesions was shown by McCance and Singer (1986) in 12 out of 15 cases. They also showed that in another four cases of early intraepithelial disease of the anal canal, there was HPV 16 positivity. The relationship between genital warts and anal cancer has also been well defined with the relative risk ranging from 3 to 32, depending on the sex of the subject (Daling et al., 1987, 1992; Holly et al., 1989).

Furthermore, many recent epidemiologic studies suggest a strong association with smoking at the time of diagnosis. Using the sensitive polymerase chain reaction (PCR), Daling et al. (1992) found that up to 69% of squamous and transitional cell anal tumors have HPV DNA, and 73% of these were of HPV type 16 (Daling et al., 1992). There have also been two case-control studies using tissue controls from the same anatomic site (Palmer et al., 1989; Scholefield et al., 1992); Palmer et al. (1989) matched 28 consecutive patients who were undergoing elective hemorrhoidectomy to 28 anal squamous cell carcinomas. They found that HPV 16 or 18 did not exist in any of the control tissues, whereas 67% (16/28) of the cases were positive for these types by Southern-blot analysis. Crook et al. (1991) have reanalyzed these tissues using PCR and have identified HPV 16 DNA to be positive in 76% of cases. Scholefield et al. (1992) have detected HPV 16 DNA in 18 (51%) out of 35 anal biopsy samples from women with anal intraepithelial neoplasia. In their control group, which was of women undergoing laparoscopic sterilization, seven (14%) out of 50 biopsies from the anus were positive for HPV 16 DNA. In three of these cases, both cervical and anal biopsies were positive for HPV 16 DNA.

A serologic association of HPV type 16 with incident anal cases has been reported by Heino et al. (1995). They showed that 55% of patients with anal cancer were seropositive for HPV 16, compared with 4% of the controls. In another prospective seroepidemiologic study by Bjorge et al. (1997), of HPV antibodies in 700000 samples in a serum bank in Finland, there was a high but not significant increase in odds ratio for seropositivity for HPV 16 in those who developed perianal skin cancer. The reason for the high proportion of seropositive controls is unclear but may relate to their over matching or to the small numbers.

In homosexual men there would seem to be a high risk of the development of anorectal intraepithelial disease. Fraser et al. (1986) showed the high incidence of cytologic signs of "dysplasia" of the anorectal epithelium and HPV infection in 61 out of 100 homosexual men in a prospective study. They concluded that HPV infections of the anorectal mucosa were frequent among homosexual men and predisposed them to epithelial abnormalities in that region. The prevalence of human immunodeficiency virus (HIV) in these men is well known and the finding of such lesions must alert the clinician to the possibility of HIV infection, whether the patient be male or female (Rutlinger et al., 1990).

Many studies have continued to show the increased risk that women with HIV have, especially if associated with HPV for the development of anal abnormalities. Melbye et al. (1996) have shown that the increased risk of anal neoplasia was significantly associated with and almost exclusively seen in the presence of HPV. Immunodeficiency and HIV positivity increased the risk of disease in HPV-positive subjects. They also concluded that a high level of HPV infection is important for the development of anal squamous intraepithelial lesions in this population.

10.3 Association with other genital intraepithelial neoplastic diseases

It has been known for many years that cervical, vaginal, and vulvar intraepithelial diseases are linked by the common etiologic factor of HPV infections. This has been alluded to many times in this text. It also seems as though women with these conditions are at increased risk for the development of anal carcinoma (Scholefield et al., 1989). However, there have been few case-control studies determining the prevalence of anal intraepithelial neoplasia in females with CIN. Sholefield et al. showed that 29 (19%) out of 152 women with CIN 3 had histologic evidence of similar anal lesions. Of these 29 patients, 11 had grade 3 anal lesions, and two of these women subsequently developed invasive anal squamous carcinoma. Only 7% (8/115) of the women with high-grade lesions of the cervix alone had evidence of anal intraepithelial neoplasia; by contrast, 57% (21/37) of those with more than one focus of intraepithelial neoplasia (cervix plus vulva, vagina, or both) had anal lesions.

HPV is common to both the etiologies of anal and cervical neoplasia and the presence of HIV would seem to accentuate this association which has been highlighted by a recent study by Melbye et al. (1996). They studied a group of 151 women at risk for HIV infection and assessed the presence of HPV and cytologic abnormalities. An equal percentage of women had abnormal cervical (12.2%) and anal (12.1%) PAP smears. HPV measured by PCR was detected in 93% of cervical squamous intraepithelial lesions (SIL) compared with 49% of normal cervical cytologies and in 100% of anal SIL and 67% of normal anal smears respectively. When they controlled for HPV-PCR status immunodeficiency as measured by a low CD4 count and HIV positivity, they found that the detection of cervical and, to some extent, anal SILs increased. They concluded that cervical SIL was associated with a more than threefold increased risk of a simultaneous abnormal smear when taken from the anal area.

10.4 Examination

Over the last few years it has become apparent that anal cytology offers a method of detecting anal neoplastic disease. A number of studies have highlighted the benefit cytologic screening of HIV infected men and women. Melbye et al. (1996) in their study of 151 women at risk of HIV found that both cervix and anal cytology were comparable, that is, 12.2% and 12.1% respectively for abnormal smears. They evaluated how precisely an HPV test could predict both cervical and anal disease, and found that the HPV-PCR test was slightly more sensitive than the HPV hybrid capture test (Hybrid Capture, Digene Corporation), (i.e. PCR: 93.3% vs. HC: 88.9%) whereas the hybrid capture test was significantly more specific (83.6% vs. 50.9%) and with a much higher positive predictive value (43.2% vs. 20.6%). HIV-positivity increased sensitivity but lowered specificity and increased the positive predictive value of these tests. As mentioned above, the diagnosis of cervical SIL was associated with more than threefold increased risk of simultaneous abnormal anal smears. They concluded that hybrid capture, which required a higher viral load than PCR to detect HPV, was clearly superior in detecting cervical and anal disease. The optimum cytologic method indeed for detecting anal neoplasia was analysed also by Sherman et al. (1995). They concluded that the thin-Prep® technique (Cytyc Corporation, Boxboro, MA, USA) was satisfactory in twice as many cases as conventional smears and detected nearly eight times as many SILs.

Although cytology and anoscopy would seem to be ideal methods, it has recently become apparent that anal neoplasia may develop deep in glands and, although detected cytologically, can exist before visible lesions are detected with the aid of the colposcope (anoscopes). Surawicz et al. (1995) screened high-risk homosexual men as part of a longitudinal study examining the effect of HIV-infection on the risk of development of high-grade anal intraepithelial neoplasia (AIN 2 and 3). They found seven individuals who had histologic evidence of AIN 2 and 3 with visually normal findings by anoscopy. Two of them were HIV seronegative, five HIV seropositive, and only one of the HIV seropositive patients had a low CD4 count below 200. However, abnormal cytology was seen over a follow-up period of 3 months to 2½ years, and suggested that the persistence of visually inapparent anal abnormalities was a reality. Indeed, two of the men had had small internal warts at earlier examinations and three of the seven men subsequently developed visually abnormal anal findings. All had HPV 16 detected at some stage during the follow-up. This led them to conclude that there were problems with the detection of high-grade anal cytology in that visible lesions could not be detected at the same time as the abnormal cytology developed. These results in respect of anal cytology would seem to be transferable to anal neoplasia of women.

An examination of this area involves use of the same techniques as those employed for the vulva, i.e. vulvoscopy. Anoscopy (use of the colposcope to examine the anal canal area) is extremely valuable in defining the extent and characteristics of intraepithelial disease of the anus, anal canal, and perianal margins. However, it must be realized that this area may be difficult to examine and prove uncomfortable for the patient. The area should be soaked with 5% acetic acid and left for at least 2 to 3 minutes to allow the tissue to stain. If it produces a burning sensation, then it should immediately be washed off with warm water. It will be evident that many areas of acetowhiteness will be visible and, as will be shown below, not all of these will be associated with intraepithelial neoplasia. Anoscopy and proctoscopy should be undertaken, and biopsy using local anesthetic can be performed.

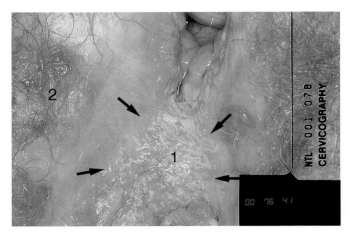

Fig. 10.1

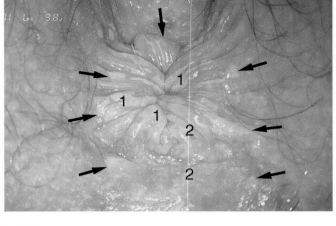

Fig. 10.3

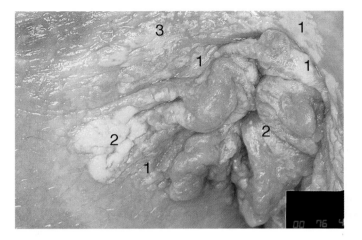

Fig. 10.2

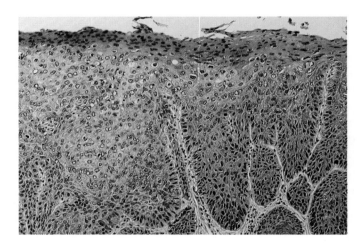

Fig. 10.4

10.5 Presentation

When considering these conditions, it is important to remember that the following three distinct sites must be examined.

1 Perineum.
2 Anus.
3 The anal canal.

Lesions involving the perineum and anal areas are similar to those involving the vulva and many will show hyperkeratotic and pigmented characteristics. The vascular patterns that are seen when colposcopy is used for a cervical examination are not commonly seen on the perianal skin but they are certainly evident within the anal canal. Typical presentations are presented in Figs 10.1–10.7. In Figs 10.1 and 10.2, a contiguous intraepithelial neoplastic lesion is seen involving both the perineum (Fig. 10.1) and the anus (Fig. 10.2); it extends to within the anal canal to the pectinate line. Biopsy of the perineal lesion (outlined by arrows in Fig. 10.1) shows grade 2 intraepithelial neoplasia in the area at (1). There is also a pigmented hyperkeratotic lesion at (2) that, on biopsy, was shown to be vulvar intraepithelial neoplasia (VIN) 3. Examination of the anal canal shown in Fig. 10.2 revealed three distinct morpho-

logic types. A biopsy taken from area (1) showed subclinical papillomavirus infection (SPI), and a biopsy taken from area (2), an area of dense hyperkeratosis that is visible clinically, showed grade 3 intraepithelial neoplasia. In area (3), the same disease as found in the perineum was present. Obviously, an examination of the anal canal must be undertaken to determine extension into that area, and this is shown in Figs 10.3–10.7. Figure 10.3 shows an extensive acetowhite area around the anus and extending into the anal canal. The outline of this area is shown by arrows. Biopsies taken from (1) in three locations in this area revealed the presence of type 3 intraepithelial neoplasia (Fig. 10.4). Examination of the specimen showed complete loss of differentiation with marked acanthosis. A biopsy taken from position (2) in Fig. 10.3 revealed the presence of subclinical wart viral infection. Figure 10.5 shows a very hyperkeratotic irregularly surfaced lesion that stained after the application of acetic acid. A punch biopsy taken from position (1) revealed grade 3 intraepithelial neoplasia (Fig. 10.6). Abnormal mitoses with occasional "corps ronds" can be seen throughout this thickened and irregular epithelium. In Fig. 10.7, a flattish fissured lesion (1) can be seen. It was localized an associated with anoscopic and histologic evidence of SPI in area (2). A biopsy taken from position (1) showed the presence of grade 3 intraepithelial neoplasia.

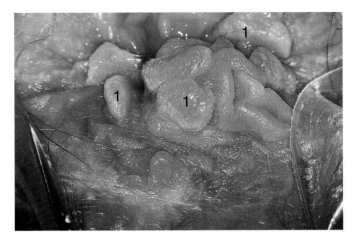

Fig. 10.5

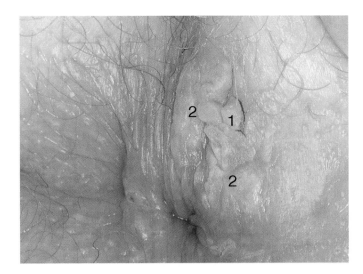

Fig. 10.7

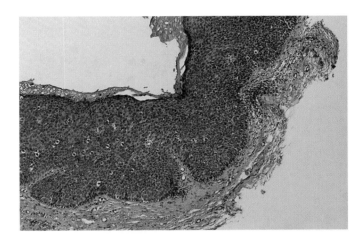

Fig. 10.6

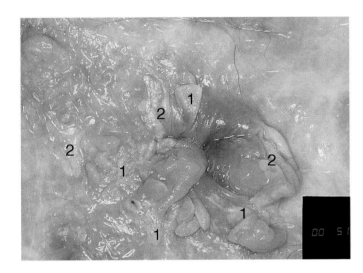

Fig. 10.8

10.6 Lesions masquerading as intraepithelial neoplasia

A number of lesions masquerade as intraepithelial neoplastic conditions; the commonest is due to condyloma acuminata. In Fig. 10.8, an acetowhite area is evident with patches of hyperkeratosis at (1) and a smooth white epithelium at (2). Biopsies taken from both these areas showed the presence of SPI. In Fig. 10.9, a view of the anus and anal canal reveals the presence of what seem like typical condyloma acuminata lesions. Multiple biopsies were taken and in positions (1) and (1) on either side of the anal canal; histologic evidence of condyloma acuminata was obtained. However, surprisingly, in the areas designated (2) and (2), grade 3 intraepithelial neoplasia was found. This illustrates the difficulty of making a diagnosis without resorting to biopsy. In Fig. 10.10, a vesicular-like surface (1) is seen on a small anal tag (2). This patient had previously had recurrent episodes of genital herpes simplex virus (HSV) 2 infection. After 1 week, the lesion had completely resolved. The initial diagnosis was of an early invasive carcinoma of the vulva. If any suspicion of HSV 2 exists, then it is prudent to observe and not to interfere. Figures 10.11 and 10.12 show the extension of the disease into the natal cleft, and biopsies taken from areas (1) in Fig. 10.11 show the presence of subclinical wart viral infection (arrowed). However, in Fig.

10.12, an area of diffuse acetowhiteness covered the perianal area and extended into the natal cleft (arrowed). Although histologic evidence of grade 3 intraepithelial neoplasia was found in the perianal area, the pattern of disease posteriorly in the natal cleft seemed of a minor grade. Punch biopsies performed at points (1) and (1) revealed the presence of SPI, but biopsies taken from (2) surprisingly showed the presence of grade 2 intraepithelial neoplasia. This again illustrates the need for local excision biopsy and the difficulty of predicting the exact nature of epithelial disease by anoscopy.

10.7 Anal canal involvement

Intraepithelial neoplasia can involve the anal canal in two ways. First, it may extend from the perianal skin inward to the pectinate line with many of the lesions being contiguous with ones in the vulvar area. The second way is for it to occur within the anal canal with no obvious connection with vulvar or perianal disease.

Evidence of any perianal papillomavirus infection must raise the possibility of intraepithelial neoplasia within the

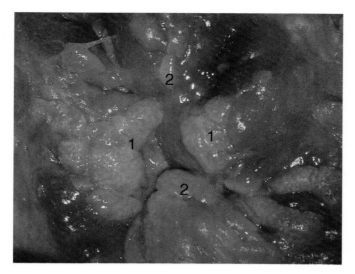

Fig. 10.9

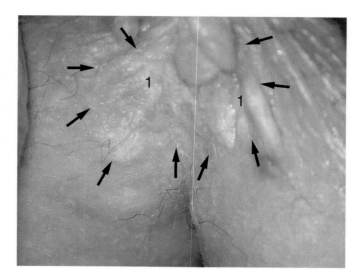

Fig. 10.11

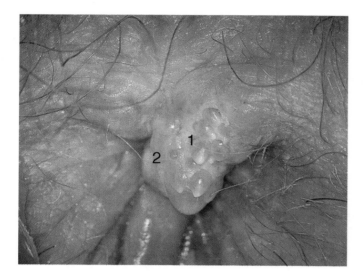

Fig. 10.10

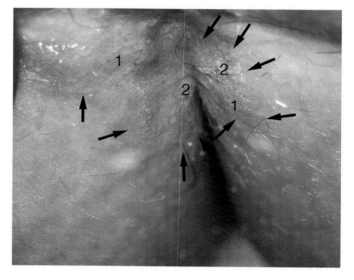

Fig. 10.12

anal canal. In Figs 10.13–10.17, these types of lesion can be seen.

In Fig. 10.13, an anoscope (1) displays the anal canal (2) with the obvious pectinate line at (3). Distal to this line is a diffuse area of acetowhite epithelium. A biopsy taken from area (4) shows it to be composed of grade 2 intraepithelial neoplasia with surrounding areas of papillomavirus infection.

Figure 10.14a shows that further examination with a proctoscope revealed a raised papular lesion (1) that is highlighted against the reddish mucosa of the anal canal. A biopsy taken from (1) shows it to be composed of a typical condylomatous tissue. In Fig. 10.14b, typical condylomata acuminata can be seen at (1), but those on the superior aspects appear more acetowhite than the former and a biopsy of them revealed the presence of intrae pithelial neoplasia of grade 1/2. Normal mucosa is visible at (3).

In Fig. 10.15, a swab stick has been used to apply acetic acid to a normal anal canal. Areas of squamous metaplastic epithelium exist within a transformation zone (2). The

dentate line is seen at (1) and large bowel mucosa is seen at (3). McCance and Singer (1986) suggest that squamous metaplasia is increased within the anal canal of homosexual men.

Figure 10.16 shows tongues of acetowhite epithelium that extend upward into the anal canal (1); an obvious condylomatous lesion exists at (2) and was proven to be so by biopsy. However, a biopsy taken from area (1) showed it to be composed of intraepithelial neoplasia of grade 1/2. Normal large bowel epithelium is shown at (3).

Figure 10.17 shows a thickened acetowhite epithelium with some punctation, mosaicism and corkscrew vessels occurring within the anal canal (1). At (2), the epithelium has become detached and formed an ulcerative lesion. A biopsy taken from point (1) showed the presence of grade 3 intraepithelial neoplasia, while at (2) an early invasive lesion is present.

A review of all these patterns illustrates the difficulty in making a diagnosis through the anoscope and proctoscope. Punch biopsy of any acetowhite lesion or, for that matter, a lesion with abnormal vascularity is recommended. After a

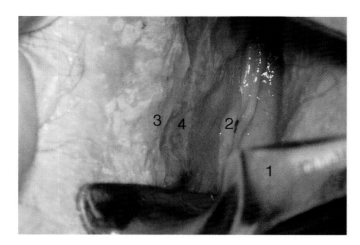

Fig. 10.13

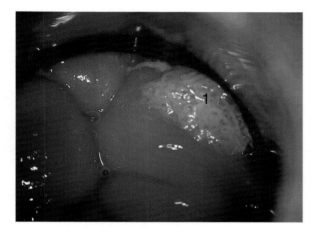

Fig. 10.14(a)

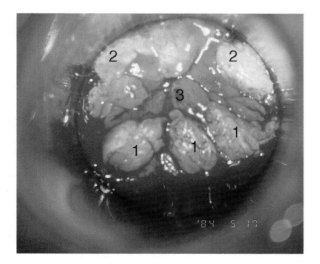

Fig. 10.14(b)

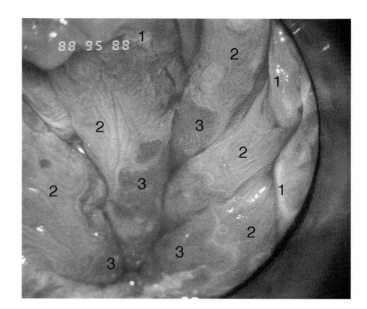

Fig. 10.15

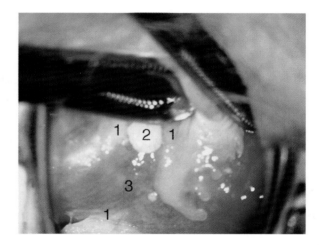

Fig. 10.16

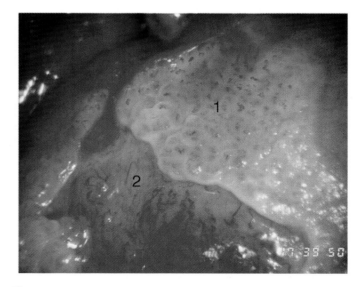

Fig. 10.17

biopsy has been taken, pressure applied with a firm swab for at least 3 minutes will stop most bleeding.

10.8 Treatment

Management of perineal, anal, and anal canal intraepithelial neoplasia depends on two factors: first, the pathology of the tissue; and second, its extent. If biopsy does not show any obvious evidence of early invasion, then one of two methods of treatment can be employed. These are: (i) laser vaporization and (ii) localized surgical excision.

Laser vaporization

Laser vaporization of small and localized areas can be undertaken. As there are no glandular elements involved, the depth of destruction can be taken to the second surgical plane, as described for treating vulvar lesions. When treating anal lesions, it is advisable to leave an epithelial skin bridge between the lasered areas so that regeneration can occur. In Fig. 10.18, a mixture of condyloma acuminata and biopsy-proven intraepithelial neoplasia of grade 1/2 existed in lesions at the entrance to the anal canal. Laser vaporization was performed. A small epithelial bridge can be seen at (1). An area of intraepithelial neoplasia had existed in the area at (2). Some carbonization is present and accounts for the darkness of the tissues. In area (3), where condyloma had existed, vaporization has been performed only to the first surgical layer and the dermal papillae with their shining surfaces can be clearly seen.

Localized surgical excision

Localized surgical excision can be undertaken for lesions that extend into the perianal and anal areas from the vulva and perineum. In Figs 10.19 and 10.20, a contiguous lesion, involving both the posterior fourchette and perineum, has extended to the anal verge. Biopsy in multiple sites showed it to be grade 3 intraepithelial neoplasia. The patient was extremely symptomatic. The technique described in Chapter 9 (p. 276), and which involves wide excision with undercutting of the vagina and its advancement, has been employed. Figure 10.19 shows the outline (arrowed) of the abnormal area, and in Fig. 10.20 the final operative result is presented. The vagina has been advanced to point (1), just distal to the site of the original posterior fourchette. A longitudinal wound (2) unites the edges of an elliptically excised area. The incision was taken to the anal verge (3). The anal canal and an accompanying hemorrhoid have been grasped in an Allis forceps and retracted downward. The labial wounds can be seen at (4).

Figures 10.21–10.23 show a very extensive lesion that involved both the labia minora and inner part of the labia majora; it has extended downward, involving the posterior fourchette and the perineum with a further extension caudally to the anal verge. The technique of a wide excision with vaginal advancement has also been employed in this case. In Fig. 10.21, the defect is obvious, and the clitoris and urethra can be seen at (1) and (2), respectively. The posterior perineal excision is obvious and the incision has been carried to the anal verge (4). In Fig. 10.22, the periclitoral and labial areas have been united, two layers having been used for this procedure. At this stage, the vagina is undercut, advanced to the perineum, and retracted down-

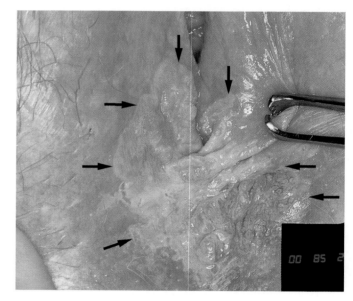

Fig. 10.19

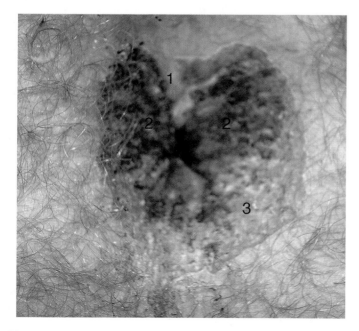

Fig. 10.18

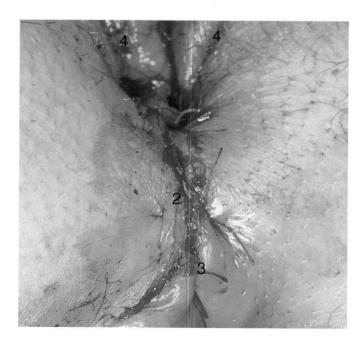

Fig. 10.20

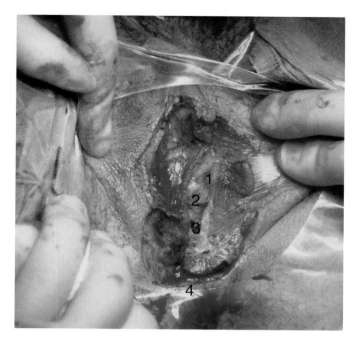

Fig. 10.21

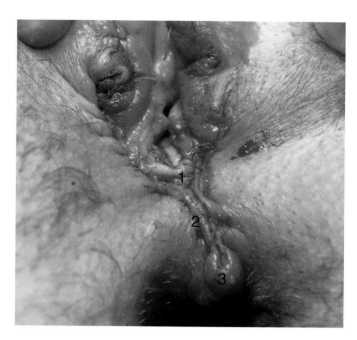

Fig. 10.23

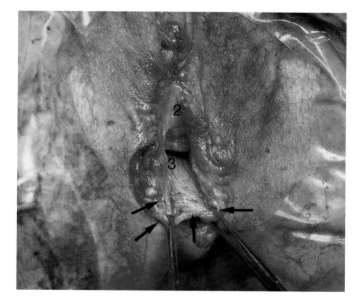

Fig. 10.22

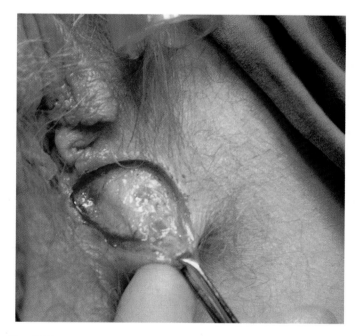

Fig. 10.24

ward. In Fig. 10.23, the final result can be seen with the vagina attached at point (1); a longitudinal incision at (2) unites the edges of the excised perineal region. The anal verge is at (3). There existed small areas of grade 3 intraepithelial neoplasia within the anal canal but these were treated by a combination of local excision and laser vaporization.

When this 26-year-old patient was seen 6 months later, there was no intraepithelial neoplasia within the genital tract and no interference with sexual function. Pathology of the excised portion showed large areas of the vulva, perineum, and perianal area to be composed of grade 3 intraepithelial neoplasia.

When an extensive but localized area extends onto the perineum, it can be widely excised using either a knife or the CO_2 laser. In Fig. 10.24, such a lesion has been cleanly excised using the CO_2 laser. The edges of the wound can be

undermined to allow primary closure. However, if this is not possible, then a bilateral rhomboid flap or local skin flaps (Hoffman et al., 1990) can be used to cover the defect. Any localized excision of lesions at the anus or in the anal canal should not necessitate resuture of the epithelial defect. A tule-gras swab or a haemostatic gelatin sponge (spongostan anal, Johnson and Johnson) should be inserted into the anal canal postoperatively.

Lesions within the anal canal, such as those shown in Figs 10.14 and 10.16, can be treated by the CO_2 laser after appropriate confirmation biopsy. It must be remembered that metal instruments need to be inserted in many of these cases for exposure purposes. For lesions lower down in the anal canal vigorous retraction of the anus can provide just as adequate exposure as the metal instrument; obviously the patient should be anesthetized. There is a theoretic risk of ignition of some lower bowel gases by the laser beam but, although anecdotal reports are forthcoming, no substantiated case has been reported. However, it is the author's (AS) practice to place a swab soaked in saline above the area to be lasered. In view of the reflection of the beam when it contacts metal instruments, it is suggested that only matted-surface instruments be used and that glasses be worn by all members of the operating team.

Intraepithelial lesions on hemorrhoids can be treated by hemorrhoidectomy. Likewise, lesions within the natal cleft are best removed by excision rather than by vaporization using the CO_2 laser.

Extensive surgical excision

In some women with multifocal intraepithelial neoplasia that involves both the perineum and anus, it is difficult to achieve removal with a localized surgical excision. This has led to more extensive surgery being performed in which a definitive vulvoperineal resection was combined with a simultaneous vulval reconstruction using meshed split skin grafts or a combination of skin grafts and local flaps. In such procedures an initial colostomy needs to be performed with closure only after achieving local control of the disease. Thomas *et al.* (1996) believe that such a staged approach achieves the objectives of eliminating disease and alleviating symptoms while preserving function and attempts to reconstruct normal anatomy without compro-

mising the principles of surgical oncology. Thomas and his group have reported on 12 women, utilizing this radical surgical approach for extensive vulval involvement with multifocal disease. Three had incomplete histopathologic clearance at the initial operation and, apart from these three patients, one had recurrence of symptoms alone, and one developed malignant squamous invasion 4 years later, which was successfully treated.

Such a procedure is seen in Figs 10.25–10.28. In Fig. 10.25, a large area of multifocal intraepithelial neoplasia is seen, involving not only the vulva and perineum but also the perianal and anal area. A colostomy has been performed and the area to be radically removed has been outlined in blue marking ink. In Fig. 10.26, the area to be covered is now exposed with complete hemostasis. Two flaps will be developed in the areas (1) and (2) by incisions along the dotted line that extends upwards and outwards. Points A eventually forming the upper part of the central band of tissue formed by the joining of these two flaps, and point B, the lower point. The incision will produce two flaps which will be brought together and united in front of the anus (3). In Fig. 10.27 this has been done and the two flaps (1) and (2) united at point B1.2. Flap 1 (1) overlaps its fellow (2) and forms the anterior margin of the anus which is at (3). The areas to be covered by the skin graft are at (4) and (5). The colostomy is closed after 10 weeks. In Fig. 10.28 the vulva and perineum/perianal area is seen at 10 weeks; the area covered by the posterior skin graft is at (5).

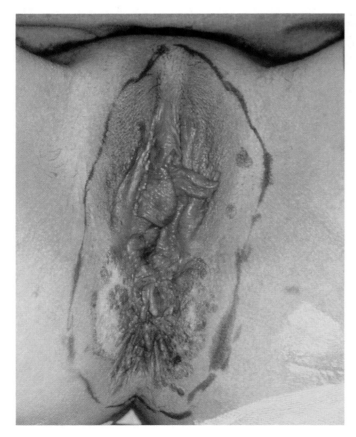

Fig. 10.25

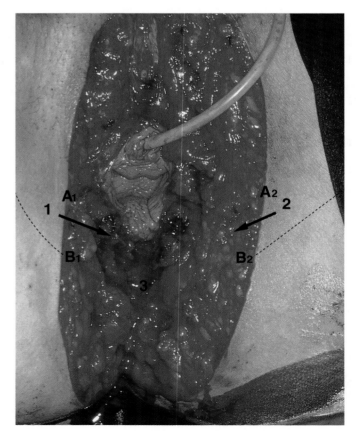

Fig. 10.26

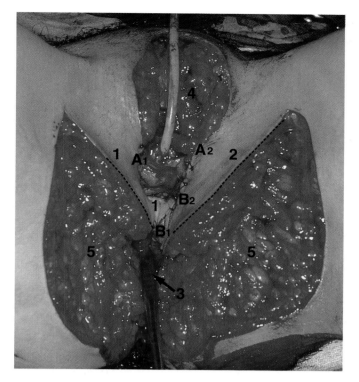

Fig. 10.27

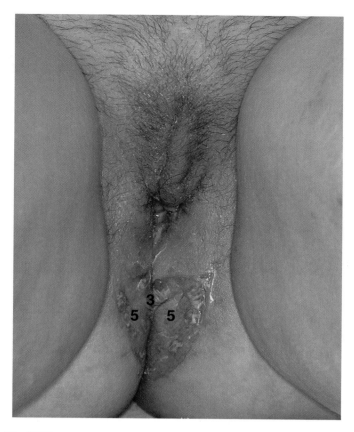

Fig. 10.28

10.9 References

Bjorge, T., Dilner, J., Anttilla, T. *et al.* (1997) Prospective sero-epidemiological study of role of human papillomavirus in non-cervical anogenital cancers. *Br Med J* **315**,646.

Crook, T., Wrede, D., Tidey, J., Scholefield, J. & Crawford, L. (1991) Status of c/myc, p53 and retinoblastoma gene in human papillomavirus positive and negative squamous cell carcinomas of the anus. *Oncogene* **6**,1251.

Daling, J.R., Sherman, K.S., Hislop, T.G. & Madden, C. (1992) Cigarette smoking and the risk of anogenital cancer. *Am J Epidemiol* **135**,180.

Daling, J.R., Weiss, N.S., Hislop, T.G. & Madden, C. (1987) Sexual practices, sexually transmitted disease, and the incidence of anal cancer. *N Engl J Med* **317**,973.

Fraser, L., Medley, G. & McKay, L. (1986) Association between anorectal dysplasia, human papillomavirus, and human immuno-deficiency virus infection in homosexual men. *Lancet* **2**,657.

Goorney, B.D., Waugh, M.A. & Clarke, J. (1987) Anal warts in heterosexual men. *Genitourin Med* **63**,216.

Heino, P., Ecklund, C., Shanazarian, F. & Goldman, S. (1995) Association of serum immunoglobulin G antibodies against human papillomavirus type 16 capsids with anal epidermoid cancer. *J Natl Cancer Inst* **87**,437.

Hoffman, M.S., La Polla, J.P., Roberts, J.S. & Kaufner, D. (1990) Use of local flaps for primary anal reconstruction following perianal resection for neoplasia. *Gynecol Oncol* **36**(3),348.

Holly, E.A., Whittemore, A.S., Aston, D.A. *et al.* (1989) Anal cancer incidence; genital warts, anal fissure or fistula, haemorrhoids, and smoking. *J Natl Cancer Inst* **81**,1726.

McCance, D. & Singer, A. (1986) The importance of HPV infection in the male and female genital tract and their relationship to cervical neoplasia. In: Peto, R. & Zur Hausen, H. (eds) *Viral Etiology of Cervical Cancer*, No. 21 Banbury Report. Cold Spring Harbor Laboratory, New York.

McIndoe, W.A., McLean, M.R., Jones, R.W. & Mullins, P.R. (1984) The invasive potential of carcinoma in situ of the cervix. *Obstet Gynecol* **64**,451.

Melbye, M., Smith, E., Walthard, J.W. *et al.* (1996) Anal and cervical abnormality in women — predilection by human papillomavirus. *Int J Cancer* **68**(5),559.

Palmer, J.G., Scholefield, J.H., Coates, P.J. *et al.* (1989) Anal cancer and human papillomavirus. *Dis Colon Rectum* **32**,1016.

Rutlinger, P., Buchman, R., Grob, F. & Colla, R. (1990) Genito-anal HPV infections in immunodeficient individuals. In: Gross, G., Jablonska, S., Pfister, H. & Stegner, H.E. (eds) *Genital Papilloma-virus Infections*, p. 249. Springer-Verlag, Berlin.

Scholefield, J.H., Hickson, W.G., Smith, J.H., Rogers, K. & Sharpe, F. (1992) Anal intraepithelial neoplasia; part of a multifocal disease process. *Lancet* **340**,1271.

Scholefield, J.H., Sonnex, C., Talbot, I. *et al.* (1989) Anal and cervical intraepithelial neoplasia: possible parallel. *Lancet* **2**,765.

Sherman, M.E., Freedman, H.B., Busseniers, A.E. *et al.* (1995) Cytologic diagnosis of anal intraepithelial neoplasia using smears and Cytyc ThinPreps. *Mod Path* **8**(3),270.

Sonnix, C., Scholefield, J.H., Kocjan, G. *et al.* (1991) Anal human papillomavirus infections in heterosexuals with genital warts; prevalence and relation with sexual behaviour. *Br Med J* **303**,1243.

Surawicz, C.M., Critchlow, C., Sayer, J. *et al.* (1995) High grade anal dysplasia and visually normal mucosa in homosexual men. *Amer J Gastroent* **10**,1776.

Thomas, S.S., Chenoy, R., Feilding, J.W. *et al.* (1996) Vulvo–perineal reconstruction after excision of ano-genital multi-focal intraepethelial neoplasia. *Br J Plast Surg* **49**,539.

Wechsner, S.D., Milsom, J.W. & Dailey, T.H. (1988) The demographics of anal cancer are changing. *Dis Colon Rectum* **30**,942.

Chapter 11
Genital Tract Adenosis

11.1 Developmental anatomy

The development of the vagina and cervix is outlined in Section 4.2 (p. 43). During the intrauterine life of the female fetus, the paired Mullerian paramesonephric ducts arise from the urogenital ridges, extend caudally, and then fuse at the urogenital sinus (Forsberg & Kalland, 1981). This column of cells is replaced by a solid core of squamous epithelium that arises from the vaginal plate. The vaginal plate grows from the urogenital sinus, extends along the paired Mullerian ducts, and develops to form the major part of the vagina and cervix. In the newly born female child, the junction between the glandular Mullerian epithelium and the squamous epithelium extending from the urogenital sinus lies close to the external os of the cervix. The position of the squamocolumnar junction is quite variable.

In the normal young girl, the vagina does not contain any glandular elements, except for occasional remnants that lie in the deep tissues and may form cystic structures (Gartner's duct cysts) at a later date.

From time to time, congenital variations of this development occur and remnants of the columnar epithelium may extend from the cervix onto the upper vagina, usually in an anteroposterior line. Later squamous metaplasia occurs in this area, producing the so-called congenital acetowhite changes (or congenital transformation zone) that are seen in a small number of individuals (Fig. 4.43a&b on p. 64). Approximately 2.5% of women will have a squamocolumnar junction that extends from the cervix onto the vagina (Nwabineli & Monaghan, 1991). Vaginal adenosis is a further variation of this development in that glandular epithelium is present in the vagina; this epithelium is of an endocervical type (Bonney & Glendinning, 1910; Sandberg *et al.*, 1965; Siders *et al.*, 1965; Sandberg, 1968; Stafl *et al.*, 1974; Robboy *et al.*, 1986). It can either be on the surface, replacing the normal squamous epithelium, or occur as mucus-secreting cystic glands and crypts in the dermis. Sandberg (1968) found that 41% of of postpubertal autopsy vaginas (nine out of 22) showed evidence of occult adenosis. No evidence of occult adenosis was found in the remaining 13 prepubertal vaginas examined. All these cases was discovered prior to 1971, when it was recognized for the first time that maternal ingestion of diethylstilbestrol (DES) could lead to the development in female offspring of extensive cervicovaginal adenosis and rarely to adenocarcinoma of the vagina. Herbst and Scully (1970) described seven cases of clear cell adenocarcinomas.

DES was first produced in 1938 and was in clinical use by the mid-1940s. Since 1971, vaginal adenosis has been reported mainly in association with prenatal exposure to DES, but still may occur in women without such exposure. Adenosis found in females born prior to the DES era is similar in type to that found in women exposed to DES.

The widespread use of colposcopy has meant that small areas of surface adenosis have been noted in asymptomatic women who have no history of DES exposure (Stafl *et al.*, 1974). The symptoms, when present, include profuse mucoid vaginal discharge, soreness, and/or postcoital bleeding resulting from the fragile and exposed glandular epithelium. The symptoms can be distressing and lead to concern about malignancy. Vaginal adenosis has already been described in Chapter 8 and illustrated in Fig. 8.25a–f p. 266. Although an uncommon condition, it has been seen by the authors with increasing frequency and in two cases, seen by one of us (AS), it has been associated with pregnancy in which a postpartum hemorrhage necessitated the use of a vaginal pack. In both women, vaginal adenosis developed within 6 months; in one such case it was associated with erosive lichen planus of the vulva and vagina. Lichen planus in association with vaginal adenosis has previously been described by Stabler (1961), Siders *et al.* (1965), Pelisse *et al.* (1982), and Ridley (1999).

Ingestion of DES and its effects on the offspring of women taking it had a profound effect on gynecology, especially in the United States, during the 1970s and 1980s. In the following section, the developmental anomalies caused by this drug will be discussed, and the clinical management will also be considered.

11.2 Developmental anomalies caused by DES

Experimental evidence

In experiments on mice it has been demonstrated that the development of the vagina can be modified by administering estrogens, such as estradiol or DES, to neonatal mice (Forsberg, 1975, 1979). The development of the mouse vagina continues into neonatal life, whereas in the human all these developmental changes occur in the intrauterine period. It has been possible to produce in the mouse model lesions that are similar to human vaginal adenosis. Other characteristics that have been noted in association with maternal ingestion of DES can be generated in the mouse. These include the vaginal and cervical ridges, which are produced by a modification in the production of connective tissue, and the hooding of the cervix, which is produced by the exuberant growth of the epithelium of the vagina. Thus, the role of DES as a teratogen has been confirmed in other species.

It has been shown that at different levels in the female genital tract the stroma can be made to undergo selective proliferation, affecting the morphology of the surrounding tissues (Mattson et al., 1989). Cunha (1976) showed that when cervical stroma was combined with uterine epithelium, cervical differentiation occurred, and when a similar combination was made with vaginal stroma and cervical epithelium, vaginal epithelium developed. Cunha suggested that DES might act on the stroma and this could result in the production of some of the morphologic deformities and epithelial abnormalities of connective tissue that were seen in women exposed to DES. The increased risk of clear cell adenocarcinoma in the offspring of such women, especially those exposed in early pregnancy, may be due to large areas of the ectopic columnar epithelium in the vagina undergoing inductive changes, as described above. For example, Faber et al. (1990) have described a case of invasive squamous carcinoma in the vagina of a DES-exposed patient; this carcinoma arose within "dysplastic vaginal adenosis." However, the mechanisms described above may be only part of an overall malignant process.

Epidemiology

After its synthesis in 1938, DES was used, especially in the late 1940s, to treat patients with habitual abortion, on the understanding that the cause of abortion was a failure by the mother and her placenta to generate adequate levels of estrogen to support the pregnancy (Dieckmann et al., 1953). It was estimated that some two to four million women in the United States were treated with DES to support such worrying pregnancies. In 1970, clear cell adenocarcinoma of the vagina was noted in females aged 14–22 years (Herbst & Scully, 1970; Herbst et al., 1971). A special register was developed and has since been maintained by Dr A.L. Herbst in Boston (Herbst et al., 1977). This register has collected data from almost 400 clear cell adenocarcinomas of the vagina and cervix from around the world. The majority of these cases occurred in the United States, but a wide-ranging geographic pattern showed cases coming from Europe, Central America, Africa, and Asia (Melnick et al., 1987). The youngest diethylstilbestrol-exposed patient to develop clear cell carcinoma was 7 years old, and a personal communication (1992) with Dr Herbst has reported a 45-year-old patient developing the disease.

Clear cell adenocarcinoma of the cervix and vagina is a rare cancer but there has been a marked increase in reports of its incidence in recent years, not only associated with DES but also in untreated patients. The natural history of these tumors is becoming better understood with the collation of figures from the Boston registry. These tumors are extremely rare in females under 14 years old; there then seems to be a rapid rise in the age–incidence curve to an irregular plateau with peak incidence rates around age 22. After this age, there seems to be a sharp decline in incidence. It is now obvious that these tumors are uncommon even in those females who have definitely been exposed to DES. It has been calculated that the risk of a clear cell adenocarcinoma developing in exposed women between birth and age 34 years is approximately one case per thousand (Melnick et al., 1987). It has been extremely difficult to calculate the rate for females in their mid-twenties and older because only a small number of cases have been reported. However, it would seem that there is a life-long risk, because before the DES problem arose it was obvious that clear cell adenocarcinoma of both vagina and cervix was a disease of older women, and it may be that younger women who are at present free of malignancies, could develop them at a later date.

Clinical findings

Following maternal ingestion of DES, the development of the fetal female genital tract is modified so that Mullerian columnar epithelium persists in the vagina, the fornices, and on the cervix. It appears that it is necessary for the fetus to be exposed to DES during the first 20 weeks of gestation for these abnormalities to develop. If DES treatment is begun after 20 weeks, the risks of generating the stigmata of DES changes are minimized. Figure 11.1 shows the characteristic features of an exuberant vaginal epithelium with a wide area of columnar epithelium present on the ectocervix (1). Figures 11.2 and 11.3 show the characteristic hooding surrounding a cervix that is entirely covered by persistent columnar epithelium; in Fig. 11.4, squamous metaplasia (1) replaces the columnar epithelium; some hypertrophied endocervical columnar epithelium exists at (2). Figure 11.5 shows the columnar epithelium (2) extending onto the anterior lip, generating a characteristic cockscomb pattern. Squamous metaplasia has occurred in areas (1). Although most patients will develop stigmata associated with the

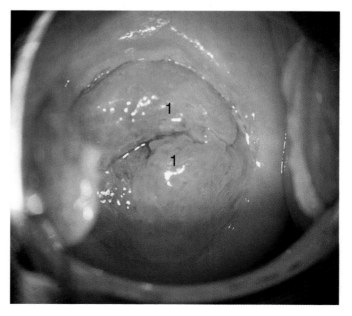

Fig. 11.1

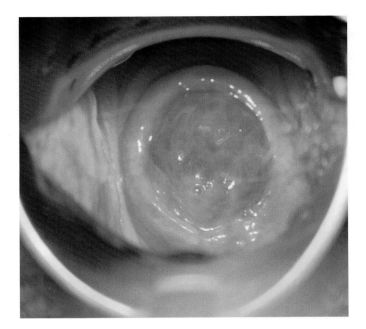

Fig. 11.2

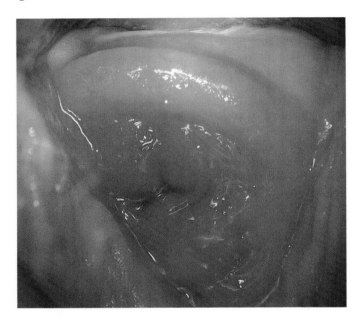

Fig. 11.3

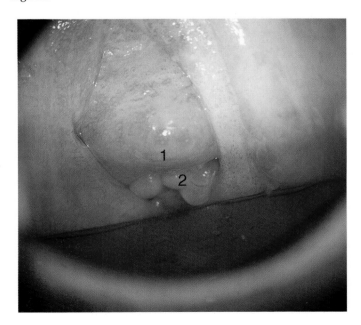

Fig. 11.4

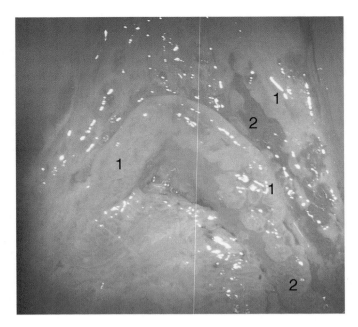

Fig. 11.5

cervix and upper vagina from time to time, patchy persistent columnar epithelium will be seen in other parts of the cervix and vagina. These patchy areas require careful monitoring.

If there is any doubt about the nature of these lesions, a wide local excision should be undertaken and the material submitted for careful histologic assessment. The risk of development of clear cell cancer of the cervix or vagina in the patient exposed to DES is markedly increased if exposure occurred during early pregnancy (i.e. before 63 days); the risk beyond 63 days is nil (Herbst *et al.*, 1977, 1979). There is also a marked increase in risk if the child is born in the autumn and if the mother has had prior spontaneous abortions. Not all fetuses will demonstrate stigmata, and the risks of development are as given above.

The characteristic appearance of the clear cell carcinoma will be either hypertrophic, as shown on the anterior cervical lip (cervical hood) in Fig. 11.6, or of an invading ulcer in the vagina or cervix (Fig. 11.7). The most common site of occurrence is in the posterior vaginal fornix. The lesion is commonly diagnosed as an incidental finding at the time of assessment of the cervix. Indeed, in the first case noted by the author (JM) in Great Britain (Monaghan & Sirisena, 1978), the lesion was covered by the speculum during the first examination but was noted at the second examination. The cancer was lying a short distance above a transverse vaginal ridge, which is a common characteristic of DES exposure. Another interesting case that presented in Great Britain was of clear cell carcinoma in a patient who had not been exposed to DES, but who had a double cervix and uterus with a septum in the vagina (Fig. 11.7). This patient developed a clear cell carcinoma in the vagina with intraepithelial neoplastic (CIN) changes in the alternate cervix. The corresponding cervicovaginal cytologic smear is shown in Fig. 11.8; some clear cell adenocarcinoma cells can be seen.

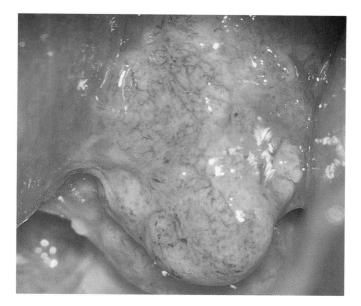

Fig. 11.6

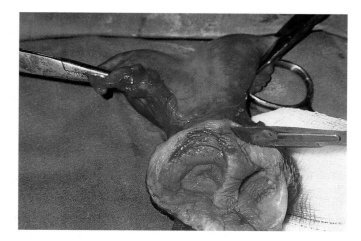

Fig. 11.7

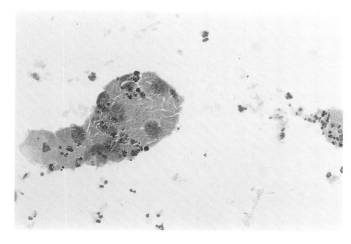

Fig. 11.8

Pathology

The characteristic histologic appearances of clear cell carcinoma are very obvious. Figures 11.9 and 11.10 show the typical hobnail clear cell carcinoma with wide open spaces. These histologic types are characterized in three groups (Scully *et al.*, 1978).

1 A tubulocystic pattern, as shown in Fig. 11.9 and the corresponding high-power morphology in Fig. 11.10.

2 The second most common pattern is of a solid tumor that contains sheets or masses of neoplastic cells with clear spaces between; these represent glycogen dissolved during the tissue processing.

3 The least frequent pattern is a papillary one with numerous papillary processes occurring within cysts or tubules.

Treatment

The treatment of clear cell adenocarcinoma is very much as for cancer of the cervix and vagina; the staging is also very similar. Survival is best among those patients who have been radically treated, either by surgery or by radiation. Attempts to practice conservative therapy have not been so successful, owing to the fact that recurrence after local therapy is much more frequent. As with carcinoma of the cervix, the 5-year survival rate of patients with a stage 1

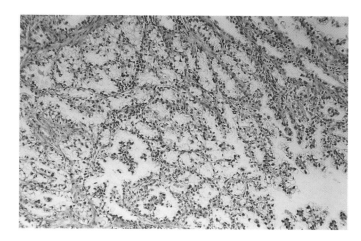

Fig. 11.9

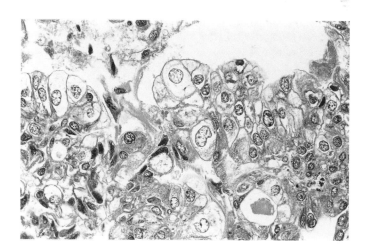

Fig. 11.10

tumor is approximately 90%; this declines to no survival in patients who have stage 4 disease. A small number of cases have been identified during a pregnancy; however, this does not appear to influence adversely the characteristics or prognosis of the disease. Similarly, no association has been found between oral contraceptive use and the development or prognosis of this disease.

There has been considerable discussion about the risk to patients with cervical vaginal adenosis of developing CIN when the columnar epithelium undergoes metaplasia. In the United States, the national collaborative diethylstilbestrol adenosis (DESAD) project was initiated, and in 1983 Noller *et al.* reported that in a series of 1580 women, there did not appear to be a substantially different risk from that of a matched cohort of unexposed women.

In 1984, Robboy *et al.* reported a further extension of the DESAD project, and concluded that in the study group the incidence of CIN, as diagnosed by biopsy or cytologic testing, was significantly increased in DES-exposed women. However, since this paper has been published no other significant studies have confirmed these findings and it must be considered that, at present, there is no conclusive evidence for an increase in the incidence of CIN within this group. This study group is now at an age where an excess amount of CIN would be evident, but this does not seem to be the case.

11.3 References

Bonney, V. & Glendinning, B. (1910) Adenomatosis vaginae: a hitherto undescribed condition. *Proc R Soc Med* **4**,18.

Cunha, G.R. (1976) Stromal induction and specification of morphogenesis and cytodifferentiation of the epithelia of the Mullerian duct and urogenital sinus during development of the uterus and vagina in mice. *J Exp Zool* **196**,361.

Dieckmann, W.J., Davis, M.D., Rynkiewiez, L.M. & Pottinger, R.E. (1953) Does administration of diethylstilbestrol during pregnancy have therapeutic value? *Am J Obstet Gynecol* **66**,1062.

Faber, K., Jones, M. & Terraza, H.M. (1990) Invasive squamous cell carcinoma of the vagina in a diethyl stilboestrol-exposed woman. *Gynecol Oncol* **37**(1),125.

Forsberg, J.G. (1975) Late effects in the vaginal and cervical epithelia after injections of diethyl stilboestrol into neonatal mice. *Am J Obstet Gynecol* **121**,101.

Forsberg, J.G. (1979) Developmental mechanisms of oestrogen-induced irreversible changes in the mouse cervico-vaginal epithelium. *Natl Cancer Inst Monogr* **54**,41.

Forsberg, J.G. & Kalland, T. (1981) Embryology of the genital tract in humans and rodents. In: Herbst, A.L. & Byrne, H.A. (eds) *Developmental Effects of Diethyl Stilboestrol (DES) in Pregnancy.* Thieme-Stratton, New York.

Herbst, A.L. & Scully, R.E. (1970) Adenocarcinoma of the vagina in adolescents. Report of seven cases including six clear cell adenocarcinomas (so-called mesonephromas). *Cancer* **25**,745.

Herbst, A.L., Cole, P., Colton, T., Robboy, S. & Scully, R.E. (1977) Age incidence and risk of diethylstilbestrol-related clear cell adenocarcinomas of the vagina and cervix. *Am J Obstet Gynecol* **128**,43.

Herbst, A.L., Cole, P., Norusis, M.J., Welsh, W.R. & Scully, R.E. (1979) Epidemiological aspects and factors related to survival of 384 cases of clear cell adenocarcinoma of the vagina and cervix. *Am J Obstet Gynecol* **135**,876.

Herbst, A., Ulfeder, H. & Poskanzer, D. (1971) Adenocarcinoma of the vagina: association of maternal stilbestrol therapy with tumor appearance in young women. *N Engl J Med* **284**,878.

Mattsson, L., Cullberg, G., Eriksson, O. & Knutsson, F. (1989) Vaginal administration of low-dose oestradiol effects on the endometrium and vaginal cytology. *Maturitas* **11**,217.

Melnick, S., Cole, P., Anderson, D. & Herbst, A.L. (1987) Rates and risks of diethylstilbestrol-related clear cell adenocarcinoma of the vagina and cervix. *N Engl J Med* **316**,514.

Monaghan, J. & Sirisena, L.A.W. (1978) Stilboestrol and vaginal clear cell adenocarcinoma. *Br Med J* **1**,1588.

Noller, K., Townsend, M., Kaufman, R. *et al.* (1983) Maturation of vaginal and cervical epithelium in women exposed to diethylstilbestrol (DESAD project). *Am J Obstet Gynecol* **146**,279.

Nwabineli, N.J. & Monaghan, J.M. (1991) Vaginal epithelial abnormalities in patients with CIN; clinical and pathological features and management. *Br J Obstet Gynaecol* **98**(1),25.

Pelisse, M., Hewitt, J. & Leibowitch, M. (1982) Le syndrome vulvo–vagino–gingival lichen plan erosif plurimuqueux. *Ann Dermatol Vénéreol* **110**,953.

Ridley, C.M. & Neill, S.M. (eds) (1999) *The Vulva*, p. 164. Blackwell Science, Oxford.

Robboy, S., Hill, E., Sandbeg, E. & Czernoblisky, B. (1986) Vaginal adenosis in women born prior to the diethylstilbestrol era. *Hum Pathol* **17**(5),488.

Robboy, S.J., Noller, K.L., O'Brien, P. *et al.* (1984). Increased incidence of cervical and vaginal dysplasia in 3980 diethylstilbestrol exposed young women; experience of the National Collaborative DES Adenosis project. *J Am Med Assoc* **252**,2979.

Sandberg, E. (1968) Incidence and distribution of occult vaginal adenosis. *Am J Obstet Gynecol* **101**,333.

Sandberg, E., Danielson, R., Cauwet, R. & Bonar, B. (1965) Adenosis vaginae. *Am J Obstet Gynecol* **93**,209.

Scully, R.E., Robboy, S.J. & Welch, W.R. (1978) Pathology and pathogenesis in diethylstilboestrol related disorders of the female genital tract. In: Herbst, A.L. (ed.) *Intrauterine Exposure to Diethylstilboestrol in the Human.* American College of Obstetrics and Gynecology, Chicago.

Siders, D., Parrot, M. & Abell, M. (1965) Gland cell prosplasia (adenosis) of the vagina. *Am J Obstet Gynecol* **91**,191.

Stabler, F. (1961) Adenomatosis vaginae. *J Obstet Gynaecol Br Commonw* **68**,857.

Stafl, A., Mattingley, R., Foley, D. & Fetherston, W. (1974) Clinical diagnosis of vaginal adenosis. *Obstet Gynecol* **43**,1.

Chapter 12
Infective and Other Conditions Causing Confusion in Diagnosis of Lower Genital Tract Precancer

12.1 Introduction

There are many infective and other conditions that cause confusion in the diagnosis of genital tract precancer and cancer. The infective conditions can be of either a protozoan, fungal, or bacterial nature, and they cause widespread inflammation to the genital tract. Viral infections, especially by human papillomavirus (HPV), have already been discussed in detail, but it is important to recognize that they, in common with other infective agents, may well present diagnostic difficulties. The development of polypoid lesions and of the specific condition of cervical vaginal adenosis in pregnancy also cause problems, and all these will be considered in the following sections.

12.2 *Trichomonas vaginalis*

This common protozoan infection is not infrequently identified in cervical smears. The characteristic appearance (Fig. 12.1) is of a small, blue–gray, ill-defined body with an elongated nucleus (arrowed).

It is important to differentiate the trichomonas from mucus and other cell debris on the smear. Although the trichomonas protozoan is easily seen on a Papanicolaou stained slide, it is probably best identified using a wet stain preparation where the active trichomonas can be easily seen. This is the most reliable method of diagnosis. Some women may be carriers of the disease and under these circumstances there is no active infection. The clinical and colposcopic appearances of the cervix are shown in Fig. 12.2,

where the characteristic strawberry patches can be seen. These strawberry patches (1) of cervicitis or vaginitis are characterized by a multitude of tiny red dots, each of which is the tip of a subepithelial capillary that reaches almost to the surface. In the worst cases, the infection is so intense that even minor trauma, such as taking a smear, produces intense bleeding. It is important that when a cervix is infected with trichomonas, lesions such as cervical intraepithelial neoplasia (CIN) should not be treated until the infection has been cleared, because gross bleeding can occur at this time. The infection is best treated using metronidazole. From time to time a male may be found to be a carrier, and in such cases it is important to deal with both partners. Usually one short course of medication will deal with the problem, though persistent change of partners will often result in reinfection. It is a condition that may be transmitted by other than sexual contact.

Figure 12.3 illustrates a difficulty that can occur when a naked-eye examination is made of the cervix and severe trichomonal cervicitis exists. Examination with the naked eye reveals a bleeding cervix that could be misinterpreted as bearing early invasive carcinoma. However, a colposcopic examination reveals the small, multiple subepithelial capillaries that have produced the generalized bleeding across the ectocervix. There is no evidence of invasive cancer.

12.3 Candidiasis

Candidiasis is the result of an overgrowth of the naturally occurring *Candida albicans* that is present in the human

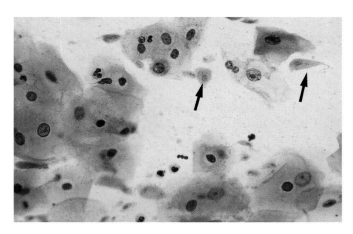

Fig. 12.1

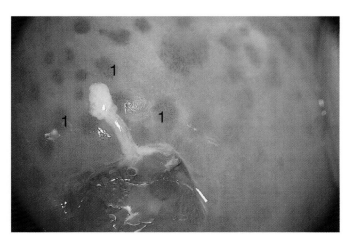

Fig. 12.2

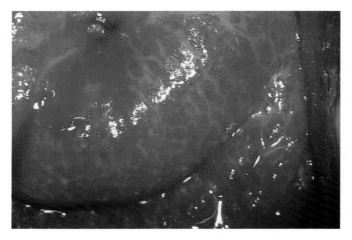

Fig. 12.3

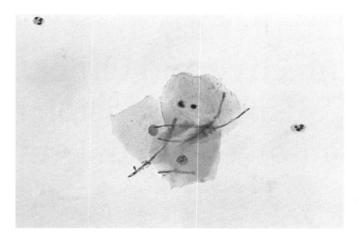

Fig. 12.4

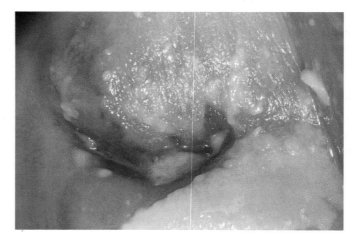

Fig. 12.5

bowel and frequently exists in the vagina. The condition tends to develop when there has been a change in the milieu or environment of the vagina. It is common in pregnancy, in association with diabetes mellitus, and following the taking of antibiotic drugs that kill the natural bacteria in the vagina that normally render the vaginal epithelium acidic. The spores and hyphae of *Candida albicans* can be easily seen as thin red lines in cervical smears (Fig. 12.4). The hyphae may occasionally be colorless or pale blue, but are more commonly orange or red. The candida produces an intense inflammatory response, and the epithelium of the cervix and vagina becomes thickened and covered with a creamy, curdy, white discharge (Fig. 12.5). This must be differentiated from changes of leukoplakia or early malignancy on the cervix and vagina, and is best demonstrated by wiping away the lesions with a swab stick. If doubt exists, then saline should be used to wash the surface, after which a colposcopic examination will reveal a normal epithelial surface.

Treatment of the condition is by the use of local agents, such as nystatin or clotrimazole in the form of a pessary or cream, or a systemic agent, such as fluconazole (150 mg taken orally). These agents will commonly remove the infection completely. Again, male partners should be treated. The condition is not uncommon among males, particularly those who have not been circumcised.

12.4 Herpes genitalis infection

Clinical presentations

Herpes genitalis is caused by infection with the herpes simplex virus type 2 (HSV 2). The disease is characterized by painful ulcers on the vulva and lower vagina, but when the lesion affects the cervix the infection is usually painless and is only found upon examination or colposcopy. When a patient presents with vulvar or lower vaginal herpes, it is important to make a simultaneous and careful assessment of the cervix, and to advise about the high risk of transference of the virus to sexual partners. In the pregnant patient there is also a significant risk of transfer of the virus to the fetus during vaginal delivery. This risk is markedly

increased during the patient's first infection with the virus but it would appear that with subsequent infections the risk is markedly reduced. In extreme cases of very active upper vaginal and cervical infection, it is recommended that a Cesarean section should be carried out.

Herpes simplex cytology

The cytologic appearance of HSV infection is easily recognized. Figure 12.6a shows the cytologic changes where the cells are characterized by large multiple nuclei that are molded together (arrowed) and show margination of chromatic and generally empty nuclei. Large intranuclear inclusions are also commonly seen. It is important to differentiate such cells from the binucleate cells that are commonly found in association with HPV infection, and from the bizarre appearances that may be associated with an invasive carcinoma and that are commonly generated following radiotherapeutic treatment of the cervix.

The cytologic changes of early infection are characterized by large intranuclear inclusions, and as the infection progresses, a nonspecific acute necrotizing cervicitis develops; this is represented cytologically by the appearance of degenerate and necrotic cells in which the ghosts of the nuclei can just be recognized. These necrotic cellular appearances have to be differentiated from those that are sometimes associated with clinical invasive squamous cell carcinoma or, indeed, occasionally with the intraepithelial stages of disease.

Colposcopic and histologic appearances of infection

The epithelial changes that occur with herpetic infection can all be recognized colposcopically; indeed, the early stages are best studied with the magnified illumination provided by colposcopy. The infection starts in the parabasal cells of the squamous epithelium; there is nuclear enlargement and the development of multinucleate cells, as described above. Vesicle formations and ulceration follows within approximately 36 hours, by which time a histologic examination of the vesicles (12.6b) shows them to be composed of giant cells at the edge (1) and in the base; polymorphonuclear leukocytes (2) are present in the surrounding epithelium. There may also be some basal cell hyperplasia present in the surrounding epithelium. Figures 12.6c & d show the colposcopic changes of this early infection with vesicles (arrowed) and epithelial "congestion" (1) caused by cellular infiltration that occurs just before ulceration. The ulceration (Fig. 12.6e) is usually associated with some secondary infection and this then leads to the nonspecific acute necrotizing cervicitis, as shown in Fig. 12.7. Not sur-

prisingly, the stroma is infiltrated with a very dense collection of acute and chronic inflammatory cells that permeate the granulation tissue at the base of the ulcer. The acute inflammatory changes surround the ulcer and generate a marked increase in blood supply; minor trauma to the ulcer commonly produces significant bleeding. The tiny vesicles seen in the initial infection do not last as long on the cervix as on the vulva (1) (Fig. 12.8), and they rapidly coalesce, producing the appearance of a single herpetic ulcer.

Again, it is important to differentiate this appearance from that of an invasive carcinoma, and at times of doubt it may be necessary, although it is generally not advised, to take a biopsy in order to confirm or refute the diagnosis of invasion. Usually, observation of the lesion over a period of 10 to 14 days will show the healing changes that occur during this time. It is normally advised not to actively treat the lesions, and although Zovirax (acyclovir) has been used, it is not so simple to apply to cervical as to vulvar or other lesions, and the results have not been consistent. The

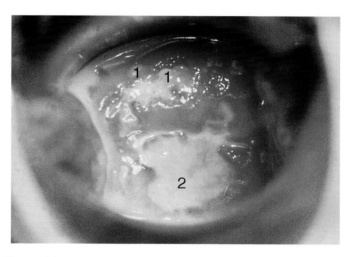

Fig. 12.6(c)

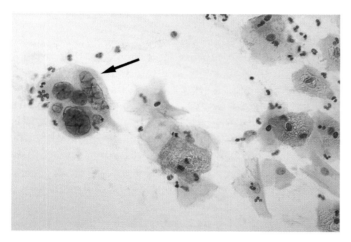

Fig. 12.6(a)

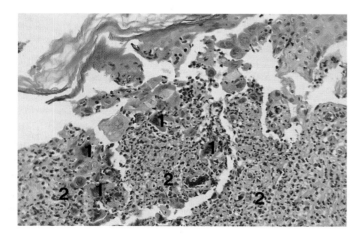

Fig. 12.6(b)

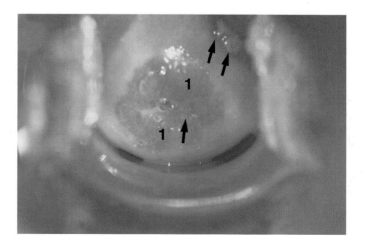

Fig. 12.6(d)

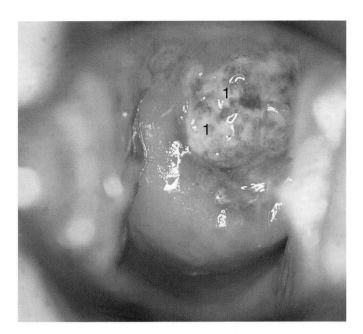

Fig. 12.6(e)

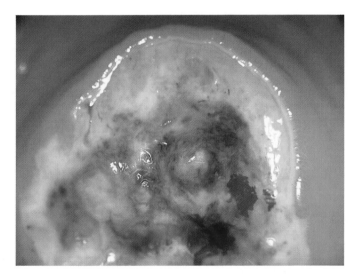

Fig. 12.7

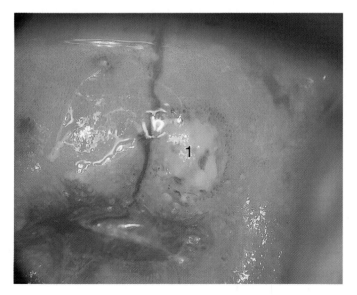

Fig. 12.8

ulcer heals spontaneously and with minimal residual damage to the cervix, as shown in Fig. 12.8 where the healed ulcer is seen at (1).

Besides HSV, another cause of necrotizing ulceration is retention of foreign materials, such as tampons and other foreign bodies, in the vagina. Usually, local cleansing will see a rapid healing of such lesions but, once more, differentiation of these lesions from invasive ulcerating carcinomas must be made. Traumatic ulceration and the healing following cervical treatment and biopsy may also give a similar appearance, but can usually be excluded by the history.

Vulvar lesions

The vulvar lesions caused by herpes can be exquisitely painful and tender (Fig. 12.9a & b). The multiple shallow ulcers that coalesce (Fig. 12.9b) and develop serpiginous red borders and pale yellow centers are classic of vulvar herpes. Extensive involvement with secondary labial edema and tender inguinal lymph glands are associated with this primary lesion. Sometimes there may be less symptomatic lesions that appear more localized (Fig. 12.10) and these are frequently seen in recurrent attacks.

The initial stages of the attack are characterized by a prodromal illness that includes malaise, fever, and swelling of the inguinal lymph glands. The vulvar lesions are characterized by small vesicles (1), as can be seen in Fig. 12.9a. These vesicles very quickly enlarge and become surrounded by an erythematous skin reaction (Fig. 12.11). They subsequently rupture and develop into shallow ulcerative lesions that are multiple, painful, and typical of the next stage. Some ulcers within the urethra, or those that are within the vestibule, may cause much distress and even lead to urinary retention. The insertion of a suprapubic catheter in these women is mandatory. The cervix and vagina are also involved in over 50% of cases in which vulvar ulcers are seen, and owing to the lack of free nerve endings in these areas, the condition may be asymptomatic.

Differentiation from malignant disease of the vulva can sometimes be difficult to determine. A single large atypical lesion may have the appearance of an early squamous cell carcinoma. Other conditions, such as secondary syphilis and Behçet's disease, should also be considered (cf. Figs 9.49 & 9.50a on p. 263).

Diagnosis is helped by obtaining smears from the ulcers; Papanicolaou staining will show the characteristic large multinucleate cells. Some will also show emargination of the chromatin and empty nuclei. Viral culture and serologic tests will also be helpful. Indeed, isolation of the virus by culture and smears is most accurate during the first 3 days of infection. When the condition is seen later with the established ulcer, negative results do not rule out herpes and it may be necessary to wait for a further episode before final confirmation can be obtained. At this stage, serologic tests will be helpful. As herpes is a very common sexually transmitted infection, other associated infections, such as syphilis and gonorrhea, must be excluded.

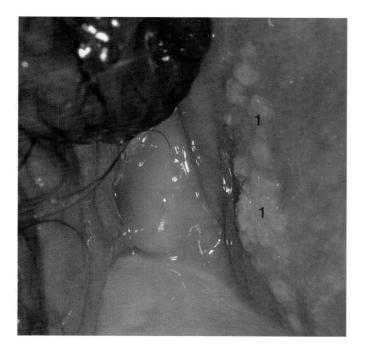

Fig. 12.9(a)

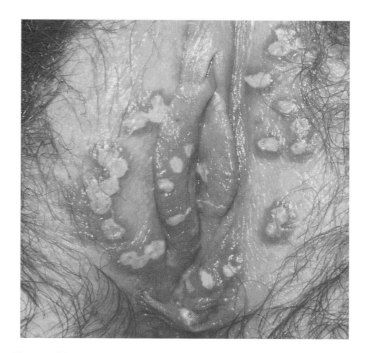

Fig. 12.9(b)

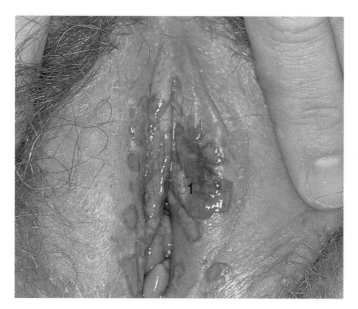

Fig. 12.10

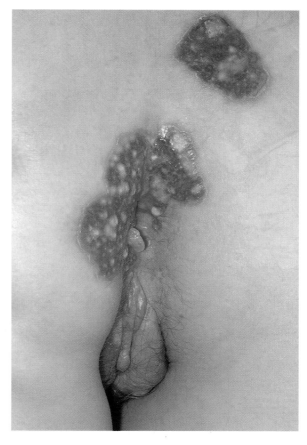

Fig. 12.11

12.5 HPV infection

HPV infection of the cervix has been discussed in detail in Chapters 2 and 6. The virus produces two types of lesion on the cervix. One is condyloma acuminata and the flat lesion that has been described as a flat wart, and the other is the noncondylomatous infection or subclinical papillomavirus infection (SPI) that can only be recognized after acetic acid application and colposcopic visualization.

Condylomata that are exophytic may be obvious to the naked eye and are usually soft pink or white, extremely vascular, and have multiple fine fingerlike projections on the surface. They involve a large area of the genital tract and when seen on the vulva are associated in about 10% of cases with coexistent cervical condyloma. Patients with this

condition are also at risk from cervical intraepithelial disease. The appearances of the condylomata are quite classic, and in Fig. 12.12 the prolific coral-like changes are shown with multiple small condyloma acuminata of the cervix. Each protuberance is a small condyloma with a central capillary. The cytologic changes, which are readily revealed by Papanicolaou staining, show the characteristic koilocyte [(1) in Fig. 12.13a]. There is nuclear enlargement, some hyperchromasia, binucleation and clearing or "cavitation" of the central part of the cell. This produces the characteristic koilocytotic appearance. The nuclear changes are indistinguishable from so-called mild dyskaryosis.

Figure 12.13(b) shows a separate field where a raft of parakeratosis (1) is present in the smear. These keratinized cells are seen in a variety of conformations and most frequently are associated with wart virus changes and low-grade lesions. Other features of HPV infection are multinucleation, dyskeratosis (individual cell keratinization) and orthokeratosis which manifests itself in smears as anucleate squamous sheets.

Figure 12.14 shows a lesion that was extremely hyperkeratotic and could have been confused with early malignancy. Even though there were no abnormal vessels or associated inflammation, the diagnosis was confirmed only after multiple biopsies had been taken. This lesion should also be differentiated from the rare condylomatous carcinoma that is an invasive squamous cell carcinoma integrated with a condyloma acuminata. Similar lesions can be found in the vulva, where they are often multifocal; these tend to occur in immunocompromised patients. In a study by Downy *et al.* (1988) of such vulvar lesions, HPV 6 and 16 were identified in two out of nine cases, while HPV 2 and HPV-related sequences were found in one lesion. This pattern resembles the situation in squamous cell carcinoma of the vulva.

Subclinical condylomatous lesions of the vagina may sometimes be confused with intraepithelial disease in that region, as discussed in Chapter 8. Obvious condylomatous lesions (Fig. 12.15) may be present not only on the cervix but also extensively in the upper vagina. Colposcopy must be performed on such patients to exclude the associated existence of intraepithelial disease of the cervix or vagina. An earlier stage of development is shown by the subclinical lesions present in Fig. 12.16; the subclinical lesions can be clearly seen on the ectocervix (1) and there is a mixture

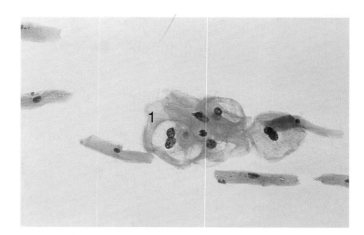

Fig. 12.13(a)

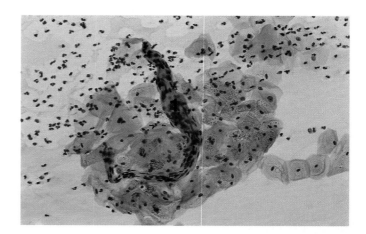

Fig. 12.13(b)

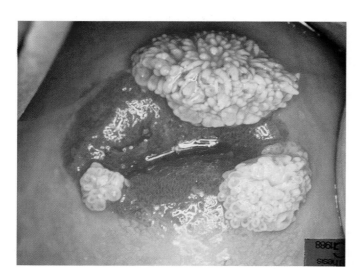

Fig. 12.12

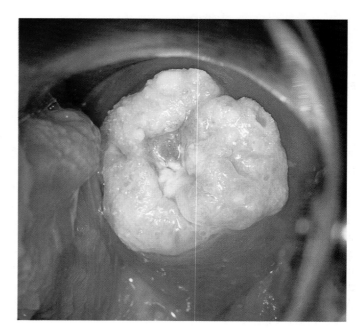

Fig. 12.14

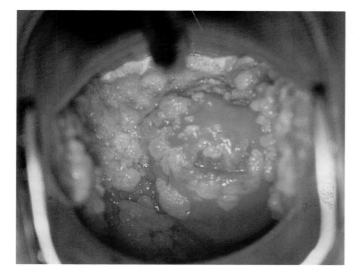

Fig. 12.15

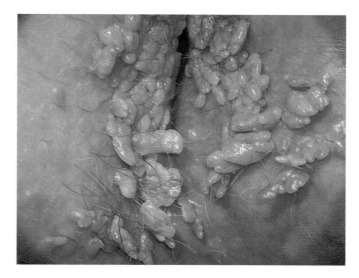

Fig. 12.17

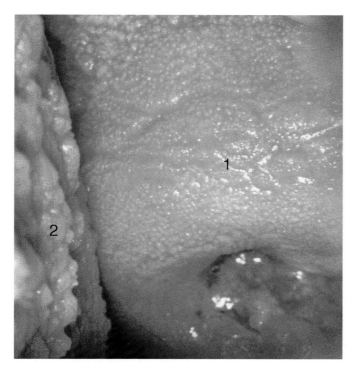

Fig. 12.16

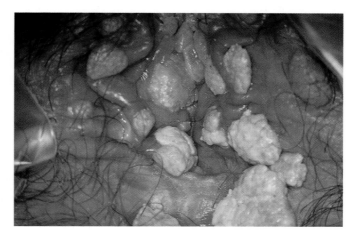

Fig. 12.18(a)

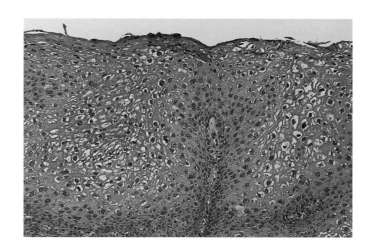

Fig. 12.18(b)

of clinical and subclinical condylomata on the vaginal wall (2) (see also Fig. 2.10, p. 19).

In Figs 12.17 and 12.18a, two types of condylomatous lesion are shown; it is important in cases with such extensive disease to inspect not only the anal canal but also the vagina and particularly the cervix. As has been pointed out before, HPV infections are associated with CIN and it is well known that vulvar warts may precede or accompany the Bowenoid type of vulvar intraepithelial neoplasia (VIN), or even invasive cancer (Shafeek et al., 1979; Wade et al., 1979). Figure 12.18b shows the characteristic histologic pattern of condyloma; the epithelium contains multi-

ple koilocytes with slightly enlarged and irregular nuclei, some exhibiting active mitosis and others demonstrating hyperkeratosis or individual cell keratinization. It is important to differentiate this histologic lesion from CIN, which it can mimic.

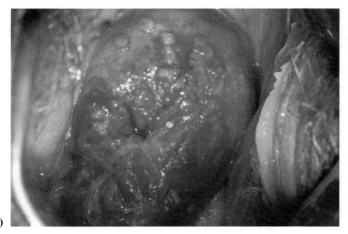

Fig. 12.19(a)

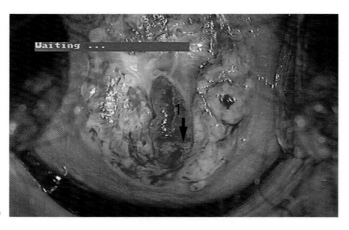

Fig. 12.19(b)

Fig. 12.19 (a) Deciduosis at 20 weeks gestation. Large areas of edematous columnar epithelium are mixed with regions of squamous metaplasia.

(b) This shows the striking elevated, often bizarre changes associated with decidualisation caused by pregnancy. An incidental finding of an endocervical polyp is seen at (1) with metaplasia apparent at its tip (arrowed). This is consistent with the most distal portion of the polyp having been exposed to the vaginal pH before pregnancy, but with the eversion of the cervical os that occurs in pregnancy, the remainder of the polyp has been exposed. The columnar tissue on its surface will eventually undergo metaplasia.

12.6 Cervical deciduosis in pregnancy

Sometimes, colposcopic examination of a patient during pregnancy will reveal gross cervical changes that may be misinterpreted as early invasive carcinoma. They are caused by hypertrophy and hyperplasia of the cervical glandular tissue. Obviously, in a diethylstilbestrol (DES)-exposed individual, the increased amounts of glandular tissue on the ectocervix will also undergo hypertrophy, leading to possible confusion with malignancy.

The uncommon condition of cervical deciduosis also has appearances which may be very suspicious of malignancy, such as those shown in Figs 12.19–12.21 in which areas of edematous epithelial elevations are visible on the ecto-cervix. High-power views of such lesions show the markedly bizarre changes that can present in this condition. These lesions bear a striking similarity to the early-stage adenocarcinomas described in Chapter 6. If the

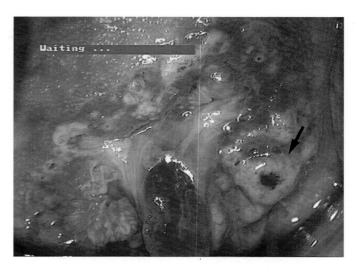

Fig. 12.20 This is a high magnification view of that seen in Fig. 12.19b. The gland openings often become large and prominent, giving the appearance of a raised lesion with a central dimple or depression (arrowed), that is characteristic of deciduosis.

clinician is uncertain of this diagnosis, a biopsy is indicated. The usual great care must be taken not to generate hemorrhage in the pregnant cervix.

Figure 12.22 shows the characteristic cytologic changes of cervical deciduosis in pregnancy; there are edematous superficial squames that are essentially normal but contain considerable amounts of fluid. The characteristic histologic changes can be seen in Fig. 12.23 under low-power magnification and in Fig. 12.24 under high-power magnification; widely expanded cells underlie a superficial single layer of cuboidal cells that are present on the upper surface of these elevated protrusions. The lesion is entirely benign and no action need be taken.

12.7 Polypoid lesions of the cervix

As with all glandular epithelium, the endocervix has a tendency to generate polypoid lesions. These are caused by expansion of the cervical glands, the surfaces of which become blocked, and the epithelium expands to cover the increase in discharge that collects beneath the surface. These expansions may manifest themselves initially as small focal spots on the cervix (Nabothian follicles), but in certain circumstances, particularly just within the endo-cervix, these small mucous cysts become polypoid, elongated, and develop into mucous polyps of the cervix. As can be seen in Figs 12.25–12.27, some polyps are quite prolonged and have a long stalk. Such a polyp is shown in Fig. 12.26, whereas others are rather more sessile (Fig. 12.27) and are clearly associated with expanding mucous glands beneath the surface. From time to time, the stroma of the polyp may increase so that the mucous element is markedly reduced.

Clinical presentation and management

Most polyps are found incidentally during a cervical smear

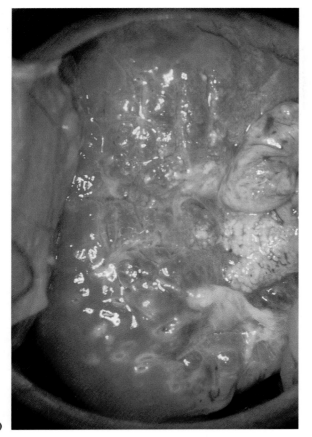

Fig. 12.21(a)

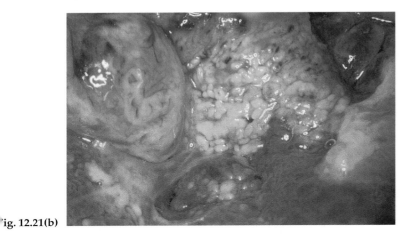

ig. 12.21(b)

Fig. 12.21 (a & b) (*High power*) Typical deciduosis at 14 weeks gestation. Edematous epithelium, both squamous and columnar, are seen.

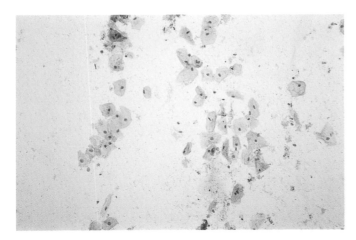

Fig. 12.22

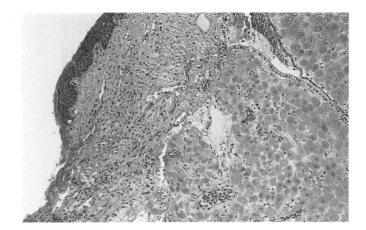

Fig. 12.23

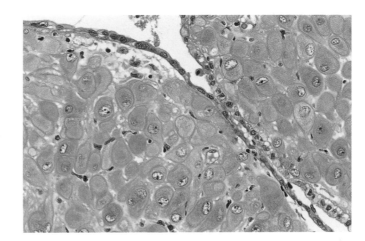

Fig. 12.24

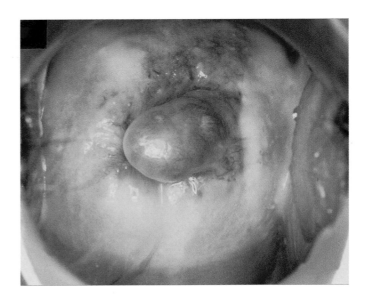

Fig. 12.25

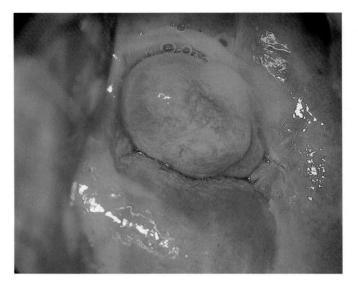

Fig. 12.26

examination. If the polyp is tiny and asymptomatic, no further action is necessary, but many patients feel uncomfortable knowing that they have an abnormality on the cervix; simple removal and a histopathologic examination of the polyp often solves the problem completely. However, all other polypoid lesions must be removed and analyzed histologically. Many bear a resemblance to malignancy and this must be excluded.

Polyps have been noted to occur frequently following treatment of the cervix with laser or loop diathermy; a button of columnar epithelium becomes polypoid in the base of the treated area. Figures 12.28 and 12.29 show cases where women had been treated by laser (Fig. 12.28) or loop diathermy (Fig. 12.29) within the preceding 2 years.

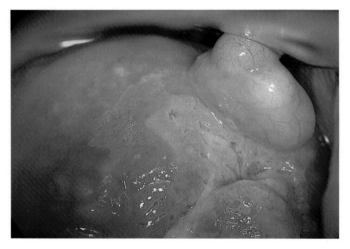

Fig. 12.27

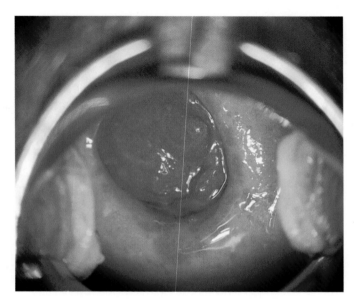

Fig. 12.29

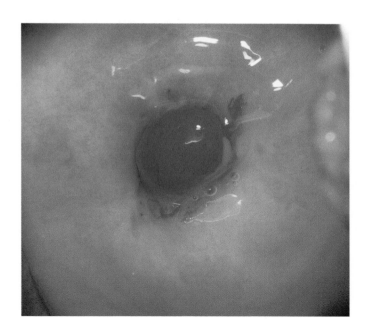

Fig. 12.28

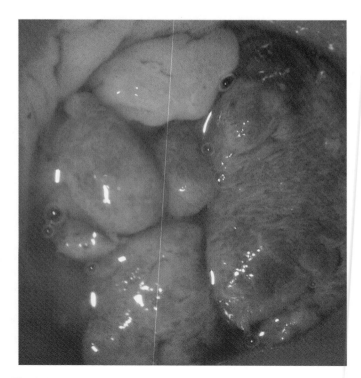

Fig. 12.30

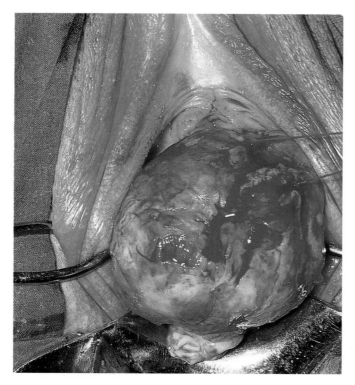

Fig. 12.31

From time to time, polyps may be multiple and become quite large, such as those shown in Figs 12.30 and 12.31. In these instances endocervical adenocarcinoma must be excluded by excision biopsy, usually with the patient under general anesthetic. A hysteroscopic examination of the uterine cavity should be performed. In Fig. 12.30, there were present not only extensive endocervical polyps but large endometrial polyps. In Fig. 12.31, a large endometrial fibroid polyp has presented at the cervix, and been removed *per vaginum*.

12.8 References

Downy, G.O., Okpagaki, T., Ostrow, R.S. *et al.* (1988) Condylomatous carcinoma of the vulva with special reference to human papillomavirus DNA. *Obstet Gynecol* **72**,68.

Shafeek, M.A., Osman, M.I. & Hussain, M.A. (1979) Carcinoma of the vulva arising in condylomata acuminata. *Obstet Gynecol* **52**,120.

Wade, T.R., Kopf, A.W. & Ackerman, A.B. (1979) Bowenoid papulosis of the genitalia. *Arch Dermatol* **115**,306.

Index

cervical cancer mortality, 84
    impact of screening, 84–5
cervical cancer screening, 84–94
    accuracy, 85
    adjunctive tests, 85, 88–92
    automation, 86–7
    cervicography, 89–90, 90
    cytology accuracy improvement, 85–6
    cytology interpretation, 86
    cytotechnician proficiency, 86
    effectiveness, 84–5
    fluorescence spectroscopy, 91–2
    historical background, 84
    HPV-DNA testing, 88–9, 89
        triage schemes, 88–9
    postmenopausal women, 92–4
    speculoscopy, 91
    TruScan* (PolarProbe), 90–1, 91
    visual inspection-based techniques, 91
cervical deciduosis in pregnancy, 312–3, 312
cervical early invasive cancer, 203–4
    adenocarcinoma, 8–9, 10
    adenosquamous differentiation, 8, 10
    atypical vessels, 105–7, 107–8, 141–2, 143
    colposcopic diagnosis, 141–7, 142–3, 145–6
    confluence, 205
    definition, 7–9
    depth of invasion, 10, 204–5
    diagnostic loop diathermy excision, 187
    FIGO staging, 203–4, **204**
    fungating/ulcerated lesions, 10
    histologic features, 7–8, 8, 204
    lymphovascular space involvement, 8, 8,
        204–5
    management, 203–9
        cone biopsy, 205, 209
        conservative treatment methods, 206
        hysterectomy, 205–6, 209
        protocol, 205–6
        recommended treatment, 205–6, 209
    microinvasion, 7–9, 7–8, 81, 203–4
        topography of lesions, 98
    pathology, 143–4, 146–7, 146
    recurrence, 9, **208–9**, 208–9
    size of lesion, 7, 10, 141, **142**
    tufted glands within abnormal (atypical)
        epithelium, 143, 144
cervical epithelium
    colposcopic appearances, 46–7
    fetal development, 43, 44
    menopause, 59, 61, 62–3
    metaplastic transformation, 43–4
        see also transformation zone
    natural history, 43–4
    pregnancy, 43–4, 56–9
    topography, 44–6
    see also abnormal (atypical) epithelium
cervical glandular intraepithelial neoplasia
    (CGIN), 6–7
    cone biopsy diagnosis, 81, 82–3
    cytodiagnosis, 81–3
    high-grade lesions, 81, 81
        histologic criteria, 6, 6–7
        see also adenocarcinoma-in-situ (AIS)
    histologic criteria, 6, 6–7
    human papilloma virus (HPV), 2
    low-grade lesions, 6, 6, 7
    tubal metaplasia, 82–3, 83
cervical intraepithelial glandular neoplasia
    (CIGN) see cervical glandular
        intraepithelial neoplasia (CGIN)
cervical intraepithelial neoplasia (CIN)
    atypical vessels, 105–6
    colposcopy, 34, 34–5, 161–3
        abnormal (atypical) epithelium, 161–2
        acetic acid technique (acetowhite change),
            37–8, 99

cytologic grade–area correlation, 134–5, 135,
    140
cytological classifications, 2, 71–2
    dyskaryosis relationship, 135, 135–6
    endocervical extension see endocervical
        extension of CIN
    glandular involvement, 162, 162
    histopathological features, 3–5, 4, 49
    HIV-positive patient, 201–2
    human papilloma virus (HPV), 2, 15
        cytopathic effects (CPE), 2
    long-term treatment complications, 190–7
        stenosis/constriction, 190–4
    management, 161–209
        algorithm, 189
        assessment, 161–3
        excision techniques, 173–87, 190
        follow-up, 190
        high-grade lesions, 164
        HPV-DNA testing, 164–5
        hysterectomy, 188–90
        indications for excision, 165
        indications for local destruction, 165
        local destructive treatments, 165–73, 190
        low-grade lesions, 164–5
        treatment rationale, 161
        treatment techniques, 163, 163
    mixed adenocarcinoma-in-situ (AIS) lesions,
        153
    natural history, **24**, 24
    in pregnancy, 197–201
    recurrence, 194–7, 195–6
        follow-up surveillance, 194–6
        treatment, 196–7
    terminology, 2
    topography of lesions, 98
    vaginal extension/vaginal intraepithelial
        neoplasia (VAIN), 214–16, 216
    vulval intraepithelial neoplasia (VIN)
        association, 234–5, 234–5
    see also CIN 1; CIN 2; CIN 3
cervical invasive cancer, 1
    acetowhite change, 99
    atypical vessels, 103, 104
        early invasion, 105–7, 107–8, 141–2, 143
    FIGO staging, 203–4, **204**
    HIV-positive patient, 201
    human papilloma virus (HPV), 15
        case reports/case series, 23
        cohort studies, 23
    microinvasion see cervical early invasive
        cancer
    post-CIN conservative treatment, 196, 196
    in pregnancy, 197, 197, 201
    referral for colposcopy, 97
    stage Ib management, 207–8
    topography of lesions, 98
    trachelectomy, 204, 207
cervical microinvasive carcinoma see cervical
    early invasive cancer
cervical polypoid lesions, 312–15, 313–14
    clinical presentation, 312, 314–15
    following local cervical treatments, 314, 314
    management, 314–15
    multiple, 314, 315
cervical ripening, 58
cervical smear see cytology
cervical stenosis, 190–4, 191–2
    cervical dilatation, 192, 192
    surgical treatment, 192–3, 193–4
cervicography, 89–90, 90
cervicoscope
    adenocarcinoma-in-situ (AIS), 149–50
    endocervical canal examination, 117, 123,
        124–5, 125
    screening, 91
chemotherapy, vulval intraepithelial neoplasia

(VIN), 284
Chlamydia trachomatis, 236
CIN 1, 2, 113
    cytological classifications, 71–2
    diagnostic method correlations, 136, 136–7
    dyskaryosis, 77–8, 78–9
    histopathological features, 3–4, 4, 49
    human papilloma virus (HPV)-related
        changes (HPV-CIN 1), 3–4, 4, 49
    management, 164–5
    natural history, 24, 25
    see also LSIL (low-grade squamous
        intraepithelial lesion)
CIN 2, 2, 113
    cytological classifications, 72
    diagnostic method correlations, 138, 139
    dyskaryosis, 77, 78–9, 79
    histopathological features, 3–5, 4, 49
    human papilloma virus (HPV)-related
        changes, 3
    management, 164
    natural history, 24, 25
    see also HSIL (high-grade squamous
        intraepithelial lesion)
CIN 3, 2, 113
    colposcopy, 109, 111
        atypical vessels, 105
    comedo-like crypt lesions, 79, 80
    cytological classifications, 72
    diagnostic method correlations, 138–9, 139
    dyskaryosis, 76, 76–7, 78–80, 79
    early invasive cancer, 141, **142**
    glandular involvement, 162
    histopathologic features, 3–5, 4, 49
    human papilloma virus (HPV)-related
        changes, 3
    management, 164
    natural history, 24, 25
    small lesion within large CIN 1 area, 139–40,
        140–1, 141
    see also HSIL (high-grade squamous
        intraepithelial lesion)
clinical referral, cytologic report guidelines, 80,
    97
clotrimazole, 306
cohort studies, 23–4, **24**, 25
cold coagulation treatment, 167–8
    follow-up, 168
    pregnancy outcome following, 168
    results, 168
    Semm cold coagulator, 167, 167
    technique, 167–8, 168
cold knife cone biopsy, 174–8
    anesthesia, 175
    cervical defect repair, 176–7, 177
    colposcopic lesion assessment, 175
    early invasive cancer, 205
    endocervical extension, 176
    hemostasis, 175
    indications, 175
    results, 177–8, 180
    technique, 175–6, 176
Collins toluidine blue test, 243–4, 243–4
colposcope, 35, 36
colposcopy, 34–41, 43–69, 97–159, 161–3
    adenocarcinoma diagnosis, 149–50, 150–2,
        152
    adolescent cervix, 52, 55–6
    assessment for excisional techniques, 175
    atypical (abnormal) cervical epithelium
        appearances, 98–108, 161–2
        acetowhite change, 99, 99
        atypical vessels, 104, 107–8
        margins, 99–100, 100
        surface contour, 100–1, 101
        vascular patterns, 100–1, 101–3, 102–3
    atypical (abnormal) cervical epithelium

epidemiology
  anal/perianal intraepithelial neoplasia, 290
  cervical adenocarcinoma, 149
  diethylstilbestrol-associated developmental
    anomalies, 301
  human papilloma virus (HPV) infection, 15
    cervical cancer/precancer risk, 23
    genital infection populations studies, 21–2,
      22
  vulval intraepithelial neoplasia (VIN), 233–4
Eppendorfer biopsy forceps, *120*, 221
erosion, 43
erythroplakia, 43
erythroplasia of Queyrat, 233
eversion of transformation zone, 49, 50, *51*
excisional techniques, 173–87, 190
  cervical early invasive cancer, 205
  endocervical extension, *174*, 174, 176
  indications, 165
  local destructive techniques comparisons,
    173–4
  methods, 174
  results, 177–8
exophytic genital wart *see* condylomata
    acuminata
extensive surgical excision, anal/perianal
    intraepithelial neoplasia, 298, *298–9*

fetal development, 43, *44*, 300
FIGO classification, 142
  cervical early invasive cancer, 203–4, **204**
  cervical invasive cancer, **9**
  vaginal carcinomas, 222
flat condyloma, 17, 18, *19–20*, *129*, 129, 137, *138*
  cervical lesions, 309
fluconazole, 306
fluorescence spectroscopy, 91–2
5-fluorouracil chemotherapy, vulval lesions, 284

Gardnerella vaginalis, 236
Gartner's duct cysts, 300
genital warts *see* condyloma acuminata
giant condylomata acuminata
    (Buschke–Löwenstein tumor), 17
glandular intraepithelial neoplasia (GIN) *see*
    cervical glandular intraepithelial
    neoplasia (CGIN)
glandular lesions, colposcopy, 97, *162*, 162
gluteraldehyde disinfection, 40
gonorrhea, 236
granuloma inguinale, 265, *267*
Graves' speculum, 178, 183
gynoscopic screening, 91

healing epithelium, acetowhite change, 99
herpes genitalis (HSV-2) infection, 306–10
  anal/perianal lesions, 293
  colposcopy, *307*, 307–8, *308*
  cytology, 306, *307*
  transmission, 306
  vulval intraepithelial neoplasia (VIN)
    associations, 236
  vulval lesions, 308, *309*
high-grade squamous intraepithelial lesion *see*
    HSIL
HIV-positive patient, 201–3
  abnormal smears, 201–3
  anal/perianal intraepithelial neoplasia, 290–1
    cytological screening, 291
  cervical intraepithelial neoplasia (CIN), 201–2
    recurrence, *202*, 203
    treatment, 203
  colposcopic screening, 203
  condylomatous lesions, 201
  human papilloma virus (HPV) coinfection,
    202–3
  invasive cervical cancer, 201

vaginal intraepithelial neoplasia (VAIN), 214
vulval intraepithelial neoplasia (VIN 3),
    236–7
HPV 6, 17
HPV 11, 17
HPV 16, 15, 17
  anal/perianal intraepithelial neoplasia, 290
  E6/E7 proteins, 16, 27–8
  genome, *16*
  host DNA synthesis induction, 16, 27
  oncogenetic mechanism, 27–8
  persistent infections, 30
  screening, 28
  vaginal cancer association, 215
  variants, 30
  vulval intraepithelial neoplasia (VIN), 235–7
  vulval lesions, 264
HPV 18, 15, 17
  persistent infections, 30
  screening, 28
  variants, 30
  vulval lesions, 264
HPV 31, 28
HPV 33, 28
HSIL (high-grade squamous intraepithelial
    lesion), 3, 72
  correlation of diagnostic methods, 138–9, *139*
  dyskaryosis, *76*, 76, *78–80*
  histopathological features, 4–5, *5–6*
  management, 164
  natural history, 24
  referral for colposcopy, 97
human papilloma virus (HPV), 2–3, 15–30
  anal/perianal intraepithelial neoplasia, 290–1
  cervical adenocarcinoma, 149
  cervical lesions, 308, 309–11, *310*, 310–11, *313*
  classification, 16
  clinical infections, 17–18
    diagnostic criteria, **17**
  condylomatous lesions, 128–9, *128–30*
    colposcopic appearances, 131–2
    flat condylomatous change, 3
  cytopathic effects (CPE), 2–5, *4*, 15, 17, 71
    continuum of biological changes, 3
    prevalence, 21
  diagnostic methods correlations, 136–7, *137*
  epidemiological studies, 15
    cervical cancer/cancer precursors risk, 23
    genital infection populations studies, 21–2,
      22
    PCR technology, 21–2
  genome, 15–16, *16*
  high-risk types, 15–17, **17**, 88
    DNA testing, 29, 164–5
    screening, 28–9
    variants, 30
  HIV coinfection, 202–3
  HPV-DNA testing, 28–9, 164–5
    cervical cancer screening, 88–9, **89**
    methods, 29, 88
    triage schemes, 88–9
  infection process, 16–17
    early HPV protein synthesis, 16
    host DNA synthesis, 16
  infection "without dyskaryosis", 72
  infection-associated acetowhite change, 99
  latent infections, 16–17, 20–1
  lower genital tract neoplastic syndrome, 222
  natural history, 15, **24**, 24, *25*
    progression, **24**, 24, *25*
    regression, **24**, 24, *25*
  nomenclature, 3
  nuclear atypia cytologic classification, 71–2,
    75
  oncogenetic molecular pathways, 26–8, *28*
  precursor lesions causation, 2–3, 15, 128–33
  risk factors, 22–3

sexual transmission, 15, 22
subclinical infection *see* subclinical
    papillomavirus infections (SPI)
types, 16, **17**
  see also HPV types
vaginal intraepithelial neoplasia (VAIN), *10*,
    11
vaginal lesions, 215, 310–11, *311*
vertical transmission, 15, 22
virus characteristics, 15–16, *16*
vulval early invasive cancer recurrence, 257
vulval intraepithelial neoplasia (VIN), 11,
    233–7
vulval lesions, 264–5, 311
hybrid capture HPV-DNA testing, 29, 88–9, *89*,
    165
hyperkeratotic Wickham's striae of the buccal
    mucosa, 266
hysterectomy
  adenocarcinoma-in-situ (AIS), 206–7
  CIN management, 188–90
    indications, 188–90
    technique, 190
  early invasive adenocarcinoma, 206–7
  early invasive cancer, 205–6, 209
    recurrence, **208**
  primary vaginal malignancy following, 222,
    223–4, 224
  stage Ib invasive cancer, 207, 208
  vaginal intraepithelial neoplasia (VAIN)
    following, 214, 218–21, *219*
    cytology, 218

image management systems, 41
immunosuppression, 23
  vulval intraepithelial neoplasia (VIN)
    progression to invasive cancer, 237
infective conditions, 305–15
interferon therapy, 284
inverted condyloma, 129
iodine solution application
  Schiller's test, 98–9, 126, *127*, 128
  vaginal intraepithelial neoplasia (VAIN), 217,
    218, 219, *220*
  vaginoscopy, 215

Keyes punch, 244, *245*
Kogan's endocervical forceps, *119*, 120, 219
koilocytosis (koilocytic nuclear atypia), 2–3, *4*,
    10–11, 15, *20*, 71
  borderline nuclear change, *75*, 75
  cervical lesions, *310*, 310
  condylomatous lesions, *128–9*, 129, *134–5*,
    137, *138*
  with dyskaryosis, 78, *79*
  vulval intraepithelial neoplasia (VIN), 235,
    240
  Bowenoid papulosis, 249

large loop excision transformation zone
    (LLETZ), 182
  see also loop diathermy excision
laser cone biopsy, 178–81
  complications, 180–1, *180–1*
  early invasive cancer, 205
  equipment, *178*, 178
  excessive eversion of columnar epithelium
    following, *192*, 194
  pregnancy following, 194
  pregnancy-associated precursor lesions, 199
  results, 180
  technique, 178, *179*, 180
laser local excision
  anal/perianal intraepithelial neoplasia, *297*,
    297–8
  cervical polypoid lesions following, *314*, 314
  vaginal intraepithelial neoplasia (VAIN),